Essentials of Physical Medicine and Rehabilitation

Essentials of Physical Medicine and Rehabilitation

Editor: Esther Henson

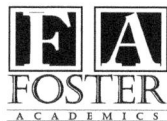

FOSTER
ACADEMICS

www.fosteracademics.com

www.fosteracademics.com

FA FOSTER
ACADEMICS

Cataloging-in-Publication Data

Essentials of physical medicine and rehabilitation / edited by Esther Henson.
    p. cm.
Includes bibliographical references and index.
ISBN 978-1-63242-472-3
1. Medicine, Physical. 2. Medical rehabilitation. 3. Physical therapy. 4. Medicine. I. Henson, Esther.
RM700 .E87 2017
615.82--dc23

Foster Academics,
118-35 Queens Blvd., Suite 400,
Forest Hills, NY 11375, USA

ISBN 978-1-63242-472-3 (Hardback)

Printed and bound in the United States of America.

Contents

Preface

This book was inspired by the evolution of our times; to answer the curiosity of inquisitive minds. Many developments have occurred across the globe in the recent past which has transformed the progress in the field.

This book on physical medicine and rehabilitation deals with the study and practice of enhancing and improving functional ability of those who suffer from physical impairments and disabilities. The various branches that fall under rehabilitation medicine are pain medicine, neuromuscular medicine, spinal cord injury medicine, sports medicine, etc. This book talks about physical and rehabilitation medicine in detail and provides knowledgeable insights about the varied branches that fall under this category. It explores all the important aspects of rehabilitation medicine in the present day scenario. For all readers who are interested in this subject, the case studies included in this text will serve as an excellent guide to develop a comprehensive understanding.

This book was developed from a mere concept to drafts to chapters and finally compiled together as a complete text to benefit the readers across all nations. To ensure the quality of the content we instilled two significant steps in our procedure. The first was to appoint an editorial team that would verify the data and statistics provided in the book and also select the most appropriate and valuable contributions from the plentiful contributions we received from authors worldwide. The next step was to appoint an expert of the topic as the Editor-in-Chief, who would head the project and finally make the necessary amendments and modifications to make the text reader-friendly. I was then commissioned to examine all the material to present the topics in the most comprehensible and productive format.

I would like to take this opportunity to thank all the contributing authors who were supportive enough to contribute their time and knowledge to this project. I also wish to convey my regards to my family who have been extremely supportive during the entire project.

Editor

Low-Educated Women with Chronic Pain Were Less Often Selected to Multidisciplinary Rehabilitation Programs

Anne Hammarström[1,2]*, Inger Haukenes[1,2,3], Anncristine Fjellman Wiklund[2,4], Arja Lehti[1,2], Maria Wiklund[2,4], Birgitta Evengård[5], Britt-Marie Stålnacke[2,6]

1 Department of Public Health and Clinical Medicine, Umeå University, Umeå, Sweden, 2 Umeå Centre for Gender Studies in Medicine, Umeå University, Umeå, Sweden, 3 Division of Mental Health, Department of Public Mental Health, Norwegian Institute of Public Health, Bergen, Norway, 4 Department of Community Medicine and Rehabilitation, Physiotherapy, Umeå University, Umeå, Sweden, 5 Department of Clinical Microbiology, Division of Infectious Diseases, Umeå University, Umeå, Sweden, 6 Department of Community Medicine and Rehabilitation, Rehabilitation Medicine, Umeå University, Umeå, Sweden

Abstract

Background: There is a lack of research about a potential education-related bias in assessment of patients with chronic pain. The aim of this study was to analyze whether low-educated men and women with chronic pain were less often selected to multidisciplinary rehabilitation than those with high education.

Methods: The population consisted of consecutive patients (n = 595 women, 266 men) referred during a three-year period from mainly primary health care centers for a multidisciplinary team assessment at a pain rehabilitation clinic at a university hospital in Northern Sweden. Patient data were collected from the Swedish Quality Registry for Pain Rehabilitation National Pain Register. The outcome variable was being selected by the multidisciplinary team assessment to a multidisciplinary rehabilitation program. The independent variables were: sex, age, born outside Sweden, education, pain severity as well as the hospital, anxiety and depression scale (HADS).

Results: Low-educated women were less often selected to multidisciplinary rehabilitation programs than high-educated women (OR 0.55, CI 0.30–0.98), even after control for age, being born outside Sweden, pain intensity and HADS. No significant findings were found when comparing the results between high- and low-educated men.

Conclusion: Our findings can be interpreted as possible discrimination against low-educated women with chronic pain in hospital referrals to pain rehabilitation. There is a need for more gender-theoretical research emphasizing the importance of taking several power dimensions into account when analyzing possible bias in health care.

Editor: Ruth Landau, University of Washington, United States of America

Funding: This work was supported by the Swedish Research Council (grant no: 344-2009-5839). The funders had no role in study design, data collection and analysis, decision to publish, or preparation of the manuscript.

Competing Interests: The authors have declared that no competing interests exist.

* E-mail: anne.hammarstrom@umu.se

Introduction

A large number of studies indicate that there is a gender bias to women's disadvantage, i.e. an unintended and systematic neglect of women, in health care [1,2]. Most of this research has been performed on coronary heart disease [3], but also in relation to other symptoms and diagnoses [1,4–6]. For example, the so-called "laundry bag project" (LBP) discovered gendered standards for dermatological treatment of common diagnoses. The study included gender-based quantitative analysis of treatment of all patients (n = 320 women, 421 men) referred to a dermatological clinic. The study showed that men with diagnoses of psoriasis or eczema received more whole-body UV treatment and more help with emollients than did women [5]. In economic terms, women patients subsidized the treatment budget of the clinic to a value of 22 per cent. In similar ways, medically unjustified differences in the availability of examination and treatment for women compared to men have been demonstrated in connection with a number of other diseases, such as irritable bowel syndrome [1], renal transplantation, HIV and pain [6,7]. Gender bias in neck pain was found when Swedish interns were asked about the diagnosis and management of this group of patients. Non-specific somatic diagnoses, psychosocial questions, drug prescriptions and the expressed need of diagnostic support from a physiotherapist and an orthopedist were more commonly proposed for women than for men [7].

Gender bias may also mean that men are disadvantaged in health care [8], which has been discussed for example in relation to the treatment of depression [9] and osteoporosis [10] in older men. In these cases, diagnostic models have been developed for women while criteria to identify risk in men are not well established. A case study of osteoporosis from Gendered Innovations [10] has developed male reference populations and identified medical conditions (especially among men) that are related to osteoporotic fracture, allowing for better evaluation of fracture risk in men. In addition, among patients with chronic pain, women participate in multidisciplinary rehabilitation programs (which are a combination of different physical and psychological interventions that is linked to teamwork) more often than men, and some studies have demonstrated that women benefit more from this kind of rehabilitation than men do [11]. Systematic reviews of treatment and rehabilitation of patients with chronic pain have shown evidence that multidisciplinary rehabilitation programs have superior effects on multidimensional outcomes compared to less intensive treatments [12–14]. However, most of the reviews do not analyze differences in treatment among men as compared to women. Thus, the question remains to study whether there is a gender bias in the treatment of chronic pain.

Increasingly important has been to analyze not only gender, but to include multiple power dimensions in the analyzes of gender bias such as socioeconomic status, ethnicity and age. For example in Swedish health care, research on gender bias has shown that it is not women as a group but older, low-educated women who have worse outcome in stroke care [15]. However, overall rather few studies have been performed within this field of intersectional gender research. To the best of our knowledge there is no research analyzing whether or not low-educated women (and men) of various ages with chronic pain are less frequently selected for multidisciplinary rehabilitation compared to high-educated.

The aim of this study was therefore to analyze whether low-educated men and women with chronic pain were less often selected for multidisciplinary rehabilitation than those with high education.

Methods

Ethical statement

The study was approved by the Regional Ethics Vetting Board in Umeå, Sweden. Informed consent was not required because we only handled unidentified register data. According to Swedish law (Swedish Ethical Review Act 2003;460, §§ 20–21, Swedish Personal Data Law 1998:204 § 19) informed consent is not required when dealing with unidentified register data (as was the case in our study).

Setting

The study was conducted in a clinical setting at the Pain Rehabilitation Clinic at Umeå University Hospital, Sweden. In order for a referred patient to be selected for assessment at the clinic the patients had to have a chronic disabling non-malignant diagnosis of chronic pain. Patients with serious somatic diagnoses (such as cancer, rheumatoid arthritis and neurological disorders that should be investigated by other specialist clinics) are excluded. The most frequent diagnostic groups at the clinic are columnar pain (50%) followed by extremity pain (18%) [16].

The selected patients were assessed during two days at the pain rehabilitation clinic by multidisciplinary diagnostic teams consisting of a specialist physician in rehabilitation medicine, a physiotherapist, a social worker, an occupational therapist and a psychologist if needed. If the multidisciplinary teams assessed that the patient was in need of multidisciplinary rehabilitation and fulfilled the inclusion criteria (described below), they were selected to participate in a rehabilitation program based on a bio-psychosocial model with cognitive behavioural principles [16]. The multidisciplinary rehabilitation program focused on pain management and education about pain and its consequences. Rehabilitation was based on collaboration within the multidisci-

plinary team with the patient as an active team member. The patient was expected to participate with the team in goal setting and reaching the decided goals. A number of core sessions were conducted, e.g. physiotherapy (swimming pool exercise and relaxation exercises), ergonomics, education about pain mechanisms and coping with pain. At the end of the program contact was established with the patient's primary care physician.

Inclusion criteria for referral to the multidisciplinary rehabilitation program were (i) disabling non-malignant chronic and complex musculoskeletal pain (on sick leave or experiencing major interference in daily life due to chronic pain); (ii) age 18–65 years; (iii) no further medical investigations needed; (iv) written consent to participate in and attend the multidisciplinary program; (v) agreement not to have parallel contacts with therapists such as physiotherapists while attending the multidisciplinary pain rehabilitation program.

Population

The population consisted of consecutive patients (n = 595 women, 266 men) referred mainly from primary health care centers to the pain rehabilitation clinic and assessed between 5 November 2007 and 13 December 2010.

Design and data collection

Patient data were collected from the Swedish Quality Registry for Pain Rehabilitation National Pain Register (SQRP) [17] and linked to the patients' individual records containing the final decision on being selected or not to multidisciplinary rehabilitation programs. The SQRP register has aggregated data since 1998 of all patients referred to the majority of Swedish rehabilitation units. The SQRP is based on patients' information from validated self-administered questionnaires completed before the first multidisciplinary assessment [17]. The patients completed the set of questionnaires at home the night before the assessment and the questions refer to pain experiences during the day before the assessment. The questionnaires were handed in on the day of assessment and were subsequently registered in SQRP.

Outcome variable

The outcome variable was being selected (= 1) for a multidisciplinary rehabilitation program as compared to not being selected (= 0).

Independent variables

The following independent variables were used: sex, age (used as a continuous variable) and country of birth (Sweden, other Nordic country, Europe (except Nordic countries) and other country) recoded as born outside of Sweden = 1, born in Sweden = 0. Education was measured with the following question: Which is your highest completed level of education? The following four answer alternatives were given: 1. Nine years of compulsory school, 2. Two- or three-year secondary high school (including both theoretical programs and vocational training), 3. University studies 4. Other education (which could mean in-service training supported by a company or organization, folk high school etc.). Low-educated was defined as having completed compulsory school (= 1) as compared to all other completed forms of education.

To adjust for depression and anxiety, the often used and validated 14-item self-reported HADS (Hospital, anxiety and depression) scale was used [18]. Due to high correlation between the anxiety and the depression scale, the two scales were combined into a continuous variable with a total range of 0–42 [19]. In the multivariate logistic regression analyzes, low HADS equals 0. The HADS has proven to be reliable and valid when used to assess symptom severity in anxiety and depression among somatic, psychiatric and primary care patients [20].

Pain severity was used as a continuous variable (range 0–6) based on a subscale from the Multidimensional Pain Inventory (MPI), Part I [21,22]. In the multivariate logistic regression analyzes, low pain severity equals 0. The MPI has demonstrated good reliability and validity for patients with chronic pain [23].

Statistical analysis

The associations between low education and referral to multidisciplinary rehabilitation programs were investigated for men and women separately by means of multivariate logistic regression analyzes, using SPSS statistical package (SPSS version 18 for Windows). The first model (Model 0) consisted of bivariate associations. The following models were age-adjusted. Model 1 included the variable 'born outside Sweden' while model 2 also included HADS and pain severity. As significance tests we used chi-square for dichotomous variables and t-test for continuous variables. The correlation between the confounders was <0.3.

Availability of data

The SQRP is a national quality registry supported by the Swedish Association of the Local Authorities and Regions and connected to the Uppsala Clinical Research Center (UCR). Our dataset has great potential for secondary analysis. The data are not freely available but collaborative ideas are welcome. Britt-Marie Stålnacke is the contact person. The website with documentation for the SQRP and detailed information about variables is available at http://www.ucr.uu/nrs/.

Results

The distribution of the dependent and independent variables for men and women are shown in Tables 1 and 2.

The tables show that significantly more women than men were selected for multidisciplinary rehabilitation. More men than women were born abroad. For the other variables, no significant differences between men and women were found. Around 15 per cent were low-educated.

Table 3 shows the logistic regression analyzes in four age-adjusted models for men and women separately with referral to multidisciplinary rehabilitation programs as outcome.

The table shows that low-educated women were less often selected for multidisciplinary rehabilitation programs as compared to high-educated women. The odds ratios for low education were significant in all models and did not particularly attenuate in the fully adjusted model (from 0.53 in the univariate to 0.55 in the last model). Among men, there were no significant odds ratios between low education and referral to multidisciplinary rehabilitation programs in any of the models. But the odds ratios pointed in the same direction as among women. None of the other independent

variables were significantly related to multidisciplinary rehabilitation among men or women.

Discussion

This study aimed to analyze whether low-educated men and women with chronic pain were less often selected for multidisciplinary rehabilitation compared to high-educated. We found that low-educated women were less often selected for multidisciplinary rehabilitation programs than high-educated women and that this relationship remained almost unchanged after control for all the covariates (including pain intensity and mental illness).

A possible explanation to these findings may be that women with lower levels of education might be less likely to fulfil the inclusion criteria. Women might for example be more likely to need further medical investigations or be less likely to agree to give up their contacts with other. However, neither low-educated nor women were overrepresented among those who needed further medical investigation (data not shown). In addition, almost everyone who was selected to the multidisciplinary rehabilitation programs agreed to participate. Thus, the fact that low-educated women were not referred to multidisciplinary rehabilitation as often as high-educated women cannot be explained by such factors.

Overall, there is a lack of international studies about possible bias in referral of low-educated patients to pain rehabilitation. However, our findings are in line with a broader scope of research, demonstrating socioeconomic bias in specialist health care [24–28]. A comprehensive study of health care utilization in 12 EU member states found consistent evidence that the wealthy and/or high-educated were more likely to have contact with medical specialists than the poor and low-educated [28]. Moreover, selection for cardiac rehabilitation has been found to favor participants with good prognosis and disfavor patients from deprived areas who tend to have poorer prognosis [24,26]. Also waiting time for carotid surgery after stroke was significantly longer for low-income patients compared with high-income patients [27,29]. However, gender differences were not analyzed in these studies.

The current finding that low-educated women with chronic musculoskeletal pain were less often selected for multidisciplinary rehabilitation programs is surprising for several reasons. First, consistent findings point to socioeconomic indicators, such as educational level, as strong predictors of musculoskeletal disorders and reporting of chronic pain conditions in both men and women [30–34]. MacFarlaine et al. found that low socioeconomic status in adulthood was associated with major regional musculoskeletal pain and chronic widespread pain [32]. Individuals in the lowest socioeconomic class had a three-fold increased risk of widespread pain, and the impact of childhood socioeconomic status was less prominent than adult socioeconomic status [32]. In addition Overland et al. found that individuals with widespread musculoskeletal pain were characterized by being women, having lower

Table 1. Prevalence of dichotomous covariates among women and men, n = 861 (per cent).

	Women n = 595	n	Men n = 266	n	p-value
Multidisciplinary rehabilitation	28.4	169	18.4	49	0.002
Low-educated	16.1	96	14.4	38	0.542
Born outside Sweden	9.4	56	14.7	39	0.026

Table 2. Prevalence of continuous covariates between women and men, n = 861 (mean (SD)).

	Women n = 595	Men n = 266	p-value
Age	39.9 (10.9)	40.8 (10.9)	0.301
HADS	14.9 (8.1)	15.0 (8.4)	0.810
Pain severity	4.4 (0.9)	4.3 (0.9)	0.402

education/lower household income, poor general health including higher prevalence of common mental disorders and higher risk for future disability pension [35]. Based on these findings one should expect that lower educated women and men with chronic musculoskeletal pain conditions were at least equally prioritized with respect to multidisciplinary treatment at specialized rehabilitation clinics [36].

Second, our findings demonstrated a limited impact of age, being born outside Sweden, pain intensity and mental illness on the relation between education and being selected for rehabilitation programs. These findings indicate that gender bias may be at stake and that the combination of gender and education play a significant role when deciding who is suitable for multidisciplinary rehabilitation.

Third, Sweden is a country well-known for its historical political engagement for achieving increased equality in society. According to Swedish law, the overall goal for health care is that it should be given on equal terms for the whole population [36]. Our findings point in the direction of discrimination against low-educated women in the rehabilitation of chronic pain which is not in accordance with the Swedish law.

More women than men were referred to rehabilitation. An explanation could be simply the fact that the prevalence of pain is higher in women than men [37,38]. Another explanation could be that men with pain are more often referred to specialist treatment and therefore get more precise diagnoses and treatment than women [7]. However, the patients in our register were assessed at a specialist clinic. Our findings cannot be interpreted as a gender bias against men because we do not know the clinical reasons behind these findings.

In general, our findings are in line with gender-theoretical research emphasizing the importance of taking several power dimensions into account when analyzing possible bias in treatment [39,40]. Thus, our findings draw attention to the importance of not viewing men and women as static groups but analyzing differences within (and similarities across) the group of men and women. Intersectional approaches mean that dimensions of inequalities do not simply accumulate. Instead one category such as 'low education' takes its meaning from another such as 'gender' and new hybrids develop as these categories are new hybrid structures which emerge at the intersections of inequality [41]. Qualitative methods could preferably be used in order to understand the meaning of such hybrids in pain rehabilitation. Thus, there is a need for more intersectional research about what happens in the meeting between patients and care-givers. In this study, we have no such measures.

Limitations and strengths

The current study is based on register data which has some limitations. Above we discuss that our findings point in the direction of discrimination of low-educated women. Discrimination can be seen to exist if high and low educated women have the same health needs but receive different treatment. However, the

lack of certain social and clinical variables in the SQRP register about health needs prohibits us from drawing firm conclusions about discrimination. Even though we assume that rehabilitation is the best treatment for the patients referred to the pain rehabilitation clinic, it could be the case that the evaluating teams concluded that the low educated women would not benefit from the programs due to for example manual workload, domestic strain and less possibility to rest. But none of these circumstances are considered contra-indicative of multidisciplinary rehabilitation, and should not be relevant when decisions are taken by multidisciplinary teams. As the rehabilitation programs take into account the individual needs of the patients and support them to set their own goals, we have no reason to believe that the needs of lower educated women are not attended to in the assessment. Since the physicians examine patients by standard procedures we do not believe that mis-diagnosis in women with low education is a problem.

Due to the limitations of the register data we do not have information on diagnoses of diseases causing the pain. However, in a previous study from the pain rehabilitation clinic (with access to diagnoses) no significant differences were found in diagnostic groups between patients being selected for multidisciplinary rehabilitation compared to all assessed patients [16]. In addition, there are strict selection criteria for the pain rehabilitation clinic in our study, which means that in order to get an initial appointment at the clinic, the patients must have a disabling non-malignant diagnosis of chronic pain and that other diagnoses (such as cancer, rheumatoid arthritis, neurological disorders) are excluded.

Co-morbidity could be the basis of different therapeutic efforts in patients with different levels of education. Our register contained information about the most important comorbid conditions, which are depression and anxiety [43,44]. We have performed sensitivity analyzes with clinical cut-off points for depression and for anxiety (with case level >10 in HADS). The inclusion of the clinical cut-off points for depression and anxiety separately did not change the overall findings. But a limitation is that we do not have information about other comorbidity, for example post-traumatic stress symptoms and fear avoidance. Earlier research shows no socioeconomic differences in post-traumatic stress symptoms [42]. Comorbid symptoms of fear avoidance are not contra-indicative of multidisciplinary pain rehabilitation and are dealt with in rehabilitation programs. A minority of the patients referred to the Pain Rehabilitation Clinic suffered from other physical diseases and were referred to other clinics. As this is a very small group we have no reason to believe that low-educated women are over-represented among them.

Due to these methodological uncertainties, we interpret our findings as a possible (in contrast to a confirmed) discrimination against low-educated women. There is a need for more empirical research about the topic with studies which have more clinical data as well as more information about the decision making process.

Table 3. Logistic regression analyzes for referral to multidisciplinary rehabilitation program among women and men in relation to low education (reference = high education) and other independent variables.

	Model 0				Model 1				Model 2			
	Women		Men		Women		Men		Women		Men	
	OR	95% CI	OR	95% CI	OR	95% CI	OR	95% CI	OR	95% CI	OR	95% CI
High-educated	1		1		1		1		1		1	
Low-educated	0.53	0.31–0.92	0.81	0.32–2.05	0.53	0.31–0.93	0.81	0.32–2.10	0.55	0.30–0.98	0.88	0.34–2.30
Born in Sweden	1		1		1		1		1		1	
Born outside Sweden	0.39	0.18–0.85	0.61	0.23–1.65	0.41	0.19–0.89	0.65	0.24–1.76	0.67	0.30–1.51	0.90	0.30–2.69
Low HADS	1		1						1		1	
High HADS	0.97	0.95–1.00	1.03	1.00–1.07					0.98	0.96–1.00	1.03	0.99–1.08
Low pain severity	1		1						1		1	
High pain severity	0.79	0.64–1.00	0.92	0.65–1.29					0.86	0.69–1.08	0.93	0.64–1.36

Model 0: bivariate associations.
Model 1: adjusted for age + born outside Sweden.
Model 2: adjusted for age, born outside Sweden + HADS and pain severity.

More women than men were referred to the rehabilitation clinic. Therefore, lack of significant findings between educational level and selection for multidisciplinary rehabilitation among men may be due to a type 2-error. Use of an already established registry (SQORP) for measures of socio-demographic data and pain indicators restricted the possibility of including other measures of interest. On the other hand, the measures included are validated and have been widely used in clinical practice for assessment of pain severity, anxiety and depression.

Low education was defined as not having education beyond compulsory school, but what is 'low' can always be discussed. Sensitivity analyzes were performed with other dichotomizations,- such as no education beyond secondary high school, which showed similar results. Therefore, we chose to use the lowest level of educational attainment.

The main strength of the present study is the relatively high number of patients included and that recruitment of participants was restricted to one specific rehabilitation clinic. During the three-year inclusion period, the procedures for multidisciplinary team assessments did not change, thus enhancing the reliability of the data. In addition the team assessment was performed by experienced professionals with high staff continuity during the data collection period. Further, SQRP is a national register for pain rehabilitation and includes approximately 80% of pain management programs in Sweden [17]. The procedure used by the multidisciplinary team for selection of patients for multidisciplinary rehabilitation is similar throughout Sweden; thus, we can assume that the generalisability of the study is good on a national level.

Moreover, since comparable multidisciplinary assessment and selection visits often precede participation in rehabilitation programs in other counties as well [16], and since the MPI and HADS questionnaires have been widely used for measuring chronic pain, depression and anxiety in a range of pain rehabilitation contexts [20], we can assume that the generalisability of the study is good to countries with similar organization for the rehabilitation of patients with chronic pain.

Our outcome measure takes account of both diagnostic (International Classification of Diseases, 10th version (ICD-10)) and functional (International Classification of Disability, Impairment and Handicap (ICIDH)) components [17]. The SQRP consists of validated scales [20,21]. Selection criteria and assessment procedures for multidisciplinary rehabilitation are relatively similar across countries that offer organized treatment of patients with chronic pain [16]; thus, we can assume that the external validity of the study is relatively good.

In this study general practitioners referred the patients to a specialist pain rehabilitation clinic. Thus, the patients represent a selected group with a more complex chronic pain condition than patients treated in primary care. More research on this topic is needed in other contexts – both other clinical contexts and various geographical locations.

Conclusions

Our findings can be interpreted as possible discrimination against low-educated women with chronic pain in hospital referrals to multidisciplinary pain rehabilitation. More research is needed to analyze whether such discrimination also occurs in other clinical settings. There is a need for more gender-theoretical research emphasizing the importance of taking several power dimensions into account when analyzing possible bias in treatment.

Acknowledgments

The authors would like to thank Vanja Nyberg and Ylva Persson for valuable assistance in collecting the data.

Author Contributions

Conceived and designed the experiments: AH BE BMS. Performed the experiments: AH BE BMS. Analyzed the data: AH IH. Contributed reagents/materials/analysis tools: AH IH BMS. Wrote the paper: AH IH AFW AL MW BE BMS.

References

1. Risberg G (2004) "I am solely a professional – neutral and genderless": on gender bias and gender awareness in the medical profession [Dissertation]: Umeå University.
2. Ruiz-Cantero MT, Vives-Cases C, Artazcoz L, Delgado A, Garcia Calvente MM, et al. (2007) A framework to analyse gender bias in epidemiological research. J Epidemiol Community Health 61 Suppl 2: ii46–53.
3. Bosner S, Haasenritter J, Hani MA, Keller H, Sonnichsen AC, et al. (2011) Gender bias revisited: new insights on the differential management of chest pain. BMC Fam Pract 12: 45.
4. Borkhoff CM, Hawker GA, Kreder HJ, Glazier RH, Mahomed NN, et al. (2008) The effect of patients' sex on physicians' recommendations for total knee arthroplasty. CMAJ 178: 681–687.
5. Nyberg F, Osika I, Evengård B (2008) "The Laundry Bag Project" – unequal distribution of dermatological healthcare resources for male and female psoriatic patients in Sweden. Int J Dermatol 47: 144–149.
6. Raine R (2000) Does gender bias exist in the use of specialist health care? J Health Serv Res Policy 5: 237–249.
7. Hamberg K, Risberg G, Johansson EE, Westman G (2002) Gender bias in physicians' management of neck pain: a study of the answers in a Swedish national examination. J Womens Health Gend Based Med 11: 653–666.
8. Noone JH, Stephens C (2008) Men, masculine identities, and health care utilisation. Sociol Health Illn 30: 711–725.
9. Apesoa-Varano EC, Hinton L, Barker JC, Unützer J (2010) Clinician Approaches and Strategies for Engaging Older Men in Depression Care. Am J Geriatr Psychiatry 18: 586–595.
10. Gendered Innovation's homepage. Available: http://genderedinnovations.stanford.edu/. Accessed 14 January 2014.
11. Jensen IB, Bergström G, Ljungquist T, Bodin L (2005) A 3-year follow-up of a multidisciplinary rehabilitation program for back and neck pain. Pain 115: 273–283.
12. SBU (2010) Chronic Pain Rehabilitation. Stockholm: Swedish Council of Health Technology Assessment.
13. SBU (2006) Methods for treatment of chronic pain. Stockholm: The Swedish Council on Technology Assessment in Health Care. Report No.177.
14. Scascighini L, Toma V, Dober-Spielmann S, Sprott H (2008) Multidisciplinary treatment for chronic pain: a systematic review of interventions and outcomes. Rheumatology (Oxford) 47: 670–678.
15. Löfmark U, Hammarström A (2007) Evidence for age-dependent education-related differences in men and women with first-ever stroke. Results from a community-based incidence study in northern Sweden. Neuroepidemiology 28: 135–141.
16. Merrick D, Sundelin G, Stålnacke BM (2012) One-year follow-up of two different rehabilitation strategies for patients with chronic pain. J Rehabil Med 44: 764–773.
17. Nyberg V, Sanne H, Sjölund BH (2011) Swedish quality registry for pain rehabilitation: purpose, design, implementation and characteristics of referred patients. J Rehabil Med 43: 50–57.
18. Zigmond AS, Snaith RP (1983) The hospital anxiety and depression scale. Acta Psychiatr Scand 67: 361–370.
19. Cosco TD, Doyle F, Ward M, McGee H (2012) Latent structure of the Hospital Anxiety and Depression Scale: a 10-year systematic review. J Psychosom Res 72: 180–184.
20. Bjelland I, Dahl AA, Haug TT, Neckelmann D (2002) The validity of the Hospital Anxiety and Depression Scale. An updated literature review. J Psychosom Res 52: 69–77.
21. Kerns RD, Turk DC, Rudy TE (1985) The West Haven-Yale Multidimensional Pain Inventory (WHYMPI). Pain 23: 345–356.
22. Pietila Holmer E, Fahlström M, Nordström A (2013) The effects of interdisciplinary team assessment and a rehabilitation program for patients with chronic pain. Am J Phys Med Rehabil 92: 77–83.
23. Dworkin RH, Turk DC, Farrar JT, Haythornthwaite JA, Jensen MP, et al. (2005) Core outcome measures for chronic pain clinical trials: IMMPACT recommendations. Pain 113: 9–19.
24. Beswick AD, Rees K, West RR, Taylor FC, Burke M, et al. (2005) Improving uptake and adherence in cardiac rehabilitation: literature review. J Adv Nurs 49: 538–555.
25. Carr JL, Moffett JA (2005) The impact of social deprivation on chronic back pain outcomes. Chronic Illn 1: 121–129.
26. Melville MR, Packham C, Brown N, Weston C, Gray D (1999) Cardiac rehabilitation: socially deprived patients are less likely to attend but patients ineligible for thrombolysis are less likely to be invited. Heart 82: 373–377.
27. van den Bos GA, Smits JP, Westert GP, van Straten A (2002) Socioeconomic variations in the course of stroke: unequal health outcomes, equal care? J Epidemiol Community Health 56: 943–948.
28. van Doorslaer E, Masseria C, Koolman X (2006) Inequalities in access to medical care by income in developed countries. CMAJ 174: 177–183.
29. Kapral MK, Wang H, Mamdani M, Tu JV (2002) Effect of socioeconomic status on treatment and mortality after stroke. Stroke 33: 268–273.
30. Björnsdottir SV, Jonsson SH, Valdimarsdottir UA (2013) Functional limitations and physical symptoms of individuals with chronic pain. Scand J Rheumatol 42: 59–70.
31. Friedrich M, Hahne J, Wepner F (2009) A controlled examination of medical and psychosocial factors associated with low back pain in combination with widespread musculoskeletal pain. Phys Ther 89: 786–803.
32. Macfarlane GJ, Norrie G, Atherton K, Power C, Jones GT (2009) The influence of socioeconomic status on the reporting of regional and widespread musculoskeletal pain: results from the 1958 British Birth Cohort Study. Ann Rheum Dis 68: 1591–1595.
33. Perruccio AV, Gandhi R, Rampersaud YR (2013) Heterogeneity in health status and the influence of patient characteristics across patients seeking musculoskeletal orthopaedic care – a cross-sectional study. BMC Musculoskelet Disord 14: 83.
34. Toivanen S (2011) Exploring the interplay between work stress and socioeconomic position in relation to common health complaints: the role of interaction. Am J Ind Med 54: 780–790.
35. Overland S, Harvey SB, Knudsen AK, Mykletun A, Hotopf M (2012) Widespread pain and medically certified disability pension in the Hordaland Health Study. Eur J Pain 16: 611–620.
36. Health and Medical Services Act [Hälso- och sjukvårdslagen] SFS 1982:763.
37. Winjhoven HA, deVet HC, Picavet HC. Prevalence of musculoskeletal disorders is systematically higher in women than in men. Clin J Pain 2006;22:717–24
38. Stubbs D, Krebs E, Bair M, Damush T, Wu J, et al. Sex-differences in pain and pain related disability among primary care patients with chronic musculoskeletal pain. Pain Med 2010;11:232–9.
39. Hankivsky O (2012) Women's health, men's health, and gender and health: implications of intersectionality. Soc Sci Med 74: 1712–1720.
40. Springer KW, Hankivsky O, Bates LM (2012) Gender and health: relational, intersectional, and biosocial approaches. Soc Sci Med 74: 1661–1666.
41. Shields S (2008) Gender: An intersectionality perspective. Sex Roles 59: 301–311.
42. Boman KK, Kjällander Y, Eksborg S, Becker J. Impact of prior traumatic life events on parental early stage reactions following a child's cancer. PLoS One. 2013;8(3):e57556.
43. Bair MJ, Robinson RL, Katon W, Kroenke K. Depression and pain comorbidity: a literature review. Arch Intern Med 2003;163: 2433–2445
44. Jordan KD, Okifuji A. Anxiety disorders: differential diagnosis and their relationship to chronic pain. J Pain Palliat Care Pharmacother 2011;25:231–245.

2

Quality of Longer Term Mental Health Facilities in Europe: Validation of the Quality Indicator for Rehabilitative Care against Service Users' Views

Helen Killaspy[1]*, Sarah White[2], Christine Wright[2], Tatiana L. Taylor[1], Penny Turton[2], Thomas Kallert[3], Mirjam Schuster[4], Jorge A. Cervilla[5], Paulette Brangier[6], Jiri Raboch[7], Lucie Kalisova[7], Georgi Onchev[8], Spiridon Alexiev[8], Roberto Mezzina[9], Pina Ridente[9], Durk Wiersma[10], Ellen Visser[10], Andrzej Kiejna[11], Patryk Piotrowski[11], Dimitris Ploumpidis[12], Fragiskos Gonidakis[12], José Miguel Caldas-de-Almeida[13], Graça Cardoso[13], Michael King[1]

1 Mental Health Sciences Unit, University College London, London, United Kingdom, 2 Division of Population Health Sciences and Education, St George's University London, London, United Kingdom, 3 Department of Psychiatry, Psychosomatic Medicine and Psychotherapy, Park Hospital Leipzig, Leipzig, Germany, 4 University Hospital Department of Psychiatry and Psychotherapy, Dresden University of Technology, Dresden, Germany, 5 San Cecilio University Hospital Mental Health Unit, University of Granada, Granada, Spain, 6 Biomedical Research Centre Mental Health Network, University of Granada, Granada, Spain, 7 Department of Psychiatry, Charles University, Prague, Czech Republic, 8 Department of Psychiatry, Medical University Sofia, Sofia, Bulgaria, 9 Department of Mental Health, Trieste Healthcare Agency, Trieste, Italy, 10 University Medical Center Groningen, University of Groningen, Groningen, The Netherlands, 11 Department of Psychiatry, Wroclaw Medical University, Wroclaw, Poland, 12 University Mental Health Research Institute, Athens, Greece, 13 Faculty of Medical Science, New University of Lisbon, Lisbon, Portugal

Abstract

Background: The Quality Indicator for Rehabilitative Care (QuIRC) is a staff rated, international toolkit that assesses care in longer term hospital and community based mental health facilities. The QuIRC was developed from review of the international literature, an international Delphi exercise with over 400 service users, practitioners, carers and advocates from ten European countries at different stages of deinstitutionalisation, and review of the care standards in these countries. It can be completed in under an hour by the facility manager and has robust content validity, acceptability and inter-rater reliability. In this study, we investigated the internal validity of the QuIRC. Our aim was to identify the QuIRC domains of care that independently predicted better service user experiences of care.

Method: At least 20 units providing longer term care for adults with severe mental illness were recruited in each of ten European countries. Service users completed standardised measures of their experiences of care, quality of life, autonomy and the unit's therapeutic milieu. Unit managers completed the QuIRC. Multilevel modelling allowed analysis of associations between service user ratings as dependent variables with unit QuIRC domain ratings as independent variables.

Results: 1750/2495 (70%) users and the managers of 213 units from across ten European countries participated. QuIRC ratings were positively associated with service users' autonomy and experiences of care. Associations between QuIRC ratings and service users' ratings of their quality of life and the unit's therapeutic milieu were explained by service user characteristics (age, diagnosis and functioning). A hypothetical 10% increase in QuIRC rating resulted in a clinically meaningful improvement in autonomy.

Conclusions: Ratings of the quality of longer term mental health facilities made by service managers were positively associated with service users' autonomy and experiences of care. Interventions that improve quality of care in these settings may promote service users' autonomy.

Editor: Michel Botbol, University of Western Brittany, France

Funding: This study was funded by a three-year grant from the European Commission's 6th Framework (SP5A–CT–2007-044088). The funders had no role in study design, data collection and analysis, decision to publish, or preparation of the manuscript.

Competing Interests: The authors have declared that no competing interests exist.

* E-mail: h.killaspy@ucl.ac.uk

Introduction

Despite the move towards community based mental health care in Europe over recent decades, many patients still reside in some form of institution [1]. Although the exact number of longer term mental health facilities is unknown, concerns have been raised about the continuing reliance on large asylums in less economically developed countries [2] and the expansion of the "virtual asylum" of smaller health and social care facilities provided by the independent sector in countries with better developed community mental health services, catering to service users with more complex needs [3]. These facilities absorb a large proportion of the mental health budget of most countries and concerns about the quality of care provided have been raised [2,4]. A review of studies that investigated the costs of care associated with deinstitutionalisation in England, Germany and Italy concluded that well managed community based care was more cost-effective than long-stay hospital care as it was able to provide better quality care that resulted in better clinical outcomes [5].

The people who reside in longer term facilities mostly have diagnoses of psychotic illnesses [6] with complications such as treatment resistance [7], cognitive impairment and negative symptoms [8], poor social functioning [9], substance misuse and challenging behaviours [10]. They are at risk of abuse of their human rights since their capacity to make informed choices and participate actively in their care may be impaired. The European Commission's Green Paper [11] on improving the mental health of the population specifically highlighted the promotion of social inclusion for this group, protection of their fundamental rights and dignity. However, until recently, there were no standardised measures available to assess the quality of care in longer term mental health facilities. The Quality Indicator for Rehabilitative Care (QuIRC) was developed to address this gap through a study funded by the European Commission involving ten European countries at different stages of deinstitutionalisation (Bulgaria, Czech Republic, Germany, Greece, Italy, Netherlands, Poland, Portugal, Spain and the UK) [12].

The QuIRC assesses seven domains of care in longer term hospital and community mental health units (Living Environment; Therapeutic Environment; Treatments and Interventions; Self-Management and Autonomy; Social Interface; Human Rights; and Recovery Based Practice). The domains of care included in the toolkit were identified through triangulation of the results of: i) a review of care standards in each country; ii) a systematic literature review of the components of care (and their effectiveness) in longer term mental health units [13]; iii) an international Delphi exercise with four stakeholder groups in each of the ten countries, involving 447 participants (service users, carers, professionals, advocates) [14]. The toolkit collects data on various aspects of the unit including: staffing; staff training and supervision; built environment; treatments and interventions offered; availability of activities for service users; care planning processes; involvement of service users in their own care and the running of the unit; promotion of service users' autonomy, independence and physical health; policies and processes relating to managing challenging behavior; facilitation of service users' access to and involvement in community activities; involvement of families and carers; policies and processes related to complaints and confidentiality; facilitation of service users' access to advocacy and legal representation. The toolkit was piloted and refined with input from an international expert panel. Its inter-rater reliability was then tested in 202 units and found to be excellent [15]. The final version comprises 145 questions that can be completed by the unit manager in less than one hour. Of these, 86 items contribute to scores on the seven QuIRC domains. A web based version of the QuIRC [16] provides a printable report on the unit's performance on the seven domains, presented as percentages for ease of interpretation by unit managers. Further details of the content of the QuIRC, its item structure and psychometric properties are published elsewhere [15].

Since the toolkit assess the quality of a facility from information provided by the unit manager, we also aimed to validate the QuIRC ratings by investigating their association with service users' ratings of the quality of care [12,15]. This paper reports on the results of this validation. Inter-rater reliability of unit manager and service user QuIRC ratings was not feasible since the QuIRC was designed for completion by the unit manager and contains many items that service users would not have been able to answer. Instead service users' assessments of the quality of care were made using standardised measures of their experiences of care, quality of life, autonomy and assessment of the facility's therapeutic milieu.

Method

Ethics Statement

The study was approved by the relevant ethics committees in each of the ten participating countries involved in developing the QuIRC (Bulgaria - Ethics Committee, Alexandrovska University Hospital; Czech Republic - General University Hospital, Prague, Ethics Committee; Germany – Ethik Kommission der Medizinischen Fakultät Carl Gustav Carus an der Technischen Universität Dresden; Greece - University Mental Health Research Institutes Medical; Italy - Comitato Etico Indipendente; the Netherlands - Medical Ethical Committee of the University Medical Centre; Poland - Commission of Bioethics, Wroclaw Medical University; Portugal - Ethical Committee of the New University of Lisbon Medical School; Spain - Comisión Etica de la Universidad de Granada; UK - City and East London Multi Region Ethics Committee).

Recruitment

At least 20 units that provided longer term care (at least six months) for adults with severe mental health problems were recruited in each of the ten countries. Units had to provide for at least six patients/residents, have communal facilities and staff on site, 24 hours per day. Units that only provided for other, specific groups (such as those with learning disability, organic brain injuries, substance misuse or dementia) were excluded. Hospital and community based units were recruited to give a range in size and geographical spread within countries. Sampling was not random; units were identified from registration lists in each country and/or were known to the lead investigator in each country. After gaining informed consent, the manager of each unit was interviewed using the QuIRC by the researcher in the relevant country.

A list of each unit's current service users was generated by the unit manager. Service users were randomly selected for potential participation from each unit with a recruitment target range of between five and 13 per unit; five was agreed by the study partners as the minimum required for a representative sample and 13 was agreed an appropriate maximum since additional participants would not add further data about that unit relevant to the study aims. In units with 13 or fewer beds, all service users were approached for potential participation. In larger units, random sampling was carried out by the research team in each country; each service user on the unit manager's list was allocated a number and a random number generator programme distributed by the lead centre (University College London) was used to identify those who the researcher should approach for potential participation. Written informed consent was then gained by the researcher before proceeding with a face to face research interview. Where fewer than five service users were recruited the unit was excluded and a further unit recruited. Service user participants were paid 10 Euros for their time in all countries except Bulgaria where such payments were not usual practice. Data were collected between February and September 2009.

Service User Measures

For each of the four standardised measures used to assess service users' assessment of the quality of care, higher scores represented better experiences. Quality of life was assessed using the Manchester Short Assessment of Quality of Life (MANSA) [17] which has been translated for use in many European countries. The service user rates 12 aspects of their life on a scale from 1 (couldn't be worse) to 7 (couldn't be better) and a total mean score between 1 and 7 is generated. The Resident Choice Scale (RCS) [18] was used to assess service users' experiences of autonomy in the unit; the freedom to choose from a range of options without any coercion to bias that choice. Although there are no measures developed specifically for the assessment of autonomy of people with long term mental health problems, the issues relevant to those in longer term mental health facilities relate to mental capacity and the degree to which the facility promotes freedom of choice and independence across all aspects of everyday living. These aspects are captured in the RCS which required only minor adaptation for our purposes (the deletion of four items). The service user rates the degree to which they have choice over various aspects of daily activities (e.g. meal times) and the running of the unit on a four point scale ("I have no choice at all about this", "I have very little choice about this", "I can express a choice about this but I do not have the final say", "I have complete choice about this"). A total score with a range 22 to 88 is generated. The degree to which service users felt involved in their treatment and care was assessed using the Your Treatment and Care (YTC) [19] questionnaire which has been used in the UK in service user led assessments of mental health services. The service user is asked to rate 25 items related to their care (e.g. "I know who my Doctor is") as "yes, "no" or "don't know". The number of "yes" answers is summed to give a total score with a possible maximum of 25. The Good Milieu Index (GMI) [20] is a five item scale that was used to assess the unit's therapeutic culture from the service user's perspective. Service users rate their general satisfaction with the unit, with staff and other residents, and the degree to which they feel the unit facilitates their confidence and abilities on a scale of one to five (from "not at all" to "very much") and a total score ranging from 5 to 25 is generated. An assessment of service user function was also made by the researcher using the Global Assessment of Function (GAF) [21] in order to take this into account as a potential mediator. All measures were translated and back translated in each centre and checked for accuracy of content at the lead centre. Researchers were trained in the use of all measures by HK. Inter-rater reliability of GAF scores was assessed at a training session for all researchers from each centre (a total of 20) using clinical vignettes and found to be 0.88 (95% CI: 0.76, 0.96).

Data Management and Analysis

A common SPSS database was developed in the lead centre and distributed to all centres. A test entry of pilot data in each centre clarified any coding queries. Double data entry was completed for 10% of the toolkit data using a separate database and the study statistician (SW) carried out data validation on the two databases for each centre. The maximum error rate was set at 5%. Any centre that had an error rate above this was required to complete double data entry for all their data.

A multilevel model was used for the analysis of associations between QuIRC ratings and service user ratings with the aim of identifying the domains of care that independently predicted better service user experiences of care. Multilevel modelling allowed analysis of associations between service user ratings (level 1 data) as dependent variables with unit QuIRC domain ratings (level 2 data) as independent variables. To be able to test for 10 predictors of a medium effect size ($R^2 = 0.35$) with 90% power at a 1.25% significance level (as four dependent variables were explored), a

minimum of 203 level 2 units were required [22]. The predictor variables were the seven QuIRC domain ratings plus an overall QuIRC score - the sum of all 86 individual items scored in the seven domains. Unit and service user variables which needed to be controlled for as potential mediators were agreed by the research partners (community or hospital based unit, service users' age, diagnosis of psychosis or not, and level of functioning as assessed by GAF) and included in the models.

The four service user (level 1, dependent) variables (MANSA, RCS, YTC and GMI) were all normally distributed. Associations with the eight unit (level 2, independent) variables, also normally distributed, were investigated (the seven QuIRC domains and the total QuIRC score). The QuIRC domain ratings and the total score were correlated with each other (21 out of the 28 pair wise correlations were above 0.5, nine correlations were above 0.8) so could not be entered simultaneously into regression models and were therefore entered separately.

Three sets of models were then fitted: in *Model A* only the indicated domain score was entered as an independent variable, a fixed effect. A random intercept term was included to adjust for the multiple service users per unit; in *Model B* the level 2 unit type variable (hospital or community) was added to *Model A*, along with the interaction between domain score and unit type; in *Model C* three level 1 service user characteristic variables were entered - age, GAF score and diagnosis (psychosis or not), in addition to the domain score and unit type. In addition to the random intercept term, random slopes were also included for age and GAF score. The interaction term added in *Model B* was removed in *Model C* as it was non-significant in all models. To illustrate the relationships found in the models the percentage of mental health unit-to-unit variation in the respective dependent variable explained by each of three models, *A*, *B* and *C* is presented. The *B-A* values represent the amount of extra variation explained by the inclusion of the unit type variable, *C-B* values show the amount of extra variation explained by the inclusion of the level 1 service user characteristic variables. *Model C* was only fitted when the domain score was significantly related to the dependent variable. In all models a country random effect was included.

Results

Response

A total of 213 units participated in the study of which 109 (51%) were in the inner city, 67 (32%) in the suburbs and 37 (17%) in a rural location. The majority (131, 62%) were in the community, 45 (21%) were hospital wards and 37 (17%) were units within the hospital grounds. Their size ranged from five to 120 beds (mean 26, median 18) and 31 (15%) units were for men only and 19 (9%) for women only. Overall, 2495 service users were randomly sampled for potential participation in the study of whom 722 (29%) were unable to give informed consent for the research interview, 23 (1%) declined to participate and 1750 (70%) were interviewed (two of whom had data missing for age). Service users were recruited from each country as follows: Bulgaria 180; Czech Republic 171; Germany 189; Greece 150; Italy 179; Netherlands 175; Poland 176; Portugal 170; Spain 210; UK 150.

Service User Characteristics

Of the 1750 service users, over one third (651, 37%) were residing in a hospital ward and the rest were coded as "community" for the purposes of our analysis. Almost two thirds (1087, 62%) were male, the mean age was 46 years (range 18 to 87), most were unemployed (547, 31%) or retired (906, 52%), with only 50 (3%) in paid employment. Two thirds (1173/1750, 67%)

had a diagnosis of psychosis and the mean length of stay in the current unit was 277 weeks (median 129, SD 838). The mean (SD) GAF score was 49 (15) and ranged from 20 to 80. In most countries, data on participants who were approached but did not agree to participate were not gathered in accordance with the guidance from the relevant ethics committee. However, data were available on 193 of the 745 non-participants; they did not differ from participants in mean age, gender or diagnosis (psychosis or not).

No centres had data entry error rates over 5% and therefore double data entry was not required.

Association between QuIRC Domain Scores and Service User Ratings

Table 1 shows the "percentage of variation explained" statistic for each of the eight independent variables and four dependent variables. Examining the *Model A* results row for each independent variable, the following can be seen: over 10% of the unit-to-unit variation in service users' mean quality of life (MANSA) scores was explained by the Living Environment and Self-Management and Autonomy domains of the QuIRC; 55% of the unit-to-unit variation in service users' mean autonomy (RCS) scores was explained by the Self-Management and Autonomy domain, and overall QuIRC score, Living Environment, Recovery Based Practice and Human Rights domains each explained 30–35% of the explainable variation; over 35% of the unit-to-unit variation in service users' mean experiences of care (YTC) scores was explained by the Self-Management and Autonomy domain and overall QuIRC score, and the Living Environment, Recovery Based Practice, Human Rights and Therapeutic Environment domains each explained 20–28%. The Self-Management and Autonomy domain explained 23% of the unit-to-unit variation in service users' mean scores of therapeutic milieu (GMI) and 16% was explained by the Living Environment domain. The Social Interface and Treatments and Interventions domains explained very little variation in any of the dependent variables.

Summary of Results for Each Dependent Variable

Quality of life (MANSA). In *Model A*, overall QuIRC score, Therapeutic Environment, Treatments and Interventions and Social Interface domain scores were not found to be associated with service users' quality of life. Whilst the other four domains were significantly associated with quality of life, Living Environment and Self-Management and Autonomy each explained only approximately 11% of unit-to-unit variation, and Recovery Based Practice and Human Rights each explained only 3–4%. Adding in type of unit in *Model B* made little or no difference to these results. In *Model C*, quality of life was found to be highly influenced by service user characteristics being included in the model, with approximately 30% more variation being explained by their inclusion. For each of the four domains explored in *Model C* (Human Rights, Recovery Based Practice, Self-Management and Autonomy, Living Environment), age, GAF and diagnosis were associated with quality of life as main effects but no interactions were significant. Age and GAF were positively associated with quality of life; those with a psychotic disorder having a slightly higher quality of life.

In summary, while there was evidence that staff ratings of their units' Living Environment and promotion of Self-Management and Autonomy explained some of the variation in service users' quality of life between units, service users' characteristics had a greater influence on this.

Autonomy (RCS). All QuIRC domain scores and overall QuIRC score were significantly associated with service users'

autonomy in *Model A*. The Self-Management and Autonomy domain score explained most of the unit-to-unit variation (55%) and the Social Interface domain explained the least (6%). Adding in the type of unit in *Model B* resulted in 9–20% more variation being explained for all domains except Self-Management and Autonomy and Living Environment. This suggests that these domains contain items which are highly related to unit type. Adding in service user characteristics in *Model C* did not result in further explanation of unit-to-unit variation. Diagnosis was not associated with autonomy. Age and GAF were significant as main effects but had few significant interactions on domain scores. Age was negatively associated with autonomy (younger people scoring higher) and GAF score was positively associated (better functioning was associated with higher autonomy scores). There was a significant interaction between GAF and Living Environment when modelled. The slope of the association for Living Environment scores and autonomy was greater for those with lower GAF scores. In other words, the association between the quality of the unit's Living Environment and its service users' autonomy was greater for those with poorer functioning.

In summary, all QuIRC domain scores were highly related to service users' autonomy, particularly the Self-Management and Autonomy domain. The type of unit was also important, users in hospital units having significantly lower levels of autonomy. User characteristics did not explain further variation between the units but age and GAF were significantly associated with autonomy.

Experiences of care (YTC). In *Model A*, all QuIRC domains were significantly associated with service users' experiences of care, with the Self-Management and Autonomy domain and overall QuIRC score each explaining over one third of the unit-to-unit variation in YTC score. The Social Interface domain explained the least variation (7%). Adding in type of unit in *Model B* increased the percentage of variation explained in all but the Self-Management and Autonomy and Living Environment domains, although this effect was minimal for the overall QuIRC score, Human Rights and Recovery Based Practice domains. For other domains (Therapeutic Environment, Treatments and Interventions, Social Interface) there was an association between type of unit and experiences of care, with service users in hospital units having lower ratings on these three domains. For all domains, age and GAF were associated with experiences of care as main effects but few interactions were significant. Diagnosis was not associated with experiences of care. Age was negatively associated with experiences of care, younger people scoring higher, and GAF was positively associated with experiences of care, with better functioning being associated with higher scores. When Social Interface was modelled the slope of the association with experiences of care was higher for older service users (borderline significant).

In summary, all QuIRC domain scores were highly related to service users' experience of care, particularly the Self-Management and Autonomy domain and the overall QuIRC score. There was some evidence that service users in hospital units had poorer experiences of care than those in community units. Service user characteristics did not explain further variation between the units but age and GAF were significantly associated with experiences of care.

Therapeutic milieu (GMI). In *Model A*, all QuIRC domain scores, apart from Social Interface and Treatments and Interventions were significantly associated with the therapeutic milieu of the unit. The Recovery Based Practice, Living Environment and Self-Management and Autonomy domains explained the most unit-to-unit variation (16–23%). Adding in unit type in *Model B* increased the amount of variation explained between units for all domains apart

Table 1. Percentage of unit-to-unit variance in service user outcomes explained by QuIRC domain scores using three models.

	Model	Quality of Life (MANSA)	Autonomy (RCS)	Experience of care (YTC)	Therapeutic Milieu (GMI)
QuIRC total	A	0.1	31.2	35.6	12.1
	B	1.7	40.6	38.2	17.4
	B–A	1.6	9.4	2.6	5.3
	C		35.7	29.1	36.0
	C–B		−4.9	−9.1	18.6
Therapeutic Environment	A	−1.0	17.2	19.8	4.8
	B	3.1	34.0	28.5	13.2
	B–A	4.1	16.7	8.7	8.4
	C		26.9	19.4	34.3
	C–B		−7.1	−9.1	21.0
Treatments and Interventions	A	−0.6	11.9	15.7	1.9
	B	3.5	28.8	24.4	10.1
	B–A	4.1	16.9	8.6	8.3
	C		22.0	15.2	
	C–B		−6.8	−9.1	
Human Rights	A	2.8	31.6	24.8	9.9
	B	3.6	40.3	28.5	16.8
	B–A	0.8	8.7	3.7	6.8
	C	10.5	39.3	21.6	40.8
	C–B	6.8	−1.0	−6.9	24.1
Recovery Based Practice	A	3.5	30.1	28.3	15.7
	B	2.8	39.6	31.5	20.0
	B–A	−0.7	9.5	3.2	4.3
	C	9.8	33.9	21.7	41.5
	C–B	7.0	−5.7	−9.8	21.5
Social Interface	A	0.1	6.4	6.8	3.0
	B	3.9	26.0	18.1	14.7
	B–A	3.7	19.6	11.2	11.7
	C		17.9	7.1	
	C–B		−8.1	−11.0	
Self-Management and Autonomy	A	10.9	55.1	36.7	23.0
	B	9.1	56.4	35.9	25.0
	B–A	−1.8	1.2	−0.8	2.1
	C	16.8	51.9	27.5	43.8
	C–B	7.7	−4.4	−8.3	18.8
Living Environment	A	11.3	35.7	27.2	16.2
	B	9.3	36.3	26.2	17.8
	B–A	−2.0	0.5	−1.0	1.6
	C	15.5	35.9	19.6	32.6
	C–B	6.2	−0.4	−6.6	14.7

QuIRC = Quality Indicator for Rehabilitative Care.
Model A: QuIRC domain score entered as the only independent variable.
Model B: unit type (hospital or community) added to Model A.
Model C: service user characteristics added to Model B (age, GAF and psychosis or not).
Differences in % variance for each model also shown: B–A, C–B.

from Self-Management and Autonomy and Living Environment. Service users in hospital units had lower GMI ratings (by just over half of one point). Adding in service user characteristics in *Model C* increased the amount of between unit variation explained in the models by between 15 and 24%, suggesting a strong relationship between service user characteristics and GMI, independent of domain scores and type of unit. The GAF scores and age were both positively associated with GMI, though diagnosis was not. However, some of the interactions between diagnosis and domain scores were significant when modelled and the slope (strength) of the associations between the Recovery Based Practice, Therapeutic Environment and overall QuIRC scores and GMI score was greater for those without a psychotic disorder.

In summary, the Self-Management and Autonomy and Living Environment domain scores explained most of the variation in service users' ratings of units' therapeutic milieu, and the Social Interface and Treatments and Interventions domains were not associated with therapeutic milieu. Service users' ratings of therapeutic milieu were highly influenced by service user characteristics, with older and better functioning service users rating the GMI higher.

Clinical Relevance

In order to illustrate the clinical relevance of changes in domain scores (change in quality of care), we calculated the impact of a 10% increase in each domain score on service users' autonomy and experiences of care. These two service user measures were chosen as they were not influenced by service user characteristics. A change of three points on the autonomy scale (RCS) was equivalent to either having complete choice on an issue (item) that the service user originally had no choice at all, or moving one point along the scale towards increased choice on three different items. On the measure of experiences of care (YTC) a change of one point was equivalent to answering 'Yes' to one further item of the 25 in this tool.

Table 2 shows the degree to which autonomy and experiences of care scores would be improved by a 10% improvement in each domain score. Results are shown for all units and for community units over hospital units.

A 10% improvement in any QuIRC domain score, except Social Interface, was associated with a statistically and clinically significant increase in service users' autonomy scores of at least three points. This effect was greater for service users in community based units than those in hospital based units for all domains except Self-Management and Autonomy, and Living Environment.

A 10% improvement in any QuIRC domain score was associated with a statistically significant increase in service users' experience of care scores of 0.3 to 1.1 points. The effect of these improvements was greater for service users in community based units compared to hospital units for all domains except Recovery Based Practice, Self-Management and Autonomy, and Living Environment.

Discussion

We found direct links between the quality of an institution (QuIRC domains) and its service users' experiences of care and autonomy. All QuIRC domains except Treatments and Interventions and Social Interface were found to be significantly positively associated with service users' assessments of the units' therapeutic milieu, though service user characteristics accounted for most of this association. The QuIRC domains Living Environment and Self-Management and Autonomy were significantly positively associated with service users' quality of life but again, service user characteristics accounted for much of the association. The associations between QuIRC domain scores and service user autonomy and experiences of care were independent of service user characteristics.

Autonomy is the freedom to choose from a range of options without any coercion to bias that choice. However, it may be affected by mental incapacity secondary to mental illness [23]. Our findings are particularly relevant therefore, since the associations we found between quality of care as assessed by QuIRC and service user autonomy were not mediated by service user function. These findings give confidence that the unit quality ratings derived from the unit manager concurred with service users' experience of the care provided and the degree to which the unit promoted their autonomy. In developing a new assessment tool, the usual approach to validation is to assess its convergence against an existing measure that assesses a similar construct, or against expert opinion. However this was not possible since there was no measure assessing the quality of longer term mental health institutions available, and expert opinion is usually used for clinical assessment tools. Given that the QuIRC is completed by the manager of the facility, we felt it was appropriate to assess its association with the experiences of care of those using the service. In other words, our results provide further validation of the toolkit domain ratings.

Ideally, staff and service users should be interviewed when assessing the quality of a facility, but in situations where service user interviews are not feasible (for example, where service users are too unwell to participate or lack capacity to give informed consent to do so), our findings suggest that the QuIRC ratings derived from the unit manager may provide a proxy indication of the overall service user experience of care and autonomy in that unit.

We demonstrated that a hypothetical, small increase in any QuIRC domain quality rating (of 10%) resulted in improvements in service user autonomy and experiences of care. This effect appeared to be more clinically meaningful for service user autonomy than experiences of care. This suggests that initiatives to improve unit quality could potentially benefit service users in achieving greater autonomy, one of the main aims of contemporary mental health services [24]. The effect on service user autonomy appeared generally greater for those in community based, rather than hospital based, units. However, increase in quality in the Living Environment and Self-Management and Autonomy domains was not associated with a significant improvement in the autonomy of service users of community based units. This may reflect a "ceiling effect" since community based facilities have been shown to be less "institutionalised" than hospital settings [25,26].

Whilst our study included over 200 units from ten countries at different stages of deinstitutionalisation across Europe, we did not randomly sample units for potential participation and therefore those that took part may not be representative of other longer term mental health units of the countries that were involved. Whilst this did not pose any systematic bias relevant to the purpose of our study (to assess the internal validity of the QuIRC), we are mindful that it is relevant to its external validity. For example, units that were willing to participate may be of higher quality than other units. However, one centre (Portugal) included all its longer term units in this study and the QuIRC has since been used to assess the quality of all mental health rehabilitation units in England without problem.

We randomly identified service users for participation in order to minimise selection bias, but almost one third were unable to give informed consent to participate. Our findings could therefore be subject to response bias since those who were least well were unable to be interviewed. However, our analyses took account of service users' global functioning in order to mitigate against this potential limitation and service user characteristics were not found

Table 2. Estimated change in service users' autonomy and experiences of care given an increase of 10% in each QuIRC domain.

QuIRC domain		Autonomy Score (RCS)		Experience of Care Score (YTC)	
		Mean Change	Significance	Mean Change	Significance
Therapeutic Environment	All units	4.2	<0.001	0.9	<0.001
	Community vs hospital	7.5	<0.001	1.1	0.003
Treatments and Interventions	All units	3.8	<0.001	0.9	<0.001
	Community vs hospital	7.5	<0.001	1.1	0.004
Human Rights	All units	4.1	<0.001	0.8	<0.001
	Community vs hospital	6.2	<0.001	0.8	0.026
Recovery Based Practice	All units	3.8	<0.001	0.7	<0.001
	Community vs hospital	5.4	<0.001	0.6	0.090
Social Interface	All units	1.5	0.001	0.3	<0.001
	Community vs hospital	7.8	<0.001	1.1	0.004
Self-Management and Autonomy	All units	4.3	<0.001	0.8	<0.001
	Community vs hospital	2.1	0.065	0.2	0.588
Living Environment	All units	3.3	<0.001	0.6	<0.001
	Community vs hospital	2.1	0.147	0.1	0.891

QuIRC = Quality Indicator for Rehabilitative Care.
RCS = Resident Choice Scale.
YTC = Your Treatment and Care.

to influence the associations we found between unit quality and service users' autonomy and experiences of care. The high non-participation rate due to lack of capacity also highlights the need for proxy assessments in this service user group.

As in all cross-sectional observational studies, our results remain open to residual confounding. For example, other, unmeasured user characteristics may have affected the associations we observed or obscured others we missed. Nevertheless, the positive associations we found between the quality of the unit and the service user experience not only support the validity of QuIRC, but also provide helpful indications for how care might be improved for the large number of people whose mental health problems necessitate their residence in longer term facilities across Europe.

In conclusion, ratings of the quality of longer term mental health facilities made by service managers using the QuIRC were positively associated with service users' ratings of their autonomy and experiences of care. In situations where service user interviews are not feasible, the QuIRC may provide a proxy indication of the overall service user experience. Interventions that improve quality of care in these settings may promote service users' autonomy.

Acknowledgments

The authors would like to thank all the unit managers who participated in the research. They would also like to acknowledge the contributions of the members of the International Expert Panel throughout the study and thank them for their valuable input: Mr Jerry Tew (social scientist, UK); social care – Mr Tony Ryan (independent consultant on out of area placements, UK), Mr Michael Clark (Care Services Improvement Partnership, UK); rehabilitation psychiatry and psychology – Professor Tom Craig (UK), Dr Frank Holloway (UK), Professor Jaap van Weeghel (Netherlands), Dr Joanna Meder (sadly, since deceased, Poland), Professor Geoff Shepherd (UK); service user perspective – Mr Maurice Arbuthnott (UK), Ms Vanessa Pinfold (Rethink, UK); human rights law - Associate Professor Luis Fernando Barrios-Flores (University of Granada, Spain); mental health law - Professor Peter Bartlett (Nottingham University, UK); disability rights – Ms Liz Sayce (Royal Association for Disability and Rehabilitation, UK); care standards – Dr Geraldine Strathdee (Healthcare Commission, UK).

Author Contributions

Conceived and designed the experiments: HK SW CW MK TK JCe JR GO RM DW AK DP JCa GC. Performed the experiments: TT PT MS PB LK SA PR EV PP FG GC. Analyzed the data: SW. Contributed reagents/materials/analysis tools: HK SW MK CW TK RM. Wrote the paper: HK SW CW MK TT PT TK MS JCe PB JR LK GO SA RM PR DW EV AK PP DP FG JCa GC.

References

1. World Health Organisation (2005) Mental Health Atlas. WHO, Geneva.
2. Muijen M (2008) Mental Health Services in Europe: An Overview. *Psychiatric Services*, **59**;5): 479–482.
3. Priebe S, Badesconyi A, Fioritti A, Hansson L, Kilian R, et al. (2005) Reinstitutionalisation in mental health care: comparison of data on service provision from six European countries. *BMJ*; 330: 123–6.
4. Killaspy H, Meier R (2010) A Fair Deal for Mental Health Rehabilitation Services. *The Psychiatrist*, 34: 265–267.

5. Knapp M, Beecham J, McDaid D, Matosevic T, Smith M (2011) The economic consequences of deinstitutionalisation of mental health services: lessons from a systematic review of European experience. *Health and Social Care in the Community* 19(2): 113–125.

6. Killaspy H, Rambarran D, Bledin K (2007) Mental health needs of clients of rehabilitation services: a survey in one Trust. *Journal of Mental Health*, 17: 207–218.

7. Meltzer H (1997) Treatment-resistant schizophrenia - the role of clozapine. *Current Medical Resident Opinion*, 14: 1–20.

8. Green MF (1996) What are the functional consequences of neurocognitive deficits in schizophrenia? *American Journal of Psychiatry*, 153: 321–330.

9. Mueser KT, Tarrier N, eds (1998) Handbook of Social Functioning in Schizophrenia. Boston, Allyn & Bacon.

10. Trieman N, Leff J (2002) Long-term outcome of long-stay psychiatric service users considered unsuitable to live in the community: TAPS Project 44. *British Journal of Psychiatry*, 181: 428–432.

11. European Commission (2005) Green Paper: Improving the Mental Health of the Population: Towards a Strategy on Mental Health for the European Union. Brussels, Commission European, eds. Health and Consumer Protection Directorate-General. Available: ec.europa.eu/health/phdeterminants/lifestyle/mental/greenpaper/mentalgpen.pdf. Accessed 9 May 2012.

12. Killaspy M, King MB, Wright C, White S, McCrone P, et al. (2009) Study Protocol for the Development of a European Measure of Best Practice for People with Long Term Mental Illness in Institutional Care (DEMoBinc). *BMC Psychiatry*, 9: 36.

13. Taylor T, Killaspy H, Wright C, Turton P, White S, et al. (2009) A systematic review of the international published literature relating to quality of institutional care for people with longer term mental health problems. *BMC Psychiatry*, 9: 55.

14. Turton P, Wright C, White S, Killaspy H, Taylor T, et al. (2010) Promoting recovery in long term mental health institutional care: an international Delphi study of stakeholder views. *Psychiatric Services*, **61**(3), 293–299.

15. Killaspy H, White S, Wright C, Taylor T, Turton P, et al. (2010) Development of the Quality Indicator for Rehabilitative Care, *BMC Psychiatry*, 11: 35.

16. The Quality Indicator for Rehabilitative Care website. Available: http://www.quirc.eu. Accessed 9 May 2012.

17. Priebe S, Huxley P, Knight S, Evans S (1999) Application and results of the Manchester Short Assessment of Quality if Life (MANSA). *International Journal of Social Psychiatry*, 45: 7–12.

18. Hatton C, Emerson E, Robertson J, Gregory N, Kessissoglou S, et al. (2004) The Resident Choice Scale: a measure to assess opportunities for self-determination in residential settings. *Journal of Intellectual Disability Research*, 48: 103–113.

19. Webb Y, Clifford P, Fowler V, Morgan C, Hanson M (2000) Comparing patients' experience of mental health services in England: a five-Trust survey. *International Journal of Health Quality Assurance*, 13(6): 273–281.

20. Røssberg JI, Friis S (2003) A suggested revision of the Ward Atmosphere Scale. *Acta Psychiatrica Scandinavica*, 108: 374–380.

21. Jones SH, Thornicroft G, Coffey M, Dunn G (1995) A brief mental health outcome scale. Reliability and validity of the Global Assessment of Functioning (GAF). *British Journal of Psychiatry*, **166**;654): 659 p.

22. Dunlap W, Xxin X, Myers L (2004) Computing aspects of power for multiple regression. *Behavior Research Methods, Instruments, & Computers*, **36**;4): 695–701.

23. Liegeois A, Van Audenove C (2005) Ethical dilemmas in community mental health care. *Journal of Medical Ethics*, 31: 452–456.

24. Rehabilitation, Social Faculty (2009) *Enabling recovery for people with complex mental health needs: a template for rehabilitation services in England*. Royal College of Psychiatrists, FR/RS/ 04.

25. Cullen D, Carson J, Holloway F, Towey A, Jumbo A, et al. (1997) Community and hospital residential care: A comparative evaluation. *Irish Journal of Psychological Medicine*, 14: 92–98.

26. Trauer T, Farhall J, Newton R, Cheung P (2001) From long-stay psychiatric hospital to Community Care Unit: evaluation at 1 year. *Social Psychiatry and Psychiatric Epidemiology*, 36: 416–419.

3

Walking Performance: Correlation between Energy Cost of Walking and Walking Participation. New Statistical Approach Concerning Outcome Measurement

Marco Franceschini[1], Anais Rampello[2], Maurizio Agosti[2], Maurizio Massucci[3], Federica Bovolenta[4], Patrizio Sale[1]*

1 Department of NeuroRehabilitation IRCCS San Raffale, Pisana, Rome, 2 Department of Rehabilitation, University Hospital of Parma, Parma, Italy, 3 Rehabilitation Unit, Hospital of Passignano, Passignano, Perugia, Italy, 4 Medicine Rehabilitation NOCSAE Hospital AUSL of Modena, Modena, Italy

Abstract

Walking ability, though important for quality of life and participation in social and economic activities, can be adversely affected by neurological disorders, such as Spinal Cord Injury, Stroke, Multiple Sclerosis or Traumatic Brain Injury. The aim of this study is to evaluate if the energy cost of walking (CW), in a mixed group of chronic patients with neurological diseases almost 6 months after discharge from rehabilitation wards, can predict the walking performance and any walking restriction on community activities, as indicated by Walking Handicap Scale categories (WHS). One hundred and seven subjects were included in the study, 31 suffering from Stroke, 26 from Spinal Cord Injury and 50 from Multiple Sclerosis. The multivariable binary logistical regression analysis has produced a statistical model with good characteristics of fit and good predictability. This model generated a cut-off value of.40, which enabled us to classify correctly the cases with a percentage of 85.0%. Our research reveal that, in our subjects, CW is the only predictor of the walking performance of in the community, to be compared with the score of WHS. We have been also identifying a cut-off value of CW cost, which makes a distinction between those who can walk in the community and those who cannot do it. In particular, these values could be used to predict the ability to walk in the community when discharged from the rehabilitation units, and to adjust the rehabilitative treatment to improve the performance.

Editor: Guglielmo Foffani, Hospital Nacional de Paraplégicos, Spain

Funding: The authors have no support or funding to report.

Competing Interests: The authors have declared that no competing interests exist.

* E-mail: patrizio.sale@gmail.com

Introduction

Walking ability can be adversely affected by neurological disorders, such as Spinal Cord Injury (SCI), Stroke, Multiple Sclerosis (MS) or Traumatic Brain Injury (TBI) [1]. Walking recovery is one of the most important goals of rehabilitation treatment for neurological and/or orthopaedic diseases [2–5]. From the perspective of the patients, walking is not more relevant than the ability to walk in the community independently [6,7] but several factors interfere with walking recovery from neurological diseases. The main one is the high energy cost of gait due to muscular weakness and consequent biomechanical inefficiency [8]. The complexity of environmental factors is another aspect [9] that makes it difficult to use skills hard earned in rehabilitation setting. The roles of the environmental factors, such as barriers of facilitators, were emphasized by the International Classification of Functioning and Disability and Health [10]. This framework distinguishes the "capacity" as the theoretical ability of walking if the environment were uniform or standard (environment without barriers or facilitators) from the "performance" that relates to what a person does in the environmental context in which he actually lives. One of the most important objectives of rehabilitation is to reduce the gap between walking capacity and walking performance. Various clinical scales were carried out to asses and

to predict the walking abilities of people suffering from neurological disease. On the basis of the gait speed and the self-reported ability to walk in the community of a group of post-stroke people, Perry and colleagues [11] have created a Walking Handicap Scale (WHS), a classification of 6 functional walking categories, 3 of which refer to community ambulation. In particular, the WHS was performed to offer quantitative method of relating the social disadvantage of patients to the impairment and disability sustained [11]. It could be important to provide community-walking performance of the patient on the basis of walking capacity acquired in the rehabilitation unit. Concerning the biomechanical aspects of walking, many works have considered that the gait velocity, the activity monitors and the spatiotemporal parameters can predict different skills of community ambulation [12–13]. Shumway-Cook and colleagues emphasize the importance of temporal factors, postural transitions, external physical load and terrain [12]. However, the energy cost of walking represents a good indicator of overall exercise performance of walking, which should be considered when evaluating a patient's functional independence [14].

The aim of this study is to evaluate if the energy cost of walking (CW) in a mixed group of patients with neurological diseases, almost 6 months after discharge from rehabilitation wards, can predict the walking performance and the walking restriction to participate in the community, as indicated by Walking Handicap Scale categories (WHS) [11].

Methods

Design

Cross-sectional study.

Sample

From January 2007 to December 2009 we recruited outpatient subjects with Stroke, Multiple Sclerosis and Spinal Cord Injury, all with walking limitations. The inclusion criteria were: (a) age >18 years at the beginning of the study; (b) almost 6 months after conclusion of a programmed rehabilitation plan; (c) return home after discharge; (d) ability to walk independently, with residual difficulty for at least 6 minutes, with or without walking aids. The exclusion criteria were: (a) presence of cardio respiratory co-morbidity; (b) presence of orthopaedic co-morbidity (c) patients who refused the consent to take part in the study.

Sample Size

Supported by literature, we calculated the power of the sample based on 15 subjects for each independent variable (predictor) used in the regression [15]. In particular, the following independent variables (Age, Sex, Etiology [Stroke, MS, SCI] and energy cost) were inserted in the regression model (binary logistic). According to these parameters, which therefore considered 6 independent variables for 15 subjects, at least 90 cases were required and we analysed 107 subjects.

Main Outcome Measures

Walking Handicap Scale (WHS) and the energy cost of walking (CW).

Testing Protocol

The local Ethics Committee approved the study. All clinical assessments and tests were performed in rehabilitation hospital and all patients gave written informed consent. A blinded examiner assessed clinical and metabolic evaluation of walking at the moment of the inclusion. The severity of MS was evaluated in accordance with EDSS scale, while for the SCI we referred to the Asia impairment scale. The Stroke group were classified in mild, moderate and severe according to FIM Score (mild >80, moderate 40–80 and severe <40). The clinical evaluation of gait ability was performed according to Walking Handicap Scale (WHS) [16], which was then dichotomized into two categories: the subjects with WHS $<=3$ (not able to perform community walking) and the subjects with WHS >3 (able to perform community walking). The Walking Handicap Scale (WHS) is an instrument that offers a quantitative method of relating the social disadvantage of walking to the impairment and disability of the patient. The metabolic test consisted of the registration of walking energy cost during a free indoor walking. For the energetic evaluation, the Body Mass Index of each subject was calculated. The energy cost of walking (CW) was measured with a portable miniature telemetry equipment (breath-by-breath-based) Oxycon Mobile (Sensormedics) [17]. Rosdahl and colleagues showed that metabolic variables, within a wide range of exercise intensities versus the Douglas bag measurements, are reliably measured with this instrument [18]. Responsiveness of Oxycon Mobile was also successfully validated in field measuring conditions, such as low temperatures, high humidity and with external wind [19]. Each test was performed in the morning, 3 hours after breakfast. The experimental procedure was the following: 5 minutes in sitting position, 6 minutes of continuous walking at a comfortable self-selected speed, and 5 minutes for recovery. All patients walked along an established route of 30 meters in length. The average speed was calculated by dividing the distance covered (m) at the time of walking. We used the term energy consumption ($mlO_2*Kg^{-1}*Kg^1$) to indicate the oxygen uptake divided by the patient's weight. Dividing this value by the speed, we obtained the energy cost per kilogram per unit of distance covered ($mlO_2*Kg^{-1}*min^{-1}$).

Statistical Methods

To predict the walking restriction of patients in community, we performed a multivariate logistic binary regression in which the dependent variable was the WHS score (dichotomized), while the independent predictors were age, sex, kind of neurological disability, speed, distance covered, energy consumption and cost of walking. Using logistic regression models, we performed multivariate analysis aimed at identifying multiple relations between a variable of interest (walking performance of patients in community) and two or more explicative variables. Inclusion of explicative variables in the models followed stepwise procedures (forward and backward), with specific motivations for each variable. The included individual variables are reported with their Odds Ratios where appropriate and the significance of each coefficient, in the model, was examined. Non-significant variables with p-value $p > 0.05$ were removed from the model one at a time, beginning with the variables having the highest probability levels. Every time a variable was eliminated, the integrity of the model was checked through Hosmer-Lemeshow test.

Once we defined a predictive model of walking in the community, we investigated whether there was a cut-off point of the energy cost of walking (the independent variables) that could predict membership of each subject in one of the two WHS categories. If a reference criterion was available, receiver-operating characteristic (ROC) analyses offered an elaborate method for the construction of cut-off points [20]. Having used a continuous variable such as Cost of Walking (CW), in which the sensitivity and specificity have for us the same statistical weight, the best cut-off point for obtaining a positive result from the test is the maximum value which can be obtained for both of these aspects of which the sum is the highest possible. This is necessary in order to identify the patients that cannot develop a walk in the context of the community. With this procedure, the determination of the cut-off point is equivalent to the achievement of the minimum value of false negative and false positive, which are dependent on mistakes in classification. The cut-off point obtained with this method has the characteristic of reaching the best expected objective, that is to say: maximize the potential for correct diagnosis and minimize the errors of classification. In the case in which c is the best cut-off point of the test results, Youden introduced the following index for ROC curve: J = sensitivity (c)+specificity (c). Moreover, finding the best cut-off point is equivalent to measuring the J of Youden Index. This index is an important synthesis of ROC curve. From the point of view of the graph, the Youden Index is the greatest vertical distance between ROC curve and the diagonal line (Fig. 1). It presents itself as having a complete and optimal potential measurement of the diagnostic capacity regarding clinical activity. ROCs describe the relation between sensitivity and specificity for different cut-off points. ROC analyses provide an evaluation of the ability of the diagnostic instruments to discriminate between health and disease.

The choice of cut-off points requires a trade-off between:

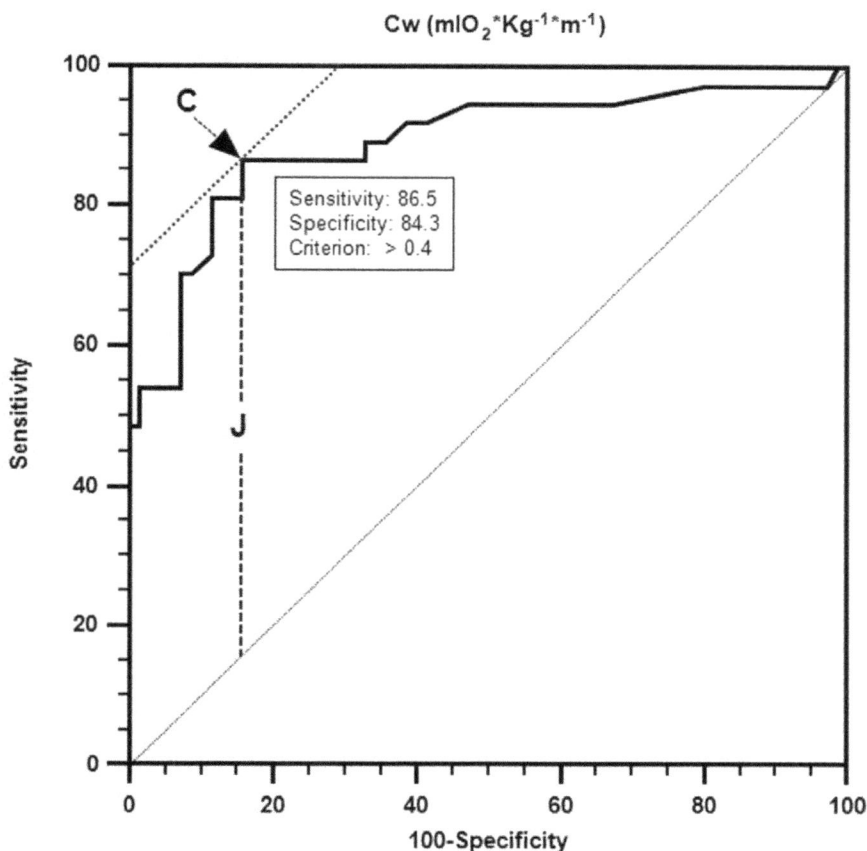

Figure 1. Model to identify a cut-off value of Energy Cost of walk (CW). The CW is the energy cost per kilogram per unit of distance covered ($mlO_2*Kg^{-1}*min^{-1}$). C is the criterion. J = sensitivity (C)+specificity (C). J finding the best cut-off point that is equivalent to measuring the J of Youden Index. Youden Index is the greatest vertical distance between ROC curve and the diagonal line.

1. High sensitivity, which means the likelihood of identifying an actual risk (i.e., "Restriction in walking participation") through a positive test result.

2. High specificity, which means the likelihood of identifying a non-existent risk (i.e., "Walking independently in the community") through a negative test result.

Assuming sensitivity and specificity are of equal importance, the maximum of the Youden Index indicates an optimal cut-off point [21]. The overall ability of a measure to discriminate between healthy and diseased subjects is indicated by the magnitude of the area under the curve (AUC). We know that it exists a correlation between the positive predictive value (PPV) and the negative predictive value (NPV), and that the prevalence, which in our sample refers to people able to "walk in a social context" in any case, is unknown. It is also noted that if the prevalence of the disease in the population is high, the results of all the tests are good but, in this case, we do not know the real prevalence of the people that walk in a social context [22–23].

The software packages "IBM SPSS version 20" and "MedCalc version 12.1.4" were used for analyses.

Results

One hundred and seven subjects were included in the study, 61 (57%) were males and 46 (43%) females: thirty-one (29%) suffering from Stroke, 26 (24.3%) from SCI and 50 (46.7%) from MS. The sample average age was 49.79±14.70 years (Stroke 62.03±11.77 years; SCI 44.92±15.56 years; MS 44.74±11.23 years), with a range of 20–84 years. Regarding clinical walking evaluation, the sample average of WHS score was 3.97±1.06 (range of 1–5), with 37 subjects whose scores were under 3, and 70 subjects whose scores were above 3 on the WHS. Walking Distance average was 203.35±129.14 meters, with a range of 12.5–528 meters; the average velocity was 33.93±21.57 m/min, with a range of 2.08–88 m/min. The mean energy consumption was 10.81±2.81 ($mlO_2*Kg^{-1}*Kg^1$) and the mean value of cost of walking was .51±.515 ($mlO_2*Kg^{-1}*min^{-1}$). For each pathology, a summary description of the collected data of the descriptive analysis of the sample and of the performance on the walking distance (WD) (m and % of predicted value), velocity (m/min), VO2 consumption, energy cost of walking (CW) with a reference to the significant range, is provided in Table 1 and Table 2. The multivariable binary logistical regression analysis has produced a statistical model with good characteristics of fit and good predictability (Table 3). The model presents a sufficient capacity of classification for each subject included in our sample (83.18% of cases). In our sample, due to the fact that both PPV and NPV are related to the sensitivity and the specificity of the test, and that they also depend on the prevalence of the disease in the population, these data, in our case, do not exist in the literature. The equation for the probability of classification model based on the measurement of energy cost (CW), which allowed us to determine the

Table 1. Descriptive analysis of the sample.

	Gender (N)	WHS (N) 1	2	3	4	5	Value	EDSS	ASIA A	ASIA B	ASIA C	ASIA D	Severe	Moderate	Mild	Time since	Brace	Cane	Rollator
Multiple Sclerosis		0	5	8	13	24											1	11	6
	Female 33						Mean	2,79								68,02			
	Male 17						SD	0,85								44,65			
							Mediane	3								66			
							Min	1								8			
							Max	4								160			
Spinal Cord Injury		1	3	8	4	10											14	8	15
	Female 6						Value				14	12							
	Male 20						Mean									35,65			
							SD									36,51			
							Mediane									14,00			
							Min									10,00			
							Max									121,00			
Stroke		0	2	10	7	12											19	21	2
	Female 7						Value						9	12	10				
	Male 24						Mean									21,06			
							SD									6,07			
							Mediane									21,00			
							Min									11,00			
							Max									33,00			

Frequency of Etiology, Gender, Walking Handicap Scale (WHS) score, Expanded Disability Status Scale (EDSS) score, International Standards for Neurological and Functional Classification of Spinal Cord Injury (ASIA) Scores, Stroke Impairment Classification (Severe, Moderate, Mild), Time since acute event (months), Walking device (Brace, Cane, Rollator).

Table 2. Descriptive analysis of the sample.

ETIOLOGY		Age (years)	BMI	WD (m)	WD (% predicted)	Speed (m/min)	VO$_2$ (mlO$_2$/min/Kg)	CW (mlO$_2$*Kg^{-1}*m^{-1})
Stroke	Mean	62.03	26.20	127.06	24.32	21.18	10.10	0.57
	Median	64.00	25.00	106.00	19.00	17.68	9.74	0.49
	SD	11.77	4.05	70.65	14.58	11.78	1.92	0.27
Spinal Cord Injury	Mean	44.92	25.32	148.50	24.35	24.72	10.60	0.62
	Median	46.50	25.15	138.00	19.50	23.00	9.95	0.42
	SD	15.57	3.75	79.74	17.90	13.28	3.49	0.48
Multiple Sclerosis	Mean	44.74	22.70	279.17	59.12	46.62	11.36	0.42
	Median	45.00	22.00	310.50	62.00	51.75	11.17	0.22
	SD	11.23	4.15	136.52	20.90	22.80	2.82	0.63
ALL	Mean	49.79	24.35	203.35	40.59	33.93	10.81	0.51
	Median	49.00	24.40	177.00	37.00	29.50	10.50	0.37
	SD	14.71	4.29	129.15	25.33	21.57	2.81	0.52

SD: standard deviation.
Age; Body Mass Index (BMI); Walking Distance (WD) expressed as meters and as percentage of predicted value; VO$_2$ consumption (VO$_2$) and energy cost of walking (CW = mlO2*Kg^{-1}*min^{-1}).

probability of "Walking Restriction in participation" for each specific value of the Energy Cost, is the following: $P(Y=1)=\dfrac{e^{\alpha+\beta X}}{1+e^{\alpha+\beta X}}$. The examples for CW = 0.39 is is the following: $P(Y=1)=\dfrac{e^{(-3.957+7.024*0.39)}}{1+e^{(-3.957+7.024*0.39)}}=\dfrac{0.296}{1+0.296}=0.228$. Finally, with the receiver-operating characteristic (ROC) analyses and Youden Index application, we have defined another model to identify a cut-off value of energy cost of walking that can predict the membership of each patient to one or other categories of dichotomy WHS. This model generated a cut-off value of .40 that is able to classify correctly the cases with a percentage of 85.05% (Fig. 1–2, table 4–5).

Discussion

The absence of definitive evidence to support the choice of the best clinical test or tests, which may be used in the examination of

neurological patient to determine the ability of walking in the community and "the walking restriction in participation", remains a matter of clinical judgement.

The literature on physical rehabilitation refers, frequently, to patient's motivation in explaining differences in outcome among patient groups with similar pathologies. Participation may involve returning to previous activities and groups which were, and still are, an important target to the stroke survivor. The goal of community re-integration or community participation is to facilitate the transformation of 'stroke survivors' to 'stroke thrivers'. Community reintegration requires an environment that empowers stroke survivors and their family/caregivers to develop personal goals and the methods to achieve them. After discharge from rehabilitation wards, it may be important to make a correlation within objective parameters of walking, the assessment of impairments and the outcome of activity and participation of individuals, and the influence on health-related quality of life. The measurement of therapeutic outcome, in relation to the social

Table 3. Multivariable binary logistical regression analysis.

	Classification table (cut-off value p = .50)		
Actual Group (WHS dichotomized)	**Predicted Group**		**Percent Correct**
	Restriction in walking participation	**Walking independently in the community**	
Restriction in walking participation	24	13	64.86%
Walking independently in the community	5	65	92.86%
Percent of cases correctly classified			**83.18%**
	Coefficients		**OR (95% CI)**
Intercept	−3.957		
CW (for one point increase)	7.024*		1123.042 (68.207−18491.073)

*P<.0001.
McFadden R^2 = .425.
Area under ROC curve = .890, 95% CI = .815−.942.

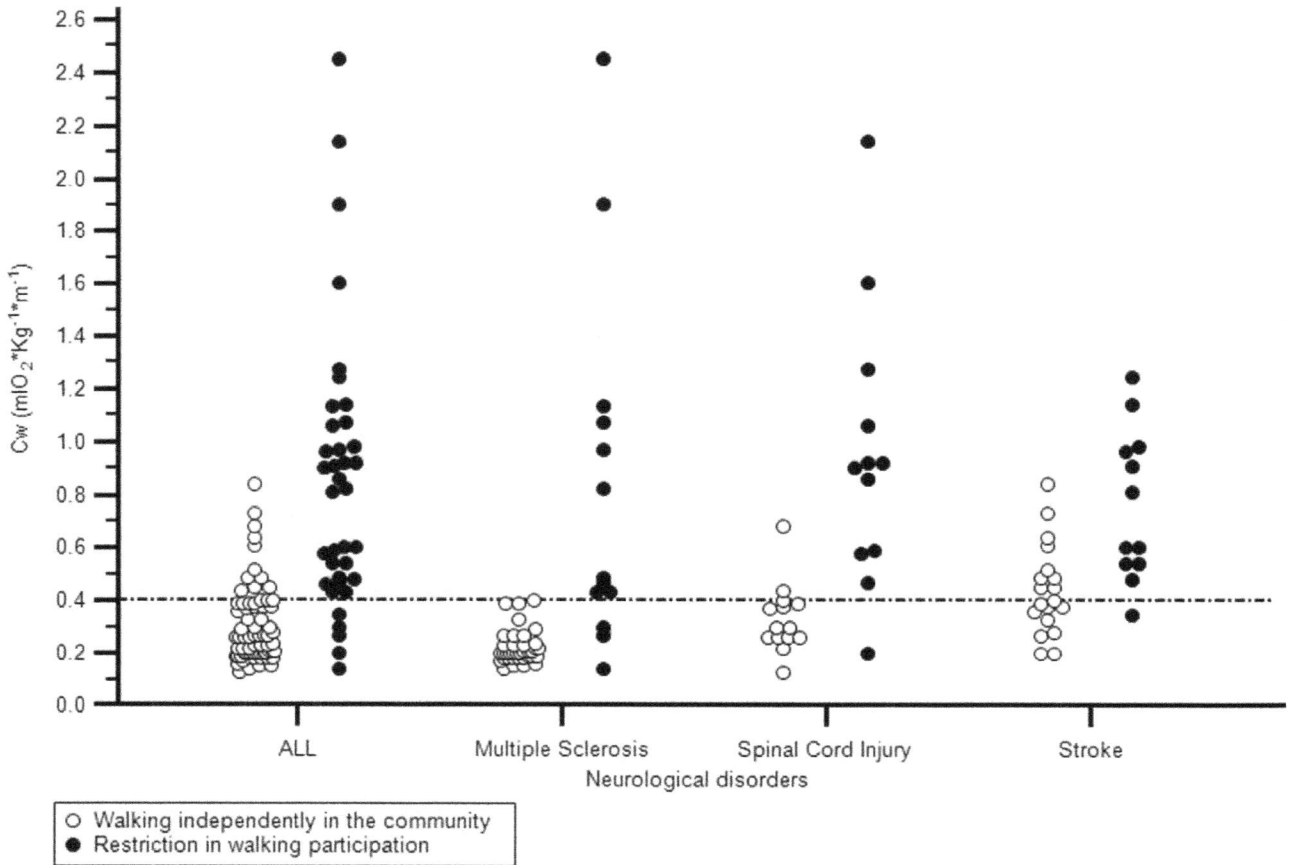

Figure 2. Interactive dot diagram of cut-off point of the energy cost of walking. (CW = Cost of walking).

advantage for the patient, would allow more efficient standardization of treatment and services but many environmental dimensions influence the walking performance in the community [24–27]. Our result could help to find out if the value of the energy cost of walking, in a mixed group of neurological patients, could predict and correlate with the walking performance in the community expressed by WHS; furthermore, these data could be used to predict the patients' outcome. The metabolic cost of walking seems to be one of the main factors that bind the stride characteristics of the individual patient with the possible performance of the road under real conditions. For this reason, reduced cardio respiratory fitness may be a secondary factor that limits the

transfer of walking skills obtained during rehabilitation back into the community environment [28]. The results of our research reveal that, for our subjects, the CW could be a good predictor of walking performance in the community, compared with the score of WHS. We have been also identifying a cut-off value of CW cost, which distinguishes between those who can walk in the community and those who cannot do it. The discriminative ability of a test, i.e. its ability to separate properly the study population into "sick" and "healthy", is proportionate to the extent of the area under the curve (ROC Area Under Curve, AUC) and is equivalent to the probability that the result of a test of an individual, chosen at random from the group of patients, is higher than the one chosen

Table 4. Cut-off value of energy cost of walking that can predict the membership of each patient to one or other categories of dichotomy WHS.

	Classification table (cut-off value CW >.40)		
Actual Group (WHS dichotomized)	**Predicted Group**		**Percent Correct**
	Restriction in walking participation	**Walking independently in the community**	
Restriction in walking participation	32	5	86.49%
Walking independently in the community	11	59	84.29%
Percent of cases correctly classified			**85.05%**

Table 5. The table below summarizes the characteristics of this second model in relation to the 3 diseases.

ETIOLOGY	CW (cut-off)	SE (95% CI)	SP (95% CI)	+PV (95% CI)	−PV (95% CI)	AUC (95% CI)
ALL	>.40	.87 (.71–.96)	.84 (.74–.92)	.74 (.59–.87)	.92 (.83–.97)	.890 (.815–.942)
Multiple Sclerosis	>.40	.77 (.46–.95)	1.00 (.91–1.00)	1.00 (.69–1.00)	.93 (.80–.98)	.902 (.785–.968)
Spinal Cord Injury	>.44	.92 (.62–1.00)	.93 (.66–1.00)	.92 (.62–1.00)	.93 (.66–1.00)	.905 (.724–.984)
Stroke	>.52	.83 (.52–.98)	.79 (.54–.94)	.72 (.42–.92)	.88 (.64–.99)	.833 (.656–.942)

CI: confidence interval.
CW: energy cost of walking.
SE: sensitivity.
SP: specificity.
+PV: positive predictive value.
−PV: negative predictive value.
AUC: area under the ROC curve (maximum = 1.0).

at random from the group of non-sufferers [21,22]. The evaluation of a test is carried out through the AUC, which gives equal importance to the sensitivity and specificity (as in our work) while, in many cases, it is necessary to differentiate the weight to be assigned to these parameters. A more suitable approach may be adopted by taking into account the relation between sensitivity and specificity, that is studying the ROC curve. The use of ROC curve represents a more "flexible" criterion as it offers the ability to view, given a choice of Specificity value, the corresponding sensitivity value and vice versa [23]. In our work, the multivariate binary logistic demonstrated the association between energy cost with the result of dichotomized WHS-score analysis. It seems that this parameter summarizes the variables of diagnosis of disease, age and sex. It is known that, in normal gait, velocity is the most important factor in determining oxygen uptake of walking and is independent of age or sex [29,30]. In addition, the literature shows that the energy cost of walking is highly related to factors that alter the biomechanics of the hand, such as paralysis, spasticity, and muscle co-contractions of the aetiology of the disease [31–33]: an indirect evidence is that the orthotic and therapeutic solutions, which try to reduce the energy expenditure of walking impairment, result from the type of pitch and biomechanical characteristics of the space-step and not from the diagnosis [34–37]. Our results of the CW in MS and SCI subjects are homogeneous but, in stroke people, the value of CW increased slightly, and this aspect could be justified with the significantly difference of ages between the groups. In post stroke patients, the elderly could reduce the motivation to have a correct participation in the community. This cut-off could be useful when discharging patients from the rehabilitation setting to define better the prognosis regarding the participation in the community and to help their families with a correct information regarding the choice of aids and home modifications. Furthermore, the result could be useful during the post-hospital rehabilitation treatment in order to intensify the work to improve walking efficiency, thus improving the performance capacity. Many people who suffered with a stroke have a low level of satisfaction in participation, after they have been discharged from the hospital and have returned to the community [38]. As many as 39% to 65% of community-dwelling people with stroke report limitations in activities and restrictions in community participation. In one study, Nancy Mayo and colleagues found out that (70%) had a restriction in travelling within and beyond the community. Also, 72% of the stroke people lacked an important and meaningful activity to fill the day, whether it be social, recreational, or occupational [39]. A first limitation of this study is secondary to single-centre that enrolled patients for this study. The second limitation could be related to the lacks of cross languages translation and validation of WHS for SCI and MS. In particular, the assessment of the CW evaluation could need an active help and motivation by the subject that performs it. The result of this study will enable the design of new observational longitudinal research through which it could be verified, on a large scale, whether these mathematical models are supported by clinical data with a long time follow-up.

Conclusion

Several Authors have shown the efficacy of gait training on improving walking function in a variety of neurological diagnoses, but the process aimed at restoring walking function is challenged by the complexity and variability inherent in these disor-ders. Many factors could interfere with walking recovery in neurological diseases. Our results reveal that the capacity and/or the inefficiency CW could interfere with walking independently in the community, furthermore, in our subjects, we have been also identifying a cut-off value of CW. These values could be used to predict the ability to walk in the community when discharged from the rehabilitation units, and to adjust the rehabilitative treatment to improve the performance. In order to confirm the present statistical approach, further multicentre clinical trials should be conducted, in the future, involving a high number of people, with a long-term follow-up.

Author Contributions

Conceived and designed the experiments: PS MF. Performed the experiments: AR FB. Analyzed the data: MA MM. Wrote the paper: MM PS MF.

References

1. Finlayson ML, Peterson EW (2010) Falls, aging, and disability Phys Med Rehabil Clin N Am. 21: 357–73.
2. Barbeau H, Fung J (2001) The role of rehabilitation in the recovery of walking in the neurological population. Curr Opin Neurol 14: 735–40.
3. Wevers L, van de Port I, Vermue M, Mead G, Kwakkel G (2009) Effects of task-oriented circuit class training on walking competency after stroke: a systematic review. Stroke 40: 2450–9.
4. Snook EM, Motl RW (2009) Effect of exercise training on walking mobility in multiple sclerosis: a meta-analysis. Neurorehabil Neural Repair 23: 108–16.

Essentials of Physical Medicine and Rehabilitation

5. van Hedel HJ, Dietz V (2010) Rehabilitation of locomotion after spinal cord injury. Restor Neurol Neurosci 28: 123–34.
6. van de Port IG, Kwakkel G, Lindeman E (2008) Community ambulation in patients with chronic stroke: how is it related to gait speed? J Rehabil Med 40: 23–7.
7. Lord SE, McPherson K, McNaughton HK, Rochester L, Weatherall M (2004) Community ambulation after stroke: how important and obtainable is it and what measures appear predictive? Arch Phys Med Rehabil 85: 234–9.
8. Zamparo P, Francescato MP, De Luca G, Lovati L, di Prampero PE (1995) The energy cost of level walking in patients with hemiplegia. Scand J Med Sci Sports 5: 348–52.
9. Corrigan R, McBurney H (2008) Community ambulation: influences on therapists and clients reasoning and decision making. Disabil Rehabil 30: 1079–87.
10. World Health Organization International Classification of Functioning Disability and Health ICF website. Avaible: http://www.who.int/classification/icf. Accessed 2013 Feb 5.
11. Perry J, Garrett M, Gronley JK, Mulroy SJ (1995) Classification of walking handicap in the stroke population. Stroke 26: 982–9.
12. Shumway-Cook A, Patla AE, Stewart A, Ferrucci L, Ciol MA, et al. (2002) Environmental demands associated with community mobility in older adults with and without mobility disabilities. Phys Ther 82: 670–81.
13. Mudge S, Stott NS (2009) Timed walking tests correlate with daily step activity in persons with stroke. Arch Phys Med Rehabil 90: 296–301.
14. Peyrot N, Thivel D, Isacco L, Morin JB, Duche P, et al. (2009) Do mechanical gait parameters explain the higher metabolic cost of walking in obese adolescents? J Appl Physiol 106: 1763–70.
15. Peduzzi P, Concato J, Kemper E, Holford TR, Feinstein AR (1996) A simulation study of the number of events per variable in logistic regression analysis. J Clin Epidemiol 49: 1373–9.
16. Perry J, Garrett M, Gronley JK, Mulroy SJ (1995) Classification of walking handicap in the stroke population. Stroke 26: 982–9.
17. Salier Eriksson J, Rosdahl H, Schantz P (2012) Validity of the Oxycon Mobile metabolic system under field measuring conditions. Eur J Appl Physiol 112: 345–55.
18. Rosdahl H, Gullstrand L, Salier-Eriksson J, Johansson P, Schantz P (2010) Evaluation of the Oxycon Mobile metabolic system against the Douglas bag method. Eur J Appl Physiol 109: 159–71.
19. Salier Eriksson J, Rosdahl H, Schantz P (2012) Validity of the Oxycon Mobile metabolic system under field measuring conditions. Eur J Appl Physiol 112: 345–55.
20. Zweig MH, Campbell G (1993) Receiver-operating characteristic (ROC) plots: a fundamental evaluation tool in clinical medicine. Clin Chem 39: 561–77.
21. YOUDEN WJ (1950) Index for rating diagnostic tests. Cancer 3: 32–5.
22. Bamber D (1975) The area above the ordinal dominance graph and the area below the receiver operating characteristic. J Math Psych 12: 387–415.
23. Schäfer H (1989) Constructing a cut-off point for a quantitative diagnostic test. Stat Med 8: 1381–91.
24. Lapointe R, Lajoie Y, Serresse O, Barbeau H (2001) Functional community ambulation requirements in incomplete spinal cord injured subjects. Spinal Cord 39: 327–35.
25. Waters RL, Adkins R, Yakura J, Vigil D (1994) Prediction of ambulatory performance based on motor scores derived from standards of the American Spinal Injury Association. Arch Phys Med Rehabil 75: 756–60.
26. Ijzerman MJ, Nene AV (2002) Feasibility of the physiological cost index as an outcome measure for the assessment of energy expenditure during walking. Arch Phys Med Rehabil 83: 1777–82.
27. Cunha IT, Lim PA, Henson H, Monga T, Qureshy H, et al. (2002) Performance-based gait tests for acute stroke patients. Am J Phys Med Rehabil 81: 848–56.
28. Kelly JO, Kilbreath SL, Davis GM, Zeman B, Raymond J (2003) Cardiorespiratory fitness and walking ability in subacute stroke patients. Arch Phys Med Rehabil 84: 1780–5.
29. Blessey RL, Hislop HJ, Waters RL, Antonelli D (1976) Metabolic energy cost of unrestrained walking. Phys Ther 56: 1019–24.
30. Waters RL, Hislop HJ, Perry J, Thomas L, Campbell J (1983) Comparative cost of walking in young and old adults. J Orthop Res 1: 73–6.
31. Bernardi M, Macaluso A, Sproviero E, Castellano V, Coratella D, et al. (1999) Cost of walking and locomotor impairment. J Electromyogr Kinesiol 9: 149–57.
32. Duffy CM, Hill AE, Graham HK (1997) The influence of flexed-knee gait on the energy cost of walking in children. Dev Med Child Neurol 39: 234–8.
33. Zamparo P, Pagliaro P (1998) The energy cost of level walking before and after hydro-kinesi therapy in patients with spastic paresis. Scand J Med Sci Sports 8: 222–8.
34. Delextrat A, Matthew D, Cohen DD, Brisswalter J (2011) Effect of stride frequency on the energy cost of walking in obese teenagers. Hum Mov Sci 30: 115–24.
35. Bregman DJ, De Groot V, Van Diggele P, Meulman H, Houdijk H, et al. (2010) Polypropylene ankle foot orthoses to overcome drop-foot gait in central neurological patients: a mechanical and functional evaluation. Prosthet Orthot Int 34: 293–304.
36. Franceschini M, Massucci M, Ferrari L, Agosti M, Paroli C (2003) Effects of an ankle-foot orthosis on spatiotemporal parameters and energy cost of hemiparetic gait. Clin Rehabil 17: 368–72.
37. Maclean N, Pound P (2000) A critical review of the concept of patient motivation in the literature on physical rehabilitation. Soc Sci Med 50: 495–506.
38. Pang MY, Eng JJ, Miller WC (2007) Determinants of satisfaction with community reintegration in older adults with chronic stroke: role of balance self-efficacy. Phys Ther 87: 282–91.
39. Mayo NE, Wood-Dauphinee S, Côté R, Durcan L, Carlton J (2002) Activity, participation, and quality of life 6 months post stroke. Arch Phys Med Rehabil 83: 1035–42.

4

Recovery in Stroke Rehabilitation through the Rotation of Preferred Directions Induced by Bimanual Movements: A Computational Study

Ken Takiyama[1], Masato Okada[1,2]*

1 Graduate School of Frontier Sciences, Department of Complex Science and Engineering, The University of Tokyo, Chiba, Tokyo, Japan, **2** RIKEN Brain Science Institute, Wako, Japan

Abstract

Stroke patients recover more effectively when they are rehabilitated with bimanual movement rather than with unimanual movement; however, it remains unclear why bimanual movement is more effective for stroke recovery. Using a computational model of stroke recovery, this study suggests that bimanual movement facilitates the reorganization of a damaged motor cortex because this movement induces rotations in the preferred directions (PDs) of motor cortex neurons. Although the tuning curves of these neurons differ during unimanual and bimanual movement, changes in PD, but not changes in modulation depth, facilitate such reorganization. In addition, this reorganization was facilitated only when encoding PDs are rotated, but decoding PDs are not rotated. Bimanual movement facilitates reorganization because this movement changes neural activities through inter-hemispheric inhibition without changing cortical-spinal-muscle connections. Furthermore, stronger inter-hemispheric inhibition between motor cortices results in more effective reorganization. Thus, this study suggests that bimanual movement is effective for stroke rehabilitation because this movement rotates the encoding PDs of motor cortex neurons.

Editor: Olivier Baud, Hôpital Robert Debré, France

Funding: This work was partially supported by a Grant-in-Aid for Japan Society for the Promotion of Science Fellows (grant no. 10J04910) and a Grant-in-Aid for Scientific Research (A) (grant no. 20240020) from the Ministry of Education, Culture, Sports, Science, and Technology of Japan. The funders had no role in study design, data collection and analysis, decision to publish, or preparation of the manuscript.

Competing Interests: The authors have declared that no competing interests exist.

* E-mail: okada@k.u-tokyo.ac.jp

Introduction

One of the challenges of rehabilitation research is to elucidate efficient method of promoting the functional recovery of upper limb movement in stroke patients. In neuroscience, a related challenge is determining the neural mechanisms of such functional recovery. Although stroke patients tend to recover lower limb movement after therapeutic intervention, the majority of these patients (65%) do not regain full movement of their upper limbs [1–3]. Recent studies have suggested that patients can recover the use of paretic upper limbs through several therapeutic methods such as constraint-induced therapy [1,4], in which patients are restricted to using only the paretic arm by immobilizing the healthy arm. Although stroke patients can recover upper limb movement after this therapy, the neural mechanisms of this recovery remain unknown.

A recent computational study suggested that constraint-induced therapy is effective because it leads to the reorganization of a damaged region in the motor cortex based on supervised and unsupervised learning [1]. The results of this computational study thus explain several aspects of the observed effects of rehabilitation; e.g., stroke patients recover upper limb movement only when they undertake more than a threshold number of rehabilitation trials [1,5]. Therefore, a computational approach will likely be effective for determining the neural mechanisms of functional recovery in recovered patients.

Although previous computational studies investigated the unimanual movements of stroke patients, individuals often move their arms bimanually. Bimanual movement is effective for the recovery of paretic arm movement [6–8]; i.e., bimanual movement facilitates recovery and retention of the recovery effect. However, it is unknown why bimanual rehabilitation is effective for stroke rehabilitation. It remains unclear what differences between unimanual and bimanual movement result in the effectiveness of bimanual rehabilitation. This study approaches this question using a computational model inspired by neurophysiological results related to bimanual movement.

Neural activities in the motor cortex differ during unimanual and bimanual movement [9–11]. In unimanual movements, when subjects move their right arms towards a radially distributed target, neural activity in the left motor cortex can be well fit by the cosine function of the target angle [12], indicating that each neuron is maximally activated when subjects reach in the preferred direction (PD) of the neuron and that neural activity is determined by the movement direction of the contralateral arm. Although neural activity is assumed to be influenced only by contralateral arm movement, this activity is also influenced also by ipsilateral arm movement [9–11,13]. Because bimanual movement is a combination of right and left arm movements, neural activity in bimanual movement appears to be well fit by a linear summation of the activities in ipsilateral and contralateral arm movement. However, this linear summation cannot explain the

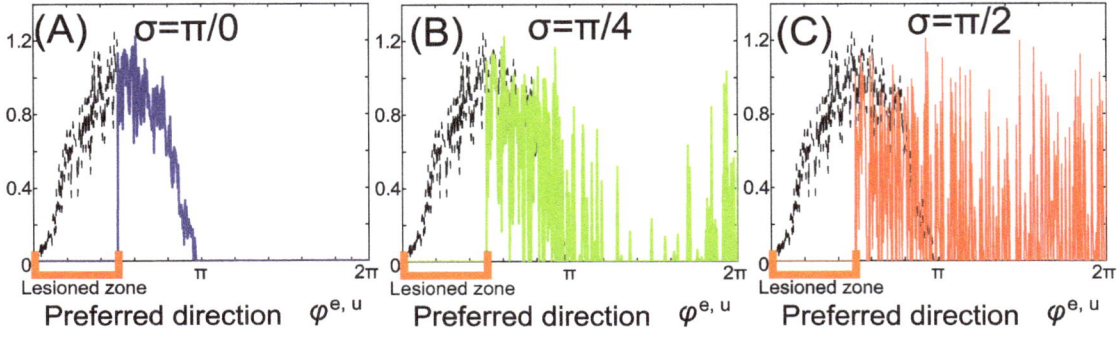

Figure 1. Neural activities in unimanual and bimanual movement after stroke. Dotted and solid lines denote the neural activities before and after stroke, respectively, when $\theta = \frac{\pi}{4}$. (A): Solid lines indicate neural activities when $\sigma = 0$. (B): Neural activities when $\sigma = \frac{\pi}{4}$. (C): Neural activities when $\sigma = \frac{\pi}{2}$.

neural activity in bimanual movement [9–11]. Furthermore, the PD and modulation depth (height of the fitted cosine function) of each neuron are different in bimanual and unimanual movement. In bimanual movement, motor cortex neurons are not maximally activated when subjects move their contralateral arms in the PD determined in unimanual movement. Thus, these differences in neural activity may explain why bimanual movement is effective for stroke rehabilitation.

Using a computational model of stroke rehabilitation [1], we investigated the following two questions: 1) what type of changes in bimanual movement affected stroke recovery or the reorganization process of the damaged motor cortex and 2) when was bimanual rehabilitation strongly effective for the reorganization process? First, we demonstrated that bimanual rehabilitation is effective because this rehabilitation causes changes in PD; changes in PD rather than in modulation depth provide a neural mechanism for the effectiveness of bimanual rehabilitation for motor cortex reorganization. Additionally, we observed the effectiveness of bimanual rehabilitation only when the PD changes were in encoding but not in decoding. Second, we confirmed that bimanual rehabilitation is strongly effective when the encoding PDs are strongly rotated. On the basis of a previous computational study [10], the present study hypothesized that bimanual rehabilitation was strongly effective when the encoding PDs undergo large changes.

Results

This study investigated how bimanual movement affected stroke recovery by modeling the different PDs and modulation depths during unimanual and bimanual movement. During bimanual movements, we invesitigated only bimanual parallel movements in which the right and left arms move in the same directions, because the neural activities during these parallel bimanual movements have been investigated previously. We describe the definitions used in the model in detail in the *Methods* section.

Initially, in simulating bimanual rehabilitation, we assume that changes occur only in the PDs. These changes are referred to as PD rotations for the remainder of this manuscript. Because PDs are rotated pseudo-randomly in bimanual movement, we modeled these rotations as

$$\phi_i^{e,b} = \phi_i^{e,u} + \varepsilon_i \qquad (1)$$

where $\phi_i^{e,b}$ and $\phi_i^{e,u}$ are the encoding PDs in bimanual and

unimanual movements, respectively $(i = 1, ..., N)$, and N is the number of neurons. The encoding PD determines the cosine-tuned neural activity, $A_i(\theta, \phi_i^{e,w})$, where θ is the angle of a reaching target and the index $w \in \{u, b\}$ indicates unimanual or bimanual movement (see the *Methods* section). The encoding PDs are rotated ε_i degree that is randomly sampled from a Gaussian distribution with a mean of 0 and a variance of σ^2. Additionally, these PDs are rotated using quenched random variables, meaning that ε_i is invariant across trials. In contrast to quenched random variables, the encoding PDs can be rotated using annealed random variables sampled from trial to trial, but this type of rotation cannot facilitate the reorganization of a damaged motor cortex (see the *Discussion* regarding the effects of the annealed random variables on the reorganization). Due to the rotations of the encoding PDs, neural activities are different in unimanual and bimanual movement as shown in figure 1. In the subsection titled *Importance of encoding PD rotations for reorganization*, we consider changes of modulation depth, i.e., $A_i(\theta, \phi_i^{e,b}) = (1 + \varepsilon_i)A_i(\theta, \phi_i^{e,b})$, but the rotations of encoding PDs are primarily investigated.

Decoding PDs are used to calculate the population vector (PV) as follows:

$$\text{PV}(\theta) \propto (\sum_i^N A_i(\theta, \phi_i^{e,w}) \cos\phi_i^{d,w}, \sum_i^N A_i(\theta, \phi_i^{e,w}) \sin\phi_i^{d,w})^T \quad (2)$$

with a direction and amplitude that model the direction and velocity of the reaching movements, respectively [12,14,15], and $\phi_i^{d,w}$ is the decoding PD. In contrast to the encoding PDs that determine neural activities, decoding PDs determine movement directions; i.e., the ith neuron generates the motor command for moving arms in the direction $\phi_i^{d,w}$. Following previous studies [14,16,17], in our simulations of unimanual movement, the decoding PD is set to equal the encoding PD ($\phi_i^{e,u} = \phi_i^{d,u}$). During bimanual movement, we assume that decoding PDs are not rotated on the basis of previous studies [10] (but see [11]), but in the section *Importance of encoding PD rotations for reorganization*, the modeling of rotations in decoding PDs is described.

We can model the upper limb movements of stroke patients using a PV by removing a fraction of the model neurons [1,18] (see also [19]). Because stroke patients have difficulty in reaching in a particular direction [20], we depleted pN neurons with encoding PDs of approximately $\pi/4$, where $p \in (0,1]$ is the fraction of depleted neurons. We refer to $\theta \in [0, \frac{\pi}{2}]$ and other θ as the movement directions of large and small errors, respectively. For this damaged motor cortex, stroke rehabilitation induced a reorganization that can be modeled using an optimization framework. In this framework, the rehabilitation modifies $\phi_i^{e,w}$ to minimize the cost function

$$E = \frac{1}{2}(1 - \cos(\theta - \theta_p)) + \frac{\lambda}{2}\sum_i^N (A_i(\theta, \phi_i^{e,w}))^2 \qquad (3)$$

where θ_p is the angle of the PV and λ is the regularization parameter [1]. We model stroke rehabilitation using two optimization terms, supervised and unsupervised learning of ϕ_i^e, which coincide to the first and the second terms in equation (3), respectively. In the rehabilitation trials, patients moved their arms towards one of eight radially distributed targets ($\theta = 2\pi\frac{k}{8}$, $k = 1,...,8$) that are selected with the same probability, i.e., $P(\theta = 2\pi\frac{k}{8}) = \frac{1}{8}$. After each rehabilitation trial, supervised learning resulted in decreased movement error between the PV and the target angle. Stroke rehabilitation also decreased the metabolic cost of neuronal activity, which was modeled by the unsupervised learning.

Reorganization due to bimanual movement

After a neuronal lesion, we investigated whether reorganization in the damaged motor cortex can be facilitated by rotations of the encoding PDs. When the encoding PDs are not rotated ($\sigma = 0$), i.e., in unimanual rehabilitation, these PDs are reorganized to increase the number of neurons with encoding PDs close to the movement directions of large errors (figure 2A). In agreement with a previous study [1], however, the encoding PDs cannot be concentrated only in just these directions, especially in the middles of these directions ($\theta = \frac{\pi}{4}$). By contrast, when the encoding PDs are rotated ($\sigma = \frac{\pi}{4}$ or $\frac{\pi}{2}$), i.e., in bimanual rehabilitation, the encoding PDs are reorganized to localize in the depleted region (figures 2B and 2C). Comparing figures 2B and 2C, larger rotations of the encoding PDs lead to better the equalization of these PDs. In the *Discussion* section, we discuss the conditions in which encoding PDs are strongly rotated. Taken together, in both unimanual and bimanual rehabilitation, encoding PDs are reorganized after the neuronal lesion, but these PDs are only reorganized in the movement directions of larger errors after bimanual rehabilitation.

Behavioral effects of bimanual rehabilitation

Bimanual rehabilitation facilitates the reorganization of damaged motor cortex, but it remains unknown how this rehabilitation affects behavioral aspects such as movement error and speed. Based on the PV model, we investigated these movement parameters in unimanual reaching after either unimanual or bimanual rehabilitation. Both unimanual and bimanual rehabilitation decreased the angular error between the target position and the PV (figure 3), suggesting that these rehabilitations can restore movement precision. Bimanual rehabilitation allows angular error to reach its minimum value when $\sigma = \frac{\pi}{2}$, indicating that when encoding PDs are strongly rotated, bimanual rehabilitation enhances movement precision.

In addition to movement error, we investigated how unimanual or bimanual rehabilitation affects movement speed by calculating the norm of the PV (figure 4). After the neuronal lesion, reaching speed becomes critically slower in the directions of large error

(figure 4A). With moderate rotations of the encoding PDs ($\sigma = \frac{\pi}{4}$), bimanual rehabilitation improved reaching speed in the movement directions of larger errors; however, this rehabilitation also resulted in reduced reaching speed in the directions of small errors (figures 4B, 4C). With strong rotations of the encoding PDs ($\sigma \neq \frac{\pi}{2}$), bimanual rehabilitation effectively improved reaching speed in the movement directions of large errors without hindering speed in those directions of small errors, suggesting that bimanual rehabilitation can be strongly recommended when bimanual movement induces strong rotations of the encoding PDs.

Importance of the rotation of encoding PDs on reorganization

This study originally modeled the rotations of encoding PDs, but we remained unsure whether these rotations are important for the reorganization of a damaged motor cortex. Bimanual movement causes changes not only in PDs but also in modulation depth, and decoding PDs may also be rotated. First, we simulated changes in modulation depth without PD rotations (figure 5); we observed no reorganization after bimanual rehabilitation. Next, we simulated the rotations of both encoding and decoding PDs, i.e., $\phi_i^{d,b} = \phi_i^{e,b} = \phi_i^{e,u} + \varepsilon_i$ (figure 6); however, after bimanual rehabilitation, we again observed no reorganization. Thus, we concluded that the rotation of encoding PDs, as opposed to changes in either modulation depth or decoding PDs, is the most important factor in reorganization via bimanual rehabilitation.

Nonuniform distribution of the target position

In the aforementioned results, motor cortex reorganization was investigated by presenting one of the eight targets with equal probability, but it remains unclear whether the reorganization still occurs when only limited targets are presented. Intuitively, this reorganization appears to effectively occur when patients repeatedly move their arms in the movement directions of large errors. We simulated this case for both unimanual and bimanual rehabilitation. In unimanual rehabilitation, excess reorganization occurred in the movement directions of larger errors, with a decrease in the number of neurons with encoding PDs approximately aligned with the directions of small errors (figure 7A). When patients did not practice reaching in the directions of large errors, effective reorganization did not with either unimanual or bimanual rehabilitation (data not shown). By contrast, in bimanual rehabilitation, uniform reorganization occurred despite a nonuniform target distribution (figures 7B and 7C). Even when a limited number of targets were presented, reorganization was facilitated during bimanual rehabilitation.

Effect of the learning rule on reorganization

Reorganization occurs due to both supervised and unsupervised learning, but it is unclear which learning rules better facilitates reorganization. With only an unsupervised learning rule, the reorganization was not facilitated independently of whether encoding PDs are rotated (figure 8). Conversely, when the only a supervised learning rule, the reorganization is facilitated when encoding PDs are rotated (figure 9). In bimanual rehabilitation, the reorganization is thus facilitated mainly by supervised learning.

Discussion

After a neuronal lesion, reorganization of a damaged motor cortex can be facilitated by the rotations of the encoding PDs; these rotations are induced by bimanual movement (figure 2). Moderate reorganization can increase the reaching velocities of

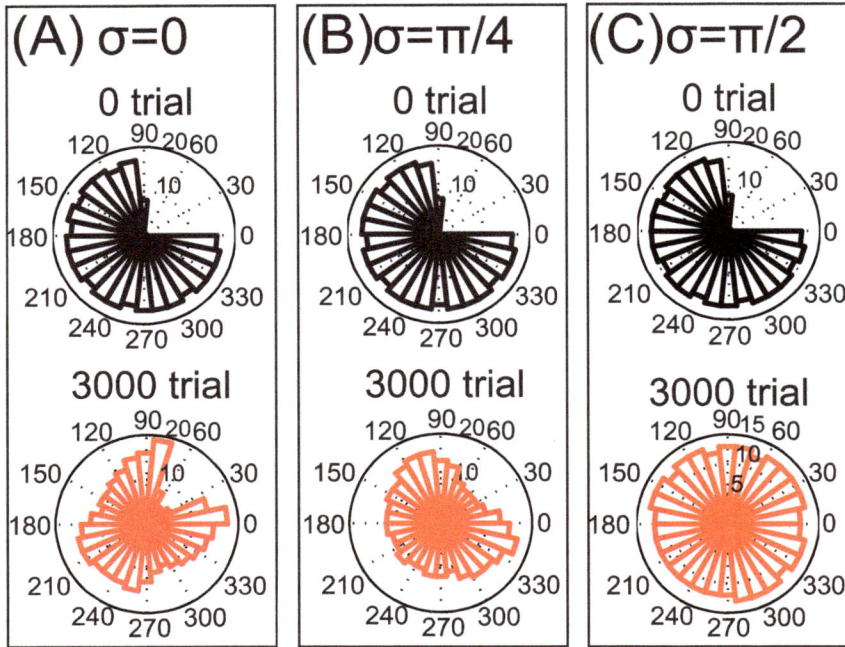

Figure 2. Reorganization of a damaged motor cortex after unimanual and bimanual rehabilitation (A): Histograms of $\phi^{e,u}$ when $\sigma = 0$. (B): The same histograms when $\sigma = \frac{\pi}{4}$. (C): The same histograms when $\sigma = \frac{\pi}{2}$.

movements in the directions of large errors but decrease the velocities in the directions of small errors (figure 4B). However, when encoding PDs are strongly rotated, the reorganization facilitates the recovery of reaching velocities in the directions of large errors without decreasing the velocities in the directions of small errors (figure 4C), which effectively facilitates the recovery of reaching precision (figure 3). The reorganization occurs only due to the rotations of encoding PDs (figures 2, 5, and 6), suggesting

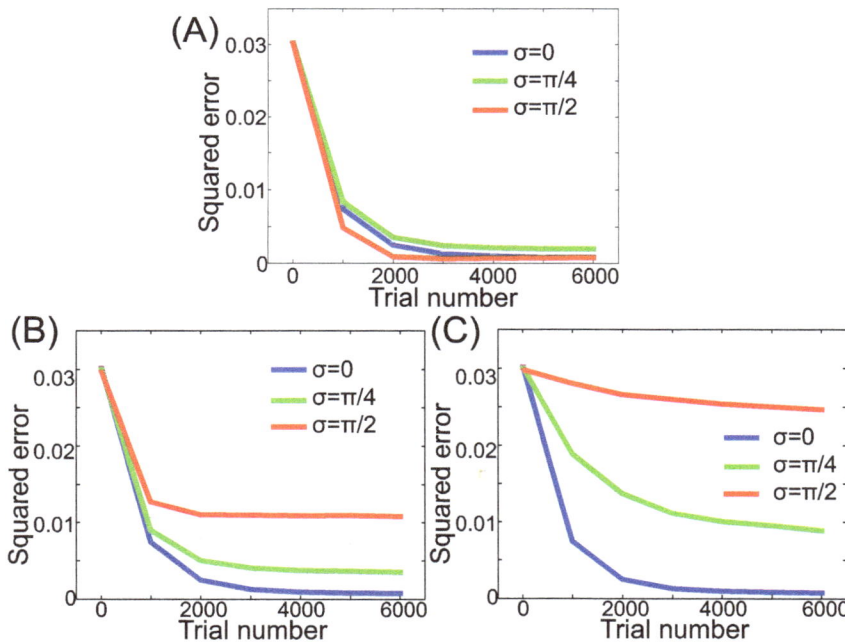

Figure 3. Angular error between the target and PV in unimanual movement. (A): The angular error between the target position and PV when the encoding PDs were rotated in bimanual movement. (B): The angular error when only modulation depth was changed in bimanual movement. (C): The angular error when both encoding and decoding PDs were rotated in bimanual movement.

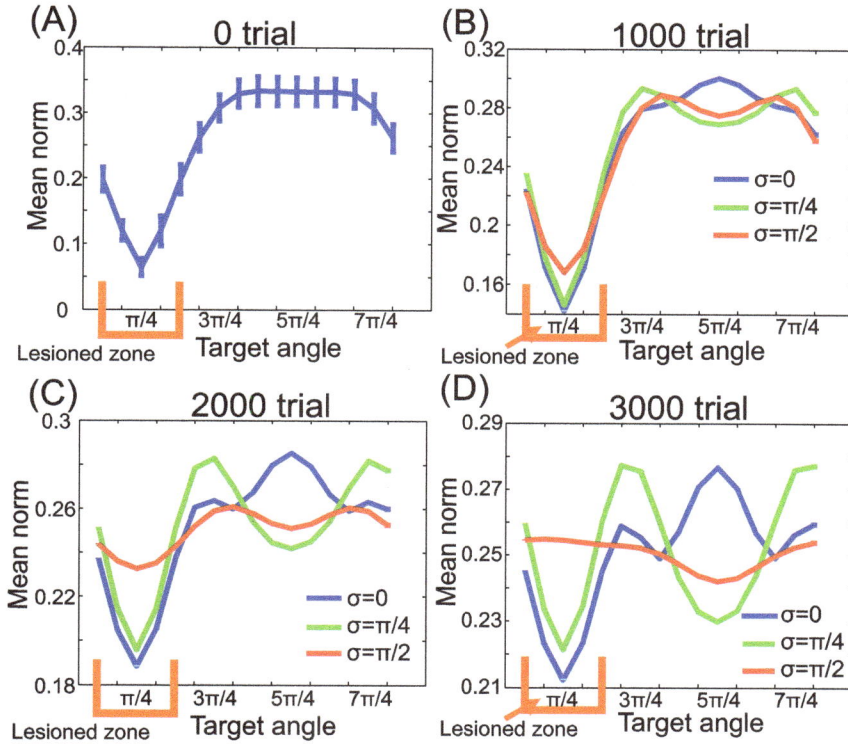

Figure 4. Norm of the PV after rehabilitation. (A): The norm of the PV immediately after the neuronal lesion. (B): The norm of the PV after 1000 rehabilitation trials. (C): The norm of the PV after 2000 rehabilitation trials. (D): The norm of the PV after 3000 rehabilitation trials.

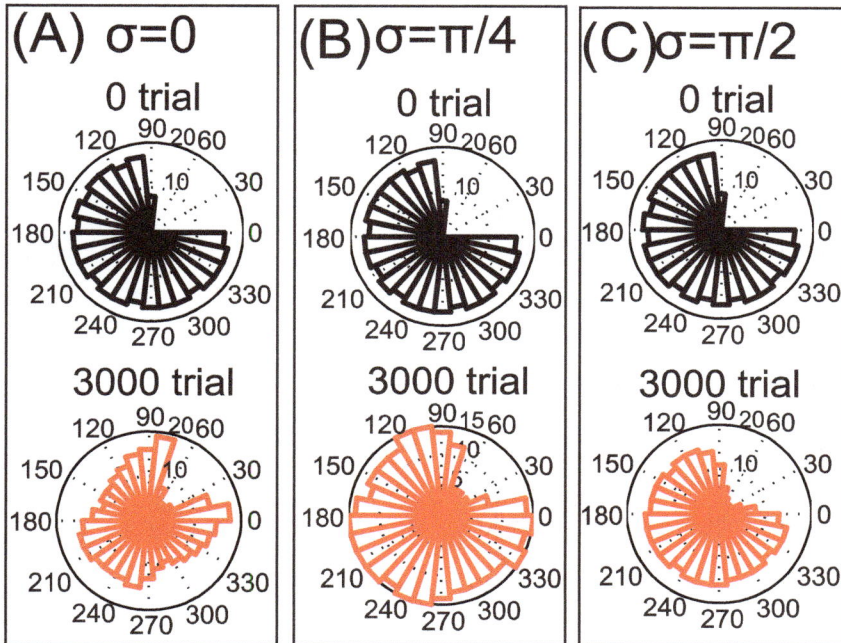

Figure 5. Reorganization of the damaged motor cortex when only modulation depth was changed in bimanual movement. (A): Histograms of $\phi^{e,u}$ when $\sigma = 0$. (B): The same histograms when $\sigma = \frac{\pi}{4}$. (C): The same histograms when $\sigma = \frac{\pi}{2}$.

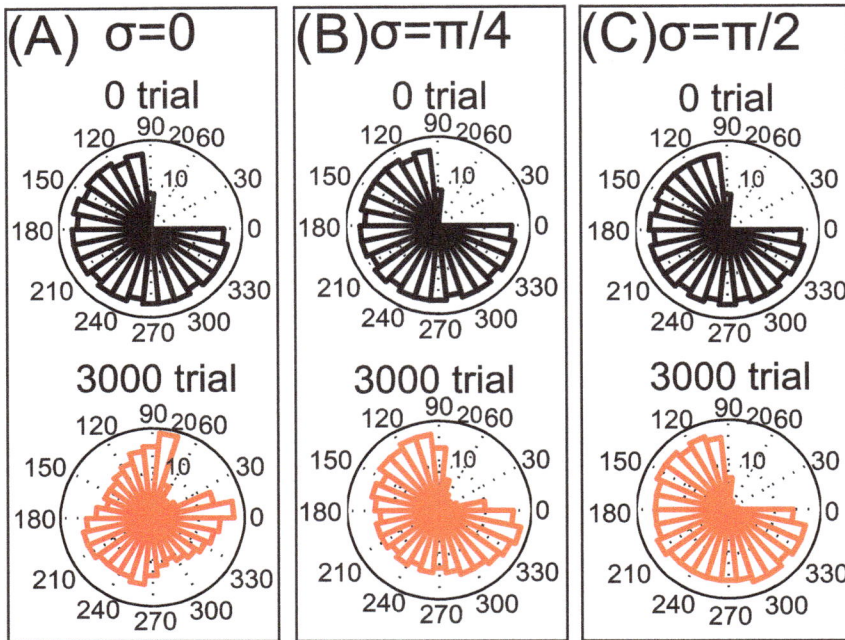

Figure 6. Reorganization of the damaged motor cortex when both encoding and decoding PDs were rotated in bimanual movement. (A): Histograms of $\phi^{e,u}$ when $\sigma=0$. (B): The same histograms when $\sigma=\frac{\pi}{4}$. (C): The same histograms when $\sigma=\frac{\pi}{2}$.

that bimanual rehabilitation is effective for stroke recovery because this movement induces the rotation of encoding PDs. We also conclude that bimanual rehabilitation is strongly effective when bimanual movement induces strong rotations of encoding PDs.

Because there are few hypothesis-driven studies in this field [3], to our knowledge, our conclusions are likely the first hypotheses regarding bimanual rehabilitation in stroke patients. However, we should note in what conditions encoding PDs are strongly rotated and in which cases bimanual rehabilitation is thus strongly

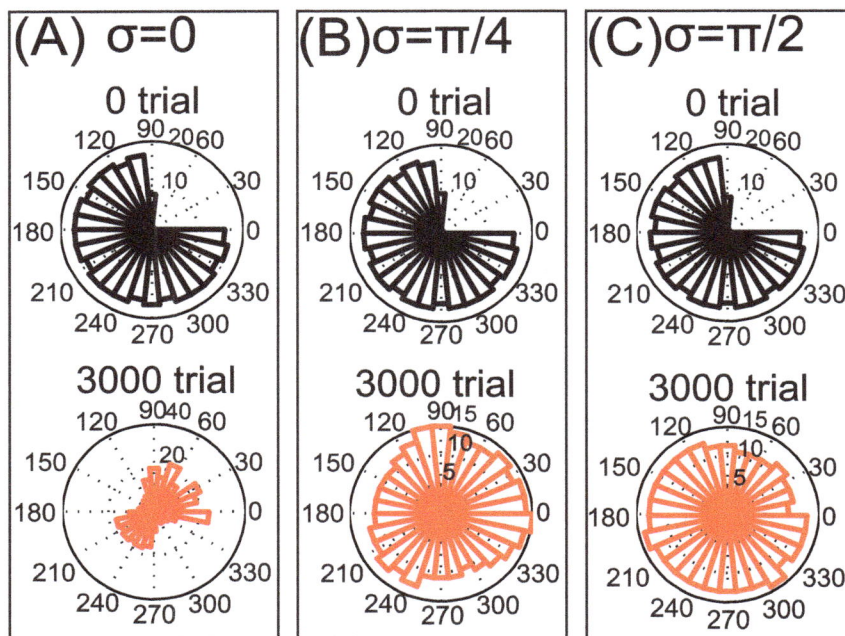

Figure 7. Reorganization of the damaged motor cortex when limited targets were presented in rehabilitation trials. (A): Histograms of $\phi^{e,u}$ when $\sigma=0$. (B): The same histograms when $\sigma=\frac{\pi}{4}$. (C): The same histograms when $\sigma=\frac{\pi}{2}$.

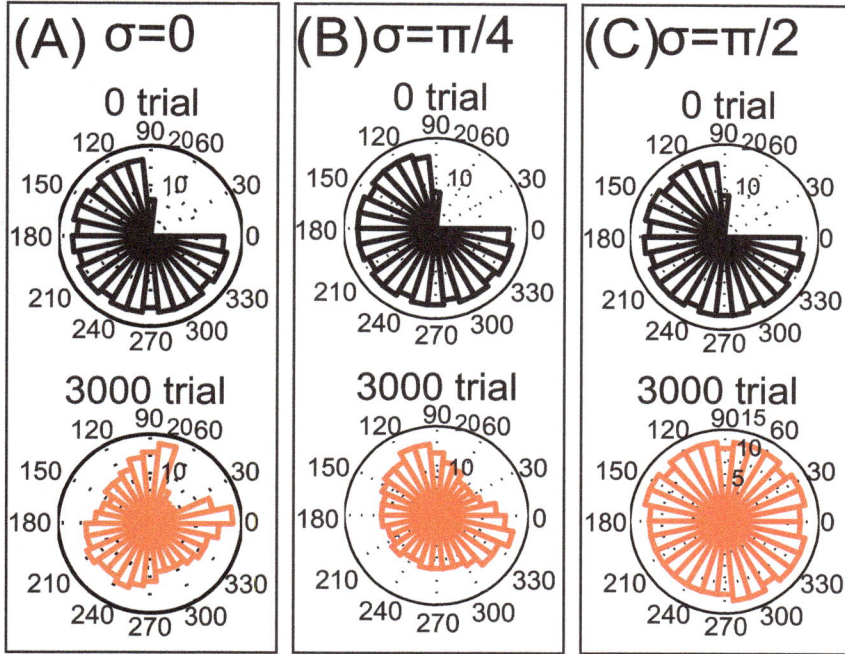

Figure 8. Reorganization of the damaged motor cortex with only supervised learning. (A): Histograms of $\phi^{e,u}$ when $\sigma=0$. (B): The same histograms when $\sigma=\frac{\pi}{4}$. (C): The same histograms when $\sigma=\frac{\pi}{2}$.

recommended. A previous computational study suggested that stronger inter-hemispheric inhibition results in stronger rotation of the encoding PDs for the following reason [10]. In unimanual movement of the right arm, the encoding PD determines the tuning curve of the ith motor cortex neuron in the left hemisphere as $A_i(\theta)=\cos(\theta-\varphi_i^{e,u})$. For simplicity, we neglected nonlinearity and neural noise here. In bimanual movement, motor cortex neurons in the right hemisphere are also activated; these neural

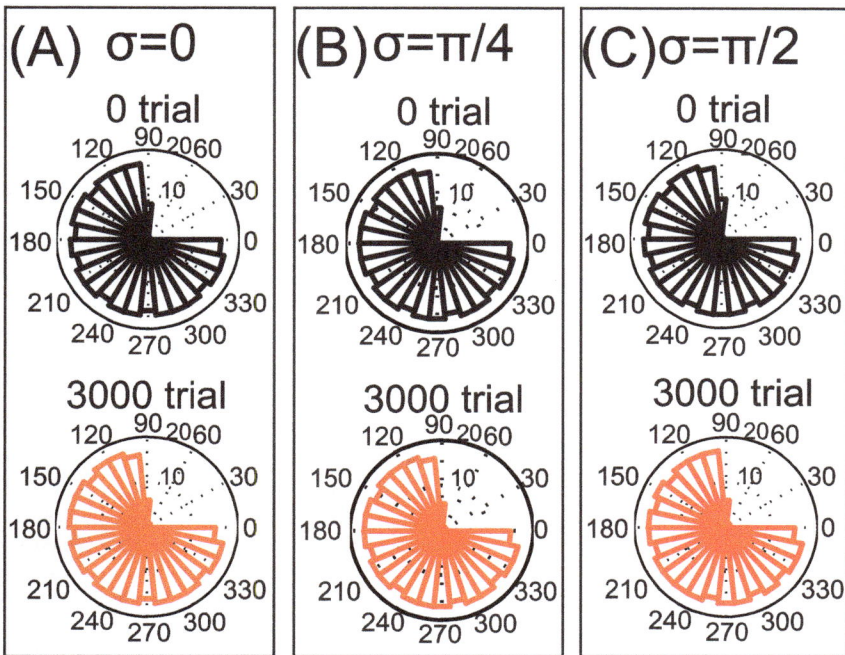

Figure 9. Reorganization of the damaged motor cortex with only unsupervised learning. (A): Histograms of $\phi^{e,u}$ when $\sigma=0$. (B): The same histograms when $\sigma=\frac{\pi}{4}$. (C): The same histograms when $\sigma=\frac{\pi}{2}$.

activations excite the inhibitory interneurons in the left hemisphere through excitatory corpus callosum connections. These interneurons inhibit the ith neuron in the left hemisphere as follows:

$$A_i(\theta) = \cos(\theta_r - \varphi_i^{e,u}) - \frac{J}{M}\sum_j^M \cos(\theta_l - \varphi_j^{e,u}) \propto \cos(\theta_r - (\varphi_i^{e,u} + \varepsilon_i))$$

where M is the number of right-hemispheric neurons projecting to the inhibitory neuron and J is the strength of inter-hemispheric inhibition determined by both the corpus callosum connections and the connections between interneurons and the ith neuron. Although the encoding PDs are not rotated ($\varepsilon_i = 0$) when $J = 0$, stronger the inter-hemispheric inhibition yields a stronger rotation of the encoding PDs. These PDs are randomly rotated only when inter-hemispheric connectivities are sparse; i.e., when M is sufficiently large, $\varepsilon_1 = \varepsilon_2 = ... = \varepsilon_N$ due to the law of large numbers. In actual rodent and primate brains, callosal connectivities are sparse in the hand region of primary motor cortex [21,22]. The strength of inter-hemispheric inhibition can be estimated from imaging data such as functional magnetic resonance imaging data [23]. In summary, our computational study suggests that we can strongly recommend bimanual rehabilitation for patients with inter-hemispheric inhibition that is stronger than a specific threshold value. Although several previous studies have suggested that unimanual and bimanual rehabilitation affect stroke recovery equivalently [3], based on our results, we observed that bimanual rehabilitation facilitates stroke recovery only when inter-hemispheric inhibition is strong. Thus, we must determine the threshold inhibition value in a future project.

Although this study distinguished between encoding and decoding processes, it is unclear why exactly we are able to separate these processes. Encoding and decoding processes are equivalent to motor planning and execution, respectively. In motor planning, the neural activities of motor cortex neurons are determined on the basis of the position of the presented target. In motor execution, these neurons send motor commands to muscles through the spinal cord. Based on a study by Georgopoulos et al. [12], because the PV models actual reaching movements well, motor cortex neurons have encoding PDs that are likely equal to or very close to decoding PDs in unimanual movement. This symmetry between encoding and decoding PDs may be broken when a perturbation is applied to the reaching movement. When adapting to a visuomotor rotation or force field, neural activities change to minimize the error between target position and actual movement. When adapting to a visuomotor rotation, neural activities change only in the motor planning phase [24], suggesting that only encoding PDs change to minimize the error. During force field adaptation, a recent computational model separately modeled encoding and decoding processes; when only the encoding process is adaptable for error minimization, this motor cortex model can explain the experimental neurophysiological data of the motor cortex [25]. To our knowledge, there is little evidence regarding whether encoding and decoding processes should be separated in bimanual movement. However, we believe that these processes should be separated on the basis of the aforementioned studies of unimanual movement.

Motor cortex neurons send motor commands to muscles [26], and thus, we should note the relationship between PDs and muscles. To our knowledge, the mechanism for the determination of encoding PDs is unknown; however, based on the PV frameworks, encoding PDs are likely to be similar to decoding PDs in unimanual movement [12]. Contrastingly, using a realistic biomechanics model, decoding PDs are suggested to be deter-

mined by the strength of the connectivities between a neuron and each muscle [27,28], i.e., the connectivities modeling cortical-spinal-muscle or direct cortical-muscle connections. When a neuron has strong connections to elbow extensors and weak or negative connections to elbow extensors, this neuron has a decoding PD in the upper-right direction in the horizontal plane. Based on these computational frameworks, a decoding PD is thus determined by the degree to which the neuron is connected to agonists or antagonists in the assumed movements. These previous studies assumed only unimanual movement, and thus, it remains for future research to determine how biomechanical properties affect decoding PDs in bimanual movement. Based on our assumptions, decoding PDs are determined in accurately generating both unimanual and bimanual movements, and rotations of the encoding PDs are responsible for generating the different motor commands in unimanual and bimanual movement. In our framework, we must thus define a biomechanics model in subsequent work.

Rotations of the encoding PDs facilitate cortical reorganization, but it remains unclear why this reorganization is facilitated by these rotations. Because we concentrated on the recovery of feedforward movements in this study, the reorganization occurs to minimize the angular error. After 3000 trials of unimanual rehabilitation, the reorganization decreased the angular error when reaching in the movement directions of larger errors by reorganizing neurons to localize in these directions. These decreases occurred because, for example, even when there is a small neuron with an encoding PD of only 45 degrees, the average PV across many trials can be directed towards 45 degrees when the neurons are reorganized as an equivalent number of neurons with encoding PDs of approximately 30 $(45-15)$ and 60 $(45+15)$ degrees. However, in this case, the norm of the PV is smaller than that of the well-equalized population; this reorganization is observed when the encoding PDs are strongly rotated. Furthermore, in well-equalized populations, more neurons are activated in generating PVs oriented at 45 degrees, and movement precision is better than that observed in the impaired populations observed after unimanual rehabilitation. In other words, in unimanual rehabilitation, the reorganization stops at one of the local solutions for which the angular error is decreased to some extent, but movement speed does not recover. When non-quenched (trial-by-trial variant) random variables are added to each rehabilitation (learning) step, these variables act as search noise and cause reorganization, thus avoiding trapping in local solutions [29]. As described in the next paragraph, it remains unclear whether such random variables are available in rehabilitation trials, but strong and quenched rotations may play similar functional roles. Thus, we suggest that strong rotations of the encoding PDs play the role of search noise, enabling the reorganization to avoid local solutions and leading the damaged motor cortex to a global solution, i.e., a well-equalized population.

This study investigated the influence of quenched (trial-by-trial invariant) rotations of encoding PDs on reorganization, but annealed (trial-by-trial variant) rotations can also be considered. However, we observed no significant reorganization when the rotations were annealed (data not shown). By contrast, when we added annealed noise to each learning step (see Methods), i.e., when we considered synaptic drift, we observed significant reorganization (figure 10). Additionally, even when the strength of this synaptic drift was moderate, we observed significant reorganization, equivalent to that observed in the case of strong and quenched rotations (figure 10B), suggesting that moderate synaptic drift enables the avoidance of local solutions and leads to a global solution. Despite the effectiveness of annealed rotations on

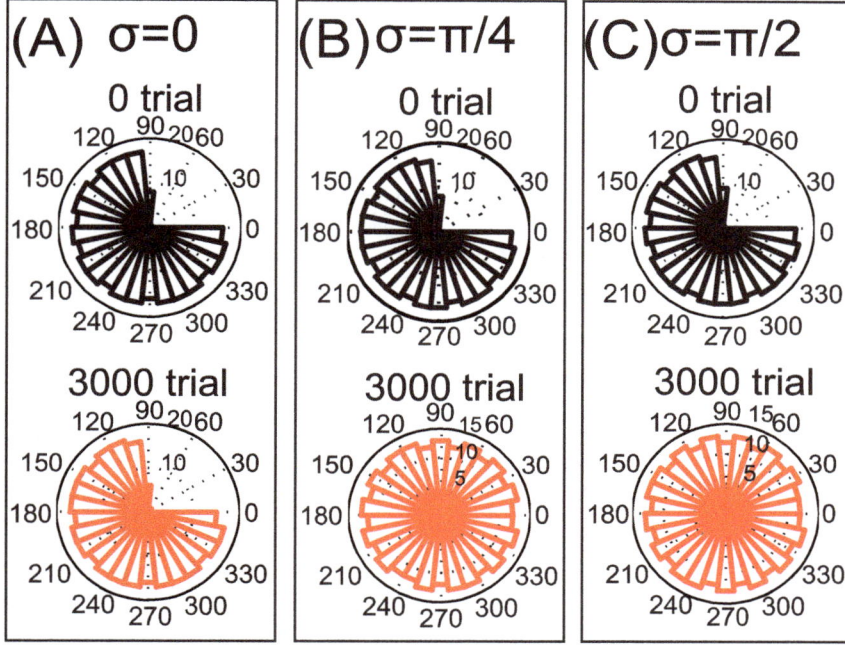

Figure 10. Reorganization of the damaged motor cortex when annealed noise was added to each learning step. (A): Histograms of $\phi_i^{e,u}$ when $\sigma_a = 0$. (B): The same histograms when $\sigma_a = \frac{\pi}{4}$. (C): The same histograms when $\sigma_a = \frac{\pi}{2}$.

reorganization, it remains unclear whether synaptic drift occurs during the reorganization process [30] (but see [25]). Conversely, quenched rotations likely occur in bimanual movement [10]. Our computational study suggests that strong and quenched PD rotations can effectively facilitate reorganization, but in future work, we plan to investigate how synaptic drift can be parsimoniously induced.

Methods

Definitions

This study assumed the following conditions: subjects move their arms towards one of eight radially distributed targets at angles of $\theta_k = 2\pi \frac{k}{8}$ ($k=1,...,8$), and the reaching movements are modeled as weighted averaging of neural activities. If the kth target is presented, then the ith neuron is activated as follows:

$$A_i(\theta_k, \phi_i^{e,w}) = [\cos(\theta_k - \phi_i^{e,w}) + \xi_i]_+ \qquad (4)$$

where ϕ_i^e is a uniformly distributed encoding PD ($i=1,...,N$), $N(=500)$ is the number of model neurons, the index $w \in \{u,b\}$ indicates unimanual or bimanual movement, and $[a]_+$ denotes a rectified nonlinearity of neural activity, where $[a]_+ = a$ if $a > 0$ and $[a]_+ = 0$ if $a < 0$. The neural activity is noisy due to signal-dependent noise, ξ_i, has a mean of 0, and its variance is determined by

$$\mathrm{Var}(\xi_i) = \sigma^2 [\cos(\theta_k - \phi_i^{e,w})]_+^2 \qquad (5)$$

where $\sigma(=0.15)$ is the strength of the noise.

Based on these neural activities, the neural population generates a population vector $PV(\theta_k)$ defined as

$$PV(\theta_k) = \frac{1}{N} \left(\sum_i^N A_i(\theta_k, \phi_i^{e,w}) \cos\phi_i^{d,w}, \sum_i^N A_i(\theta_k, \phi_i^{e,w}) \sin\phi_i^{d,w} \right)^T (6)$$

where $\phi_i^{d,w}$ is the decoding PD. Following previous studies, the decoding PD is set to equal the encoding PD in unimanual movement ($\phi_i^{e,u} = \phi_i^{d,u}$) [1,12]. Although the PV is normalized by the summation of neural activity in the standard PV algorithm, this study assumed normalized neural activity, which allows the PV to be normalized simply by using a weighted average of the neural activities, as shown in equation (6) [1].

Stroke implementation. The PV can be used to model the reaching movements of stroke patients by depleting a fraction of the model neurons [1,18]. As an initial condition, we removed model neurons with encoding PDs of approximately $\pi/4$ because stroke patients have difficulty moving their paretic limbs to targets far from their body centers [20]. We thus removed the neurons for which $\phi_i^{e,u} \in [\pi/8, 3\pi/8]$. We modeled the recovery process by defining supervised and unsupervised learning (see the following section) because these learning rules model the recovery process of post-stroke rehabilitation.

Stroke recovery implementation. After the neuron depletion we modeled the reorganization process of a damaged motor cortex as the optimization process of the following cost function:

$$E^t(\theta_t, \phi_i^{e,w}) = \frac{1}{2}(1 - \cos(\theta_t - \theta_p)) + \frac{\lambda}{2} \sum_i^N (A_i(\theta_t, \phi_i^{e,w}))^2 \qquad (7)$$

where λ is the regularization parameter and θ_p is the angle of PV at the tth trial. The reorganization process decreases the angular error between θ_p and θ by rotating PVs toward the target position; this supervised learning is modeled by the first term of equation (7). The process also decreases the total neural activation, or metabolic cost; this unsupervised learning is modeled by the second term of equation (7). After each rehabilitation trial, the reorganization occurs as follows:

$$(\phi_i^{e,w})^{t+1} = (\phi_i^{e,w})^t + \eta_s \sin(\theta - \theta_p) A_i(\theta, \phi_i^{e,w}) + \eta_u \sin(\theta - \phi_i^{e,w}) \quad (8)$$

where $\eta_s = 0.005$ and $\eta_u = 0.002$ are the learning rates for the supervised and unsupervised learning methods, respectively. The learning process is not affected by these learning rates, as shown in figures 8 and 9. The reorganization is facilitated when this learning step includes synaptic drift (figure 10); this drift is modeled by adding a random Gaussian variable ζ_i^t to this learning rule, for which the variable mean is 0 and the variance is σ_a^2.

Bimanual movement implementation. We assumed that bimanual movement induces rotations of the PDs only during encoding and not in decoding [10] (but see [11]). In other words, we assumed that bimanual movement changes neural activities through inter-hemispheric inhibition between primary motor

cortices, but this movement does not affect cortical-spinal-muscle connectivities. In bimanual movement, the encoding PDs are rotated pseudo-randomly [10]; these rotations are modeled as $\phi_i^{d,u} = \phi_i^{d,b} = \phi_i^{e,u}$ and $\phi_i^{e,b} = \phi_i^{e,u} + \varepsilon_i$, where ε_i is a random Gaussian variable with a mean of 0 and a variance of σ^2. Additionally, ε_i is a quenched random variable, meaning that this variable is invariant across trials; we assumed constant rotations of the encoding PDs in bimanual movement.

Acknowledgments

We thank H. Tanaka, Y. Naruse, and T. Omori for their helpful discussions.

Author Contributions

Conceived and designed the experiments: KT. Performed the experiments: KT. Analyzed the data: KT. Contributed reagents/materials/analysis tools: KT MO. Wrote the paper: KT MO.

References

1. Han CE, Arbib Ma, Schweighofer N (2008) Stroke rehabilitation reaches a threshold. PLoS Comput Biol 4: e1000133.
2. Dobkin BH (2004) Strategies for stroke rehabilitation. Lancet neurology 3: 528–36.
3. Rose DK, Winstein CJ (2004) Bimanual training after stroke: are two hands better than one? Topics in stroke rehabilitation 11: 20–30.
4. Taub E, Uswatte G, Elbert T (2002) New treatments in neurorehabilitation founded on basic research. Nat Rev Neurosci 3: 228–36.
5. Schweighofer N, Han CE, Wolf SL, Arbib Ma, Winstein CJ (2009) A functional threshold for longterm use of hand and arm function can be determined: predictions from a computational model and supporting data from the Extremity Constraint-Induced Therapy Evaluation (EXCITE) Trial. Physical therapy 89: 1327–36.
6. Latimer CP, Keeling J, Lin B, Henderson M, Hale LA (2010) The impact of bilateral therapy on upper limb function after chronic stroke: a systematic review. Disability and rehabilitation 32: 1221–31.
7. Mudie MH, Matyas Ta (2000) Can simultaneous bilateral movement involve the undamaged hemisphere in reconstruction of neural networks damaged by stroke? Disability and rehabilitation 22: 23–37.
8. Cunningham CL, Stoykov MEP, Walter CB (2002) Bilateral facilitation of motor control in chronic hemiplegia. Acta psychologica 110: 321–337.
9. Donchin O, Gribova a, Steinberg O, Mitz aR, Bergman H, et al. (2002) Single-unit activity related to bimanual arm movements in the primary and supplementary motor cortices. Journal of neurophysiology 88: 3498–517.
10. Rokni U, Steinberg O, Vaadia E, Sompolinsky H (2003) Cortical representation of bimanual movements. J Neurosci 23: 11577–11586.
11. Steinberg O, Donchin O, Gribova a, Cardosa de Oliveira S, Bergman H, et al. (2002) Neuronal populations in primary motor cortex encode bimanual arm movements. Eur J Neurosci 15: 1371–1380.
12. Georgopoulos A, Schwartz A, Kettner R (1986) Neuronal population coding of movement direction. Science 233: 1416–1419.
13. Ganguly K, Secundo L, Ranade G, Orsborn A, Chang EF, et al. (2009) Cortical representation of ipsilateral arm movements in monkey and man. J Neurosci 29: 12948–12956.
14. Lukashin AV, Georgopoulos AP (1994) A Neural Network for Coding of Trajectories by Time Series of Neuronal Population Vectors. Neural Comput 6: 19–28.
15. Li CS, Padoa-Schioppa C, Bizzi E (2001) Neuronal correlates of motor performance and motor learning in the primary motor cortex of monkeys adapting to an external force field. Neuron 30: 593–607.
16. Salinas E, Abbott LF (1995) Transfer of coded information from sensory to motor networks. J Neurosci 15: 6461–6474.
17. Verstynen T, Sabes PN (2011) How each movement changes the next: an experimental and theoretical study of fast adaptive priors in reaching. The Journal of neuroscience : the official journal of the Society for Neuroscience 31: 10050–9.
18. Reinkensmeyer DJ, Iobbi MG, Kahn LE, Kamper DG, Takahashi CD (2003) Modeling reaching impairment after stroke using a population vector model of movement control that incorporates neural firing-rate variability. Neural Compt 15: 2619–2642.
19. Goodall S, Reggia J, Chen Y, Ruppin E, Whitney C (1997) A computational model of acute focal cortical lesions. Stroke 28: 101–109.
20. Beer RF, Dewald JPA, Dawson ML, Rymer WZ (2004) Target-dependent differences between free and constrained arm movements in chronic hemiparesis. Exp Brain Res 156: 458–470.
21. Gould HJ, Cusick CG, Pons TP, H KJ (1986) The relationship of corpus callosum connections to electrical stimulation maps of motor, supplementary motor, and the frontal eye fields in owl monkeys. J Comp Neurol. pp 297–325.
22. Rouille EM, Babalian A, Kazennikov O, V M, H YX, et al. (1994) The relationship of corpus callosum connections to electrical stimulation maps of motor, supplementary motor, and the frontal eye fields in owl monkeys. Exp Brain Res. pp 227–243.
23. Grefkes C, Fink GR (2011) Reorganization of cerebral networks after stroke: new insights from neuroimaging with connectivity approaches. Brain. pp 1–13.
24. Paz R, Boraud T, Natan C, Bergman H, Vaadia E (2003) Preparatory activity in motor cortex reflects learning of local visuomotor skills. Nat Neurosci 6: 882–890.
25. Rokni U, Richardson A, Bizzi E, Seung H (2007) Motor learning with unstable neural representations. Neuron 54: 653–666.
26. Morrow M, Miller LE (2003) Prediction of muscle activity by populations of sequentially recorded primary motor cortex neurons. J Neurophysiol 89: 2279–2288.
27. Todorov E (2000) Direct cortical control of muscle activation in voluntary arm movements: a model. Nat Neurosci 3(4): 391–398.
28. Guigon E, Baraduc P, Desmurget M (2007) Coding of movement- and force-related information in primate primary motor cortex: a computational approach. E J Neurosci 26: 250–60.
29. Schmidt MF (2003) Pattern of interhemispheric synchronization in HVc during singing correlates with key transitions in the song pattern. J Neurophysiol 6: 3931–3949.
30. Stevenson IH, Cherian A, London BM, Sachs N, Lindberg E, et al. (2011) Statistical assessment of the stability of neural movement representations. J Neurophysiol.

5

What Is the Evidence for Physical Therapy Poststroke? A Systematic Review and Meta-Analysis

Janne Marieke Veerbeek[1], Erwin van Wegen[1], Roland van Peppen[2], Philip Jan van der Wees[3], Erik Hendriks[4], Marc Rietberg[1], Gert Kwakkel[1,5]*

1 Department of Rehabilitation Medicine, MOVE Research Institute Amsterdam, VU University Medical Center, Amsterdam, The Netherlands, 2 Department of Physiotherapy, University of Applied Sciences Utrecht, Utrecht, The Netherlands, 3 Scientific Institute for Quality of Healthcare (IQ healthcare), Radboud University Nijmegen Medical Center, Nijmegen, The Netherlands, 4 Department of Epidemiology, Maastricht University, Maastricht, The Netherlands, 5 Department of Neurorehabilitation, Reade Center for Rehabilitation and Rheumatology, Amsterdam, The Netherlands

Abstract

Background: Physical therapy (PT) is one of the key disciplines in interdisciplinary stroke rehabilitation. The aim of this systematic review was to provide an update of the evidence for stroke rehabilitation interventions in the domain of PT.

Methods and Findings: Randomized controlled trials (RCTs) regarding PT in stroke rehabilitation were retrieved through a systematic search. Outcomes were classified according to the ICF. RCTs with a low risk of bias were quantitatively analyzed. Differences between phases poststroke were explored in subgroup analyses. A best evidence synthesis was performed for neurological treatment approaches. The search yielded 467 RCTs (N = 25373; median PEDro score 6 [IQR 5–7]), identifying 53 interventions. No adverse events were reported. Strong evidence was found for significant positive effects of 13 interventions related to gait, 11 interventions related to arm-hand activities, 1 intervention for ADL, and 3 interventions for physical fitness. Summary Effect Sizes (SESs) ranged from 0.17 (95%CI 0.03–0.70; $I^2 = 0\%$) for therapeutic positioning of the paretic arm to 2.47 (95%CI 0.84–4.11; $I^2 = 77\%$) for training of sitting balance. There is strong evidence that a higher dose of practice is better, with SESs ranging from 0.21 (95%CI 0.02–0.39; $I^2 = 6\%$) for motor function of the paretic arm to 0.61 (95%CI 0.41–0.82; $I^2 = 41\%$) for muscle strength of the paretic leg. Subgroup analyses yielded significant differences with respect to timing poststroke for 10 interventions. Neurological treatment approaches to training of body functions and activities showed equal or unfavorable effects when compared to other training interventions. Main limitations of the present review are not using individual patient data for meta-analyses and absence of correction for multiple testing.

Conclusions: There is strong evidence for PT interventions favoring intensive high repetitive task-oriented and task-specific training in all phases poststroke. Effects are mostly restricted to the actually trained functions and activities. Suggestions for prioritizing PT stroke research are given.

Editor: Terence J. Quinn, University of Glasgow, United Kingdom

Funding: This research project was supported by the Royal Dutch Society for Physical Therapy (KNGF grant no. 8091.1; http://www.fysionet.nl/). The funders had no role in study design, data collection and analysis, decision to publish, or preparation of the manuscript.

Competing Interests: The authors have declared that no competing interests exist.

* E-mail: g.kwakkel@vumc.nl

Introduction

Prospective studies have estimated that about 795.000 people in the USA suffer a first or recurrent stroke each year [1]. The prevalence of chronic stroke in the USA is estimated at about 7 million [1], with about 80% of patients with stroke being over the age of 65. The prevalence of stroke is likely to increase in the future due to the aging population. Even though acute stroke care has improved, for example by large-scale application of recombinant tissue plasminogen activator (rTPA) [1,2] and organized interdisciplinary inpatient stroke care [3], and although mortality rates have been decreasing [1], a large number of patients still remain disabled regardless of the time that has elapsed poststroke. Only 12% of the patients with stroke are independent in basic activities of daily living (ADL) at the end of the first week [4]. In the long term, 25–74% of patients have to rely on human assistance for basic ADLs like feeding, self-care, and mobility [5].

Interdisciplinary complex rehabilitation interventions [6,7] are assumed to represent the mainstay of poststroke care [8]. One of the key disciplines in interdisciplinary stroke rehabilitation is physical therapy which is primarily aimed at restoring and maintaining ADLs, usually starting within the first days and often continuing into the chronic phase poststroke [8]. While the interdisciplinary character of stroke rehabilitation is paramount, the availability of specific, up-to-date, and professional evidence-based guidelines for the physical therapy profession is crucial for making adequate evidence-based clinical decisions [9–11]. The recommendations in the first Dutch evidence-based 'Clinical Practice Guideline for physical therapy in patients with stroke' were based on meta-analyses of 123 randomized controlled trials (RCTs) and date back to 2004 [12]. In view of the tremendous growth in the number of RCTs in this field, it is now necessary to re-establish the "state of the art" concerning the evidence for physical therapy interventions in stroke rehabilitation. This aim is in line with the 2006 Helsingborg Declaration on European Stroke Strategies, which states that stroke rehabilitation should be based on evidence as much as possible [13,14].

The first aim of the present systematic review was to update our previous meta-analyses of complex stroke rehabilitation interventions in the domain of physical therapy, based on RCTs with a low risk of bias (i.e. a moderate to good methodological quality) with no restrictions to the comparator. Primary outcomes, measured post intervention, were defined at the levels of body functions and/or activities and participation of the International Classification of Functioning, disability and health model (ICF) [15]. The second aim was to explore whether the timing of interventions poststroke moderated the main effects.

Methods

Definitions

In accordance with the definition used by the World Health Organization (WHO), stroke was defined as "rapidly developing clinical symptoms and/or signs of focal, and at times global, loss of cerebral function, with symptoms lasting more than 24 hours or leading to death, with no apparent cause other than that of vascular origin" [16]. We distinguished four poststroke phases: the hyper acute or acute phase (0–24 hours), the early rehabilitation phase (24 hours until 3 months), the late rehabilitation phase (3–6 months), and the chronic phase (>6 months).

A study was considered an RCT when "the individuals (or other units) followed in the trial were definitely or possibly assigned prospectively to one of two (or more) alternative forms of health care using random allocation" [17].

Physical therapy was defined as "therapeutic modalities frequently used in physical therapy specialty by physical therapists or physiotherapists to promote, maintain, or restore the physical and physiological well-being of an individual" (Medline Subject Heading; MeSH). According to the American Physical Therapy Association (APTA), "physical therapists are health care professionals who maintain, restore, and improve movement, activity, and health, enabling an individual to have optimal functioning and quality of life, while ensuring patient safety and applying evidence to provide efficient and effective care. Physical therapists evaluate, diagnose, and manage individuals of all ages who have impairments, activity limitations, and participation restrictions. In addition, physical therapists are involved in promoting health, wellness, and fitness through risk factor identification and the implementation of services to reduce risk, slow the progression of or prevent functional decline and disability, and enhance participation in chosen life situations." [18].

Exercise therapy refers to "a regimen or plan of physical activities designed and prescribed for specific therapeutic goals" (MeSH) in the field of physical therapy, intended to restore optimal functioning [19]. For the present meta-analysis, we included the use of technical applications such as robotics, electrostimulation and treadmills with body-weight support.

In line with previous reviews, we defined intensity of practice as the number of hours spent in exercise therapy [12,19,20]. Treatment contrast refers to "the amount of time spent on exercise therapy by the experimental group minus that spent by the control group" [20].

Activities of daily living (ADL) are "the daily self-care activities required to function in the home and/or outdoor environment. They may be classified as basic or extended" [21]. Basic ADL covers the ability to perform basic activities of self-care and mobility [21,22]. These activities are captured by a combination of two or more of the codes d510 (washing oneself), d530 (toileting), d550 (eating), d540 (dressing), b5253 (fecal continence) and b6202 (urinary continence), d410 (changing basic body position), d420 (transferring oneself), and d450 (walking) as listed in the ICF [22]. By contrast, extended ADL "whilst not fundamental to functioning, allow an individual to live independently, e.g. shopping, housekeeping, managing finances, preparing meals, and using transportation" [21].

Study Identification

Our previous search, covering the period up to January 29, 2004, was updated. Relevant publications were identified by searching the electronic databases PubMed (last searched June 28, 2011), EBSCO*host*/Excerpta Medica Databank (EMBASE; last searched June 9, 2011), EBSCO*host*/Cumulative Index of Nursing and Allied Health Literature (CINAHL; last searched July 14, 2011), Wiley/Cochrane Library (Cochrane Database of Systematic Reviews [CDSR], Cochrane Central Register of Controlled Trials [CENTRAL], Cochrane Methodology Register [CMR], Database of Abstracts of Reviews of Effects [DARE], Health Technology Assessment Database [HTA], NHS Economic Evaluation Database [EED]; last searched July 21, 2011), Physiotherapy Evidence Database (PEDro; last searched August 24, 2011), and SPORTDiscus[TM] (last searched August 24, 2011). This was done by J.M.V. after two researchers (J.M.V. and J.C.F.K.) had built the search string. The databases were searched by indexing terms and free-text terms used with synonyms and related terms in the title or abstract. We searched for "stroke", and "exercise" or "physical therapy" or "physiotherapy" or "rehabilitation", and "randomized controlled trials" or "reviews" (see table 1). Additional searches were performed for specified interventions. The full search strategy can be obtained from the corresponding author. One reviewer (J.M.V.), who was not blinded, screened the titles and abstracts and assessed potentially relevant publications in fulltext. In addition, references of included RCTs and relevant reviews like those of the Cochrane Collaboration and the Evidence-Based Review of Stroke Rehabilitation (EBRSR) were screened. Authors of conference abstracts were contacted for fulltext publications, if available, and experts in the field were consulted.

Studies were included if they met the following inclusion criteria: (1) the study sample analyzed consisted exclusively of patients with stroke aged 18 years or over; (2) the study was designed as an RCT including those with a two-group parallel, multi-arm parallel, crossover, cluster, or factorial designs; (3) the experimental intervention delivered fitted the domain of physical therapy and aimed to improve body functions and/or activities and participation and/or contextual factors; (4) the comparator was usual care, another intervention, the same intervention with a different dose, or no intervention; (5) the outcomes were measured post intervention and belonged to the domain of physical therapy (see the section on "Intervention categories and outcome domains"); and (6) the full-text publication was written in English, French, German, Spanish, Portuguese, or Dutch.

A review protocol was not published. An ethics statement was not required for this work.

Data Extraction

One reviewer (J.M.V.) extracted the following information from the included RCTs using two forms developed in advance: first author, year of publication, number of patients in each group, eligibility criteria, stroke characteristics including poststroke phase, intervention characteristics, outcome measures, timing of assessment, the authors' conclusions and the post intervention, and if

Table 1. Search strategy PubMed.

#1	Search "Stroke"[Mesh] OR cva[tiab] OR cvas[tiab] OR poststroke*[tiab] OR stroke*[tiab] OR apoplex*[tiab]
#2	Search (((brain*[tiab] OR cerebr*[tiab] OR cerebell*[tiab] OR intracran*[tiab] OR intracerebral[tiab] OR vertebrobasilar[tiab]) AND vascular*[tiab]) OR cerebrovascular*[tiab]) AND (disease[tiab] OR diseases[tiab] OR accident*[tiab] OR disorder*[tiab])
#3	Search (brain*[tiab] OR cerebr*[tiab] OR cerebell*[tiab] OR intracran*[tiab] OR intracerebral[tiab] OR vertebrobasilar[tiab]) AND (haemorrhag*[tiab] OR hemorrhag*[tiab] OR ischemi*[tiab] OR ischaemi*[tiab] OR infarct*[tiab] OR haematoma*[tiab] or hematoma*[tiab] or bleed*[tiab])
#4	Search "Hemiplegia"[Mesh] OR "Paresis"[Mesh] OR (hemipleg*[tiab] OR hemipar*[tiab] OR paresis[tiab] OR paretic[tiab])
#5	Search #1 OR #2 OR #3 OR #4
#6	Search "Occupational Therapy"[MeSH] OR "Physical Therapy Modalities"[MeSH] OR "Rehabilitation"[MeSH] OR "Exercise Therapy"[Mesh] OR "Exercise Movement Techniques"[Mesh] OR "Physical Therapy (Specialty)"[MeSH] OR "Recovery of Function"[Mesh] OR "rehabilitation"[SH] OR rehabilitati*[tiab] OR physiotherap*[tiab] OR (physical[tiab] AND (therapy[tiab] OR therapies[tiab] OR activity[tiab] OR activities[tiab])) OR exercis*[tiab] OR training[tiab] OR (occupational[tiab] AND (therapy[tiab] OR therapies[tiab]))
#7	Search (review*[tiab] OR search*[tiab] OR survey*[tiab] OR handsearch*[tiab] OR hand-search*[tiab]) AND (databa*[tiab] OR data-ba*[tiab] OR bibliograph*[tiab] OR electronic*[tiab] OR medline*[tiab] OR pubmed*[tiab] OR embase*[tiab] OR Cochrane[tiab] OR cinahl[tiab] OR psycinfo[tiab] OR psychinfo[tiab] OR cinhal[tiab] OR "web of science"[tiab] OR "web of knowledge"[tiab] OR ebsco[tiab] OR ovid[tiab] OR mrct[tiab] OR metaregist*[tiab] OR meta-regist*[tiab] OR ((predetermined[tiab] OR pre-determined[tiab]) AND criteri*[tiab]) OR apprais*[tiab] OR inclusion criteri*[tiab] OR exclusion criteri*[tiab]) OR (review[pt] AND systemat*[tiab]) OR "systematic review"[tiab] OR "systematic literature"[tiab] OR "integrative review"[tiab] OR "integrative literature"[tiab] OR "evidence-based review"[tiab] OR "evidence-based overview"[tiab] OR "evidence-based literature"[tiab] OR "evidence-based survey"[tiab] OR "literature search"[tiab] OR ((systemat*[ti] OR evidence-based[ti]) AND (review*[ti] OR literature[ti] OR overview[ti] OR survey[ti])) OR "data synthesis"[tiab] OR "evidence synthesis"[tiab] OR "data extraction"[tiab] OR "data source"[tiab] OR "data sources"[tiab] OR "study selection"[tiab] OR "methodological quality"[tiab] OR "methodologic quality"[tiab] OR cochrane database syst rev[ta] OR meta-analy*[tiab] OR metaanaly*[tiab] OR metanaly*[tiab] OR meta-analysis[pt] OR meta-synthesis[tiab] OR metasynthesis[tiab] OR meta-study[tiab] OR metastudy[tiab] OR metaethnograph*[tiab] OR meta-ethnograph*[tiab] OR Technology Assessment, Biomedical[mh] OR hta[tiab] OR health technol assess [ta] OR evid rep technol assess summ[ta] OR health technology assessment[tiab]
#8	Search randomized controlled trial[pt] OR controlled clinical trial[pt] OR randomized[tiab] OR placebo[tiab] OR drug therapy[sh] OR randomly[tiab] OR trial[tiab] OR groups[tiab] OR "cross over"[tiab] OR "Cross-Over Studies"[Mesh]
#9	Search #7 OR #8
#10	Search #5 AND #6 AND #9 NOT (animal[mh] NOT human [mh])

applicable follow-up, point measures and measures of variability for each of the reported outcomes. Study authors were contacted in case the published results could not be used in the meta-analyses, e.g. when ranges were given instead of standard deviations (SDs) or interquartile ranges (IQRs), or results were only presented in graphs. The extracted data for the meta-analyses were cross-checked in random order. Duplicate publications were included, but counted as one RCT.

Intervention Categories and Outcome Domains

Based on consensus between the authors, physical therapy interventions for the rehabilitation of patients with stroke were divided into: (1) interventions related to gait and mobility-related functions and activities, including novel methods focusing on efficient resource use, such as circuit class training and caregiver-mediated exercises; (2) interventions related to arm-hand activities; (3) interventions related to activities of daily living; (4) interventions related to physical fitness; and (5) other interventions which could not be classified into one of the other categories. In addition, attention was paid to (6) intensity of practice and (7) neurological treatment approaches.

The ICF [15,23] was used to classify the outcome measures into the following domains: **muscle and movement functions** (e.g. muscle power functions [b730], control of voluntary movement functions [b760], muscle tone functions [b735]), **joint and bone functions** (e.g. mobility of joint functions [b710]), **sensory functions** (e.g. proprioceptive function [b260], touch function [b365], sensory functions related to temperature and other stimuli [b720]), **gait pattern functions** [b770] (e.g. gait speed, stride length), **functions of the cardiovascular and respiratory systems** (e.g. heart functions [b410], blood pressure functions [b420], respiration functions [b440], respiratory muscle functions

[b445], exercise tolerance functions [b455]), **mental functions** (e.g. quality of life, depression), **balance** (e.g. changing basic body position [d410], maintaining a body position [d415]), **walking** [d450] (e.g. distance, independence, falls), **arm-hand activities** (e.g. fine hand use [d440], hand and arm use [d445]), **basic ADL** (e.g. washing oneself [d510], toileting [d520], dressing [d540], eating [d550], urination functions [d620]), **extended ADL** (e.g. acquisition of goods and services [d620], preparing meals [d630], doing housework [d640], recreation and leisure [d920]), and **attitudes** (e.g. individual attitudes of immediate or extended family members, like caregiver strain [e410 and e425 respectively]). The primary outcomes were at the body functions and activities and participation levels, while secondary outcomes included contextual factors.

Quality Appraisal

The PEDro checklist was used to assess the risk of bias in the included RCTs [24,25]. This 11-item list estimates the internal and external validity of an RCT based on 11 items. The items concern eligibility criteria, random allocation, concealment of allocation, group similarity at baseline, blinding of subjects, blinding of therapists, blinding of assessors, availability of key outcome measures of more than 85% of the subjects, intention-to-treat analysis, between-group statistical comparisons, and point measures and measures of variability [24,25]. Except for item 1, which assesses the generalizability, one point is awarded if a criterion is satisfied. The maximum score is 10 points. For the purpose of this study, we considered RCTs with a score of ≥4 to have a low risk of bias [12]. One reviewer (J.M.V.) scored all RCTs identified in the updated search unblinded and cross-checked the scores with the PEDro database (www.pedro.org.au). In case of disagreement, another reviewer (E.v.W) made the final decision. For RCTs not listed in the PEDro database, two reviewers (J.M.V. and E.v.W.) independently assessed the risk of bias and disagreements were resolved in a consensus meeting.

Analyses

Data from identified RCTs are reported in the results section. Our quantitative analyses only included RCTs with a PEDro score of ≥ 4. Aggregated data of individual RCTs were pooled when at least two RCTs with a measure in the same outcome category were available for an intervention. Interventions for which pooling was possible were automatically indicated as "strong evidence", regardless of the direction of the results, because only RCTs with a low risk of bias were included (Level 1) [26]. A "strong evidence" label was also assigned when only one phase III trial was available for a particular intervention. Analogous to our 2004 review, a qualitative analysis was performed for the intervention category "neurological treatment approaches". Based on an adaptation of the criteria established by Van Tulder et al. [26] the following four levels of evidence were distinguished:

Level 1. Strong evidence – provided by generally consistent findings in multiple, relevant, high-quality RCTs.

Level 2. Moderate evidence – provided by findings in one relevant, high-quality RCT.

Level 3. Limited evidence – provided by generally consistent findings in one or more relevant low-quality RCTs.

Level 4. No or conflicting evidence – if there were no RCTs or if the results were conflicting.

RCTs with a PEDro score of ≥ 4 are considered to be of high-quality, while a score of < 4 is considered as low-quality.

Quantitative Analysis

Studies with a crossover design were considered RCTs. Measurements up to the crossover point were used as post intervention outcomes. Single-session experiments were not included in the quantitative analyses.

Meta-analyses were performed for each intervention for which at least two RCTs with comparable outcomes were identified. Based on post intervention outcomes (means and SDs), the individual effect sizes with their 95% confidence intervals (CI) were calculated as Hedges' g. The individual Hedges' g values were pooled to determine the summary effect size (SES; number of SD units) and 95%CI. The I^2 statistic was used to determine statistical consistency (between-study variation) [17]. An I^2 of $> 50.0\%$ was considered to reflect substantial heterogeneity [17] and in that case a random-effects model was applied, while a fixed-effect model was applied in case of statistical homogeneity. A significant positive SES indicates that the experimental intervention is beneficial for patients when compared to a comparator. In the same vein, a significant negative SES indicates that the intervention has unfavorable effects for patients when compared to a comparator.

We pre-specified that in case of differences between RCTs in the timing of the interventions after stroke, a possible moderator effect of timing after stroke would be explored (in accordance with the phases described in the "*Definitions*" section) [27]. The variance between the subgroups was statistically tested in a "fixed-effect or random-effects within, fixed-effects between" model by applying the Q-test based on analysis of variance (ANOVA). Since the number of studies within each subgroup was five or less in nearly all meta-analyses, a pooled estimate of τ^2 (variance of the distribution of the true effect sizes within subgroups) across subgroups was used, as separate estimates of τ^2 for each subgroup are likely to be imprecise [27]. The SES (95%CI) and number of RCTs for each subgroup were only reported if there were significant differences between the poststroke phases.

In all analyses, the null hypothesis was rejected when the probability value was < 0.05 (2-tailed). Following Cohen, the effect sizes were classified into small (< 0.2), medium (0.2–0.8), and large (> 0.8) [28]. All analyses were performed using Comprehensive Meta-analysis (Biostat, Englewood, New Jersey).

The statistical power of each meta-analysis was calculated post hoc, based on the number of RCTs included, the within-study sample size, the SES, the between-studies variance, and 2-tailed p-value [29]. A power of ≥ 0.8 was regarded as satisfactory.

Results

Study Identification

The search for relevant RCTs is visualized in figure 1. The final selection of RCTs consisted of 467 studies involving 25 373 patients with stroke; 123 RCTs from the 2004 search and an additional 344 RCTs from the updated search. Most studies included patients in the early rehabilitation phase (n = 198) or chronic phase (n = 202). Three RCTs included patients in the hyper acute or acute rehabilitation phase. For details see tables S1A–S1G in file S1.

Quality Appraisal

The risk of bias in RCTs has decreased over time, as shown by the increase in PEDro scores from a median of 5 (IQR 4–6) points for RCTs published till 2004 [12] to 6 (IQR 5–7) for the RCTs published from 2004 to 2011. The median PEDro score of all 467 RCTs was 6 (IQR 5–7).

Analyses

Pooling was possible for 23 physical therapy interventions related to gait and mobility-related functions and activities, for 23 interventions related to arm-hand activities, for two interventions related to ADL in general, for four interventions related to physical fitness, and for inspiratory muscle training which did not fit the other categories (see tables S1A–S1E in file S1). Meta-analyses were also performed for intensity of practice (for details see table S1F in file S1).

Quantitative Analysis

Physical therapy interventions related to gait and mobility-related functions and activities. The results of the meta-analyses for interventions related to gait and mobility-related functions and activities are summarized in figure 2 (for details see table S2A in file S1). Pooling was not possible for bilateral leg training with rhythmic gait cueing [30], mirror therapy for the paretic leg [31], mental practice with motor imagery [32], limb overloading with external weights [33], systematic verbal feedback on gait speed [34], maintenance of ankle dorsiflexion by using a standing frame or night splint [35], manual passive mobilization of the ankle [36], range of motion exercises of the ankle with specially designed equipment [37], ultrasound for the paretic leg [38], segmental muscle vibration for a drop foot [39], whole body vibration [40], and wheel chair propulsion [41].

1. Early mobilization

Early mobilization out of bed within 24 hours poststroke and stimulating the patient to exercise outside the bed [42] was investigated in two RCTs (N = 103, PEDro score 8) [43,44], including patients in the hyper acute or acute phase.

A nonsignificant SES was found for complications, neurological deterioration early poststroke, fatigue, independence in basic ADL at 3 months, and discharge home.

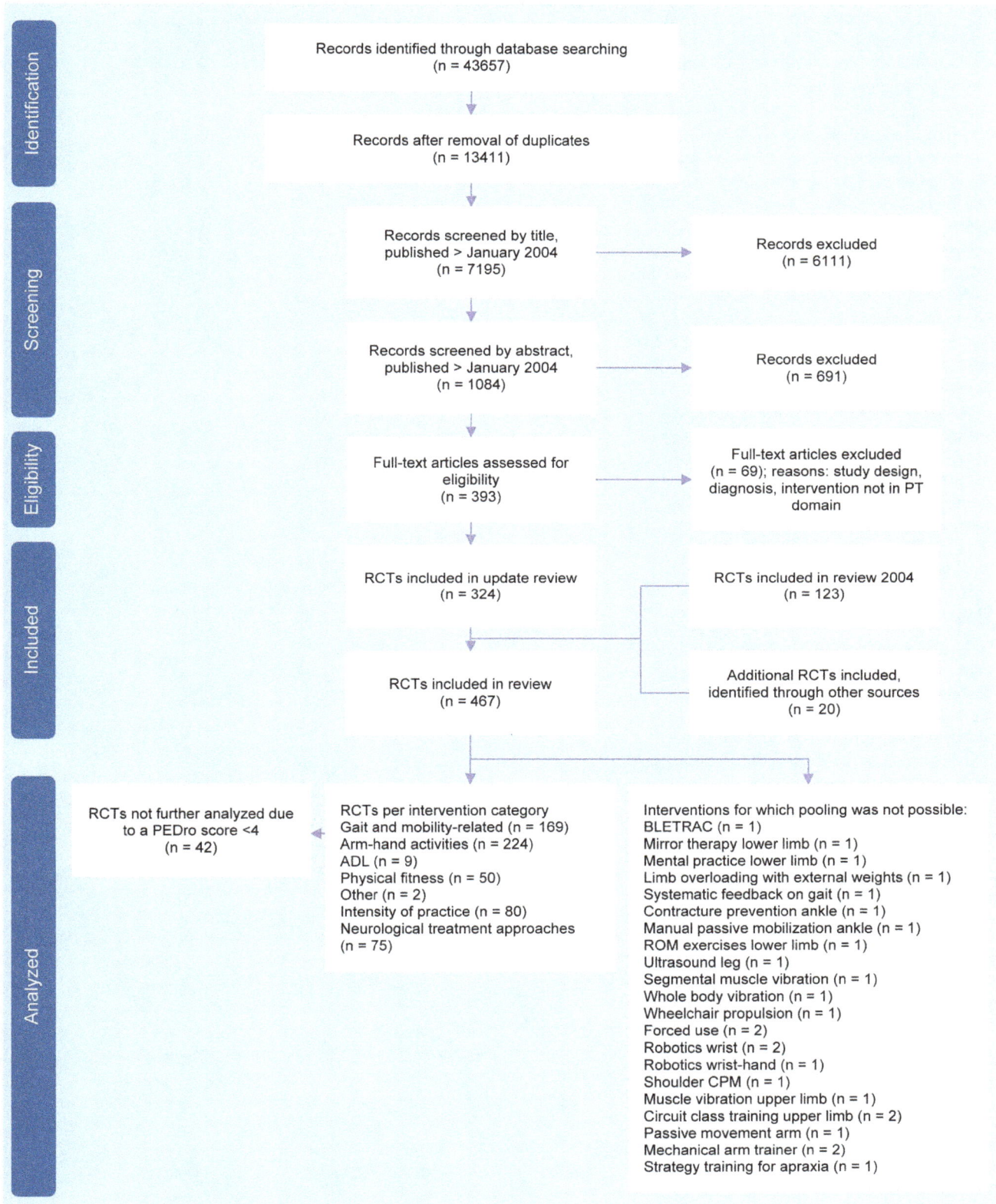

Figure 1. PRISMA Flow diagram. Legend: ADL, Activities of daily living; BLETRAC, Bilateral leg training with rhythmic auditory cueing; CPM, Continuous passive motion; PEDro, Physiotherapy evidence database; PT, Physical therapy; RCTs, Randomized controlled trials; ROM, Range of motion.

Intervention	Compari-sons (n) / Patients (N)	I² (%)	Hedges' g (95%CI)	Power
Outcome: walking ability				
Early mobilization	NA			
Sitting balance training	4 / 59	0		0.058
Sit-to-stand training	NA			
Standing balance training without BF	2 / 148	0		0.134
Standing balance training with BF	9 / 251	60		0.051
Balance training (various activities)	7 / 271	24		0.162
Body-weight supported TT	9 / 357	42		0.422
Electromechanical-assisted GT	16 / 669	82		0.550
Electromechanical-assisted GT (FES)	2 / 72	0		0.955
Speed dependent TT	4 / 133	73		0.877
Overground walking	12 / 576	82		0.787
Rhythmic gait cueing	NA			
Community walking	NA			
Virtual reality mobility training	2 / 30	0		0.069
Circuit class training	6 / 259	0		0.496
Caregiver-mediated exercises	NA			
Water-based exercises	NA			
Orthosis for walking	NA			
Interventions somatosensory functions	NA			
NMS	9 / 237	65		0.141
EMG-NMS	NA			
TENS	5 / 195	0		0.958
EMG-BF	NA			
Outcome: comfortable gait speed				
Early mobilization	NA			
Sitting balance training	NA			
Sit-to-stand training	NA			
Standing balance training without BF	NA			
Standing balance training with BF	6 / 184	0		0.248
Balance training (various activities)	2 / 88	0		0.244
Body-weight supported TT	15 / 858	82		1.000
Electromechanical-assisted GT	4 / 122	58		0.235
Electromechanical-assisted GT (FES)	NA			
Speed dependent TT	7 / 192	0		0.050
Overground walking	11 / 541	56		0.771
Rhythmic gait cueing	2 / 118	97		0.717
Community walking	NA			
Virtual reality mobility training	2 / 42	54		0.262
Circuit class training	4 / 181	58		0.790
Caregiver-mediated exercises	NA			
Water-based exercises	NA			
Orthosis for walking	2 / 84	55		0.770
Interventions somatosensory functions	2 / 51	0		0.068
NMS	9 / 215	59		0.581
EMG-NMS	NA			
TENS	6 / 170	0		0.257
EMG-BF	2 / 34	52		0.247

-1   0   1   2

Favors control   Favors treatment

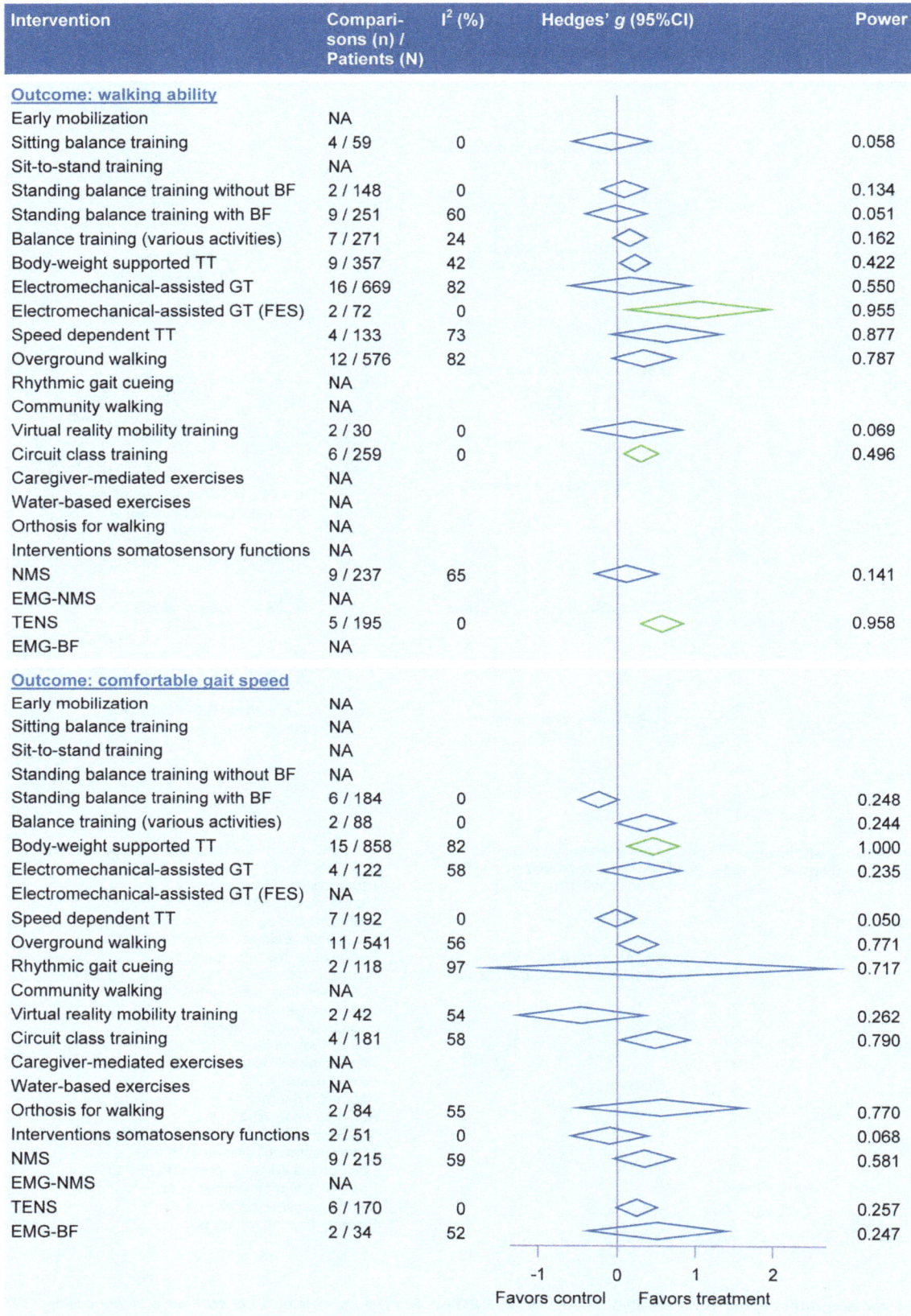

Figure 2. Summary effect sizes for physical therapy interventions – gait and mobility-related functions and activities. Legend: A green colored diamond indicates that the summary effect size is significant, while a blue colored diamond indicates that the summary effect size is

nonsignificant; CI, Confidence interval; EMG-BF, Electromyographic biofeedback; EMG-NMS, Electromyography-triggered neuromuscular stimulation; FES, Functional electrostimulation; GT, Gait training; NA, Not applicable; NMS, Neuromuscular stimulation; TENS, Transcutaneous electrical nerve stimulation; TT, Treadmill training.

2. Sitting balance training

Training of balance (i.e. maintaining, achieving, or restoring balance) during sitting [45] was investigated in six RCTs (N = 150, PEDro score range 4 [46] to 8 [47]) [46–51], including patients in the early rehabilitation phase [46,47,49–51] or chronic phase [48].

Overall, pooling of data showed a nonsignificant SES for symmetry while sitting and standing, balance, walking ability, and basic ADL. However, pooling only data of RCTs which investigated training of sitting balance while reaching beyond arm's length yielded a significant heterogeneous positive SES for sitting balance. Nonsignificant SESs were found for ground reaction force while sitting and hand movement time. Subgroup analyses revealed no significant differences between poststroke phases.

3. Sit-to-stand training

Training the transfer from sit-to-stand and vice versa while maintaining balance [52] was investigated in five RCTs (N = 163, PEDro score range 4 [53] to 6 [54–56]) [53–57], including patients who were unable to perform a sit-to-stand without help in the early rehabilitation phase [53,54,56,57] or chronic phase [55].

Nonsignificant SESs were found for body weight distribution, sit-to-stand, and balance. Subgroup analyses revealed no significant differences between poststroke phases.

4. Standing balance training without biofeedback

Training of balance (i.e. maintaining, achieving, or restoring balance) during standing [45] without the use of biofeedback was investigated in four RCTs (N = 199, PEDro score range 4 [58] to 8 [59]) [58–61], including patients in the early rehabilitation phase [59–61] or chronic phase [58]. The training consisted of standing on surfaces of different compliance with eyes open, optionally combined with eyes closed, or standing in a frame.

Nonsignificant SESs were found for postural sway, sit-to-stand, balance, and walking ability. Subgroup analyses revealed no significant differences between poststroke phases.

5. Standing balance training with biofeedback – force and position feedback

The use of a force platform with force sensors to measure the weight on each foot and the center of pressure to subsequently give visual or auditory feedback to the patient [8] was investigated in 12 RCTs (N = 333, PEDro score range 3 [62] to 6 [56,63–67]) [56,62–73], including patients in the early rehabilitation phase [56,68–70,72,73], late rehabilitation phase [62–64,67,71], or chronic phase [66]. In most of the RCTs, patients had to be able to get from a seated to a standing position and be able to stand with or without physical support.

A significant homogeneous positive SES was found for postural sway. Subgroup analyses showed that the effect size was only significant in the chronic phase (n = 1), while the SES for the early rehabilitation phase (n = 6) was not. Nonsignificant SESs were found for motor function of the paretic leg (synergy), comfortable gait speed, step length, cadence, monopedal and bipedal phase, balance, walking ability, and basic ADL. Subgroup analyses revealed no significant differences between poststroke phases for these outcomes.

6. Balance training during various activities

Training of balance (i.e. maintaining, achieving, or restoring balance) during various activities [45] was investigated in 11 RCTs (N = 419, PEDro score range 4 [74] to 8 [75,76]) [74–84], including patients in the early rehabilitation phase [76,77,80,83,84], late rehabilitation phase [74,75,82], or chronic phase [78,79,81].

Pooling resulted in a significant homogeneous positive SES for basic ADL and a significant heterogeneous positive SES for balance. Nonsignificant SESs were found for comfortable gait speed, falls-efficacy, walking ability, and quality of life. Subgroup analyses revealed no significant differences between poststroke phases.

7. Body-weight supported treadmill training

Treadmill training with the patient's body-weight partially supported by a harness [8] was investigated in 18 RCTs (N = 1158, PEDro score range 4 [85–87] to 8 [88–91]) [85–105], including patients in the early rehabilitation phase [85–91,94,96,98,101,103,105] or chronic phase [90,92,93,95,97,99,100,102,104]. The patients had to be restricted in their walking ability, except in one study [90].

Meta-analyses showed significant heterogeneous positive SESs for comfortable gait speed and walking distance. Nonsignificant SESs were found for motor function of the paretic leg (synergy), maximum gait speed, stride length, cadence, aerobic capacity, energy expenditure, balance, walking ability, and quality of life. Subgroup analyses revealed no significant differences between poststroke phases.

8. Electromechanical-assisted gait training

Gait training using an apparatus which guides the walking cycle by electromechanical driven footplates or exoskeleton [8,106,107] was investigated in 16 RCTs (N = 766, PEDro score range 4 [108,109] to 8 [110,111]) [96,102,108–123], including patients in the early rehabilitation phase [96,110,113–115,118–123], late rehabilitation phase [109], or chronic phase [102,108,112,116]. For the purpose of this review, the meta-analyses for electromechanical-assisted gait training were subdivided into two groups: (a) without functional electrostimulation and (b) with functional electrostimulation.

a. Electromechanical-assisted gait training without functional electrostimulation

Electromechanical-assisted gait training without functional electrostimulation was investigated in 16 RCTs (N = 766) [96,102,108–110,112–123].

Pooling resulted in significant homogeneous positive SESs for maximum gait speed, walking distance, peak heart rate, and basic ADL. Nonsignificant SESs were found for neurological functions, motor function of the paretic leg (synergy), muscle strength, comfortable gait speed, cadence, step length, heart rate at rest, balance, walking ability, extended ADL, and quality of life. Subgroup analyses showed significant differences between poststroke phases. The analysis for comfortable gait speed showed that only patients in the early rehabilitation phase who were dependent in walking benefited from electromechanical-assisted gait training.

As regards balance, a significant homogeneous positive SES was found for the early rehabilitation phase (n = 4), a significant negative effect size for the late rehabilitation phase (n = 1), and a nonsignificant SES for the chronic phase (n = 4). As regards walking ability, a significant homogeneous positive SES was found for patients in the early rehabilitation phase (n = 12), a significant negative effect size for the late rehabilitation phase (n = 1), and a nonsignificant homogeneous negative SES for the chronic phase (n = 3).

b. Electromechanical-assisted gait training with functional electrostimulation

Electromechanical-assisted gait training with functional electrostimulation was investigated in three RCTs (N = 149) [112,113,118].

When data of these RCTs were pooled, significant homogeneous positive SESs were found for balance and walking ability (only for patients in the early rehabilitation phase). The statistical analyses for maximum gait speed and basic ADL resulted in nonsignificant SESs. Subgroup analyses for maximum gait speed revealed that patients in the early rehabilitation phase (dependent in walking; n = 1) significantly benefitted from electromechanical-assisted gait training with functional electrostimulation, while a nonsignificant effect was found for patients with chronic stroke (independent in walking; n = 1).

9. Speed dependent treadmill training (without body-weight support)

Speed dependent treadmill training without a harness to partially support the body-weight was investigated in 13 RCTs (N = 610, PEDro score range 4 [124,125] to 8 [126,127]) [92,124–136], including patients in the early rehabilitation phase [127,129,136]; late rehabilitation phase [130], or chronic phase [92,124–126,128,131,132,134,135].

Pooling the results of individual RCTs showed significant homogeneous positive SESs for maximum gait speed and step width. For comfortable gait speed, gait speed endurance, stride length, cadence, VO_2max, balance, and walking ability nonsignificant SESs were found. Subgroup analyses revealed no significant differences between poststroke phases.

10. Overground walking

Overground walking [137] was investigated in 19 RCTs (N = 1008, PEDro score range 2 [138] to 8 [89,103,139–143]) [86,87,89,103,109,112,119,122,123,125,138–150], including patients in the early rehabilitation phase [86,89,119,122,123], late rehabilitation phase [109,140,148,150], or chronic phase [112,125,138,139,142,144–147,149].

The meta-analyses resulted in a significant homogeneous positive SES for anxiety in independently walking patients and a significant homogeneous negative SES for aerobic capacity in patients unable to walk dependently. Nonsignificant SESs were found for comfortable gait speed, maximum gait speed, walking distance, stride length, stride time, cadence, gait pattern symmetry, peak heart rate (patients unable to walk dependently), diastolic blood pressure (independently walking patients), systolic blood pressure (independent walking patients), balance, number of falls (independently walking patients), depression (independently walking patients), walking ability, and basic and extended ADL. Subgroup analyses revealed a significant difference in effects between poststroke phases for walking distance, cadence, stride length, balance, and walking ability. As regards walking distance, a

significant homogeneous positive SES was found for independently walking patients in the chronic phase (n = 4) and a significant homogeneous negative SES for patients in the early rehabilitation phase who were unable to walk independently (n = 5). As regards cadence, a nonsignificant SES was found in the late rehabilitation phase (n = 2) and a significant negative effect size in the chronic phase (n = 1). As regards stride length, a nonsignificant effect size was found in the early rehabilitation phase, and a significant positive effect size was found in the late rehabilitation phase and chronic phase (all n = 1). As regards balance, a significant positive effect size was found in the late rehabilitation phase (n = 1) and a nonsignificant SES in the chronic phase (n = 4). As regards walking ability, a nonsignificant SES was found in the early rehabilitation phase (n = 6), a significant positive effect size in the late rehabilitation phase (n = 1), and a significant homogeneous positive SES in the chronic phase (n = 5).

11. Rhythmic gait cueing

Rhythmic auditory cueing to improve the gait pattern [8,151] was investigated in six RCTs (N = 231, PEDro score range 3 [151–153] to 7 [154]) [151–156], including patients in the early rehabilitation phase [151,153–155] or chronic phase [152,156].

Only the RCTs including patients in the early rehabilitation phase could be pooled. Nonsignificant SESs were found for gait speed, cadence, stride length, and gait pattern symmetry.

12. Community walking

Training of walking in a community environment like a shopping mall or park [157] was investigated in three RCTs (N = 94, PEDro score range 6 [157,158] to 8 [126]) [126,157,158], including patients in the early rehabilitation phase [157] or chronic phase [126,158].

Pooling the data from the individual RCTs resulted in nonsignificant SESs for maximum gait speed, walking distance, and balance confidence. Subgroup analyses revealed no significant differences between poststroke phases.

13. Virtual reality mobility training

Training of mobility in a virtual environment using computer technology which enables patients to interact with this environment and receive feedback about the performance of movements and activities [159,160] was investigated in six RCTs (N = 150, PEDro score range 5 [161,162] to 7 [163]) [161–167], including patients in the early rehabilitation phase.

The meta-analyses showed nonsignificant SESs for comfortable gait speed, maximum gait speed, step length, and walking ability.

14. Circuit class training

Supervised circuit class training focused on gait and mobility-related functions and activities, in which patients train in groups in various work stations [168,169], was investigated in eight RCTs (N = 359, PEDro score range 5 [146] to 8 [75,142,149,170,171]) [75,81,142,143,146,170–173], including patients in the early rehabilitation phase [170], late rehabilitation phase [75,171, 173], or chronic phase [81,142,146,172].

Pooling resulted in significant homogeneous positive SESs for walking distance, balance, walking ability, and physical activity. Nonsignificant SESs were found for muscle strength, gait speed, self-efficacy, depression, number of falls, basic and extended ADL, and quality of life. Subgroup analyses revealed no significant differences between poststroke phases.

15. Caregiver-mediated exercises

Training of gait and mobility-related functions and activities with a caregiver under the auspices of a physical therapist [174] was investigated in three RCTs (N = 350, PEDro score range 4 [144] to 8 [174,175]) [144,174,175], including patients in the early rehabilitation phase [174,175] or chronic phase [144].

The meta-analyses resulted in significant homogeneous positive SESs for basic ADL and caregiver strain. A nonsignificant SES was found for extended ADL. Subgroup analyses revealed no significant differences between poststroke phases.

16. Orthosis for walking

The use of a splint or orthosis (ankle foot orthosis [AFO] or knee ankle foot orthosis [KEVO]) for walking was investigated in four RCTs (N = 137, PEDro score range 2 [176] to 7 [177]) [85,176–178], which included patients in the early rehabilitation phase [85] or chronic phase [177,178]. The poststroke phase was unclear for one RCT [176].

After pooling, a nonsignificant SES for comfortable gait speed was found when comparing walking with an orthosis with walking without an orthosis. Subgroup analyses revealed no significant differences between poststroke phases.

17. Water-based exercises

Water-based exercises are defined as "a therapy programme using the properties of water, designed by a suitably qualified physical therapist, to improve function, ideally in a purpose-built and suitably heated hydrotherapy pool" [179]. These exercises were investigated in three RCTs (N = 65, PEDro score range 5 [180,181] to 6 [182]) [180–182], which all included patients in the chronic phase.

A significant homogeneous positive SES was found for muscle strength and a nonsignificant SES for balance.

18. Interventions for somatosensory functions of the paretic leg

Interventions designed to decrease or resolve impairments of the somatosensory functions of the paretic leg by e.g. electrostimulation or exposure to different stimuli such as texture, shape, temperature, or position [183,184] were investigated in six RCTs (N = 151, PEDro score range 5 [185] to 8 [186]) [60,185–189], including patients in the early rehabilitation phase [60,187,189], late rehabilitation phase [186,188], or chronic phase [185].

The meta-analyses resulted in nonsignificant SESs for motor function of the paretic leg (synergy), gait speed, and balance. Subgroup analyses revealed no significant differences between poststroke phases.

19. Electrostimulation of the paretic leg

Electrostimulation of peripheral nerves and muscles with external electrodes [190] can be applied during training of activities, but also when just functions, like ankle dorsiflexion, are trained in a non-functional manner. For the purpose of this review, electrostimulation was divided into (a) neuromuscular stimulation (NMS); (b) electromyography-triggered neuromuscular stimulation (EMG-NMS); and (c) transcutaneous electrical nerve stimulation (TENS). Electrostimulation of the paretic leg was investigated in 26 RCTs (N = 814, PEDro score range 2 [176] to 8 [186,191,192]) [113,118,176,186,191–213], including patients in the early rehabilitation phase [113,118,192,195,196,199–201,203,204,206,208, 212], late rehabilitation phase [186,193,197,209], or chronic phase [194,198,202,205,207,210,213]. The RCT investigating the

combination of EMG-NMS and NMS was not included in the meta-analyses [195]. The electrostimulation was not applied when outcomes were measured.

a. NMS

NMS of the paretic leg was investigated in 18 RCTs (N = 551) [113,118,176,191–194,196–198,201–204,206–208,213].

Pooling resulted in significant homogeneous positive SESs for motor function of the paretic leg (synergy), muscle strength, and muscle tone. Nonsignificant SESs were found for active range of motion, gait speed, cadence, step and stride length, gait symmetry, balance, walking ability, and basic ADL. Subgroup analyses revealed no significant differences between poststroke phases.

b. EMG-NMS

EMG-NMS of the paretic leg was investigated in two RCTs (N = 68) [199,209].

The meta-analyses resulted in nonsignificant SESs for muscle tone and basic ADL. Subgroup analyses revealed no significant differences between phases poststroke.

c. TENS

TENS of the paretic leg was investigated in five RCTs (N = 349) [186,200,205,210–212].

Meta-analyses showed significant homogeneous positive SESs for muscle strength and walking ability, while nonsignificant SESs were found for muscle tone, active range of motion, gait speed, and walking distance. Subgroup analyses revealed no significant differences between poststroke phases.

20. Electromyographic biofeedback for the paretic leg

Electromyographic biofeedback (EMG-BF) involves registering the muscle activity by surface electrodes that are applied to the skin covering the muscles of interest [214,215]. A biofeedback apparatus converts the recorded muscle activity (EMG) into visual or auditory information. EMG-BF for the paretic leg was investigated in 11 RCTs (N = 254, PEDro score range 2 [216] to 7 [217]) [152,194,216–224], including patients in the early rehabilitation phase [216,219,224] or chronic phase [152,194,217, 218,220,222,223].

Pooling resulted in nonsignificant SESs for range of motion, gait speed, step and stride length, and EMG activity. Subgroup analyses revealed no significant differences between poststroke phases.

Physical therapy interventions related to arm-hand activities. The results of the meta-analyses for interventions related to arm-hand activities are summarized in figure 3 (for details see table S2B in file S1). Pooling was not possible for immobilization of the paretic arm (i.e. "forced-use") [225,226], wrist robotics [227,228], wrist-hand robotics [229], continuous passive motion for the paretic shoulder [230], subsensory threshold electrical and vibration stimulation of the paretic arm [231], circuit class training [143,182], passive bilateral arm training [232], and using a mechanical arm trainer [233,234].

1. Therapeutic positioning of the paretic arm

Therapeutic positioning of the paretic arm, without the use of splints, with the purpose of maintaining range of motion and preventing harmful positions of the paretic arm [8] was investigated in five RCTs (N = 140, PEDro score range 6

Intervention	Comparisons (n) / Patients (N)	I^2 (%)	Hedges' g (95%CI)	Power
Outcome: arm-hand activities				
Therapeutic positioning arm	NA			
Reflex-inhibiting/immobilization	NA			
Air-splints	3 / 180	0		0.050
Techniques and devices GHS/HSP	NA			
Bilateral arm training	10 / 417	40		0.061
Original CIMT	1 / 222	0		0.927
High-intensity mCIMT	16 / 348	11		0.676
Low-intensity mCIMT	16 / 337	41		0.997
Robotics—unilateral shoulder-elbow	10 / 261	0		0.335
Robotics—bilateral elbow-wrist	NA			
Robotics—shoulder-elbow-wrist-hand	NA			
Mental practice with motor imagery	15 / 246	63		0.954
Mirror therapy	4 / 104	82		0.252
Virtual reality training	6 / 89	0		0.098
NMS wrist/finger extensors	3 / 82	79		0.090
NMS wrist/finger flexors/extensors	2 / 41	13		0.341
NMS shoulder	NA			
EMG-NMS wrist/finger extensors	14 / 162	49		0.971
EGM-NMS wrist/finger flexors/extensors	2 / 31	22		0.284
TENS	NA			
EMG-BF	5 / 102	0		0.149
Trunk restraint	3 / 58	0		0.056
Interventions somatosensory functions	12 / 266	0		0.308
Outcome: motor function arm				
Therapeutic positioning arm	NA			
Reflex-inhibiting/immobilization	NA			
Air-splints	5 / 205	68		0.056
Techniques and devices GHS/HSP	4 / 140	20		0.162
Bilateral arm training	9 / 274	80		0.281
Original CIMT	NA			
High-intensity mCIMT	4 / 50	67		0.097
Low-intensity mCIMT	15 / 333	39		0.887
Robotics—unilateral shoulder-elbow	17 / 327	0		0.343
Robotics—bilateral elbow-wrist	4 / 62	0		0.841
Robotics—shoulder-elbow-wrist-hand	2 / 36	75		0.053
Mental practice with motor imagery	11 / 149	29		0.154
Mirror therapy	3 / 112	52		0.434
Virtual reality training	8 / 158	0		0.183
NMS wrist/finger extensors	2 / 49	84		0.053
NMS wrist/finger flexors/extensors	2 / 41	0		0.657
NMS shoulder	2 / 32	33		0.219
EGM-NMS wrist/finger extensors	3 / 49	0		0.398
EMG-NMS wrist/finger flexors/extensors	2 / 31	0		0.315
TENS	NA			
EMG-BF	2 / 69	0		0.282
Trunk restraint	NA			
Interventions somatosensory functions	4 / 170	51		0.716

-1   0   1   2

Favors control   Favors treatment

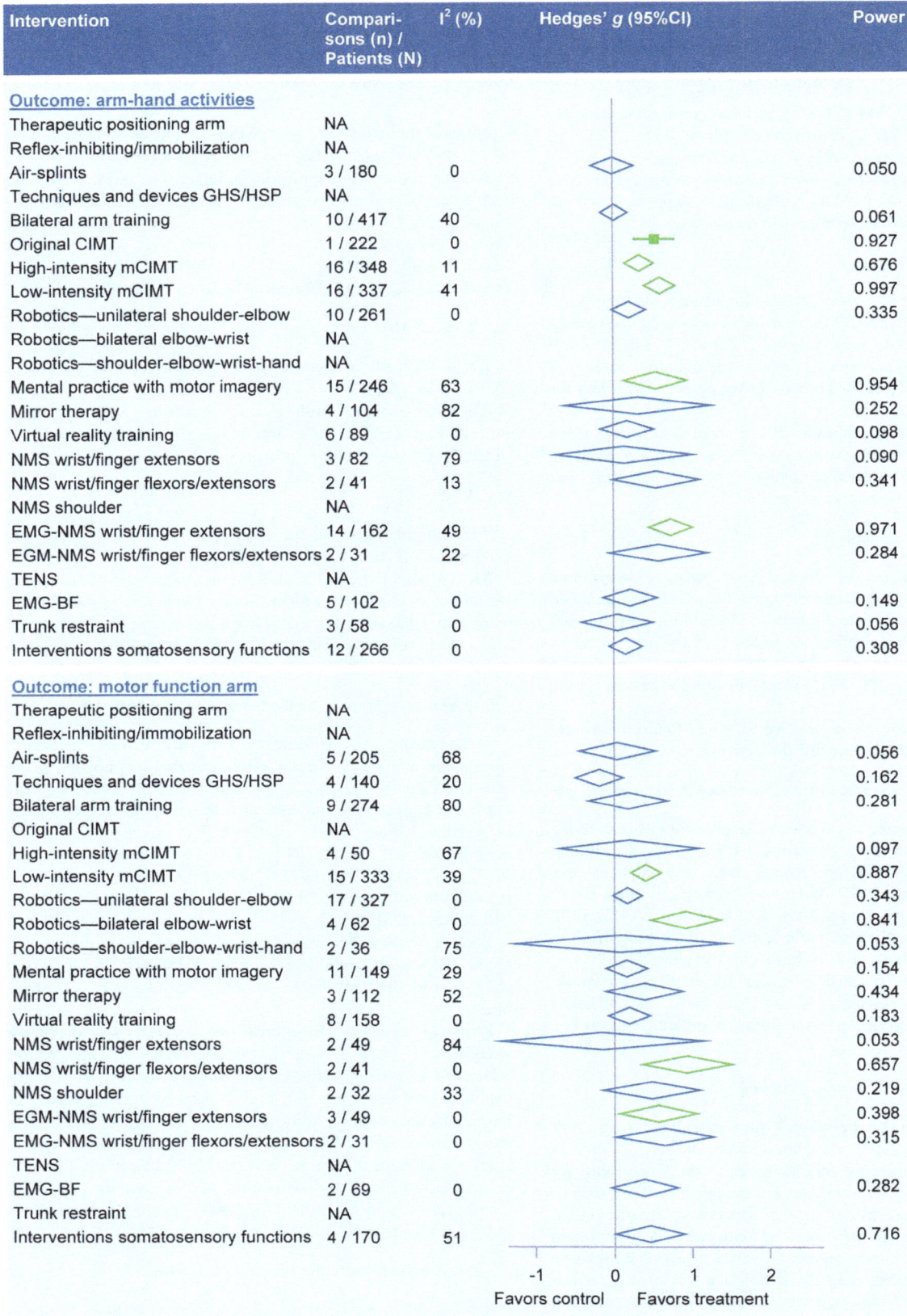

Figure 3. Summary effect sizes for physical therapy interventions – arm-hand activities. Legend: A green colored diamond indicates that the summary effect size is significant, while a blue colored diamond indicates that the summary effect size is nonsignificant; CI, Confidence Interval;

CIMT, Constraint-induced movement therapy; EMG-BF, Electromyographic biofeedback; EMG-NMS, Electromyography-triggered neuromuscular stimulation; GHS, Glenohumeral subluxation; HSP, Hemiplegic shoulder pain; mCIMT, modified Constraint-induced movement therapy; NA, Not applicable; NMS, Neuromuscular stimulation; TENS, Transcutaneous electrical nerve stimulation.

[235,236] to 7 [237–239]) [235–239], which all included patients in the early rehabilitation phase.

A significant homogeneous positive SES was found for passive range of motion of shoulder external rotation. Nonsignificant SESs were found for passive range of motion of shoulder internal rotation, external rotation contracture of the shoulder, pain at rest and while moving, and basic ADL.

2. Reflex-inhibiting positions and immobilization techniques for the paretic wrist and hand

The use of reflex-inhibiting positions or local immobilization of the wrist and hand by splints or plaster to (1) prevent or decrease an increased muscle tone or (2) to maintain or increase the range of motion of wrist and/or finger extension [8] were investigated in eight RCTs (N = 197, PEDro score range 3 [240] to 8 [241,242]) [240–247], including patients in the early rehabilitation phase [241,242], late rehabilitation phase [240], or chronic phase [243–247].

Meta-analyses resulted in nonsignificant SESs for passive range of motion, muscle tone, and pain. Subgroup analyses revealed no significant differences between poststroke phases.

3. Air-splints around the paretic arm

Air-splints give external pressure around the paretic limb and are primarily used to reduce an increased muscle tone [248,249] and/or hand edema. Five RCTs investigated the effect of air-splints (N = 285, PEDro score range 4 [250,251] to 8 [252]) [250–255], including patients in the early rehabilitation phase [250,252,254] or late rehabilitation phase [255]. The poststroke phase was unclear in one RCT [253].

Pooling resulted in nonsignificant SESs for motor function of the paretic arm (synergy), muscle tone, somatosensory functions, pain, and arm-hand activities. However, subgroup analyses revealed a significant homogeneous negative SES for muscle tone for patients in the early rehabilitation phase (n = 1, with 2 comparisons) and a significant homogeneous positive effect size for patients in the late rehabilitation phase (n = 1).

4. Supportive techniques or devices for the prevention or treatment of glenohumeral subluxation and/or hemiplegic shoulder pain

Supportive techniques – like strapping – or devices – like a sling or arm orthosis – for the prevention or treatment of glenohumeral subluxation and/or hemiplegic shoulder pain [256] were investigated in three RCTs (N = 142, PEDro score range from 4 [257] to 7 [258,259]) [257–259], including patients in the early rehabilitation phase.

In the meta-analyses, nonsignificant SESs were found for motor function of the paretic arm and for pain.

5. Bilateral arm training

During bilateral arm training, movement patterns or activities are performed with both hands simultaneously but independent from each other and could be cyclic [8,260]. This type of training was investigated in 22 RCTs (N = 823, PEDro score range 2 [261,262] to 8 [263]) [261–282], including patients in the early rehabilitation phase [263,265,272], late rehabilitation phase [273],

or chronic phase [261,262,264,265,267–271,274–282]. The poststroke phase was unknown for one RCT [266].

The meta-analyses yielded nonsignificant SESs for motor function of the paretic arm (synergy), muscle strength, arm-hand activities, self-reported arm-hand use in daily life, and basic ADL. Subgroup analyses revealed no significant differences between poststroke phases.

6. Original or modified Constraint-induced movement therapy

Original or modified Constraint-Induced Movement Therapy (CIMT or mCIMT respectively) consists of immobilization of the non-paretic arm and is combined with repetitive task-specific training of the paretic arm, including shaping techniques [8].

(m)CIMT was investigated in 41 RCTs (N = 1342, PEDro score range 2 [261,262,283–285] to 8 [286]) [225,226,261,262,264, 270,278,282–318], including patients in the early rehabilitation phase [225,226,288,293,295,299,305,309,310,312,318], late rehabilitation phase [284,289,297], or chronic phase [261,262,264, 270,278,282,283,285–287,290–292,294,296,300–304,307,308,313–317].

Different categories can be distinguished, depending on the duration of the immobilization of the paretic arm and the intensity of task-specific practice: (a) original CIMT, (b) high-intensity mCIMT, (c) low-intensity mCIMT, and (d) immobilization of the non-paretic arm (i.e. "forced-use").

a. Original CIMT

Original CIMT is applied for 2 to 3 weeks and consists of (1) immobilization of the non-paretic arm with a padded mitt for 90% of the waking hours; (2) task-oriented training with a high number of repetitions for 6 hours a day; and (3) behavioral strategies to improve both compliance and transfer of the activities practiced from the clinical setting to the patient's home environment. Original CIMT was investigated in one RCT (N = 222) [297,298], which included patients in the late rehabilitation phase.

Significant positive effect sizes were found for arm-hand activities, self-reported amount of arm-hand use in daily life, and self-reported quality of arm-hand movement in daily life. Due to the size of the study sample and the low risk of bias, this result is classified as level 1 evidence.

b. High-intensity mCIMT

High-intensity mCIMT consists of (1) immobilization of the non-paretic arm with a padded mitt during 90% of the waking hours and (2) between 3 and 6 hours of task-oriented training a day. High-intensity mCIMT was investigated in 17 RCTs (N = 512) [261,270,285–287,290,291,295,296,299,304,305,308, 310–312,314,318], including patients in the early rehabilitation phase [295,299,305,310,312,318] or chronic phase [261,270,285–287,290,291,296,304,308,314].

Pooling resulted in significant homogeneous positive SESs for arm-hand activities and self-reported quality of arm-hand movement in daily life. In addition, a significant heterogeneous positive SES was found for self-reported amount of the arm-hand use in daily life. Nonsignificant SESs were found for motor function of the paretic arm (synergy) and basic ADL. Subgroup analyses revealed a significant difference between poststroke phases for basic ADL. A significant positive effect size was found for the early rehabilitation phase (n = 1) and a nonsignificant effect size for the chronic phase (n = 1).

c. Low-intensity mCIMT

Low-intensity mCIMT consists of (1) immobilization of the non-paretic arm with a padded mitt during >0% to <90% of the waking hours and (2) between 0 and 3 hours of task-oriented training a day. Low-intensity mCIMT was investigated in 23 RCTs (N = 627) [262,264,278,280,282–284,288,289,292–294,300–303,307,309–313,315,317], including patients in the early rehabilitation phase [288,293,309,312], late rehabilitation phase [284,289], or chronic phase [262,264,278,282,283,292,294,300–303,307,313,315–317].

The meta-analyses yielded significant homogeneous positive SESs for motor function of the paretic arm (synergy), arm-hand activities, self-reported amount of arm-hand use in daily life, self-reported quality of arm-hand movement in daily life, and basic ADL. A nonsignificant SES was found for arm-related quality of life. Subgroup analyses for motor function of the paretic arm (synergy) showed that the positive effects were significant for the early rehabilitation phase (n = 1) and chronic phase (n = 12), but not for the late rehabilitation phase (n = 2).

7. Robot-assisted arm training

Robotic devices allow repetitive, interactive, high intensity training of the paretic arm and/or hand [8,319]. Training with robotic devices was investigated in 22 RCTs (N = 648, PEDro score range 4 [227,320–322] to 8 [323]) [227–229,273,320–338], including patients in the early rehabilitation phase [321,322,324, 325,329,331,332,336,337], late rehabilitation phase [273], or chronic phase [227–229,320,323,326–328,330,333–335,338].

For the purpose of this review, robotic devices are classified on the basis of the joints they target: (a) shoulder-elbow robots; (b) elbow-wrist robots; and (c) shoulder-elbow-wrist-hand robots.

a. Shoulder-elbow robotics

Shoulder-elbow robots used in a unilateral mode were applied in 15 RCTs (N = 546) [273,322,324,326–328,330–338].

Pooling resulted in significant homogeneous positive SESs for motor function of the proximal part of the paretic arm (synergy), muscle strength, and pain. Nonsignificant SESs were found for motor function of the paretic arm, motor function of the distal part of the paretic arm, muscle tone, arm-hand activities, basic ADL, and quality of life. Subgroup analyses revealed no significant differences between poststroke phases.

b. Elbow-wrist robotics

Elbow-wrist robots used in a bilateral mode were investigated in two RCTs (N = 62) [323,329].

Meta-analyses showed significant homogeneous positive SESs for motor function of the paretic arm (synergy) and muscle strength. Subgroup analyses revealed no significant differences between phases poststroke.

c. Shoulder-elbow-wrist-hand robotics

Shoulder-elbow-wrist-hand robots were investigated in two RCTs (N = 39) [320,321].

Pooling the data resulted in nonsignificant SESs for both motor function of the paretic arm (synergy) and muscle strength of the distal part of the arm. Subgroup analyses revealed no significant differences between poststroke phases.

8. Mental practice with motor imagery

Mental practice of motor actions and/or activities for the purpose of improving their performance [8,339] combined with physical practice, was investigated in 14 RCTs (N = 424, PEDro score range 4 [340,341] to 7 [342–345]) [340–352], including patients in the early rehabilitation phase [340–342,344,345,351] or chronic phase [346–350,352,353].

The meta-analyses showed a significant heterogeneous positive SES for arm-hand activities and nonsignificant SESs for motor function of the paretic arm (synergy), muscle strength, and basic ADL. Subgroup analyses revealed no significant differences between poststroke phases.

9. Mirror therapy for the paretic arm

During mirror therapy, the patient looks in a mirror placed perpendicular to the body. Looking in the mirror creates the suggestion that the patient is observing movements of the affected arm. Mirror therapy was investigated in seven RCTs (N = 255, PEDro score range 5 [349,354] to 8 [355]) [349,354–359], including patients in the early rehabilitation phase [359], late rehabilitation phase [357,358], or chronic phase [349,354–356].

Pooling resulted in nonsignificant SESs for motor function of the paretic arm (synergy), muscle tone, pain, and arm-hand activities. Subgroup analyses revealed a significant positive effect size for arm-hand activities in the late rehabilitation phase (n = 1) and a nonsignificant SES in the chronic phase (n = 2).

10. Virtual reality training for the paretic arm

Training of the arm and hand in a virtual environment using computer technology which enables patients to interact with this environment and receive feedback about the performance of movements and activities [159,360] was investigated in 15 RCTs (N = 357, PEDro score range 3 [361–365] to 8 [366]) [360–375], including patients in the early rehabilitation phase [360,363,364, 373,375], late rehabilitation phase [369,370], or chronic phase [361,362,365–368,371,372,374].

Pooling resulted in a significant homogeneous positive SES for basic ADL and a significant homogeneous negative SES for muscle tone. Nonsignificant SESs were found for motor function of the paretic arm (synergy) and arm-hand activities. Subgroup analyses revealed no significant differences between poststroke phases.

11. Electrostimulation of the paretic arm

Electrostimulation of peripheral nerves and muscles with external electrodes [190] can be applied during training of activities, but also when just functions, like wrist extension, are trained in a non-functional manner. For the purpose of the present review, electrostimulation was divided into (a) neuromuscular stimulation (NMS); (b) electromyography-triggered neuromuscular stimulation (EMG-NMS); and (c) transcutaneous electrical nerve stimulation (TENS). Electrostimulation of the paretic arm was investigated in 49 RCTs (N = 1521, PEDro score range 3 [376–379] to 8 [380]) [200,267,271,321,328,376–423], including patients in the early rehabilitation phase [200,321,376,380,381,383,384,386,387,389–392,395,402,404,405,407,413,415–417,419,420,422], late rehabilitation phase [382,398–400,406,418], or chronic phase [267,271,328,377–379,393,394,396,397,401,403,408–412,414,421,423].

The electrostimulation was not applied when outcomes were measured.

a. NMS

NMS of the paretic arm was investigated in 22 RCTs (N = 894) [376,380,381,383–386,389–392,396,398,400,402,404,406,407,410, 417–421].

a1. Wrist and finger extensors

Meta-analyses showed nonsignificant SESs for motor function of the paretic arm (synergy), active range of motion, muscle strength, and arm-hand activities. Subgroup analyses revealed no significant differences between poststroke phases.

a2. Wrist and finger flexors and extensors

The meta-analyses yielded significant homogeneous positive SESs for motor function of the paretic arm (synergy) and muscle strength, while the SES for arm-hand activities was nonsignificant.

a3. Shoulder muscles

Pooling resulted in a significant heterogeneous positive SES for shoulder subluxation, while nonsignificant SESs were found for motor function of the paretic arm (synergy), range of motion, and pain. Subgroup analyses revealed no significant differences between poststroke phases.

b. EMG-NMS

EMG-NMS of the paretic arm was investigated in 25 RCTs (N = 492) [267,271,321,328,378,379,387,393–395,397,399,401, 403–405,408–414,416,422,423].

b1. Wrist and finger extensors

The meta-analyses resulted in significant homogeneous positive SESs for motor function of the paretic arm (synergy) and arm-hand activities. A significant heterogeneous positive SES was found for active range of motion. The SESs for muscle strength and muscle tone were nonsignificant. Subgroup analyses revealed no significant differences between poststroke phases.

b2. Wrist and finger flexors and extensors

Pooling showed nonsignificant SESs for motor function of the paretic arm (synergy) and arm-hand activities. Subgroup analyses revealed no significant differences between poststroke phases.

c. TENS

TENS of the paretic arm was investigated in four RCTs (N = 484) [200,377,382,388,415].
Pooling resulted in nonsignificant SESs for both muscle tone and basic ADL. Subgroup analyses revealed no significant differences between poststroke phases.

12. Electromyographic biofeedback of the paretic arm

Electromyographic biofeedback (EMG-BF) involves the muscle activity being registered by surface electrodes which are applied to the skin covering the muscles of interest [214,215]. A biofeedback apparatus converts the recorded muscle activity (EMG) into visual or auditory information. EMG-BF for the paretic arm was investigated in 11 RCTs (N = 317, PEDro score range 2 [424] to 7 [425,426]) [219,424–433], including patients in the early

rehabilitation phase [219,425,430], late rehabilitation phase [426,429,432,433], or chronic phase [427,428,431]. The phase poststroke was unclear for one RCT [424].
Meta-analyses resulted in nonsignificant SESs for motor function of the paretic arm (synergy), active range of motion, and arm-hand activities. Subgroup analyses revealed no significant differences between poststroke phases.

13. Trunk restraint

Fixing the trunk externally during reaching and grasping prevents compensatory movements of the trunk [434]. Trunk restraint was investigated in four RCTs (N = 86, PEDro score range 4 [435] to 8 [436]) [314,434–436], which all included patients in the chronic phase.
The meta-analyses showed a significant homogeneous negative SES for self-reported amount of arm-hand use in daily life. A nonsignificant SES was found for active range of motion and arm-hand activities.

14. Interventions for somatosensory functions of the paretic arm

Interventions designed to decrease or resolve impairments in somatosensory functions of the paretic arm by e.g. electrostimulation or exposure to different stimuli like texture, shape, temperature or position [183,184] were investigated in 12 RCTs (N = 580, PEDro score range 3 [377,388] to 9 [437]) [188, 250,251,255,377,388,398,437–443], including patients in the early rehabilitation phase [250,440,443], late rehabilitation phase [188,255,398,437], or chronic phase [377,438,439,441,442].
Meta-analyses showed significant homogeneous positive SESs for somatosensory functions and muscle tone. The analyses resulted in nonsignificant SESs for motor function of the paretic arm (synergy), muscle strength, pain, arm-hand activities, and basic ADL. Subgroup analyses revealed no significant differences between poststroke phases.

Physical therapy interventions for physical fitness. Planned and structured physical exercises aiming to improve physical fitness can be divided into programs primarily targeting (1) strength of the paretic leg; (2) strength of the paretic arm; (3) aerobic capacity; and (4) a combination of strength and aerobic capacity [8,444,445]. The results of the meta-analyses are summarized in figure 4 (for details see table S2C in file S1).

1. Strength exercises for the paretic leg

Progressive active exercises against resistance for the paretic leg were investigated in 19 RCTs (N = 786, PEDro score range 2 [446] to 8 [172,447]) [172,446–464], including patients in the early rehabilitation phase [448,452,456,457,461,463,464], late rehabilitation phase [449], or chronic phase [172,446,447, 450,451,453–455,458,460,462].
Pooling resulted in significant homogeneous positive SESs for muscle strength, muscle tone, and spatiotemporal gait pattern parameters like cadence, stride length, and symmetry. Nonsignificant SESs were found for motor function of the paretic leg (synergy), comfortable gait speed, maximum gait speed, walking distance, aerobic capacity, heart rate work, workload, physical cost index, walking ability, basic ADL, and quality of life. Subgroup analyses revealed no significant differences between poststroke phases.

2. Strength exercises for the paretic arm

Progressive active exercises against resistance for the paretic arm were investigated in nine RCTs (N = 327, PEDro score range

Intervention	Comparisons (n) / Patients (N)	I^2 (%)	Hedges' g (95%CI)	Power
Outcome: muscle strength (leg)				
Strength exercises paretic leg	12 / 328	31		0.788
Cardiorespiratory exercises	5 / 106	43		0.200
Mixed strength/cardiorespiratory exercises	8 / 313	29		0.810
Outcome: muscle strength (arm)				
Strength exercises paretic arm	4 / 88	0		0.061
Cardiorespiratory exercises	NA			
Mixed strength/cardiorespiratory exercises	4 / 156	0		0.149
Outcome: aerobic capacity				
Strength exercises paretic leg	3 / 48	0		0.099
Strength exercises paretic arm	NA			
Cardiorespiratory exercises	10 / 313	0		0.775
Mixed strength/cardiorespiratory exercises	7 / 256	20		0.863
Outcome: comfortable gait speed				
Strength exercises paretic leg	13 / 390	27		0.116
Strength exercises paretic arm	NA			
Cardiorespiratory exercises	10 / 321	0		0.388
Mixed strength/cardiorespiratory exercises	10 / 344	0		0.701
Outcome: walking ability				
Strength exercises paretic leg	8 / 373	0		0.169
Strength exercises paretic arm	NA			
Cardiorespiratory exercises	6 / 228	0		0.150
Mixed strength/cardiorespiratory exercises	5 / 190	0		0.226
Outcome: arm-hand activities				
Strength exercises paretic leg	NA			
Strength exercises paretic arm	6 / 88	0		0.103
Cardiorespiratory exercises	NA			
Mixed strength/cardiorespiratory exercises	2 / 29	0		0.119

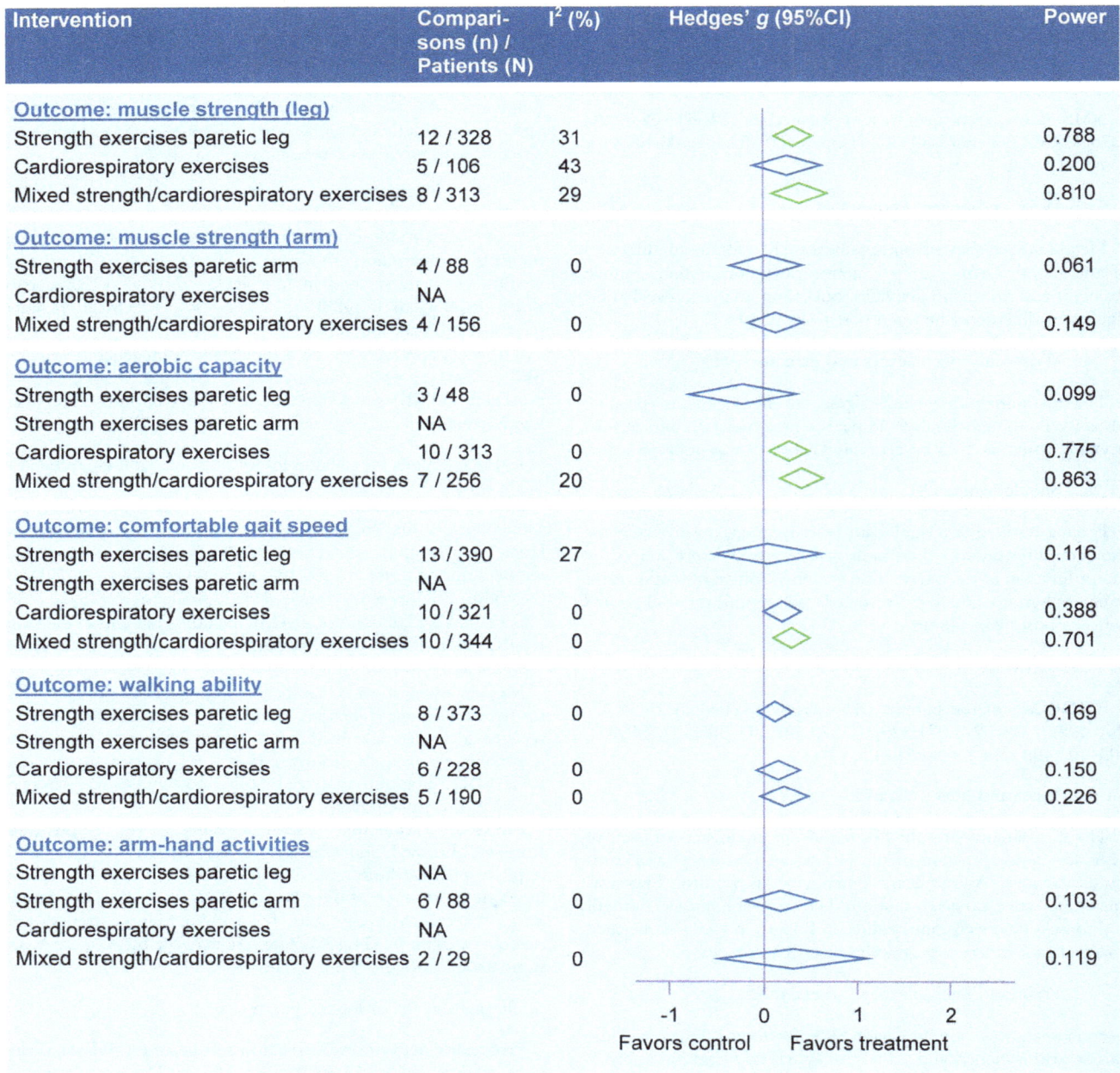

Figure 4. Summary effect sizes for physical therapy interventions – physical fitness. Legend: A green colored diamond indicates that the summary effect size is significant, while a blue colored diamond indicates that the summary effect size is nonsignificant; CI, Confidence interval; NA, Not applicable.

2 [465] to 7 [99,466]) [99,446,451,462,465–469], including patients in the early rehabilitation phase [465,466,468] or chronic phase [99,446,451,462,467,469].

Pooling the data resulted in nonsignificant SESs for motor function of the paretic arm (synergy), muscle strength, range of motion, and pain. Subgroup analyses revealed no significant differences between poststroke phases.

3. Cardiorespiratory exercises

Interventions focusing on maintenance or improvement of the aerobic capacity by training large muscle groups, for example

while walking overground or on a treadmill, or cycling on an ergometer, were investigated in 13 RCTs (N = 531, PEDro score range 4 [470,471] to 8 [88,127,447,459]) [88,104,124,127,132–135,182,447,459,470–477], including patients in the early rehabilitation phase [88,127,472,477] or chronic phase [104,132,182,447,470,471,474–476].

Pooling resulted in significant homogeneous positive SESs for aerobic capacity and workload, and significant heterogeneous positive SESs for respiratory functions such as forced expiratory volume in 1 second (FEV_1). Nonsignificant SESs were found for motor function of the paretic leg (synergy), muscle strength, comfortable gait speed, maximum gait speed, heart rate at rest and during work, diastolic and systolic blood pressure, physical cost index, body composition, blood variables, sitting and standing balance, and walking ability. Subgroup analyses showed significant differences between poststroke phases for resting heart rate: a significant SES was found for the early rehabilitation phase (n = 2) and a nonsignificant SES for the chronic phase (n = 2).

4. Mixed strength and cardiorespiratory exercises

Training regimes which combined both strength and cardiorespiratory exercises were investigated in 13 RCTs (N = 608, PEDro score range 3 [478] to 8 [140,447,479]) [140,142,143,146, 171,447,459,478–487], including patients in the early rehabilitation phase [479–481,486,487], late rehabilitation phase [140,171], or chronic phase [142,146,447,478,482,485].

Significant homogeneous positive SESs were found for motor function of the paretic leg (synergy), muscle strength of the leg, comfortable gait speed, maximum gait speed, walking distance, aerobic capacity, heart rate during work, balance, physical activity, and quality of life. Nonsignificant SESs were found for motor function of the paretic arm (synergy), muscle strength of the arm, physical cost index, depression, walking ability, arm-hand activities, and basic and extended ADL. Subgroup analyses revealed no significant differences between poststroke phases.

Physical therapy interventions related to activities of daily living. The results of the meta-analyses for interventions related to activities of daily living are summarized in figure 5 (for details see table S2D in file S1). Pooling was not possible for strategy training for apraxia [488].

1. Interventions for apraxia: gestural training

Gestural training has been developed for patients with apraxia to teach them to regain tasks and handling of objects by using gestures [489]. This training method was investigated in two RCTs (N = 46) [489,490], including patients in the chronic phase.

Pooling showed a significant homogeneous positive SES for gesture comprehension. Nonsignificant SESs were found for ideational and ideomotor apraxia.

2. Leisure therapy

Leisure therapy focuses on the execution of individual and social activities at home or in the home environment [491,492]. This therapy was investigated in five RCTs (N = 641) [491–496], including patients who were to be discharged home or were already living at home in the early rehabilitation phase [492,495], late rehabilitation phase [494], or chronic phase [491,496].

The meta-analyses resulted in a significant heterogeneous positive SES for participation in leisure activities, while nonsignificant SESs were found for depression, mood, and quality of life. Subgroup analyses revealed significant differences between groups for participation in leisure activities: there was a significant homogeneous positive SES for the early rehabilitation phase (n = 1, with 2 comparisons), a nonsignificant SES size for the late rehabilitation phase (n = 1, with 2 comparisons), and a nonsignificant effect size for the chronic phase (n = 1).

Other physical therapy interventions. The results of the meta-analyses for other physical therapy interventions are summarized in figure 6 (for details see table S2E in file S1).

1. Inspiratory muscle training

Inspiratory muscle training was investigated in two RCTs (N = 66, PEDro score range 4 [497] to 7 [498]) [497,498], including patients in the late rehabilitation phase [498] or chronic phase [497].

Pooling was possible for maximal inspiratory pressure, which resulted in a nonsignificant SES. Subgroup analyses revealed a difference between poststroke phases. A significant positive effect size was found in the chronic phase (n = 1) and a nonsignificant SES in the late rehabilitation phase (n = 1, with 2 comparisons).

Intensity of practice. The analyses of high-intensity exercise therapy involved pooled data of the RCTs reporting on a treatment contrast between the experimental and control groups in terms of time spent in exercise therapy without the use of extensive equipment [19,20]. The results of the meta-analyses for high-intensity exercise therapy are summarized in figure 7 (for details see table S2F in file S1).

High-intensity exercise therapy. In total, 80 RCTs were identified which used a treatment contrast in terms of time (N = 5776, PEDro score range 2 [465] to 8 [43,44,75,127, 139,171,172,174,175,443,479,499–509]) [43,44,51,53–55,60,61, 74,75,80,83,84,119,127,139,144,145,147–149,152,156,158,171,

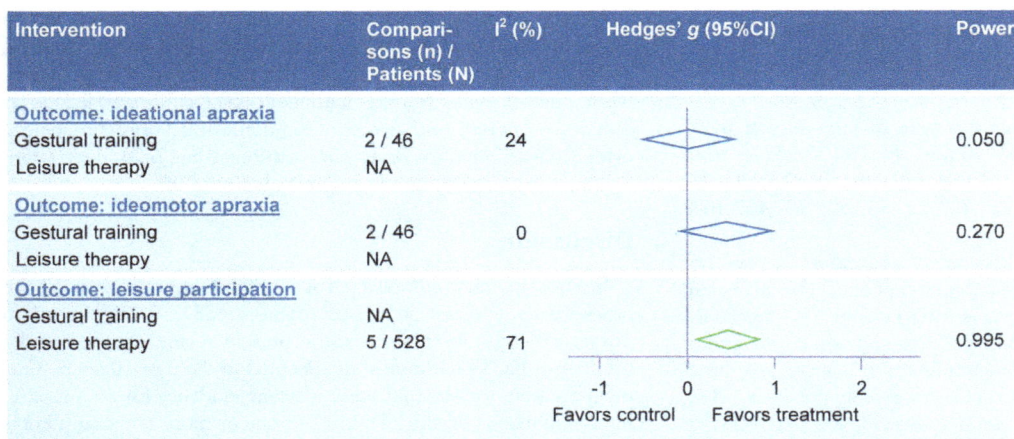

Intervention	Comparisons (n) / Patients (N)	I² (%)	Hedges' g (95%CI)	Power
Outcome: ideational apraxia				
Gestural training	2 / 46	24		0.050
Leisure therapy	NA			
Outcome: ideomotor apraxia				
Gestural training	2 / 46	0		0.270
Leisure therapy	NA			
Outcome: leisure participation				
Gestural training	NA			
Leisure therapy	5 / 528	71		0.995

-1 0 1 2
Favors control   Favors treatment

Figure 5. Summary effect sizes for physical therapy interventions – activities of daily living. Legend: A green colored diamond indicates that the summary effect size is significant, while a blue colored diamond indicates that the summary effect size is nonsignificant; CI, Confidence interval; NA, Not applicable.

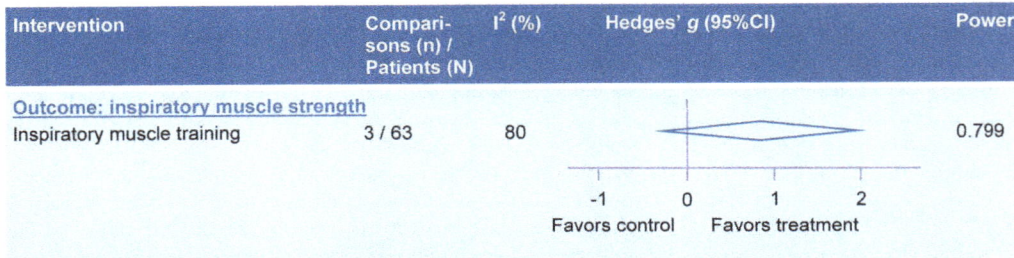

Figure 6. Summary effect sizes for physical therapy interventions – other: inspiratory muscle training. Legend: C, Control group; CI, Confidence interval; E, Experimental group.

172,174,175,178,180,189,250,307,439,440,443,458,463–466,468, 471–474,477–482,486,494,499–526], including patients in the hyper acute or acute rehabilitation phase, early rehabilitation phase, late rehabilitation phase, or chronic phase. In most of the RCTs, the interventions focused on the lower limb (n = 78). The mean treatment contrast amounted 17 hours over 10 weeks, indicating that on average the experimental groups received an additional therapy time of 17 hours when compared to the control groups.

Pooling the data resulted in significant homogeneous positive SESs for motor function of the paretic leg (synergy), motor function of the paretic arm (synergy), muscle strength of the leg, comfortable gait speed, maximum gait speed, muscle tone, and quality of life. Significant heterogeneous SESs were found for depression and anxiety, balance, and basic ADL. Meta-analyses for muscle strength of the arm, mental health of the patient, falls efficacy, walking ability, arm-hand activities, extended ADL, number of falls, and mental health of the caregiver resulted in nonsignificant SESs. The subgroup analysis for walking distance showed significantly different effects between phases, with a significant homogeneous positive SES for the chronic phase (n = 4), a nonsignificant SES for the early rehabilitation phase (n = 5), and a nonsignificant effect size for a group including patients regardless of timing poststroke (n = 1).

Neurological treatment approaches. Neurodevelopmental Treatment (NDT/Bobath) was delivered in 75 RCTs (N = 3502). For the purpose of the present review, the effects of NDT were analyzed in three different categories: (a) NDT vs. another intervention; (b) NDT vs. NDT plus another intervention; and (c) NDT vs. augmented NDT (for details see table S1G in file S1).

1. NDT vs. another intervention

NDT was compared with another type of intervention in 37 RCTs (N = 1670, PEDro score range 4 [108,276,527] to 8 [323,366,505]) [50,82,108,118,154,264,269,270,272,273,276,278, 280–282,301–303,305,313,315,316,323,326,333,366,432,457,468, 505,527–534].

Strong evidence for *equal effectiveness* compared to another intervention was found for muscle strength of the arm and depression. In addition, there was strong evidence for *unfavorable effects* of NDT on motor function (synergy), gait speed, spatiotemporal gait pattern functions, kinematics of the arm, arm-hand activities, self-reported arm-hand activities in daily life, basic ADL, and quality of life. There was moderate evidence that NDT is *equally effective* as another intervention regarding strength of the knee muscles, maximal weight bearing on the paretic leg, coordination, stability of the shoulder joint, shoulder pain, health beliefs, walking distance, and balance. Moderate evidence was found for an *unfavorable effect* of NDT on length of stay. Insufficient

evidence was found for muscle strength of the leg, grip strength, muscle tone, brain activity, walking ability, and extended ADL.

2. NDT vs. NDT plus another intervention

NDT was compared with NDT plus another intervention in 33 RCTs (N = 1106, PEDro score range 2 [138] to 8 [88,186,191]) [49,51,59,64,66,80,88,96,123,129,138,148,151,158,186,191,199, 203,217,246,331,357,390,395,399,400,413,419,433,524,535,536].

There was strong evidence that NDT alone has *unfavorable effects* compared to NDT plus another intervention as regards motor function (synergy), muscle strength of the arm, walking speed, spatiotemporal gait pattern functions like stride length, muscle tone, range of motion, balance, walking ability, arm-hand activities, and basic ADL. Strong evidence was found that they are *equally effective* for gait kinematics. Moderate evidence was found for *unfavorable effect* of NDT when compared to NDT plus another intervention on muscle strength of the leg, walking distance, coordination, EMG contraction, shoulder subluxation, neglect, and aerobic capacity. Moderate evidence was found for *equal effectiveness* regarding symmetry while sitting, standing, performing sit-to-stand and reaching; depression; and ability to change posture from sit to stand and vice versa.

3. NDT vs. augmented NDT

The effect of more time spent in NDT versus less time spent in NDT was investigated in 6 RCTs (N = 786, PEDro score range 6 [513,517] to 8 [503–505]) [503–505,513,517,519].

There was strong evidence that NDT is *equally effective* as augmented NDT for the outcomes muscle strength, walking ability, arm-hand activities, basic ADL, and extended ADL. There was moderate evidence that augmented NDT is *beneficial* for motor function (synergy) and range of motion. In addition, moderate evidence was found for *equal effectiveness* regarding pain, depression, balance, sit-to-stand, handicap, and quality of life.

Discussion

Interdisciplinary complex stroke rehabilitation is one of the fastest growing fields in stroke research [537]. With regard to physical therapy interventions, the present review shows that the number of RCTs has almost quadrupled in the past 10 years. Our meta-analyses suggest that there is strong evidence for 30 out of 53 interventions for beneficial effects on one or more outcomes. For a large proportion of the outcomes there is strong evidence that experimental interventions accomplish equal results when compared to 'conventional therapy', suggesting that the same results can be obtained with the control intervention, while no adverse events were reported. The generally small to medium SESs,

Study	Patients (N) Total (E / C)	Hedges' g (95%CI)	Random effects model

Outcome: basic ADL

Study	Patients (N) Total (E / C)	Hedges' g (95%CI)	
Smith 1981 (1)	68 (46 / 22)	-0.001 (-0.504, 0.501)	
Smith 1981 (2)	65 (43 / 22)	0.043 (-0.465, 0.551)	
Sivenius 1985	77 (42 / 35)	1.851 (1.320, 2.383)	
Young 1991	107 (57 / 50)	0.277 (-0.102, 0.656)	
Wade 1992	89 (48 / 41)	-0.158 (-0.571, 0.256)	
Sunderland 1992	64 (34 / 30)	0.164 (-0.322, 0.650)	
Sunderland 1992	57 (27 / 30)	0.072 (-0.441, 0.585)	
Werner 1996	40 (28 / 12)	0.634 (-0.043, 1.311)	
Feys 1998	100 (50 / 50)	0.183 (-0.207, 0.572)	
Baskett 1999	110 (46 / 44)	0.212 (-0.199, 0.623)	
Lincoln 1999 (1)	152 (94 / 48)	-0.154 (-0.500, 0.192)	
Lincoln 1999 (2)	140 (93 / 47)	-0.134 (-0.483, 0.215)	
Kwakkel 1999 (1)	50 (31 / 19)	0.627 (0.051, 1.202)	
Kwakkel 1999 (2)	52 (33 / 19)	0.187 (-0.370, 0.744)	
Walker 1999	163 (84 / 79)	0.856 (0.537, 1.176)	
Gilbertson 2000	138 (67 / 71)	0.224 (-0.109, 0.557)	
Parker 2001 (1)	235 (156 / 79)	0.000 (-0.270, 0.270)	
Parker 2001 (2)	232 (153 / 79)	0.269 (-0.002, 0.541)	
Green 2002	161 (81 / 80)	0.000 (-0.307, 0.307)	
Di Lauro 2003	53 (26 / 27)	0.000 (-0.531, 0.531)	
Duncan 2003	93 (44 / 49)	0.594 (0.182, 1.007)	
Katz-Leurer 2003	90 (46 / 44)	0.305 (-0.107, 0.717)	
Rodgers 2003	105 (54 / 51)	0.000 (-0.380, 0.380)	
Fang 2003	128 (50 / 78)	0.018 (-0.335, 0.371)	
Lin 2004	19 (9 / 10)	0.303 (-0.563, 1.168)	
GAPS 2004	65 (32 / 33)	0.161 (-0.320, 0.642)	
Davidson 2005	36 (19 / 17)	-0.330 (-0.975, 0.315)	
Katz-Leurer 2006	24 (10 / 14)	0.190 (-0.596, 0.975)	
Mead 2007	66 (32 / 34)	-0.027 (-0.504, 0.450)	
Langhammer	63 (32 / 31)	-0.238 (-0.727, 0.252)	
Askim 2010	62 (30 / 32)	-0.110 (-0.602, 0.383)	
Holmgren 2010	34 (15 / 19)	0.466 (-0.204, 1.136)	
Letombe 2010	18 (9 / 9)	0.713 (-0.197, 1.623)	
Galvin 2011	40 (20 / 20)	0.381 (-0.232, 0.995)	
Hesse 2011	50 (25 / 25)	0.361 (-0.189, 0.911)	
Merkert 2011	48 (25 / 23)	0.674 (0.101, 1.247)	
	3064 (1691 / 1373)	*0.217 (0.094, 0.339)*	

I^2=62%

Favors control   Favors treatment

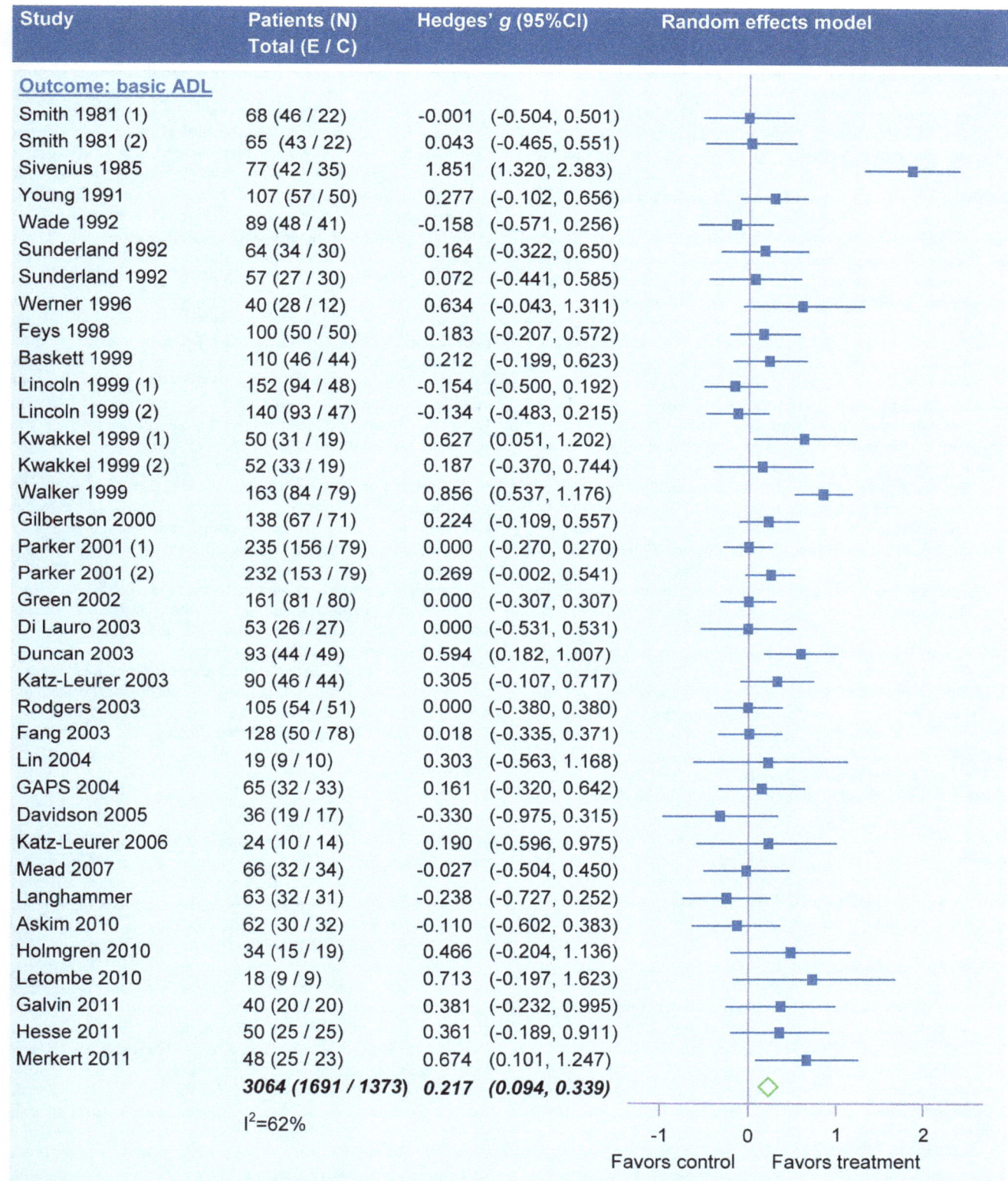

Figure 7. Summary effect sizes for physical therapy interventions – intensity of practice. Legend: ADL, Activities of daily living; C, Control group; CI, Confidence interval; E, Experimental group.

indicating differential effects between 5 and 15%, mainly relate to those functions and activities specifically trained in the intervention, and are restricted to the period of intervention alone. While these findings were – globally – similar to the review from 2004, a comparison of the present results with the results of our previous review shows clear changes [12]. The main change lies in the increased number of interventions to which 'strong evidence' could be assigned and an increase in the number of outcomes for which the findings are statistically significant. In addition, shifts are observed for a few 'strong evidence' interventions with significant positive effects in 2004. For example, speed dependent treadmill training now shows neutral results for walking ability; rhythmic auditory cueing of gait currently shows neutral results for gait speed and stride length; and training of standing balance now also shows neutral results. In contrast to the 2004 review which reported no significant effects at the participation level, now mixed strength and cardiovascular exercises and leisure therapy show a favorable effect at the participation level. In general, exploring the possible moderator effect of poststroke timing largely did not show significant differences in effects. Higher intensity of practice proves to be an important aspect of effective physical therapy. This review also highlights that well controlled, dose-matched trials with significant effects in favor of the experimental intervention have been rather scarce (e.g. [76,81,110]). The above findings suggest that intensity of practice is a key factor in meaningful training after stroke, and that more practice is better [8]. This implies that our previous conclusion that high-intensity practice is better still holds [12], and that an additional therapy time of 17 hours over 10 weeks is necessary to find significant positive effects at both the body function level and activities and participation level of the ICF. In national clinical guidelines for stroke in the United Kingdom and the Netherlands, it is recommended that patients should be enabled to exercise at least 45 minutes on each weekday as long as there are rehabilitation goals and the patient tolerates this intensity [184,538]. However, there is a big contrast between the recommended and actual applied therapy time. A survey in the Netherlands showed that patients with stroke admitted to a hospital stroke unit only received a mean of 22 minutes of physical therapy on weekdays [539]. Similarly, in the United Kingdom inpatients received 30.6 minutes physical therapy per day on which this therapy was given [540]. Contrary to previous reviews which concluded that neurological treatment approaches (NDT/Bobath) were not superior [12,541], the present review demonstrates that neurological treatment approaches are less effective when compared to focused interventions such as mCIMT, bilateral arm training, or strengthening when applied in a task-specific way.

Repetition is an important principle in motor learning which reflects the Hebbian learning rule that connections between neurons are strengthened when they are simultaneously active (i.e., long term potentiation) [542]. An earlier review has shown that repetitive task training is a key modality of effective training in stroke [543]. This repetition aspect relates to "an active motor sequence performed repetitively within a single training session, with practice aiming towards a clear functional goal" [543]. However, this does not mean that each repetition should be identical to the previous ones. Instead, is suggested that implementing slight variation between repetitions is more successful [544]. Although we did not analyze 'repetition' separately, this modality is a feature included in many focused interventions for which strong evidence was found in the present review. For example, CIMT and gait training are both characterized by a high number of repetitions executed within a single treatment session, serving a functional goal.

To facilitate application of the findings presented in the current review in daily practice, it is necessary to further specify for which interventions there is strong evidence that patients benefit from this therapeutic intervention and for which outcome this evidence is valid. Therefore, figure 8 graphically displays the outcomes classified according to the ICF, with corresponding interventions for which is strong evidence that they significantly affect those outcomes. It should be noted that the clinical applicability of some interventions like electromechanical-assisted gait training and robot-assisted arm training is questionable, due to the accompanying high costs of the equipment. For these interventions, there are often alternative 'strong evidence' interventions available.

The large number of interventions and outcomes for which nonsignificant SESs were found in the meta-analyses (i.e. neutral results) suggests that for many forms of exercise therapy the same patient outcomes can be obtained with the control intervention. This implies that the physical therapist, in cooperation with the patient, has to decide for each individual patient which of these interventions is the optimal treatment option. In this clinical decision-making process, that preferably should be based on existing knowledge about the functional prognosis for outcome [22,545], also resource use and possible alternative interventions should be taken into account.

It should also be noted that we found three significant negative SESs. The first being for overground walking (aerobic capacity; for dependent walking patients in the early rehabilitation phase when compared to electromechanical-assisted gait training or body-weight supported treadmill training), the second for virtual reality training for the paretic arm (muscle tone), and the third for trunk restraint (self-reported amount of arm-hand use in daily life). However, the meta-analysis for all these outcomes showed insufficient statistical power, suggesting that more trials are needed. Furthermore, although a negative SES was found for both overground walking and virtual reality training for the upper paretic limb, these interventions also show beneficial effects on one or more other outcomes. Therefore, we recommend that when physical therapists select one of these interventions, they should regularly monitor the outcomes which are at risk for being adversely affected by the intervention.

(In)stability of Results in Trials

A comparison between the current results and those of our previous meta-analyses [12] shows that some interventions for which strong evidence was reported in 2004, such as rhythmic auditory cueing of gait, no longer have the same level of evidence, whereas other interventions with initially only indicative findings or no evidence, such as EMG-NMS for the paretic arm, now show significant positive small to moderate effect sizes. This finding reflects a lack of robustness of existing evidence favoring or disfavoring an intervention when new trials are added to the current pool of studies. In our opinion, this (in)stability of current evidence depends on several factors. First, differential effects seem to be largely dependent on the content and dose-matching of the therapy given in the control group [6,546]. In a number of trials, the content and dosage of therapy applied in the control group is poorly defined. 'Usual care' frequently reflects the existing guidelines, suggesting that the patients in the control group received treatment according to the best available evidence at that moment. Obviously, researchers hypothesize that the added value of the experimental intervention will considerably exceed the existing standards of care, acknowledging that comparison of an experimental intervention with a real 'sham' or placebo intervention is not desirable in stroke rehabilitation, and is in most Western countries not allowed for medical ethical reasons. Second, many

Body functions	
Motor function leg	NMS of the paretic leg ●
	Mixed strength and cardiorespiratory exercises ●
	High-intensity practice ●
Motor function arm	Low-intensity mCIMT ●
	Bilateral elbow-wrist robotics ●
	NMS wrist/finger flexors/extensors ●
	EMG-NMS wrist/finger extensors ●
	High-intensity practice ●
Motor function arm (prox.)	Unilateral shoulder-elbow robotics ●
Muscle strength leg	Water-based exercises ●
	NMS of the paretic leg ●
	TENS ●
	Strength training paretic leg ●
	Mixed strength and cardiorespiratory exercises ●
	High-intensity practice ●
Muscle strength arm	Unilateral shoulder-elbow robotics ●
	Bilateral elbow-wrist robotics ●
	NMS wrist/finger flexors/extensors ●
	High-intensity practice ●
Muscle tone leg	NMS of the paretic leg ●
	Strength training paretic leg ●
	High-intensity practice ●
Muscle tone arm	Interventions for somatosensory functions ●
	High-intensity practice ●
	Virtual reality training for the paretic arm ●
Pain	Unilateral shoulder-elbow robotics ●
Active range of motion	EMG-NMS wrist/finger extensors ●
Passive range of motion *	Therapeutic positioning of the paretic arm ●
Shoulder subluxation	NMS shoulder ●
Comfortable gait speed	BWSTT ●
	Mixed strength and cardiorespiratory exercises ●
	High-intensity practice ●
Maximum gait speed	Electromechanical-assisted gait training ● **
	Speed dependent treadmill training ●
	Mixed strength and cardiorespiratory exercises ●
	High-intensity practice ●
Walking distance	BWSTT ●
	Electromechanical-assisted gait training ● **
	Circuit class training ●
	Mixed strength and cardiorespiratory exercises ●
Spatiotemporal gait pattern parameters	Speed dependent treadmill training ●
	Strength training paretic leg ●
Postural sway	Standing balance training with biofeedback ●
Aerobic capacity	Cardiorespiratoiry exercises ●
	Mixed strength and cardiorespiratory exercises ●
	Overground walking ● △
Peak heart rate	Electromechanical-assisted gait training ● **
Heart rate work	Mixed strength and cardiorespiratory exercises ●
Workload	Cardiorespiratory exercises ●
Respiratory functions	Cardiorespiratory exercises ●
Hand movement time	Sitting balance training ●
Anxiety	Overground walking ● □
	High-intensity practice ●
Depression	High-intensity practice ●
Gesture comprehension	Gestural training ●

Activities	
Sitting balance	Sitting balance training ●
Sitting and standing balance	Balance training during various activities ●
	Electromechanical-assisted gait training with ES ●
	Circuit class training ●
	Mixed strength and cardiorespiratory exercises ●
	High-intensity practice ●
Walking ability	Electromechanical-assisted gait training with ES ●
	Circuit class training ●
	TENS ●
Arm-hand activities	Original CIMT ●
	High-intensity mCIMT ●
	Low-intensity mCIMT ●
	Mental practice with motor imagery ●
	EMG-NMS wrist/finger extensors ●
Self-reported amount of arm-hand use in daily life	Original CIMT ●
	High-intensity mCIMT ●
	Low-intensity mCIMT ●
	Trunk restraint ●
Self-reported quality of arm-hand movement in daily life	Original CIMT ●
	High-intensity mCIMT ●
	Low-intensity mCIMT ●
Basic ADL	Balance training during various activities ●
	Electromechanical-assisted gait training ●
	Caregiver-mediated exercises ●
	Low-intensity mCIMT ●
	Virtual reality training for the paretic arm ●
	High-intensity practice ●
Physical activity	Circuit class training ●
	Mixed strength and cardiorespiratory exercises ●

Participation	
Quality of life	Mixed strength and cardiorespiratory exercises ●
	High-intensity practice ●
Leisure participation	Leisure therapy ●

Environmental factors	
Caregiver strain	Caregiver-mediated exercises ●

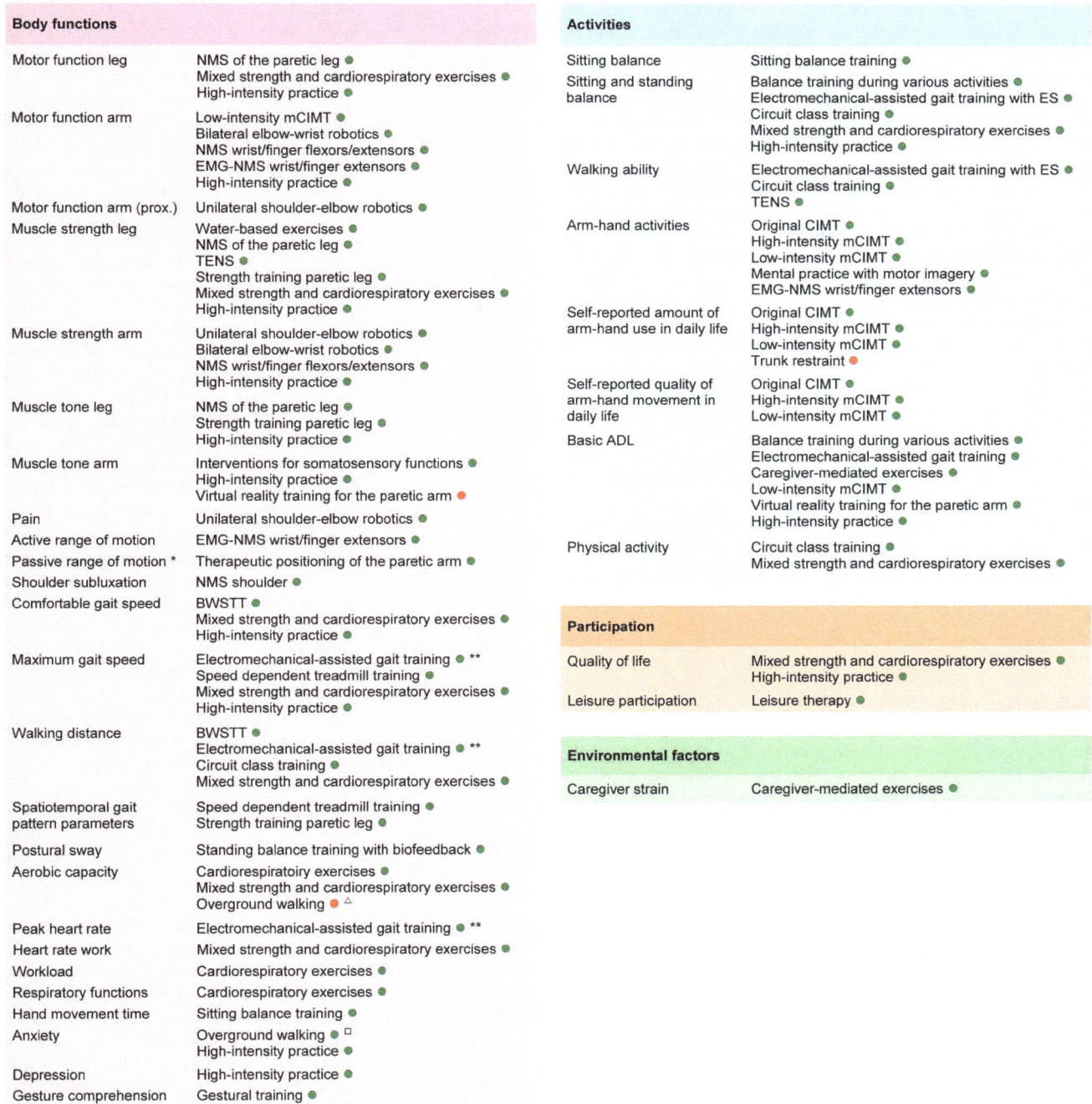

Figure 8. Overview of outcomes for which interventions are available with significant summarized effects. Legend: A green point indicates that the intervention has a significant positive effect on the outcome, while a red point indicates that the intervention has a significant negative effect on the outcome; *, shoulder external rotation; **, dependent walking patients in the early rehabilitation phase; △, dependent walking patients when compared to electromechanical-assisted gait training or BWSTT; □, independent walking patients; BWSTT, Body-weight supported treadmill training; CIMT, Constraint-induced movement therapy; EMG-NMS, Electromyography-triggered neuromuscular stimulation; ES, Electrostimulation; mCIMT, modified Constraint-induced movement therapy; NMS, Neuromuscular stimulation; prox., Proximal; TENS, Transcutaneous electrical nerve stimulation.

primary outcome measures do not appropriately reflect the underlying biological rationale for the content of the experimental therapy [547], whereas other outcomes may be rather insensitive to the changes introduced by physical therapy [548]. To improve comparability between trials applying the same intervention, international consensus about outcomes and timing of (follow-up) measurements is urgently needed [8,549]. Third, of the 326 meta-analyses we performed, the statistical power was sufficient for only 58 meta-analyses divided over 28 interventions (e.g. training of sitting balance and (m)CIMT) and intensity of practice. The instability of SESs over time and hence the current level of evidence is mainly due to the low number of small-sized phase II trials [550]. The dominance of rather positive phase II trials in physical therapy may well reflect publication bias, since low-powered negative trials are less likely to be published [551]. In contrast, recent sufficiently powered phase III and IV trials in physical therapy, such as those on the impact of shoulder-elbow robotics [335] and body-weight supported treadmill training [91] yielded less positive findings than the previously published phase II trials on these type of interventions [552]. However, one may also argue that in small numbered monocenter trials, therapists are more committed to the trial than in multicenter trials. Fourth, heterogeneity of patient samples could have played a role [553–555]. Not only can differences between studies in inclusion criteria, resulting in between-study heterogeneity, play a role, but also within-study heterogeneity, especially in larger trials which tend to have less strict inclusion criteria. As referred to above, the therapeutic content of the experimental intervention applied was often poorly defined, since most journals do not allow publication of treatment protocols [556], preventing researchers from properly reporting on treatment content due to word limitations, replicating studies, or judging if interventions are sufficiently comparable to allow meta-analyses. Finally, the observed shifts in evidence may reflect the improved methodological quality of studies due to the introduction of the CONSORT Statement for reporting RCTs [557]. In the present review, the median PEDro score was found to have increased from 5 (IQR 4–6) for RCTs published before 2004 [12] to 6 (IQR 5–7) in the subsequent period. This finding suggests increased efforts by researchers to reduce bias in clinical trials [558,559].

Deficiencies in the Focus of Trials

Remarkably, only three RCTs started their intervention within the first days poststroke, despite evidence that most patients are physical inactive early poststroke [560] as well as the growing evidence of a greater potential for neuroplasticity in the first three to four weeks poststroke [561]. One may assume that giving appropriate training within this window of increased homeostatic neuroplasticity may enhance motor recovery. Although our subgroup analyses suggest that timing poststroke is only a significant moderator of effect sizes in a small number of interventions, this is based on very few trials that started in this critical phase of the first days or weeks poststroke.

While the strength of evidence is growing for certain physical therapy interventions, the cost-effectiveness of these interventions has so far hardly been subject of investigation [562,563], and long-term outcomes have often not been systematically measured at fixed times post intervention. In addition, even though the main effects of intensity of practice are in favor of high-intensity training, there is still a paucity of well-controlled dose-response RTCs in the field of physical therapy directly investigating the impact of intensity of practice [19,353].

How to Proceed?

While acknowledging that interdisciplinary collaboration is a key aspect of stroke rehabilitation [3], we think it is important that each discipline should take responsibility to further extend the specific contribution of different types of therapy in the interdisciplinary care, in terms of evidence and implementation. Therefore, a roadmap is needed to prioritize research in the domain of physical therapy. In determining research priorities, different perspectives ought to be considered, like those of patients and their caregivers, clinicians, researchers and policy-makers [564,565].

In our opinion, this roadmap should contain the following elements: (1) investigating dose-response relations in exercise therapy, in which the experimental and control groups receive the same type of intervention but with different dosage [566]; (2) investigating resource-efficient interventions to augment physical therapy and allow early supported discharge such as telerehabilitation [567] and caregiver-mediated exercises [174]; (3) investigating the benefits of an (very) early start of physical therapy poststroke [560] and continuation of poststroke therapy in the weekends; (4) investigating the cost-effectiveness of interventions and numbers needed to treat; (5) investigating the effectiveness of interventions which have so far only been investigated in phase II trials and from which patients may benefit; (6) investigating interventions that are used by physical therapists but have not been investigated in RCTs, like the effectiveness of falls prevention programs and physical fitness training in the context of secondary prevention. Finally, (7) investigating the mechanisms behind motor learning and stroke recovery, which are still poorly understood. Only translational research is able to bridge the gap between the effects of an intervention that have been found and the underlying mechanisms that may contribute to therapy-induced poststroke recovery. In order to understand what actually changes during stroke recovery, we need to discriminate between recovery of body functions (restitution) and learning to use compensation strategies in accomplishing tasks [568,569]. In this respect, new therapeutic approaches in which physical exercise is combined with innovative treatments enhancing neuroplasticity in crucial (early) time windows, such as transcranial Direct Current Stimulation [570,571], repetitive Transcranial Magnetic Stimulation [572], or neuropharmacological interventions [573], may be promising.

Stroke rehabilitation intervention research in the domain of physical therapy can be organized using a step-wise approach [6,546]: interventions with positive effects in the first explorative stages on relevant consensus-based outcomes should become the subject of high-quality phase III and IV trials. In all cases, subgroups of patients should be selected which, from a biological perspective, would benefit the most from the intervention, while taking into account "the sensitive period for response to intervention" [574].

Implementation of research findings into daily practice is essential to improve quality of care, but is also challenging. First of all, because physical therapy as part of complex interdisciplinary stroke rehabilitation, contains several interrelated components that may be targeted at different levels (i.e., at service, operator, and/or treatment level) [8,575,576]. Second, physical therapy typically entails a cyclical process involving (1) assessment, to identify and quantify the patient's needs; (2) goal setting, to define realistic and attainable goals for improvement; (3) intervention, to assist in the achievement of goals; and (4) reassessment, to assess progress against agreed goals [8]. For all of these four steps, a broad scientific base is available but the evidence is dynamic. Due to this complexity and it's dynamics, a country wide postbachelor physical therapy course was started in 2008 in the Netherlands in which the different aspects of evidence-based practice in stroke are educated [541]. This one year course includes themes such as: (1) how to make clinical decisions; (2) how to measure outcome and clinical change; (3) how to estimate the individual prognosis for outcome at the activities level; and (4) how to select the best intervention. In addition, in this course special attention is paid to assumed pathophysiology and underlying working mechanisms of recovery poststroke. However, effective but efficient methods for physical therapists to keep their knowledge and skill level up-to-date in the long term needs further investigation.

Limitations

Although this systematic review was performed with the greatest of care, there are some methodological limitations like the language restriction, not hand-searching conference proceedings, missing outcome data [577], not performing meta-analyses of individual patient data [578], and the lack of both a correction for multiple testing and systematic investigation of reporting bias. In addition, the observational nature of the subgroup analyses means they should be interpreted with caution, as it is known that subgroup analyses in meta-analyses can be less highly powered than analyses for main effects [29,579,580].

Conclusion

In summary, the body of knowledge about physical therapy in stroke rehabilitation is still growing. This is evident both from the increased number of published RCTs with a low risk of bias, resulting in strong evidence for many physical therapy modalities, and from the exploration of innovative ways for efficient use of resources like circuit class training. This endorses the central role of physical therapy in interdisciplinary evidence-based stroke rehabilitation. Further confirmation of the evidence for physical therapy after stroke, and facilitating the transfer to clinical practice, requires a better understanding of (neurophysiological) mechanisms, including neuroplasticity, that drive stroke recovery, as well as the impact of physical therapy interventions on these underlying mechanisms. Thus, well-designed RCTs should address questions like: Which patients benefit most from a specific intervention? At what time poststroke should interventions be initiated? What are the underlying mechanisms that drive improvement of sensorimotor control? What are the preferred intervention characteristics, including the optimal dosage? And are interventions cost-effective? Subsequent meta-analyses should analyze the evidence using individual participant data. Finally, implementation strategies should be further explored in order to optimize the transfer of scientific knowledge into clinical practice.

The high growth in the number of RCTs on physical therapy stroke rehabilitation makes it virtually impossible for individual physical therapists to identify and ascertain the content of each relevant science citation indexed study. There is therefore a need for a worldwide continuing – online – update of the summarized evidence, discussed in the context of interdisciplinary stroke care.

Supporting Information

File S1 Contains Supporting Tables. TABLE S1A. Title: Summary of physical therapy interventions – gait and mobility-related functions and activities. Legend: +, significant positive SES; =, nonsignficant SES; –, significant negative SES; ADL, Activities of daily living; C, Chronic phase; d, day(s); ER, Early rehabilitation phase; EMG, Electromyographic (H)AR, (hyper)-acute rehabilitation phase; min, minutes; LR, Late rehabilitation phase; mos, months; RCTs, Randomized controlled trials; SES, Summary effect size; wk, week(s). TABLE S1B. Title: Summary of physical therapy interventions – arm-hand activities. Legend: +, significant positive SES; =, nonsignficant SES; –, significant negative SES; ?, unclear; ADL, Activities of daily living; C, Chronic phase; d, day(s); CIMT, Constraint-induced movement therapy; ER, Early rehabilitation phase; (H)AR, (hyper)acute rehabilitation phase; LR, Late rehabilitation phase; min, minutes; mCIMT, modified Constraint-induced movement therapy; mos, months; RCTs, Randomized controlled trials; wk, week(s); SES, Summary effect size. TABLE S1C. Title: Summary of physical therapy interventions – physical fitness. Legend: +, significant

positive SES; =, nonsignficant SES; ?, unclear; ADL, Activities of daily living; C, Chronic phase; d, day(s); ER, Early rehabilitation phase; (H)AR, (hyper)acute rehabilitation phase; LR, Late rehabilitation phase; RCTs, Randomized controlled trials; min, minutes; mos, months; SES, Summary effect size; wk, week(s). TABLE S1D. Title: Summary of physical therapy interventions – activities of daily living. Legend: +, significant positive SES; =, nonsignficant SES; C, Chronic phase; d, day(s); ER, Early rehabilitation phase; (H)AR, (hyper)acute rehabilitation phase; LR, Late rehabilitation phase; min, minutes; mos, months; RCTs, Randomized controlled trials; SES, Summary effect size; wk, week(s). TABLE S1E. Title: Summary of physical therapy interventions – other. Legend: =, nonsignficant SES; C, Chronic phase; d, day(s); ER, Early rehabilitation phase; (H)AR, (hyper)-acute rehabilitation phase; LR, Late rehabilitation phase; min, minutes; mos, months; RCTs, Randomized controlled trials; SES, Summary effect size; wk, week(s). TABLE S1F. Title: Summary of physical therapy interventions – intensity of practice. Legend: ?, unclear; +, significant positive SES; =, nonsignficant SES; ADL, Activities of daily living; C, Chronic phase; ER, Early rehabilitation phase; (H)AR, (hyper)acute rehabilitation phase; h, hours; LR, Late rehabilitation phase; RCTs, Randomized controlled trials; SES, Summary effect size; wk, weeks. TABLE S1G. Title: Summary of physical therapy interventions – neurological treatment approaches. Legend: +, significant positive effect; =, nonsignficant effect; –, significant negative effect; ?, unclear; ADL, Activities of daily living; BWSTT, Body-weight supported treadmill training; C, Chronic phase; EMG-BF, Electromyographic biofeedback; EMG, Electromyograpic; EMG-NMS, Electromyography-triggered neuromuscular stimulation; ER, Early rehabilitation phase; (H)AR, (hyper)acute rehabilitation phase; LR, Late rehabilitation phase; mCIMT, modified Constraint-induced movement therapy; NDT, Neurodevelopmental treatment; NMS, Neuromuscular stimulation; RCTs, Randomized controlled trials; SES, Summary effect size; TENS, Transcutaneous electrical nerve stimulation. TABLE S2A. Title: Summary of the evidence for physical therapy interventions – gait and mobility-related functions and activities. Legend: 10MWT, 10-meter walk test; 12MWT, 12-minute walk test; 3MWT, 3-minute walk test; 5MWT, 5-meter walk test; 6MWT, 6-minute walk test; 8MWT, 8-meter walk test; AAP, Adelaide activities profile; ABC, Activities-specific balance confidence scale; ADL, Activities of daily living; BBA, Brunel balance assessment; BBS, Berg balance scale; BI, Barthel index; BP, Blood pressure; BWD, Body-weight distribution; C, Chronic phase; CI, Confidence interval; CSS, Composite spasticity scale; CNS, Canadian neurological scale; DB, Dynamic balance; DST, Double support time; EFAP, Emory functional ambulation profile; EMS, Elderly mobility scale; ER, Early rehabilitation phase; FAC, Functional ambulation categories; FAI, Frenchay activities index; FES-I, Falls-efficacy scale; FIM, Functional independence measure; FMA, Fugl-meyer assessment; FR, Functional reach; FSST, Four square step test; GDS-15, Geriatric depression scale - 15;GRF, Ground reaction force; HADS, Hospital anxiety and depression scale; HR, Heart rate; LLFDI, Late life function and disability instrument; LR, Late rehabilitation phase; LRT, Lateral reach test; MAS, Modified ashworth scale; MAS*, Motor assessment scale; mEFAP, modified Emory functional ambulation profile; MI, Motricity index; MMAS*, modified Motor assessment scale; MRC, Medical research council; mRS, modified Rankin scale; NA, Not applicable; NEADL, Nottingham extended ADL index; NHP, Nottingham health profile; NIHSS, National institutes of health stroke scale; NS, Not significant; PADS, Physical activity and disability scale; PASIPD, Physical activity scale for individuals with physical disabilities; PASS, Postural assessment scale for stroke; QoL, Quality of life; RMI, Rivermead mobility index; RMA, Rivermead motor assessment; RMA GF, RMA gross function; RMA LT, RMA leg and trunk; ROM, Range of motion; RPE, Rating of perceived exertion; S, Significant; SA-SIP30, Stroke-adapted 30-item version of the sickness impact profile; SAS, Stroke activities scale; SES, Summary effect size; SF-36, 36-Item short form health survey; SB, Static balance; SI, Spasticity index; SIS, Stroke impact scale; SPPB, Short physical performance battery; SST, Single-support time; ST, Step test; STREAM, Stroke rehabilitation assessment of movement instrument; STS, Sit-to-stand; TCT, Trunk control test; TIS, Trunk impairment scale; TMS, Toulouse motor scale; TUG, Timed up and go test; WAQ, Walking ability questionnaire; WD, Walking distance; WQ, Walking quality; WS, Walking speed gait analysis. TABLE S2B. Title: Summary of the evidence for physical therapy interventions – arm-hand activities. Legend: 10CMT, 10-cup moving test; ADL, Activities of daily living; AFT, Arm function test; AMAT, Arm motor ability test; ARAT, Action research arm test; BBT, Box and block test; BI, Barthel index; C, Chronic phase; CAHAI, Chedoke arm and hand activity inventory; CI, Confidence interval; CMMSA, Chedoke-McMaster stroke assessment; ER, Early rehabilitation phase; FE, Functional evaluation; FIM, Functional independence measure; FMC, Fine motor control; FMA, Fugl-meyer assessment; FTHUE, Functional test for the hemiplegic upper extremity; GP, Grip power; GS, Grip strength; JTHFT, Jebsen-Taylor hand function test; LR, Late rehabilitation phase; MAL, Motor activity log; MAS, Modified ashworth scale; MAS*, Motor assessment scale; mFMA, modified Fugl-meyer assessment; MP, Motor power; MRC, Medical research council; MSS, Motor status scale; mBI, modified Barthel index; NA, Not applicable; NS, Not significant; NSA, Nottingham sensory assessment; PPT, Perdue pegboard test; PS, Pinch strength; ROM, Range of motion; S, Significant; SES, Summary effect size; SIS, Stroke impact scale; TEMPA, Test d'evaluation des membres supérieurs de personnes agéés; UEFT, Upper extremity function test; VAS, Visual analogue scale; WFMT, Wolf motor function test. TABLE S2C. Title: Summary of the evidence for physical therapy interventions – physical fitness. Legend: 10MWT, 10-meter walk test; 12MWT, 12-minute walk test; 5MWT, 5-meter walk test; 6MWT, 6-minute walk test; ADL, Activities of daily living; ARAT, Action research arm test; BBS, Berg balance scale; BI, Barthel index; BMI, Body mass index; BP, Blood pressure; C, Chronic phase; CI, Confidence interval; CMMSA, Chedoke-McMaster stroke assessment; EQ, EuroQoL 5D; ER, Early rehabilitation phase; FAP, Functional ambulation profile; FEV1, Forced expiratory volume in 1 second; FIM, Functional independence measure; FMA, Fugl-meyer assessment; FR, Functional reach; FSST, Four square step test; FTHUE, Functional test for the hemiplegic upper extremity; GF, Grip force; GS, Grip strength; HADS, Hospital anxiety and depression scale; HR, Heart rate; IADL, Instrumental ADL; JTHFT, Jebsen-Taylor hand function test; LLFDI, Late life function and disability instrument; LR, Late rehabilitation phase; MAS, Modified ashworth scale; NA, Not applicable; NEADL, Nottingham extended ADL index; NHPT, Nine hole peg test; NS, Not significant; O2cost, Oxygen cost; PADS, physical activities and disability scale; PASIPD, Physical activity scale for individuals with physical disabilities; PF, Pinch force; PPT, Perdue pegboard test; RER, Respiratory exchange ratio; RMA GF, Rivermead motor assessment gross function; RMI, Rivermead mobility index; S, Significant; SES, Summary effect size; SF-36, 36-item Short form health survey; SLC90, Symptom checklist-90-R; STS, Sit-to-stand; TMS, Tolouse motor scale; TUG, Timed up and go test; VE, Ventilatory exchange;

VO2max, Ventilatory oxygen uptake, WD, Walking distance; WS, WQ, Walking questionnaire; Walking speed gait analysis. TABLE S2D. Title: Summary of the evidence for physical therapy interventions – activities of daily living. Legend: *1 RCT with 2 comparisons; NLQ, Nottingham leisure questionnaire; BDI, Beck depression inventory; C, Chronic phase; CES-D, Centre for epidemiologic studies for depression scale; CI, Confidence interval; ER, Early rehabilitation phase; GHQ, General health questionnaire; GWBS, General well-being scale; LR, Late rehabilitation phase; NA, Not applicable; NS, Not significant; TLAS, Total leisure activities score; TLS, Total leisure score; S, Significant; SES, Summary effect size; SIP, Stroke impact profile; SA-SIP30, Stroke-adapted 30-item version of the sickness impact profile; WDI, Wakefield depression inventory. TABLE S2E. Title: Summary of the evidence for physical therapy interventions – other. Legend: CI, Confidence interval; C, Chronic phase; LR, Late rehabilitation phase; MIP, Maximal inspiratory pressure; S, Significant; SES, Summary effect size. TABLE S2F. Title: Summary of the evidence for physical therapy interventions – intensity of practice. Legend: 10MWT, 10-meter walk test; 5MWT, 5-meter walk test; ABC, Activities-specific balance confidence scale; ADL, Activities of daily living; ARAT, Action research arm test; BBS, Berg balance scale; BDI, Beck depression inventory; BI, Barthel index; C, Chronic phase; CI, Confidence interval; COOP scale, Dartmouth primary care cooperative information functional health assessment; ER, Early rehabilitation phase; FAC, Functional ambulation categories; FAI, Frenchay activities index; FES-I, Falls-efficacy scale; FIM, Functional independence measure; FMA, Fugl-meyer assessment; FR, Functional reach; FSST, Four square step test; FTHUE, Functional test for the hemiplegic upper extremity; GDS, Geriatric depression scale –15; GHQ, General health questionnaire; GS, Grip strength; HADS, Hospital anxiety and depression scale; IADL, Instrumental ADL; LHS, London handicap scale; LR, Late rehabilitation phase; MAS, Modified ashworth scale; mBI, modified Barthel index; MI, Motricity index; mRMI, modified Rivermead mobility index; NA, Not applicable; NEADL, Nottingham extended ADL index; NHP, Nottingham health profile; NHPT, Nine hole peg test; NS, Not significant; PASS, Postural assessment scale for stroke; POR, profile of recovery; PS, Pinch strength; RMA, Rivermead motor assessment; RMI, Rivermead mobility index; S, Significant; SCL-90, Symptom checklist-90-R; SES, Summary effect size; SF-36, 36-item Short form health survey; SIP, Stroke impact scale, SIS, Stroke impact scale; ST, Step test; STREAM, Stroke rehabilitation assessment of movement instrument; WD, Walking distance; WS, Walking speed gait analysis.

Acknowledgments

We would like to thank Hans Ket, medical information specialist at the VU University library, for his contribution to the literature search, and Frank van Hartingsveld MSc, teacher at Amsterdam School of Health Professions ASHP, for supervising students who crosschecked the data extracted for the meta-analyses. Also, we would like to thank Karin Heijblom as representative and clinical guidelines portfolio holder of the Royal Dutch Society for Physical Therapy and Jan Klerkx for language editing.

Author Contributions

Analyzed the data: JMV EVW GK. Wrote the paper: JMV EVW RVP PJVDW EH MR GK.

References

1. Roger V, Go A, Lloyd-Jones D, Adams R, Berry J, et al. (2011) Heart disease and stroke statistics–2011 update: a report from the American Heart Association. Circulation 123: e18–e209.
2. Wardlaw J, Murray V, Berge E, Del Zoppo G (2009) Thrombolysis for acute ischaemic stroke. Cochrane Database Syst Rev: CD000213.
3. Stroke Unit Trialists' Collaboration (2007) Organised inpatient (stroke unit) care for stroke. Cochrane Database Syst Rev: CD000197.
4. Wade D, Hewer R (1987) Functional abilities after stroke: measurement, natural history and prognosis. J Neurol Neurosurg Psychiatry 50: 177–182.
5. Miller E, Murray L, Richards L, Zorowitz R, Bakas T, et al. (2010) Comprehensive overview of nursing and interdisciplinary rehabilitation care of the stroke patient: a scientific statement from the American Heart Association. Stroke 41: 2402–2448.
6. Medical Research Council (2000) A framework for development and evaluation of RCTs for complex interventions to improve health.
7. Langhorne P, Legg L (2003) Evidence behind stroke rehabilitation. J Neurol Neurosurg Psychiatry 74 Suppl 4: iv18–iv21.
8. Langhorne P, Bernhardt J, Kwakkel G (2011) Stroke rehabilitation. Lancet 377: 1693–1702.
9. Grimshaw J, Eccles M, Russell I (1995) Developing clinically valid practice guidelines. J Eval Clin Pract 1: 37–48.
10. Grimshaw J, Freemantle N, Wallace S, Russell I, Hurwitz B, et al. (1995) Developing and implementing clinical practice guidelines. Qual Health Care 4: 55–64.
11. Grol R, Grimshaw J (2003) From best evidence to best practice: effective implementation of change in patients' care. Lancet 362: 1225–1230.
12. Van Peppen R, Kwakkel G, Wood-Dauphinee S, Hendriks H, Van der Wees P, et al. (2004) The impact of physical therapy on functional outcomes after stroke: what's the evidence? Clin Rehabil 18: 833–862.
13. Kjellström T, Norrving B, Shatchkute A (2007) Helsingborg Declaration 2006 on European stroke strategies. Cerebrovasc Dis 23: 231–241.
14. Norrving B (2007) The 2006 Helsingborg Consensus Conference on European Stroke Strategies: Summary of conference proceedings and background to the 2nd Helsingborg Declaration. Int J Stroke 2: 139–143.
15. World Health Organization (2001) International Classification of Functioning, Disability and Health: ICF. Geneva.
16. Hatano S (1976) Experience from a multicentre stroke register: a preliminary report. Bull World Health Organ 54: 541–553.
17. Higgins J, Green S (2011) Cochrane Handbook for Systematic Reviews of Interventions. Version 5.1.0 [updated March 2011]: The Cochrane Collaboration.
18. American Physical Therapy Association (2011) Today's Physical Therapist: A Comprehensive Review of a 21st-Century Health Care Profession.
19. Veerbeek J, Koolstra M, Ket J, Van Wegen E, Kwakkel G (2011) Effects of augmented exercise therapy on outcome of gait and gait-related activities in the first 6 months after stroke: a meta-analysis. Stroke 42: 3311–3315.
20. Kwakkel G, Van Peppen R, Wagenaar R, Wood-Dauphinee S, Richards C, et al. (2004) Effects of augmented exercise therapy time after stroke: a meta-analysis. Stroke 35: 2529–2539.
21. World Confederation for Physical Therapy (2013) World Confederation for Physical Therapy (WCPT) Glossary. Available: http://wwwwcptorg/glossary.
22. Veerbeek J, Kwakkel G, Van Wegen E, Ket J, Heymans M (2011) Early prediction of outcome of activities of daily living after stroke: a systematic review. Stroke 42: 1482–1488.
23. Geyh S, Cieza A, Schouten J, Dickson H, Frommelt P, et al. (2004) ICF Core Sets for stroke. J Rehabil Med 36: 135–141.
24. Moseley A, Herbert R, Sherrington C, Maher C (2002) Evidence for physiotherapy practice: a survey of the Physiotherapy Evidence Database (PEDro). Aust J Physiother 48: 43–49.
25. Sherrington C, Herbert R, Maher C, Moseley A (2000) PEDro. A database of randomized trials and systematic reviews in physiotherapy. Man Ther 5: 223–226.
26. Van Tulder M, Cherkin D, Berman B, Lao L, Koes B (1999) The effectiveness of acupuncture in the management of acute and chronic low back pain. A systematic review within the framework of the Cochrane Collaboration Back Review Group. Spine (Phila Pa 1976) 24: 1113–1123.
27. Borenstein M, Hedges L, Higgins J, Rothstein R (2009) Subgroup analyses. Introduction to meta-analysis. New Jersey: John Wiley & Sons, Ltd. 149–186.
28. Cohen J (1977) Statistical power analysis for the behavioural sciences. New York: Academic Press.
29. Hedges L, Pigott T (2001) The power of statistical tests in meta-analysis. Psychol Methods 6: 203–217.
30. Johannsen L, Wing A, Pelton T, Kitaka K, Zietz D, et al. (2010) Seated bilateral leg exercise effects on hemiparetic lower extremity function in chronic stroke. Neurorehabil Neural Repair 24: 243–253.
31. Sütbeyaz S, Yavuzer G, Sezer N, Koseoglu B (2007) Mirror therapy enhances lower-extremity motor recovery and motor functioning after stroke: a randomized controlled trial. Arch Phys Med Rehabil 88: 555–559.
32. Malouin F, Richards C, Durand A, Doyon J (2009) Added value of mental practice combined with a small amount of physical practice on the relearning of rising and sitting post-stroke: a pilot study. J Neurol Phys Ther 33: 195–202.
33. Pomeroy V, Evans B, Falconer M, Jones D, Hill E, et al. (2001) An exploration of the effects of weighted garments on balance and gait of stroke patients with residual disability. Clin Rehabil 15: 390–397.
34. Dobkin B, Plummer-D'Amato P, Elashoff R, Lee J (2010) International randomized clinical trial, stroke inpatient rehabilitation with reinforcement of walking speed (SIRROWS), improves outcomes. Neurorehabil Neural Repair 24: 235–242.
35. Robinson W, Smith R, Aung O, Ada L (2008) No difference between wearing a night splint and standing on a tilt table in preventing ankle contracture early after stroke: a randomised trial. Aust J Physiother 54: 33–38.
36. Kluding P, Santos M (2008) Effects of ankle joint mobilizations in adults poststroke: a pilot study. Arch Phys Med Rehabil 89: 449–456.
37. Rydwik E, Eliasson S, Akner G (2006) The effect of exercise of the affected foot in stroke patients–a randomized controlled pilot trial. Clin Rehabil 20: 645–655.
38. Ansari N, Naghdi S, Bagheri H, Ghassabi H (2007) Therapeutic ultrasound in the treatment of ankle plantarflexor spasticity in a unilateral stroke population: a randomized, single-blind, placebo-controlled trial. Electromyogr Clin Neurophysiol 47: 137–143.
39. Paoloni M, Mangone M, Scettri P, Procaccianti R, Cometa A, et al. (2010) Segmental muscle vibration improves walking in chronic stroke patients with foot drop: a randomized controlled trial. Neurorehabil Neural Repair 24: 254–262.
40. Van Nes I, Latour H, Schils F, Meijer R, Van Kuijk A, et al. (2006) Long-term effects of 6-week whole-body vibration on balance recovery and activities of daily living in the postacute phase of stroke: a randomized, controlled trial. Stroke 37: 2331–2335.
41. Barrett J, Watkins C, Plant R, Dickinson H, Clayton L, et al. (2001) The COSTAR wheelchair study: a two-centre pilot study of self-propulsion in a wheelchair in early stroke rehabilitation. Collaborative Stroke Audit and Research. Clin Rehabil 15: 32–41.
42. Bernhardt J, Indredavik B, Dewey H, Langhorne P, Lindley R, et al. (2007) Mobilisation 'in bed' is not mobilisation. Cerebrovasc Dis 24: 157–158.
43. Bernhardt J, Dewey H, Thrift A, Collier J, Donnan G (2008) A very early rehabilitation trial for stroke (AVERT): phase II safety and feasibility. Stroke 39: 390–396.
44. Langhorne P, Stott D, Knight A, Bernhardt J, Barer D, et al. (2010) Very early rehabilitation or intensive telemetry after stroke: a pilot randomised trial. Cerebrovasc Dis 29: 352–360.
45. Pollock A, Durward B, Rowe P, Paul J (2000) What is balance? Clin Rehabil 14: 402–406.
46. Ibrahim N, Tufel S, Singh H, Maurya M (2010) Effect of sitting balance training under varied sensory input on balance and quality of life in stroke patients. Ind J Physiother Occup Ther 4: 40–45.
47. Dean C, Channon E, Hall J (2007) Sitting training early after stroke improves sitting ability and quality and carries over to standing up but not to walking: a randomised trial. Aust J Physiother 53: 97–102.
48. Dean C, Shepherd R (1997) Task-related training improves performance of seated reaching tasks after stroke. A randomized controlled trial. Stroke 28: 722–728.
49. De Sèze M, Wiart L, Bon-Saint-Côme A, Debelleix X, De Sèze M, et al. (2001) Rehabilitation of postural disturbances of hemiplegic patients by using trunk control retraining during exploratory exercises. Arch Phys Med Rehabil 82: 793–800.
50. Mudie M, Winzeler-Mercay U, Radwan S, Lee L (2002) Training symmetry of weight distribution after stroke: a randomized controlled pilot study comparing task-related reach, Bobath and feedback training approaches. Clin Rehabil 16: 582–592.
51. Pollock A, Durward B, Rowe P, Paul J (2002) The effect of independent practice of motor tasks by stroke patients: a pilot randomized controlled trial. Clin Rehabil 16: 473–480.
52. Janssen W, Bussmann H, Stam H (2002) Determinants of the sit-to-stand movement: a review. Phys Ther 82: 866–879.
53. Britton E, Harris N, Turton A (2008) An exploratory randomized controlled trial of assisted practice for improving sit-to-stand in stroke patients in the hospital setting. Clin Rehabil 22: 458–468.
54. Barreca S, Sigouin C, Lambert C, Ansley B (2004) Effects of extra training on the ability of stroke survivors tp perform an independent ist-to-stand: a randomized controlled trial. J Geriatr Phys Ther 27: 59–68.
55. Tung F, Yang Y, Lee C, Wang R (2010) Balance outcomes after additional sit-to-stand training in subjects with stroke: a randomized controlled trial. Clin Rehabil 24: 533–542.
56. Varoqui D, Froger J, Pelissier J, Bardy B (2011) Effect of coordination biofeedback on (re)learning preferred postural patterns in post-stroke patients. Motor Control 15: 187–205.
57. Engardt M, Ribbe T, Olsson E (1993) Vertical ground reaction force feedback to enhance stroke patients' symmetrical body-weight distribution while rising/sitting down. Scand J Rehabil Med 25: 41–48.
58. Bayouk J, Boucher J, Leroux A (2006) Balance training following stroke: effects of task-oriented exercises with and without altered sensory input. Int J Rehabil Res 29: 51–59.

59. Bagley P, Hudson M, Forster A, Smith J, Young J (2005) A randomized trial evaluation of the Oswestry Standing Frame for patients after stroke. Clin Rehabil 19: 354–364.

60. Morioka S, Yagi F (2003) Effects of perceptual learning exercises on standing balance using a hardness discrimination task in hemiplegic patients following stroke: a randomized controlled pilot trial. Clin Rehabil 17: 600–607.

61. Allison R, Dennett R (2007) Pilot randomized controlled trial to assess the impact of additional supported standing practice on functional ability post stroke. Clin Rehabil 21: 614–619.

62. Chen I, Cheng P, Chen C, Chen S, Chung C, et al. (2002) Effects of balance training on hemiplegic stroke patients. Chang Gung Med J 25: 583–590.

63. Sackley C, Lincoln N (1997) Single blind randomized controlled trial of visual feedback after stroke: effects on stance symmetry and function. Disabil Rehabil 19: 536–546.

64. Yavuzer G, Eser F, Karakus D, Karaoglan B, Stam H (2006) The effects of balance training on gait late after stroke: a randomized controlled trial. Clin Rehabil 20: 960–969.

65. Eser F, Yavuzer G, Karakus D, Karaoglan B (2008) The effect of balance training on motor recovery and ambulation after stroke: a randomized controlled trial. Eur J Phys Rehabil Med 44: 19–25.

66. Gok H, Alptekin N, Geler-Kulcu D, Dincer G (2008) Efficacy of treatment with a kinaesthetic ability training device on balance and mobility after stroke: a randomized controlled study. Clin Rehabil 22: 922–930.

67. Goljar N, Burger H, Rudolf M, Stanonik I (2010) Improving balance in subacute stroke patients: a randomized controlled study. Int J Rehabil Res 33: 205–210.

68. Shumway-Cook A, Anson D, Haller S (1988) Postural sway biofeedback: its effect on reestablishing stance stability in hemiplegic patients. Arch Phys Med Rehabil 69: 395–400.

69. Grant T, Brouwer B, Culham E (1997) Balance retraining following acute stroke: a comparison of two methods. Can J Rehabil 11: 69–73.

70. Walker C, Brouwer B, Culham E (2000) Use of visual feedback in retraining balance following acute stroke. Phys Ther 80: 886–895.

71. Geiger R, Allen J, O'Keefe J, Hicks R (2001) Balance and mobility following stroke: effects of physical therapy interventions with and without biofeedback/forceplate training. Phys Ther 81: 995–1005.

72. Kerdoncuff V, Durufle A, Petrilli S, Nicolas B, Robineau S, et al. (2004) [Interest of visual biofeedback training in rehabilitation of balance after stroke]. Ann Readapt Med Phys 47: 169–176.

73. Heller F, Beuret-Blanquart F, Weber J (2005) [Postural biofeedback and locomotion reeducation in stroke patients]. Ann Readapt Med Phys 48: 187–195.

74. Merkert J, Butz S, Nieczaj R, Steinhagen-Thiessen E, Eckardt R (2011) Combined whole body vibration and balance training using Vibrosphere(R): Improvement of trunk stability, muscle tone, and postural control in stroke patients during early geriatric rehabilitation. Z Gerontol Geriatr 44: 256–261.

75. Holmgren E, Gosman-Hedström G, Lindström B, Wester P (2010) What is the benefit of a high-intensive exercise program on health-related quality of life and depression after stroke? A randomized controlled trial. Adv Physiother 12: 115–124.

76. Karthikbabu S, Nayak A, Vijayakumar K, Misri Z, Suresh B, et al. (2011) Comparison of physio ball and plinth trunk exercises regimens on trunk control and functional balance in patients with acute stroke: a pilot randomized controlled trial. Clin Rehabil 25: 709–719.

77. Cheng P, Wu S, Liaw M, Wong A, Tang F (2001) Symmetrical body-weight distribution training in stroke patients and its effect on fall prevention. Arch Phys Med Rehabil 82: 1650–1654.

78. Bonan I, Yelnik A, Colle F, Michaud C, Normand E, et al. (2004) Reliance on visual information after stroke. Part II: Effectiveness of a balance rehabilitation program with visual cue deprivation after stroke: a randomized controlled trial. Arch Phys Med Rehabil 85: 274–278.

79. McClellan R, Ada L (2004) A six-week, resource-efficient mobility program after discharge from rehabilitation improves standing in people affected by stroke: placebo-controlled, randomised trial. Aust J Physiother 50: 163–167.

80. Howe T, Taylor I, Finn P, Jones H (2005) Lateral weight transference exercises following acute stroke: a preliminary study of clinical effectiveness. Clin Rehabil 19: 45–53.

81. Marigold D, Eng J, Dawson A, Inglis J, Harris J, et al. (2005) Exercise leads to faster postural reflexes, improved balance and mobility, and fewer falls in older persons with chronic stroke. J Am Geriatr Soc 53: 416–423.

82. Yelnik A, Le Breton F, Colle F, Bonan I, Hugeron C, et al. (2008) Rehabilitation of balance after stroke with multisensorial training: a single-blind randomized controlled study. Neurorehabil Neural Repair 22: 468–476.

83. Verheyden G, Vereeck L, Truijen S, Troch M, Lafosse C, et al. (2009) Additional exercises improve trunk performance after stroke: a pilot randomized controlled trial. Neurorehabil Neural Repair 23: 281–286.

84. Askim T, Morkved S, Engen A, Roos K, Aas T, et al. (2010) Effects of a community-based intensive motor training program combined with early supported discharge after treatment in a comprehensive stroke unit: a randomized, controlled trial. Stroke 41: 1697–1703.

85. Kosak M, Reding M (2000) Comparison of partial body weight-supported treadmill gait training versus aggressive bracing assisted walking post stroke. Neurorehabil Neural Repair 14: 13–19.

86. Teixeira da Cunha Filho I, Lim P, Qureshy H, Henson H, Monga T, et al. (2001) A comparison of regular rehabilitation and regular rehabilitation with supported treadmill ambulation training for acute stroke patients. J Rehabil Res Dev 38: 245–255.

87. Da Cunha Jr I, Lim P, Qureshy H, Henson H, Monga T, et al. (2002) Gait outcomes after acute stroke rehabilitation with supported treadmill ambulation training: a randomized controlled pilot study. Arch Phys Med Rehabil 83: 1258–1265.

88. Eich H, Mach H, Werner C, Hesse S (2004) Aerobic treadmill plus Bobath walking training improves walking in subacute stroke: a randomized controlled trial. Clin Rehabil 18: 640–651.

89. Dean C, Ada L, Bampton J, Morris M, Katrak P, et al. (2010) Treadmill walking with body weight support in subacute non-ambulatory stroke improves walking capacity more than overground walking: a randomised trial. J Physiother 56: 97–103.

90. Yang Y, Chen I, Liao K, Huang C, Wang R (2010) Cortical reorganization induced by body weight-supported treadmill training in patients with hemiparesis of different stroke durations. Arch Phys Med Rehabil 91: 513–518.

91. Duncan PW, Sullivan KJ, Behrman AL, Azen SP, Wu SS, et al. (2011) Body-weight-supported treadmill rehabilitation after stroke. N Engl J Med 364: 2026–2036.

92. Visintin M, Barbeau H, Korner-Bitensky N, Mayo N (1998) A new approach to retrain gait in stroke patients through body weight support and treadmill stimulation. Stroke 29: 1122–1128.

93. Barbeau H, Visintin M (2003) Optimal outcomes obtained with body-weight support combined with treadmill training in stroke subjects. Arch Phys Med Rehabil 84: 1458–1465.

94. Nilsson L, Carlsson J, Danielsson A, Fugl-Meyer A, Hellström K, et al. (2001) Walking training of patients with hemiparesis at an early stage after stroke: a comparison of walking training on a treadmill with body weight support and walking training on the ground. Clin Rehabil 15: 515–527.

95. Sullivan K, Knowlton B, Dobkin B (2002) Step training with body weight support: effect of treadmill speed and practice paradigms on poststroke locomotor recovery. Arch Phys Med Rehabil 83: 683–691.

96. Werner C, Von Frankenberg S, Treig T, Konrad M, Hesse S (2002) Treadmill training with partial body weight support and an electromechanical gait trainer for restoration of gait in subacute stroke patients: a randomized crossover study. Stroke 33: 2895–2901.

97. Suputtitada A, Yooktanan P, Rarerng-Ying T (2004) Effect of partial body weight support treadmill training in chronic stroke patients. J Med Assoc Thai 87 Suppl 2: S107–S111.

98. Yagura H, Hatakenaka M, Miyai I (2006) Does therapeutic facilitation add to locomotor outcome of body weight–supported treadmill training in nonambulatory patients with stroke? A randomized controlled trial. Arch Phys Med Rehabil 87: 529–535.

99. Sullivan K, Brown D, Klassen T, Mulroy S, Ge T, et al. (2007) Effects of task-specific locomotor and strength training in adults who were ambulatory after stroke: results of the STEPS randomized clinical trial. Phys Ther 87: 1580–1602.

100. Yen C, Wang R, Liao K, Huang C, Yang Y (2008) Gait training induced change in corticomotor excitability in patients with chronic stroke. Neurorehabil Neural Repair 22: 22–30.

101. Franceschini M, Carda S, Agosti M, Antenucci R, Malgrati D, et al. (2009) Walking after stroke: what does treadmill training with body weight support add to overground gait training in patients early after stroke?: a single-blind, randomized, controlled trial. Stroke 40: 3079–3085.

102. Westlake K, Patten C (2009) Pilot study of Lokomat versus manual-assisted treadmill training for locomotor recovery post-stroke. J Neuroeng Rehabil 6: 18.

103. Ada L, Dean C, Morris M, Simpson J, Katrak P (2010) Randomized trial of treadmill walking with body weight support to establish walking in subacute stroke: the MOBILISE trial. Stroke 41: 1237–1242.

104. Moore J, Roth E, Killian C, Hornby T (2010) Locomotor training improves daily stepping activity and gait efficiency in individuals poststroke who have reached a "plateau" in recovery. Stroke 41: 129–135.

105. Takami A, Wakayama S (2010) Effects of partial body weight support while training acute stroke patients to walk backwards on a treadmill - a controlled clinical trial using randomized allocation. J Phys Ther Sci 22: 177–187.

106. Mehrholz J, Werner C, Kugler J, Pohl M (2007) Mechanical-assisted training for walking after stroke. Cochrane Database Syst Rev: CD006185.

107. Mehrholz J, Pohl M (2012) Electromechanical-assisted gait training after stroke: a systematic review comparing end-effector and exoskeleton devices. J Rehabil Med 44: 193–199.

108. Dias D, Lains J, Pereira A, Nunes R, Caldas J, et al. (2007) Can we improve gait skills in chronic hemiplegics? A randomised control trial with gait trainer. Eura Medicophys 43: 499–504.

109. Hidler J, Nichols D, Pelliccio M, Brady K, Campbell D, et al. (2009) Multicenter randomized clinical trial evaluating the effectiveness of the Lokomat in subacute stroke. Neurorehabil Neural Repair 23: 5–13.

110. Pohl M, Werner C, Holzgraefe M, Kroczek G, Mehrholz J, et al. (2007) Repetitive locomotor training and physiotherapy improve walking and basic activities of daily living after stroke: a single-blind, randomized multicentre trial (DEutsche GAngtrainerStudie, DEGAS). Clin Rehabil 21: 17–27.

111. Mehrholz J, Werner C, Hesse S, Pohl M (2008) Immediate and long-term functional impact of repetitive locomotor training as an adjunct to conventional physiotherapy for non-ambulatory patients after stroke. Disabil Rehabil 30: 830–836.

112. Peurala S, Tarkka I, Pitkänen K, Sivenius J (2005) The effectiveness of body weight-supported gait training and floor walking in patients with chronic stroke. Arch Phys Med Rehabil 86: 1557–1564.

113. Tong R, Ng M, Li L (2006) Effectiveness of gait training using an electromechanical gait trainer, with and without functional electric stimulation, in subacute stroke: a randomized controlled trial. Arch Phys Med Rehabil 87: 1298–1304.

114. Husemann B, Muller F, Krewer C, Heller S, Koenig E (2007) Effects of locomotion training with assistance of a robot-driven gait orthosis in hemiparetic patients after stroke: a randomized controlled pilot study. Stroke 38: 349–354.

115. Mayr A, Kofler M, Quirbach E, Matzak H, Frohlich K, et al. (2007) Prospective, blinded, randomized crossover study of gait rehabilitation in stroke patients using the Lokomat gait orthosis. Neurorehabil Neural Repair 21: 307–314.

116. Hornby T, Campbell D, Kahn J, Demott T, Moore J, et al. (2008) Enhanced gait-related improvements after therapist- versus robotic-assisted locomotor training in subjects with chronic stroke: a randomized controlled study. Stroke 39: 1786–1792.

117. Lewek M, Cruz T, Moore J, Roth H, Dhaher Y, et al. (2009) Allowing intralimb kinematic variability during locomotor training poststroke improves kinematic consistency: a subgroup analysis from a randomized clinical trial. Phys Ther 89: 829–839.

118. Ng M, Tong R, Li L (2008) A pilot study of randomized clinical controlled trial of gait training in subacute stroke patients with partial body-weight support electromechanical gait trainer and functional electrical stimulation: six-month follow-up. Stroke 39: 154–160.

119. Peurala S, Airaksinen O, Huuskonen P, Jakala P, Juhakoski M, et al. (2009) Effects of intensive therapy using gait trainer or floor walking exercises early after stroke. J Rehabil Med 41: 166–173.

120. Schwartz I, Sajin A, Fisher I, Neeb M, Shochina M, et al. (2009) The effectiveness of locomotor therapy using robotic-assisted gait training in subacute stroke patients: a randomized controlled trial. PM R 1: 516–523.

121. Fisher S, Lucas L, Thrasher T (2011) Robot-assisted gait training for patients with hemiparesis due to stroke. Top Stroke Rehabil 18: 269–276.

122. Morone G, Bragoni M, Iosa M, De Angelis D, Venturiero V, et al. (2011) Who may benefit from robotic-assisted gait training? A randomized clinical trial in patients with subacute stroke. Neurorehabil Neural Repair 25: 636–644.

123. Chang W, Kim M, Huh J, Lee P, Kim Y (2012) Effects of robot-assisted gait training on cardiopulmonary fitness in subacute stroke patients: a randomized controlled study. Neurorehabil Neural Repair 26: 318–324.

124. Ivey F, Hafer-Macko C, Ryan A, Macko R (2010) Impaired leg vasodilatory function after stroke: adaptations with treadmill exercise training. Stroke 41: 2913–2917.

125. Olawale O, Jaja S, Anigbogu C, Appiah-Kubi K, Jones-Okai D (2011) Exercise training improves walking function in an African group of stroke survivors: a randomized controlled trial. Clin Rehabil 25: 442–450.

126. Langhammer B, Stanghelle J (2010) Exercise on a treadmill or walking outdoors? A randomized controlled trial comparing effectiveness of two walking exercise programmes late after stroke. Clin Rehabil 24: 46–54.

127. Kuys S, Brauer S, Ada L (2011) Higher-intensity treadmill walking during rehabilitation after stroke is feasible and not detrimental to walking pattern or quality: a pilot randomized trial. Clin Rehabil 25: 316–326.

128. Liston R, Mickelborough J, Harris B, Hann A, Tallis R (2000) Conventional physiotherapy and treadmill re-training for higher-level gait disorders in cerebrovascular disease. Age Ageing 29: 311–318.

129. Laufer Y, Dickstein R, Chefez Y, Marcovitz E (2001) The effect of treadmill training on the ambulation of stroke survivors in the early stages of rehabilitation: a randomized study. J Rehabil Res Dev 38: 69–78.

130. Pohl M, Mehrholz J, Ritschel C, Ruckriem S (2002) Speed-dependent treadmill training in ambulatory hemiparetic stroke patients: a randomized controlled trial. Stroke 33: 553–558.

131. Ada L, Dean C, Hall J, Bampton J, Crompton S (2003) A treadmill and overground walking program improves walking in persons residing in the community after stroke: a placebo-controlled, randomized trial. Arch Phys Med Rehabil 84: 1486–1491.

132. Macko R, Ivey F, Forrester L, Hanley D, Sorkin J, et al. (2005) Treadmill exercise rehabilitation improves ambulatory function and cardiovascular fitness in patients with chronic stroke: a randomized, controlled trial. Stroke 36: 2206–2211.

133. Ivey F, Ryan A, Hafer-Macko C, Goldberg A, Macko R (2007) Treadmill aerobic training improves glucose tolerance and indices of insulin sensitivity in disabled stroke survivors: a preliminary report. Stroke 38: 2752–2758.

134. Luft A, Macko R, Forrester L, Villagra F, Ivey F, et al. (2008) Treadmill exercise activates subcortical neural networks and improves walking after stroke: a randomized controlled trial. Stroke 39: 3341–3350.

135. Ivey F, Ryan A, Hafer-Macko C, Macko R (2011) Improved cerebral vasomotor reactivity after exercise training in hemiparetic stroke survivors. Stroke 42: 1994–2000.

136. Lau K, Mak M (2011) Speed-dependent treadmill training is effective to improve gait and balance performance in patients with sub-acute stroke. J Rehabil Med 43: 709–713.

137. States R, Pappas E, Salem Y (2009) Overground physical therapy gait training for chronic stroke patients with mobility deficits. Cochrane Database Syst Rev: CD006075.

138. Patil P, Rao S (2011) Effects of Thera-Band elastic resistance-assisted gait training in stroke patients: a pilot study. Eur J Phys Rehabil Med 47: 427–433.

139. Green J, Forster A, Bogle S, Young J (2002) Physiotherapy for patients with mobility problems more than 1 year after stroke: a randomised controlled trial. Lancet 359: 199–203.

140. Salbach N, Mayo N, Wood-Dauphinee S, Hanley J, Richards C, et al. (2004) A task-orientated intervention enhances walking distance and speed in the first year post stroke: a randomized controlled trial. Clin Rehabil 18: 509–519.

141. Salbach N, Mayo N, Robichaud-Ekstrand S, Hanley J, Richards C, et al. (2005) The effect of a task-oriented walking intervention on improving balance self-efficacy poststroke: a randomized, controlled trial. J Am Geriatr Soc 53: 576–582.

142. Pang M, Eng J, Dawson A, McKay H, Harris J (2005) A community-based fitness and mobility exercise program for older adults with chronic stroke: a randomized, controlled trial. J Am Geriatr Soc 53: 1667–1674.

143. Pang M, Harris J, Eng J (2006) A community-based upper-extremity group exercise program improves motor function and performance of functional activities in chronic stroke: a randomized controlled trial. Arch Phys Med Rehabil 87: 1–9.

144. Wall J, Turnbull G (1987) Evaluation of out-patient physiotherapy and a home exercise program in the management of gait asymmetry in residual stroke. Neurorehabil Neural Repair 1: 115–123.

145. Wade D, Collen F, Robb G, Warlow C (1992) Physiotherapy intervention late after stroke and mobility. BMJ 304: 609–613.

146. Dean C, Richards C, Malouin F (2000) Task-related circuit training improves performance of locomotor tasks in chronic stroke: a randomized, controlled pilot trial. Arch Phys Med Rehabil 81: 409–417.

147. Lin J, Hsieh C, Lo S, Chai H, Liao L (2004) Preliminary study of the effect of low-intensity home-based physical therapy in chronic stroke patients. Kaohsiung J Med Sci 20: 18–23.

148. Yang Y, Yen J, Wang R, Yen L, Lieu F (2005) Gait outcomes after additional backward walking training in patients with stroke: a randomized controlled trial. Clin Rehabil 19: 264–273.

149. Yang Y, Wang R, Chen Y, Kao M (2007) Dual-task exercise improves walking ability in chronic stroke: a randomized controlled trial. Arch Phys Med Rehabil 88: 1236–1240.

150. Sungkarat S, Fisher B, Kovindha A (2011) Efficacy of an insole shoe wedge and augmented pressure sensor for gait training in individuals with stroke: a randomized controlled trial. Clin Rehabil 25: 360–369.

151. Thaut M, McIntosh G, Rice R (1997) Rhythmic facilitation of gait training in hemiparetic stroke rehabilitation. J Neurol Sci 151: 207–212.

152. Mandel A, Nymark J, Balmer S, Grinnell D, O'Riain M (1990) Electromyographic versus rhythmic positional biofeedback in computerized gait retraining with stroke patients. Arch Phys Med Rehabil 71: 649–654.

153. Schauer M, Mauritz K (2003) Musical motor feedback (MMF) in walking hemiparetic stroke patients: randomized trials of gait improvement. Clin Rehabil 17: 713–722.

154. Thaut M, Leins A, Rice R, Argstatter H, Kenyon G, et al. (2007) Rhythmic auditory stimulation improves gait more than NDT/Bobath training in near-ambulatory patients early poststroke: a single-blind, randomized trial. Neurorehabil Neural Repair 21: 455–459.

155. Argstatter H, Hillecke T, Thaut M, Bolay H (2007) Music therapy in motor rehabilitation. Evaluation of a musicomedical gait training programfor hemiparetic stroke patients [Musiktherapie in der neurologischen Rehabilitation. Evaluation eines musikmedizinischen Behandlungskonzepts für die Gangrehabilitation von hemiparetischen Patienten nach Schlaganfall]. Neurol Rehabil 13: 159–165.

156. Jeong S, Kim M (2007) Effects of a theory-driven music and movement program for stroke survivors in a community setting. Appl Nurs Res 20: 125–131.

157. Lord S, McPherson K, McNaughton H, Rochester L, Weatherall M (2008) How feasible is the attainment of community ambulation after stroke? A pilot randomized controlled trial to evaluate community-based physiotherapy in subacute stroke. Clin Rehabil 22: 215–225.

158. Park H, Oh D, Kim S, Choi J (2011) Effectiveness of community-based ambulation training for walking function of post-stroke hemiparesis: a randomized controlled pilot trial. Clin Rehabil 25: 451–459.

159. Henderson A, Korner-Bitensky N, Levin M (2007) Virtual reality in stroke rehabilitation: a systematic review of its effectiveness for upper limb motor recovery. Top Stroke Rehabil 14: 52–61.

160. Saposnik G, Levin M (2011) Virtual reality in stroke rehabilitation: a meta-analysis and implications for clinicians. Stroke 42: 1380–1386.

161. Jaffe D, Brown D, Pierson-Carey C, Buckley E, Lew H (2004) Stepping over obstacles to improve walking in individuals with poststroke hemiplegia. J Rehabil Res Dev 41: 283–292.

162. You S, Jang S, Kim Y, Hallett M, Ahn S, et al. (2005) Virtual reality-induced cortical reorganization and associated locomotor recovery in chronic stroke: an experimenter-blind randomized study. Stroke 36: 1166–1171.

163. Kim J, Jang S, Kim C, Jung J, You J (2009) Use of virtual reality to enhance balance and ambulation in chronic stroke: a double-blind, randomized controlled study. Am J Phys Med Rehabil 88: 693–701.

164. Lam Y, Man D, Tam S, Weiss P (2006) Virtual reality training for stroke rehabilitation. NeuroRehabilitation 21: 245–253.

165. Yang Y, Tsai M, Chuang T, Sung W, Wang R (2008) Virtual reality-based training improves community ambulation in individuals with stroke: a randomized controlled trial. Gait Posture 28: 201–206.

166. Mirelman A, Bonato P, Deutsch J (2009) Effects of training with a robot-virtual reality system compared with a robot alone on the gait of individuals after stroke. Stroke 40: 169–174.

167. Mirelman A, Patritti B, Bonato P, Deutsch J (2010) Effects of virtual reality training on gait biomechanics of individuals post-stroke. Gait Posture 31: 433–437.

168. Wevers L, Van de Port I, Vermue M, Mead G, Kwakkel G (2009) Effects of task-oriented circuit class training on walking competency after stroke: a systematic review. Stroke 40: 2450–2459.

169. English C, Hillier S (2010) Circuit class therapy for improving mobility after stroke. Cochrane Database Syst Rev: CD007513.

170. Blennerhassett J, Dite W (2004) Additional task-related practice improves mobility and upper limb function early after stroke: a randomised controlled trial. Aust J Physiother 50: 219–224.

171. Mead G, Greig C, Cunningham I, Lewis S, Dinan S, et al. (2007) Stroke: a randomized trial of exercise or relaxation. J Am Geriatr Soc 55: 892–899.

172. Yang Y, Wang R, Lin K, Chu M, Chan R (2006) Task-oriented progressive resistance strength training improves muscle strength and functional performance in individuals with stroke. Clin Rehabil 20: 860–870.

173. Mudge S, Barber P, Stott N (2009) Circuit-based rehabilitation improves gait endurance but not usual walking activity in chronic stroke: a randomized controlled trial. Arch Phys Med Rehabil 90: 1989–1996.

174. Galvin R, Cusack T, O'Grady E, Murphy T, Stokes E (2011) Family-mediated exercise intervention (FAME): evaluation of a novel form of exercise delivery after stroke. Stroke 42: 681–686.

175. Kalra L, Evans A, Perez I, Melbourn A, Patel A, et al. (2004) Training carers of stroke patients: randomised controlled trial. BMJ 328: 1099.

176. Wright P, Mann G, Swain I (2004) A comparison of electrical stimulation and the conventional ankle foot orthosis in the correction of a dropped foot following stroke. Final report to funder.

177. Beckerman H, Becher J, Lankhorst G, Verbeek A, Vogelaar T (1996) The efficacy of thermocoagulation of the tibial nerve and a polypropylene ankle-foot orthosis on spasticity of the leg in stroke patients: results of a randomized clinical trial. Clin Rehabil 10: 112–120.

178. Erel S, Uygur F, Engin Simsek I, Yakut Y (2011) The effects of dynamic ankle-foot orthoses in chronic stroke patients at three-month follow-up: a randomized controlled trial. Clin Rehabil 25: 515–523.

179. Mehrholz J, Kugler J, Pohl M (2011) Water-based exercises for improving activities of daily living after stroke. Cochrane Database Syst Rev: CD008186.

180. Aidar F, Silva A, Reis V, Carneiro A, Carneiro-Cotta S (2007) A study of the quality of life in ischemic vascular accidents and its relation to physical activity [Estudio de la calidad de vida en el accidente vascular isquémico y sur relación con la actividad física]. Rev Neurol 45: 518–522.

181. Noh D, Lim J, Shin H, Paik N (2008) The effect of aquatic therapy on postural balance and muscle strength in stroke survivors–a randomized controlled pilot trial. Clin Rehabil 22: 966–976.

182. Chu K, Eng J, Dawson A, Harris J, Ozkaplan A, et al. (2004) Water-based exercise for cardiovascular fitness in people with chronic stroke: a randomized controlled trial. Arch Phys Med Rehabil 85: 870–874.

183. Doyle S, Bennett S, Fasoli S, McKenna K (2010) Interventions for sensory impairment in the upper limb after stroke. Cochrane Database Syst Rev: CD006331.

184. Intercollegiate Stroke Working Party (2012) National clinical guideline for stroke, 4th edition. London: Royal College of Physicians.

185. Torriani C, Mota E, Moreira Sales A, Ricci M, Nishida P, et al. (2008) Effect of foot motor and sensorial stimulation hemiparetic in stroke patients. Rev Neurocienc 16: 25–29.

186. Yavuzer G, Oken O, Atay M, Stam H (2007) Effects of sensory-amplitude electric stimulation on motor recovery and gait kinematics after stroke: a randomized controlled study. Arch Phys Med Rehabil 88: 710–714.

187. Lynch E, Hillier S, Stiller K, Campanella R, Fisher P (2007) Sensory retraining of the lower limb after acute stroke: a randomized controlled pilot trial. Arch Phys Med Rehabil 88: 1101–1107.

188. Wu H, Lin Y, Hsu M, Liu S, Hsieh C, et al. (2010) Effect of thermal stimulation on upper extremity motor recovery 3 months after stroke. Stroke 41: 2378–2380.

189. Chen J, Lin C, Wei Y, Hsiao J, Liang C (2011) Facilitation of motor and balance recovery by thermal intervention for the paretic lower limb of acute stroke: a single-blind randomized clinical trial. Clin Rehabil 25: 823–832.

190. Pomeroy V, King L, Pollock A, Baily-Hallam A, Langhorne P (2006) Electrostimulation for promoting recovery of movement or functional ability after stroke. Cochrane Database Syst Rev: CD003241.

191. Bakhtiary A, Fatemy E (2008) Does electrical stimulation reduce spasticity after stroke? A randomized controlled study. Clin Rehabil 22: 418–425.

192. Ambrosini E, Ferrante S, Pedrocchi A, Ferrigno G, Molteni F (2011) Cycling induced by electrical stimulation improves motor recovery in postacute hemiparetic patients: a randomized controlled trial. Stroke 42: 1068–1073.

193. Merletti R, Zelaschi F, Latella D, Galli M, Angeli S, et al. (1978) A control study of muscle force recovery in hemiparetic patients during treatment with functional electrical stimulation. Scand J Rehabil Med 10: 147–154.

194. Cozean C, Pease W, Hubbell S (1988) Biofeedback and functional electric stimulation in stroke rehabilitation. Arch Phys Med Rehabil 69: 401–405.

195. Winchester P, Montgomery J, Bowman B, Hislop H (1983) Effects of feedback stimulation training and cyclical electrical stimulation on knee extension in hemiparetic patients. Phys Ther 63: 1096–1103.

196. Macdonell R, Triggs W, Leikauskas J, Bourque M, Robb K, et al. (1994) Functional electrical stimulation to the affected lower limb and recovery after cerebral infarction. J Stroke Cerebrovasc Dis 4: 155–160.

197. Bogataj U, Gros N, Kljajic M, Acimovic R, Malezic M (1995) The rehabilitation of gait in patients with hemiplegia: a comparison between conventional therapy and multichannel functional electrical stimulation therapy. Phys Ther 75: 490–502.

198. Burridge J, Taylor P, Hagan S, Wood D, Swain I (1997) The effects of common peroneal stimulation on the effort and speed of walking: a randomized controlled trial with chronic hemiplegic patients. Clin Rehabil 11: 201–210.

199. Heckmann J, Mokrusch T, Krockel A, Warnke S, Neundorfer B (1997) EMG-triggered electrical muscle stimulation in the treatment of central hemiparesis after a stroke. Eur J Phys Med Rehabil 7: 138–141.

200. Tekeoglu Y, Adak B, Goksoy T (1998) Effect of transcutaneous electrical nerve stimulation (TENS) on Barthel Activities of Daily Living (ADL) index score following stroke. Clin Rehabil 12: 277–280.

201. Newsam C, Baker L (2004) Effect of an electric stimulation facilitation program on quadriceps motor unit recruitment after stroke. Arch Phys Med Rehabil 85: 2040–2045.

202. Chen S, Chen Y, Chen C, Lai C, Chiang W, et al. (2005) Effects of surface electrical stimulation on the muscle-tendon junction of spastic gastrocnemius in stroke patients. Disabil Rehabil 27: 105–110.

203. Yan T, Hui-Chan C, Li L (2005) Functional electrical stimulation improves motor recovery of the lower extremity and walking ability of subjects with first acute stroke: a randomized placebo-controlled trial. Stroke 36: 80–85.

204. Yavuzer G, Geler-Kulcu D, Sonel-Tur B, Kutlay S, Ergin S, et al. (2006) Neuromuscular electric stimulation effect on lower-extremity motor recovery and gait kinematics of patients with stroke: a randomized controlled trial. Arch Phys Med Rehabil 87: 536–540.

205. Ng S, Hui-Chan C (2007) Transcutaneous electrical nerve stimulation combined with task-related training improves lower limb functions in subjects with chronic stroke. Stroke 38: 2953–2959.

206. Ferrante S, Pedrocchi A, Ferrigno G, Molteni F (2008) Cycling induced by functional electrical stimulation improves the muscular strength and the motor control of individuals with post-acute stroke. Europa Medicophysica-SIMFER 2007 Award Winner. Eur J Phys Rehabil Med 44: 159–167.

207. Janssen T, Beltman J, Elich P, Koppe P, Konijnenbelt H, et al. (2008) Effects of electric stimulation-assisted cycling training in people with chronic stroke. Arch Phys Med Rehabil 89: 463–469.

208. Kojovic J, Djuric-Jovicic M, Dosen S, Popovic M, Popovic D (2009) Sensor-driven four-channel stimulation of paretic leg: functional electrical walking therapy. J Neurosci Methods 181: 100–105.

209. Mesci N, Ozdemir F, Kabayel D, Tokuc B (2009) The effects of neuromuscular electrical stimulation on clinical improvement in hemiplegic lower extremity rehabilitation in chronic stroke: a single-blind, randomised, controlled trial. Disabil Rehabil 31: 2047–2054.

210. Ng SS, Hui-Chan CW (2009) Does the use of TENS increase the effectiveness of exercise for improving walking after stroke? A randomized controlled clinical trial. Clin Rehabil 23: 1093–1103.

211. Hui-Chan C, Ng S, Mak M (2009) Effectiveness of a home-based rehabilitation programme on lower limb functions after stroke. Hong Kong Med J 15: 42–46.

212. Yan T, Hui-Chan C (2009) Transcutaneous electrical stimulation on acupuncture points improves muscle function in subjects after acute stroke: a randomized controlled trial. J Rehabil Med 41: 312–316.

213. Cheng J, Yang Y, Cheng S, Lin P, Wang R (2010) Effects of combining electric stimulation with active ankle dorsiflexion while standing on a rocker board: a pilot study for subjects with spastic foot after stroke. Arch Phys Med Rehabil 91: 505–512.

214. Moreland J, Thomson M, Fuoco A (1998) Electromyographic biofeedback to improve lower extremity function after stroke: a meta-analysis. Arch Phys Med Rehabil 79: 134–140.

215. Woodford H, Price C (2007) EMG biofeedback for the recovery of motor function after stroke. Cochrane Database Syst Rev: CD004585.

216. John J (1986) Failure of electrical myofeedback to augment the effects of physiotherapy in stroke. Int J Rehabil Res 9: 35–45.

217. Jonsdottir J, Cattaneo D, Recalcati M, Regola A, Rabuffetti M, et al. (2010) Task-oriented biofeedback to improve gait in individuals with chronic stroke: motor learning approach. Neurorehabil Neural Repair 24: 478–485.

218. Basmajian J, Kukulka C, Narayan M, Takebe K (1975) Biofeedback treatment of foot-drop after stroke compared with standard rehabilitation technique: effects on voluntary control and strength. Arch Phys Med Rehabil 56: 231–236.

219. Hurd W, Pegram V, Nepomuceno C (1980) Comparison of actual and simulated EMG biofeedback in the treatment of hemiplegic patients. Am J Phys Med 59: 73–82.

220. Binder S, Moll C, Wolf S (1981) Evaluation of electromyographic biofeedback as an adjunct to therapeutic exercise in treating the lower extremities of hemiplegic patients. Phys Ther 61: 886–893.

221. Mulder T, Hulstijn W, Van der Meer J (1986) EMG feedback and the restoration of motor control. A controlled group study of 12 hemiparetic patients. Am J Phys Med 65: 173–188.

222. Colborne G, Olney S, Griffin M (1993) Feedback of ankle joint angle and soleus electromyography in the rehabilitation of hemiplegic gait. Arch Phys Med Rehabil 74: 1100–1106.

223. Intiso D, Santilli V, Grasso M, Rossi R, Caruso I (1994) Rehabilitation of walking with electromyographic biofeedback in foot-drop after stroke. Stroke 25: 1189–1192.

224. Bradley L, Hart B, Mandana S, Flowers K, Riches M, et al. (1998) Electromyographic biofeedback for gait training after stroke. Clin Rehabil 12: 11–22.

225. Ploughman M, Corbett D (2004) Can forced-use therapy be clinically applied after stroke? An exploratory randomized controlled trial. Arch Phys Med Rehabil 85: 1417–1423.

226. Hammer A, Lindmark B (2009) Is forced use of the paretic upper limb beneficial? A randomized pilot study during subacute post-stroke recovery. Clin Rehabil 23: 424–433.

227. Hu X, Tong K, Song R, Zheng X, Leung W (2009) A comparison between electromyography-driven robot and passive motion device on wrist rehabilitation for chronic stroke. Neurorehabil Neural Repair 23: 837–846.

228. Kutner N, Zhang R, Butler A, Wolf S, Alberts J (2010) Quality-of-life change associated with robotic-assisted therapy to improve hand motor function in patients with subacute stroke: a randomized clinical trial. Phys Ther 90: 493–504.

229. Takahashi C, Der-Yeghiaian L, Le V, Motiwala R, Cramer S (2008) Robot-based hand motor therapy after stroke. Brain 131: 425–437.

230. Lynch D, Ferraro M, Krol J, Trudell C, Christos P, et al. (2005) Continuous passive motion improves shoulder joint integrity following stroke. Clin Rehabil 19: 594–599.

231. Stein J, Hughes R, D'Andrea S, Therrien B, Niemi J, et al. (2010) Stochastic resonance stimulation for upper limb rehabilitation poststroke. Am J Phys Med Rehabil 89: 697–705.

232. Stinear C, Barber P, Coxon J, Fleming M, Byblow W (2008) Priming the motor system enhances the effects of upper limb therapy in chronic stroke. Brain 131: 1381–1390.

233. Wang T, Wang X, Wang H, He X, Su J, et al. (2007) Effects of ULEM apparatus on motor function of patients with stroke. Brain Inj 21: 1203–1208.

234. Hesse S, Werner C, Pohl M, Merholz J, Puzich U, et al. (2008) Mechanical arm trainer for the treatment of the severely affected arm after a stroke: a single-blinded randomized trial in two centers. Am J Phys Med Rehabil 87: 779–788.

235. Turton A, Britton E (2005) A pilot randomized controlled trial of a daily muscle stretch regime to prevent contractures in the arm after stroke. Clin Rehabil 19: 600–612.

236. Gustafsson L, McKenna K (2006) A programme of static positional stretches does not reduce hemiplegic shoulder pain or maintain shoulder range of motion–a randomized controlled trial. Clin Rehabil 20: 277–286.

237. Dean C, Mackey F, Katrak P (2000) Examination of shoulder positioning after stroke: A randomised controlled pilot trial. Aust J Physiother 46: 35–40.

238. Ada L, Goddard E, McCully J, Stavrinos T, Bampton J (2005) Thirty minutes of positioning reduces the development of shoulder external rotation contracture after stroke: a randomized controlled trial. Arch Phys Med Rehabil 86: 230–234.

239. De Jong L, Nieuwboer A, Aufdemkampe G (2006) Contracture preventive positioning of the hemiplegic arm in subacute stroke patients: a pilot randomized controlled trial. Clin Rehabil 20: 656–667.

240. Rose V, Shah S (1980) A comparative study on the immediate effects of hand orthosis on reduction of hypertonus. Aust Occup Ther J 34: 59–64.

241. Lannin N, Cusick A, McCluskey A, Herbert H (2007) Effects of splinting on wrist contracture after stroke: a randomized controlled trial. Stroke 38: 111–116.

242. Bürge E, Kupper D, Finckh A, Ryerson S, Schnider A, et al. (2008) Neutral functional realignment orthosis prevents hand pain in patients with subacute stroke: a randomized trial. Arch Phys Med Rehabil 89: 1857–1862.

243. Carey J (1990) Manual stretch: effect on finger movement control and force control in stroke subjects with spastic extrinsic finger flexor muscles. Arch Phys Med Rehabil 71: 888–894.

244. Langlois S, Pederson L, MacKinnon J (1991) The effects of splinting on the spastic hemiplegic hand: report of a feasible study. Can J Occup Ther 58: 17–25.

245. Sheehan J, Winzeler-Mercay U, Mudie M (2006) A randomized controlled pilot study to obtain the best estimate of the size of the effect of a thermoplastic resting splint on spasticity in the stroke-affected wrist and fingers. Clin Rehabil 20: 1032–1037.

246. Heidari M, Eghlidi Z, About Talebi S, Hosseini S, Rahimifard H, et al. (2011) Comparison of mobilizing and immobilizing splints on hand motor function in stroke patients: a randomized clinical trial. QOM University Med Sci J 4: 48–53.

247. Suat E, Engin S, Nilgun B, Yavuz Y, Fatma U (2011) Short- and long-term effects of an inhibitor hand splint in poststroke patients: a randomized controlled trial. Top Stroke Rehabil 18: 231–237.

248. Robichaud J, Agostinucci J, Van der Linden D (1992) Effect of air-splint application on soleus muscle motoneuron reflex excitability in nondisabled subjects and subjects with cerebrovascular accidents. Phys Ther 72: 176–183.

249. Johnstone M (1989) Current advances in the use of pressure splints in the management of adult hemiplegia. Physiotherapy 75: 381–384.

250. Feys H, De Weerdt W, Selz B, Cox Steck G, Spichiger R, et al. (1998) Effect of a therapeutic intervention for the hemiplegic upper limb in the acute phase after stroke: a single-blind, randomized, controlled multicenter trial. Stroke 29: 785–792.

251. Feys H, De Weerdt W, Verbeke G, Steck G, Capiau C, et al. (2004) Early and repetitive stimulation of the arm can substantially improve the long-term outcome after stroke: a 5-year follow-up study of a randomized trial. Stroke 35: 924–929.

252. Platz T, Van Kaick S, Mehrholz J, Leidner O, Eickhof C, et al. (2009) Best conventional therapy versus modular impairment-oriented training for arm paresis after stroke: a single-blind, multicenter randomized controlled trial. Neurorehabil Neural Repair 23: 706–716.

253. Poole J, Whitney S, Hangeland N, Baker C (1990) The effectiveness of inflatable pressure splints on motor function in stroke patients. Occup Ther J Res 10: 360–366.

254. Roper T, Redford S, Tallis R (1999) Intermittent compression for the treatment of the oedematous hand in hemiplegic stroke: a randomized controlled trial. Age Ageing 28: 9–13.

255. Cambier D, De Corte E, Danneels L, Witvrouw E (2003) Treating sensory impairments in the post-stroke upper limb with intermittent pneumatic compression. Results of a preliminary trial. Clin Rehabil 17: 14–20.

256. Ada L, Foongchomcheay A, Canning C (2005) Supportive devices for preventing and treating subluxation of the shoulder after stroke. Cochrane Database Syst Rev: CD003863.

257. Appel C, Mayston M, Perry J (2011) Feasibility study of a randomized controlled trial protocol to examine clinical effectiveness of shoulder strapping in acute stroke patients. Clin Rehabil 25: 833–843.

258. Hanger H, Whitewood P, Brown G, Ball M, Harper J, et al. (2000) A randomized controlled trial of strapping to prevent post-stroke shoulder pain. Clin Rehabil 14: 370–380.

259. Griffin A, Bernhardt J (2006) Strapping the hemiplegic shoulder prevents development of pain during rehabilitation: a randomized controlled trial. Clin Rehabil 20: 287–295.

260. Mudie M, Matyas T (2000) Can simultaneous bilateral movement involve the undamaged hemisphere in reconstruction of neural networks damaged by stroke? Disabil Rehabil 22: 23–37.

261. Hayner K, Gibson G, Giles G (2010) Comparison of constraint-induced movement therapy and bilateral treatment of equal intensity in people with chronic upper-extremity dysfunction after cerebrovascular accident. Am J Occup Ther 64: 528–539.

262. Wu C, Hsieh Y, Lin K, Chuang L, Chang Y, et al. (2010) Brain reorganization after bilateral arm training and distributed constraint-induced therapy in stroke patients: a preliminary functional magnetic resonance imaging study. Chang Gung Med J 33: 628–638.

263. Morris J, Van Wijck F, Joice S, Ogston S, Cole I, et al. (2008) A comparison of bilateral and unilateral upper-limb task training in early poststroke rehabilitation: a randomized controlled trial. Arch Phys Med Rehabil 89: 1237–1245.

264. Van der Lee J, Wagenaar R, Lankhorst G, Vogelaar T, Deville W, et al. (1999) Forced use of the upper extremity in chronic stroke patients: results from a single-blind randomized clinical trial. Stroke 30: 2369–2375.

265. Mudie M, Matyas T (2001) Responses of the densely hemiplegic upper extremity to bilateral training. Neurorehabil Neural Repair 15: 129–140.

266. Platz T, Bock S, Prass K (2001) Reduced skilfulness of arm motor behaviour among motor stroke patients with good clinical recovery: does it indicate reduced automaticity? Can it be improved by unilateral or bilateral training? A kinematic motion analysis study. Neuropsychologia 39: 687–698.

267. Cauraugh J, Kim S (2002) Two coupled motor recovery protocols are better than one: electromyogram-triggered neuromuscular stimulation and bilateral movements. Stroke 33: 1589–1594.

268. Cauraugh J, Kim S (2003) Progress toward motor recovery with active neuromuscular stimulation: muscle activation pattern evidence after a stroke. J Neurol Sci 207: 25–29.

269. Luft A, McCombe-Waller S, Whitall J, Forrester L, Macko R, et al. (2004) Repetitive bilateral arm training and motor cortex activation in chronic stroke: a randomized controlled trial. JAMA 292: 1853–1861.

270. Suputtitada A, Suwanwela N, Tumvitee S (2004) Effectiveness of constraint-induced movement therapy in chronic stroke patients. J Med Assoc Thai 87: 1482–1490.

271. Cauraugh J, Kim S, Duley A (2005) Coupled bilateral movements and active neuromuscular stimulation: intralimb transfer evidence during bimanual aiming. Neurosci Lett 382: 39–44.

272. Desrosiers J, Bourbonnais D, Corriveau H, Gosselin S, Bravo G (2005) Effectiveness of unilateral and symmetrical bilateral task training for arm during the subacute phase after stroke: a randomized controlled trial. Clin Rehabil 19: 581–593.

273. Lum P, Burgar C, Van der Loos M, Shor P, Majmundar M, et al. (2006) MIME robotic device for upper-limb neurorehabilitation in subacute stroke subjects: A follow-up study. J Rehabil Res Dev 43: 631–642.

274. Summers J, Kagerer F, Garry M, Hiraga C, Loftus A, et al. (2007) Bilateral and unilateral movement training on upper limb function in chronic stroke patients: A TMS study. J Neurol Sci 252: 76–82.

275. Cauraugh J, Kim S, Summers J (2008) Chronic stroke longitudinal motor improvements: cumulative learning evidence found in the upper extremity. Cerebrovasc Dis 25: 115–121.

276. McCombe Waller S, Liu W, Whitall J (2008) Temporal and spatial control following bilateral versus unilateral training. Hum Mov Sci 27: 749–758.

277. Cauraugh J, Coombes S, Lodha N, Naik S, Summers J (2009) Upper extremity improvements in chronic stroke: coupled bilateral load training. Restor Neurol Neurosci 27: 17–25.

278. Lin K, Chang Y, Wu C, Chen Y (2009) Effects of constraint-induced therapy versus bilateral arm training on motor performance, daily functions, and quality of life in stroke survivors. Neurorehabil Neural Repair 23: 441–448.

279. Stoykov M, Lewis G, Corcos D (2009) Comparison of bilateral and unilateral training for upper extremity hemiparesis in stroke. Neurorehabil Neural Repair 23: 945–953.

280. Lin K, Chen Y, Chen C, Wu C, Chang Y (2010) The effects of bilateral arm training on motor control and functional performance in chronic stroke: a randomized controlled study. Neurorehabil Neural Repair 24: 42–51.

281. Whitall J, Waller S, Sorkin J, Forrester L, Macko R, et al. (2011) Bilateral and unilateral arm training improve motor function through differing neuroplastic mechanisms: a single-blinded randomized controlled trial. Neurorehabil Neural Repair 25: 118–129.

282. Wu C, Chuang L, Lin K, Chen H, Tsay P (2011) Randomized trial of distributed constraint-induced therapy versus bilateral arm training for the rehabilitation of upper-limb motor control and function after stroke. Neurorehabil Neural Repair 25: 130–139.

283. Page S, Sisto S, Levine P, Johnston M, Hughes M (2001) Modified constraint induced therapy: a randomized feasibility and efficacy study. J Rehabil Res Dev 38: 583–590.

284. Atteya A (2004) Effects of modified constraint induced therapy on upper limb function in subacute stroke patients. Neurosciences (Riyadh) 9: 24–29.

285. Kim D, Cho Y, Hong J, Song J, Chung H, et al. (2008) Effect of constraint-induced movement therapy with modified opposition restriction orthosis in chronic hemiparetic patients with stroke. NeuroRehabilitation 23: 239–244.

286. Dahl A, Askim T, Stock R, Langorgen E, Lydersen S, et al. (2008) Short- and long-term outcome of constraint-induced movement therapy after stroke: a randomized controlled feasibility trial. Clin Rehabil 22: 436–447.

287. Taub E, Miller N, Novack T, Cook 3rd E, Fleming W, et al. (1993) Technique to improve chronic motor deficit after stroke. Arch Phys Med Rehabil 74: 347–354.

288. Dromerick A, Edwards D, Hahn M (2000) Does the application of constraint-induced movement therapy during acute rehabilitation reduce arm impairment after ischemic stroke? Stroke 31: 2984–2988.

289. Page S, Sisto S, Johnston M, Levine P (2002) Modified constraint-induced therapy after subacute stroke: a preliminary study. Neurorehabil Neural Repair 16: 290–295.

290. Wittenberg G, Chen R, Ishii K, Bushara K, Eckloff S, et al. (2003) Constraint-induced therapy in stroke: magnetic-stimulation motor maps and cerebral activation. Neurorehabil Neural Repair 17: 48–57.

291. Alberts J, Butler A, Wolf S (2004) The effects of constraint-induced therapy on precision grip: a preliminary study. Neurorehabil Neural Repair 18: 250–258.

292. Page S, Sisto S, Levine P, McGrath R (2004) Efficacy of modified constraint-induced movement therapy in chronic stroke: a single-blinded randomized controlled trial. Arch Phys Med Rehabil 85: 14–18.

293. Page S, Levine P, Leonard A (2005) Modified constraint-induced therapy in acute stroke: a randomized controlled pilot study. Neurorehabil Neural Repair 19: 27–32.

294. Yen J, Wang R, Chen H, Hong C (2005) Effectiveness of modified constraint-induced movement therapy on upper limb function in stroke subjects. Acta Neurol Taiwan 14: 16–20.

295. Ro T, Noser E, Boake C, Johnson R, Gaber M, et al. (2006) Functional reorganization and recovery after constraint-induced movement therapy in subacute stroke: case reports. Neurocase 12: 50–60.

296. Brogardh C, Sjolund B (2006) Constraint-induced movement therapy in patients with stroke: a pilot study on effects of small group training and of extended mitt use. Clin Rehabil 20: 218–227.

297. Wolf S, Winstein C, Miller J, Taub E, Uswatte G, et al. (2006) Effect of constraint-induced movement therapy on upper extremity function 3 to 9 months after stroke: the EXCITE randomized clinical trial. JAMA 296: 2095–2104.

298. Wolf S, Thompson P, Winstein C, Miller J, Blanton S, et al. (2010) The EXCITE stroke trial: comparing early and delayed constraint-induced movement therapy. Stroke 41: 2309–2315.

299. Boake C, Noser E, Ro T, Baraniuk S, Gaber M, et al. (2007) Constraint-induced movement therapy during early stroke rehabilitation. Neurorehabil Neural Repair 21: 14–24.

300. Lin K, Wu C, Wei T, Lee C, Liu J (2007) Effects of modified constraint-induced movement therapy on reach-to-grasp movements and functional performance after chronic stroke: a randomized controlled study. Clin Rehabil 21: 1075–1086.

301. Wu C, Chen C, Tang S, Lin K, Huang Y (2007) Kinematic and clinical analyses of upper-extremity movements after constraint-induced movement therapy in patients with stroke: a randomized controlled trial. Arch Phys Med Rehabil 88: 964–970.

302. Wu C, Chen C, Tsai W, Lin K, Chou S (2007) A randomized controlled trial of modified constraint-induced movement therapy for elderly stroke survivors: changes in motor impairment, daily functioning, and quality of life. Arch Phys Med Rehabil 88: 273–278.

303. Wu C, Lin K, Chen H, Chen I, Hong W (2007) Effects of modified constraint-induced movement therapy on movement kinematics and daily function in patients with stroke: a kinematic study of motor control mechanisms. Neurorehabil Neural Repair 21: 460–466.

304. Gauthier L, Taub E, Perkins C, Ortmann M, Mark V, et al. (2008) Remodeling the brain: plastic structural brain changes produced by different motor therapies after stroke. Stroke 39: 1520–1525.

305. Myint J, Yuen G, Yu T, Kng C, Wong A, et al. (2008) A study of constraint-induced movement therapy in subacute stroke patients in Hong Kong. Clin Rehabil 22: 112–124.

306. Myint M, Yuen F, Yu K, Kng P, Wong M, et al. (2008) Use of constraint-induced movement therapy in Chinese stroke patients during the sub-acute period. Hong Kong Med J 14: 40–42.

307. Page S, Levine P, Leonard A, Szaflarski J, Kissela B (2008) Modified constraint-induced therapy in chronic stroke: results of a single-blinded randomized controlled trial. Phys Ther 88: 333–340.

308. Sawaki L, Butler A, Leng X, Wassenaar P, Mohammad Y, et al. (2008) Constraint-induced movement therapy results in increased motor map area in subjects 3 to 9 months after stroke. Neurorehabil Neural Repair 22: 505–513.

309. Azab M, Al-Jarrah M, Nazzal M, Maayah M, Sammour M, et al. (2009) Effectiveness of constraint-induced movement therapy (CIMT) as home-based therapy on Barthel Index in patients with chronic stroke. Top Stroke Rehabil 16: 207–211.

310. Brogardh C, Vestling M, Sjolund B (2009) Shortened constraint-induced movement therapy in subacute stroke - no effect of using a restraint: a randomized controlled study with independent observers. J Rehabil Med 41: 231–236.

311. Brogardh C, Lexell J (2010) A 1-year follow-up after shortened constraint-induced movement therapy with and without mitt poststroke. Arch Phys Med Rehabil 91: 460–464.

312. Dromerick A, Lang C, Birkenmeier R, Wagner J, Miller J, et al. (2009) Very Early Constraint-Induced Movement during Stroke Rehabilitation (VEC-TORS): a single-center RCT. Neurology 73: 195–201.

313. Lin K, Wu C, Liu J, Chen Y, Hsu C (2009) Constraint-induced therapy versus dose-matched control intervention to improve motor ability, basic/extended daily functions, and quality of life in stroke. Neurorehabil Neural Repair 23: 160–165.

314. Woodbury M, Howland D, McGuirk T, Davis S, Senesac C, et al. (2009) Effects of trunk restraint combined with intensive task practice on poststroke upper extremity reach and function: a pilot study. Neurorehabil Neural Repair 23: 78–91.

315. Abu Tariah H, Almalty A, Sbeih, Al-Oraibi S (2010) Constraint induced movement therapy for stroke survivors in Jordon: a home-based model. Int J Ther Rehab 17: 638–646.

316. Lin K, Chung H, Wu C, Liu H, Hsieh Y, et al. (2010) Constraint-induced therapy versus control intervention in patients with stroke: a functional magnetic resonance imaging study. Am J Phys Med Rehabil 89: 177–185.

317. Sun S, Hsu C, Sun H, Hwang C, Yang C, et al. (2010) Combined botulinum toxin type A with modified constraint-induced movement therapy for chronic stroke patients with upper extremity spasticity: a randomized controlled study. Neurorehabil Neural Repair 24: 34–41.

318. Wang Q, Zhao J, Zhu Q, Li J, Meng P (2011) Comparison of conventional therapy, intensive therapy and modified constraint-induced movement therapy to improve upper extremity function after stroke. J Rehabil Med 43: 619–625.

319. Mehrholz J, Platz T, Kugler J, Pohl M (2008) Electromechanical and robot-assisted arm training for improving arm function and activities of daily living after stroke. Cochrane Database Syst Rev: CD006876.

320. Housman S, Scott K, Reinkensmeyer D (2009) A randomized controlled trial of gravity-supported, computer-enhanced arm exercise for individuals with severe hemiparesis. Neurorehabil Neural Repair 23: 505–514.

321. Mayr A, Kofler M, Saltuari L (2008) [ARMOR: an electromechanical robot for upper limb training following stroke. A prospective randomised controlled pilot study]. Handchir Mikrochir Plast Chir 40: 66–73.

322. Volpe B, Krebs H, Hogan N, Edelstein OTR L, Diels C, et al. (2000) A novel approach to stroke rehabilitation: robot-aided sensorimotor stimulation. Neurology 54: 1938–1944.

323. Hsieh Y, Wu C, Liao W, Lin K, Wu K, et al. (2011) Effects of treatment intensity in upper limb robot-assisted therapy for chronic stroke: a pilot randomized controlled trial. Neurorehabil Neural Repair 25: 503–511.

324. Aisen M, Krebs H, Hogan N, McDowell F, Volpe B (1997) The effect of robot-assisted therapy and rehabilitative training on motor recovery following stroke. Arch Neurol 54: 443–446.

325. Volpe B, Krebs H, Hogan N, Edelsteinn L, Driels C, et al. (1999) Robot training enhances motor outcome in patients with stroke maintained over 3 years. Neurology 53: 1874–1876.

326. Lum P, Burgar C, Shor P, Majmundar M, Van der Loos M (2002) Robot-assisted movement training compared with conventional therapy techniques for the rehabilitation of upper-limb motor function after stroke. Arch Phys Med Rehabil 83: 952–959.

327. Stein J, Krebs H, Frontera W, Fasoli S, Hughes R, et al. (2004) Comparison of two techniques of robot-aided upper limb exercise training after stroke. Am J Phys Med Rehabil 83: 720–728.

328. Daly J, Hogan N, Perepezko E, Krebs H, Rogers J, et al. (2005) Response to upper-limb robotics and functional neuromuscular stimulation following stroke. J Rehabil Res Dev 42: 723–736.

329. Hesse S, Werner C, Pohl M, Rueckriem S, Mehrholz J, et al. (2005) Computerized arm training improves the motor control of the severely affected arm after stroke: a single-blinded randomized trial in two centers. Stroke 36: 1960–1966.

330. Kahn L, Zygman M, Rymer W, Reinkensmeyer D (2006) Robot-assisted reaching exercise promotes arm movement recovery in chronic hemiparetic stroke: a randomized controlled pilot study. J Neuroeng Rehabil 3: 12.

331. Masiero S, Celia A, Rosati G, Armani M (2007) Robotic-assisted rehabilitation of the upper limb after acute stroke. Arch Phys Med Rehabil 88: 142–149.

332. Rabadi M, Galgano M, Lynch D, Akerman M, Lesser M, et al. (2008) A pilot study of activity-based therapy in the arm motor recovery post stroke: a randomized controlled trial. Clin Rehabil 22: 1071–1082.

333. Volpe B, Lynch D, Rykman-Berland A, Ferraro M, Galgano M, et al. (2008) Intensive sensorimotor arm training mediated by therapist or robot improves hemiparesis in patients with chronic stroke. Neurorehabil Neural Repair 22: 305–310.

334. Ellis M, Sukal-Moulton T, Dewald J (2009) Progressive shoulder abduction loading is a crucial element of arm rehabilitation in chronic stroke. Neurorehabil Neural Repair 23: 862–869.

335. Lo A, Guarino P, Richards L, Haselkorn J, Wittenberg G, et al. (2010) Robot-assisted therapy for long-term upper-limb impairment after stroke. N Engl J Med 362: 1772–1783.

336. Masiero S, Armani M, Rosati G (2011) Upper-limb robot-assisted therapy in rehabilitation of acute stroke patients: focused review and results of new randomized controlled trial. J Rehabil Res Dev 48: 355–366.

337. Burgar C, Lum P, Scremin A, Garber S, Van der Loos H, et al. (2011) Robot-assisted upper-limb therapy in acute rehabilitation setting following stroke: Department of Veterans Affairs multisite clinical trial. J Rehabil Res Dev 48: 445–458.

338. Conroy S, Whitall J, Dipietro L, Jones-Lush L, Zhan M, et al. (2011) Effect of gravity on robot-assisted motor training after chronic stroke: a randomized trial. Arch Phys Med Rehabil 92: 1754–1761.

339. Barclay-Goddard R, Stevenson T, Poluha W, Thalman L (2011) Mental practice for treating upper extremity deficits in individuals with hemiparesis after stroke. Cochrane Database Syst Rev: CD005950.

340. Müller K, Bütefisch C, Seitz R, Hömberg V (2007) Mental practice improves hand function after hemiparetic stroke. Restor Neurol Neurosci 25: 501–511.

341. Liu K (2009) Use of mental imagery to improve task generalisation after a stroke. Hong Kong Med J 15: 37–41.

342. Liu K, Chan C, Lee T, Hui-Chan C (2004) Mental imagery for promoting relearning for people after stroke: a randomized controlled trial. Arch Phys Med Rehabil 85: 1403–1408.

343. Page S, Levine P, Leonard A (2007) Mental practice in chronic stroke: results of a randomized, placebo-controlled trial. Stroke 38: 1293–1297.

344. Braun S, Beurskens A, Kleynen M, Oudelaar B, Schols J, et al. (2012) A multicenter randomized controlled trial to compare subacute 'treatment as usual' with and without mental practice among persons with stroke in Dutch nursing homes. J Am Med Dir Assoc 13: e1–7.

345. Ietswaart M, Johnston M, Dijkerman HC, Joice S, Scott CL, et al. (2011) Mental practice with motor imagery in stroke recovery: randomized controlled trial of efficacy. Brain 134: 1373–1386.

346. Page S (2000) Imagery improves upper extremity motor function in chronic stroke patients: a pilot study. Occup Ther J Res 20: 200–215.

347. Page S, Levine P, Sisto S, Johnston M (2001) Mental practice combined with physical practice for upper-limb motor deficit in subacute stroke. Phys Ther 81: 1455–1462.

348. Page S, Levine P, Leonard A (2005) Effects of mental practice on affected limb use and function in chronic stroke. Arch Phys Med Rehabil 86: 399–402.

349. Cacchio A, De Blasis E, Necozione S, Di Orio F, Santilli V (2009) Mirror therapy for chronic complex regional pain syndrome type 1 and stroke. N Engl J Med 361: 634–636.

350. Page S, Szaflarski J, Eliassen J, Pan H, Cramer S (2009) Cortical plasticity following motor skill learning during mental practice in stroke. Neurorehabil Neural Repair 23: 382–388.

351. Riccio I, Iolascon G, Barillari MR, Gimigliano R, Gimigliano F (2010) Mental practice is effective in upper limb recovery after stroke: a randomized single-blind cross-over study. Eur J Phys Rehabil Med 46: 19–25.

352. Ferreira H, Leite Lopes M, Luiz R, Cardoso L, Andre C (2011) Is visual scanning better than mental practice in hemispatial neglect? Results from a pilot study. Top Stroke Rehabil 18: 155–161.

353. Page S, Dunning K, Hermann V, Leonard A, Levine P (2011) Longer versus shorter mental practice sessions for affected upper extremity movement after stroke: a randomized controlled trial. Clin Rehabil 25: 627–637.

354. Altschuler E, Wisdom S, Stone L, Foster C, Galasko D, et al. (1999) Rehabilitation of hemiparesis after stroke with a mirror. Lancet 353: 2035–2036.

355. Michielsen M, Selles R, Van der Geest J, Eckhardt M, Yavuzer G, et al. (2011) Motor recovery and cortical reorganization after mirror therapy in chronic stroke patients: a phase II randomized controlled trial. Neurorehabil Neural Repair 25: 223–233.

356. Rothgangel A, Morton A, Van der Hout J, Beurskens A (2004) Phantoms in the brain: spiegeltherapie bij chronische CVA-patiënten: een pilot-study. Ned Tijdschr Fysiother 114: 36–40.

357. Yavuzer G, Selles R, Sezer N, Sutbeyaz S, Bussmann JB, et al. (2008) Mirror therapy improves hand function in subacute stroke: a randomized controlled trial. Arch Phys Med Rehabil 89: 393–398.

358. Cacchio A, De Blasis E, De Blasis V, Santilli V, Spacca G (2009) Mirror therapy in complex regional pain syndrome type 1 of the upper limb in stroke patients. Neurorehabil Neural Repair 23: 792–799.

359. Dohle C, Pullen J, Nakaten A, Kust J, Rietz C, et al. (2009) Mirror therapy promotes recovery from severe hemiparesis: a randomized controlled trial. Neurorehabil Neural Repair 23: 209–217.

360. Saposnik G, Teasell R, Mamdani M, Hall J, McIlroy W, et al. (2010) Effectiveness of virtual reality using Wii gaming technology in stroke rehabilitation: a pilot randomized clinical trial and proof of principle. Stroke 41: 1477–1484.

361. Carey J, Kimberley T, Lewis S, Auerbach E, Dorsey L, et al. (2002) Analysis of fMRI and finger tracking training in subjects with chronic stroke. Brain 125: 773–788.

362. Carey J, Durfee W, Bhatt E, Nagpal A, Weinstein S, et al. (2007) Comparison of finger tracking versus simple movement training via telerehabilitation to alter hand function and cortical reorganization after stroke. Neurorehabil Neural Repair 21: 216–232.

363. Piron L, Tonin P, Atzori A, Zucconi C, Massaro C, et al. (2003) The augmented-feedback rehabilitation technique facilitates the arm motor recovery in patients after a recent stroke. Stud Health Technol Inform 94: 265–267.

364. Piron L, Tombolini A, Turolla C, Zucconi C, Agostini M, et al. (2007) Reinforced feedback in virtual environment facilitates the arm motor recovery in patients after a recent stroke. IEEE Xplore: 121–123.

365. Sucar L, Luis R, Leder R, Hernandez J, Sanchez I (2010) Gesture therapy: a vision-based system for upper extremity stroke rehabilitation. Conf Proc IEEE Eng Med Biol Soc 2010: 3690–3693.

366. Piron L, Turolla A, Agostini M, Zucconi CS, Ventura L, et al. (2010) Motor learning principles for rehabilitation: a pilot randomized controlled study in poststroke patients. Neurorehabil Neural Repair 24: 501–508.

367. Jang S, You S, Hallett M, Cho Y, Park C, et al. (2005) Cortical reorganization and associated functional motor recovery after virtual reality in patients with chronic stroke: an experimenter-blind preliminary study. Arch Phys Med Rehabil 86: 2218–2223.

368. Broeren J, Claesson L, Goude D, Rydmark M, Sunnerhagen K (2008) Virtual rehabilitation in an activity centre for community-dwelling persons with stroke. The possibilities of 3-dimensional computer games. Cerebrovasc Dis 26: 289–296.

369. Crosbie J, Lennon S, McDonough S (2007) Virtual reality in the rehabilitation of the upper limb following hemiplegic stroke: a pilot randomised controlled trial (RCT). UK Stroke Forum Conference 2007: 9.

370. Piron L, Turolla A, Tonin P, Piccione F, Lain L, et al. (2008) Satisfaction with care in post-stroke patients undergoing a telerehabilitation programme at home. J Telemed Telecare 14: 257–260.

371. Yavuzer G, Senel A, Atay M, Stam H (2008) "Playstation eyetoy games" improve upper extremity-related motor functioning in subacute stroke: a randomized controlled clinical trial. Eur J Phys Rehabil Med 44: 237–244.

372. Piron L, Turolla A, Agostini M, Zucconi C, Cortese F, et al. (2009) Exercises for paretic upper limb after stroke: a combined virtual-reality and telemedicine approach. J Rehabil Med 41: 1016–1102.

373. Da Silva Cameirao M, Bermúdez I Badia S, Duarte E, Verschure P (2011) Virtual reality based rehabilitation speeds up functional recovery of the upper extremities after stroke: a randomized controlled pilot study in the acute phase of stroke using the Rehabilitation Gaming System. Restor Neurol Neurosci 29: 287–298.

374. Fischer H, Stubblefield K, Kline T, Luo X, Kenyon R, et al. (2007) Hand rehabilitation following stroke: a pilot study of assisted finger extension training in a virtual environment. Top Stroke Rehabil 14: 1–12.

375. Carmeli E, Peleg S, Bartur G, Elbo E, Vatine J (2010) HandTutor(TM) enhanced hand rehabilitation after stroke - a pilot study. Physiother Res Int 16: 191–200.

376. Bowman B, Baker L, Waters R (1979) Positional feedback and electrical stimulation: an automated treatment for the hemiplegic wrist. Arch Phys Med Rehabil 60: 497–502.

377. Sonde L, Gip C, Fernaeus S, Nilsson C, Viitanen M (1998) Stimulation with low frequency (1.7 Hz) transcutaneous electric nerve stimulation (low-tens) increases motor function of the post-stroke paretic arm. Scand J Rehabil Med 30: 95–99.

378. Cauraugh J, Light K, Kim S, Thigpen M, Behrman A (2000) Chronic motor dysfunction after stroke: recovering wrist and finger extension by electromyography-triggered neuromuscular stimulation. Stroke 31: 1360–1364.

379. Gabr U, Levine P, Page S (2005) Home-based electromyography-triggered stimulation in chronic stroke. Clin Rehabil 19: 737–745.

380. Church C, Price C, Pandyan A, Huntley S, Curless R, et al. (2006) Randomized controlled trial to evaluate the effect of surface neuromuscular electrical stimulation to the shoulder after acute stroke. Stroke 37: 2995–3001.

381. Baker L, Parker K (1986) Neuromuscular electrical stimulation of the muscles surrounding the shoulder. Phys Ther 66: 1930–1937.

382. Leandri M, Parodi C, Corrieri N, Rigardo S (1990) Comparison of TENS treatments in hemiplegic shoulder pain. Scand J Rehabil Med 22: 69–71.

383. Faghri P, Rodgers M, Glaser R, Bors J, Ho C, et al. (1994) The effects of functional electrical stimulation on shoulder subluxation, arm function recovery, and shoulder pain in hemiplegic stroke patients. Arch Phys Med Rehabil 75: 73–79.

384. Faghri P (1997) The effects of neuromuscular stimulation-induced muscle contraction versus elevation on hand edema in CVA patients. J Hand Ther 10: 29–34.

385. King T (1996) The effect of neuromuscular electrical stimulation in reducing tone. Am J Occup Ther 50: 62–64.

386. Chae J, Bethoux F, Bohine T, Dobos L, Davis T, et al. (1998) Neuromuscular stimulation for upper extremity motor and functional recovery in acute hemiplegia. Stroke 29: 975–979.

387. Francisco G, Chae J, Chawla H, Kirshblum S, Zorowitz R, et al. (1998) Electromyogram-triggered neuromuscular stimulation for improving the arm function of acute stroke survivors: a randomized pilot study. Arch Phys Med Rehabil 79: 570–575.

388. Sonde L, Kalimo H, Fernaeus S, Viitanen M (2000) Low TENS treatment on post-stroke paretic arm: a three-year follow-up. Clin Rehabil 14: 14–19.

389. Linn S, Granat M, Lees K (1999) Prevention of shoulder subluxation after stroke with electrical stimulation. Stroke 30: 963–968.

390. Powell J, Pandyan A, Granat M, Cameron M, Stott D (1999) Electrical stimulation of wrist extensors in poststroke hemiplegia. Stroke 30: 1384–1389.

391. Wang R, Chan R, Tsai M (2000) Functional electrical stimulation on chronic and acute hemiplegic shoulder subluxation. Am J Phys Med Rehabil 79: 385–390.

392. Wang R, Yang Y, Tsai M, Wang W, Chan R (2002) Effects of functional electric stimulation on upper limb motor function and shoulder range of motion in hemiplegic patients. Am J Phys Med Rehabil 81: 283–290.

393. Cauraugh J, Kim S (2003) Chronic stroke motor recovery: duration of active neuromuscular stimulation. J Neurol Sci 215: 13–19.

394. Cauraugh J, Kim S (2003) Stroke motor recovery: active neuromuscular stimulation and repetitive practice schedules. J Neurol Neurosurg Psychiatry 74: 1562–1566.

395. Popovic M, Popovic D, Sinkjaer T, Stefanovic A, Schwirtlich L (2003) Clinical evaluation of functional electrical therapy in acute hemiplegic subjects. J Rehabil Res Dev 40: 443–453.

396. De Kroon J, IJzerman M, Lankhorst G, Zilvold G (2004) Electrical stimulation of the upper limb in stroke: stimulation of the extensors of the hand vs. alternate stimulation of flexors and extensors. Am J Phys Med Rehabil 83: 592–600.

397. Kimberley T, Lewis S, Auerbach E, Dorsey L, Lojovich J, et al. (2004) Electrical stimulation driving functional improvements and cortical changes in subjects with stroke. Exp Brain Res 154: 450–460.

398. Mann G, Burridge J, Malone L, Strike P (2005) A pilot study to investigate the effects of electrical stimulation on recovery of hand function and sensation in subacute stroke patients. Neuromodulation 8: 193–202.

399. Popovic M, Thrasher T, Zivanovic V, Takaki J, Hajek V (2005) Neuroprosthesis for retraining reaching and grasping functions in severe hemiplegic patients. Neuromodulation 8: 58–72.

400. Ring H, Rosenthal N (2005) Controlled study of neuroprosthetic functional electrical stimulation in sub-acute post-stroke rehabilitation. J Rehabil Med 37: 32–36.

401. Hara Y, Ogawa S, Muraoka Y (2006) Hybrid power-assisted functional electrical stimulation to improve hemiparetic upper-extremity function. Arch Phys Med Rehabil 85: 977–985.

402. Alon G, Levitt A, McCarthy P (2007) Functional electrical stimulation enhancement of upper extremity functional recovery during stroke rehabilitation: a pilot study. Neurorehabil Neural Repair 21: 207–215.

403. Bhatt E, Nagpal A, Greer K, Grunewald T, Steele J, et al. (2007) Effect of finger tracking combined with electrical stimulation on brain reorganization and hand function in subjects with stroke. Exp Brain Res 182: 435–447.

404. Hemmen B, Seelen H (2007) Effects of movement imagery and electromyography-triggered feedback on arm hand function in stroke patients in the subacute phase. Clin Rehabil 21: 587–594.

405. Kowalczewski J, Gritsenko V, Ashworth N, Ellaway P, Prochazka A (2007) Upper-extremity functional electric stimulation-assisted exercises on a workstation in the subacute phase of stroke recovery. Arch Phys Med Rehabil 88: 833–839.

406. McDonnell M, Hillier S, Miles T, Thompson P, Ridding M (2007) Influence of combined afferent stimulation and task-specific training following stroke: a pilot randomized controlled trial. Neurorehabil Neural Repair 21: 435–443.

407. Alon G, Levitt A, McCarthy P (2008) Functional electrical stimulation (FES) may modify the poor prognosis of stroke survivors with severe motor loss of the upper extremity: a preliminary study. Am J Phys Med Rehabil 87: 627–636.

408. Barker R, Brauer S, Carson R (2008) Training of reaching in stroke survivors with severe and chronic upper limb paresis using a novel nonrobotic device: a randomized clinical trial. Stroke 39: 1800–1807.

409. Barker R, Brauer S, Carson R (2009) Training-induced changes in the pattern of triceps to biceps activation during reaching tasks after chronic and severe stroke. Exp Brain Res 196: 483–496.

410. De Kroon J, IJzerman M (2008) Electrical stimulation of the upper extremity in stroke: cyclic versus EMG-triggered stimulation. Clin Rehabil 22: 690–697.

411. Hara Y, Ogawa S, Tsujiuchi K, Muraoka Y (2008) A home-based rehabilitation program for the hemiplegic upper extremity by power-assisted functional electrical stimulation. Disabil Rehabil 30: 296–304.

412. Shin H, Cho S, Jeon H, Lee Y, Song J, et al. (2008) Cortical effect and functional recovery by the electromyography-triggered neuromuscular stimulation in chronic stroke patients. Neurosci Lett 442: 174–179.

413. Thrasher T, Zivanovic V, McIlroy W, Popovic M (2008) Rehabilitation of reaching and grasping function in severe hemiplegic patients using functional electrical stimulation therapy. Neurorehabil Neural Repair 22: 706–714.

414. Chan M, Tong R, Chung K (2009) Bilateral upper limb training with functional electric stimulation in patients with chronic stroke. Neurorehabil Neural Repair 23: 357–365.

415. Klaiput A, Kitisomprayoonkul W (2009) Increased pinch strength in acute and subacute stroke patients after simultaneous median and ulnar sensory stimulation. Neurorehabil Neural Repair 23: 351–356.

416. Mangold S, Schuster C, Keller T, Zimmermann-Schlatter A, Ettlin T (2009) Motor training of upper extremity with functional electrical stimulation in early stroke rehabilitation. Neurorehabil Neural Repair 23: 184–190.

417. Hsu S, Hu M, Wang Y, Yip P, Chiu J, et al. (2010) Dose-response relation between neuromuscular electrical stimulation and upper-extremity function in patients with stroke. Stroke 41: 821–824.

418. Koyuncu E, Nakipoglu-Yüzer G, Dogan A, Ozgirgin N (2010) The effectiveness of functional electrical stimulation for the treatment of shoulder subluxation and shoulder pain in hemiplegic patients: A randomized controlled trial. Disabil Rehabil 32: 560–566.

419. Fil A, Armutlu K, Atay A, Kerimoglu U, Elibol B (2011) The effect of electrical stimulation in combination with Bobath techniques in the prevention of shoulder subluxation in acute stroke patients. Clin Rehabil 25: 51–59.

420. Lin Z, Yan T (2011) Long-term effectiveness of neuromuscular electrical stimulation for promoting motor recovery of the upper extremity after stroke. J Rehabil Med 43: 506–510.

421. Sentandreu Mano T, Salom Terradez J, Tomas J, Melendez Moral J, Fuente Fernandez T, et al. (2011) [Electrical stimulation in the treatment of the spastic hemiplegic hand after stroke: a ramdomized study]. Med Clin (Barc) 137: 297–301.

422. Shindo K, Fujiwara T, Hara J, Oba H, Hotta F, et al. (2011) Effectiveness of hybrid assistive neuromuscular dynamic stimulation therapy in patients with subacute stroke: a randomized controlled pilot trial. Neurorehabil Neural Repair 25: 830–837.

423. Tarkka I, Pitkänen K, Popovic D, Vanninen R, Könönen M (2011) Functional electrical therapy for hemiparesis alleviates disability and enhances neuroplasticity. Tohoku J Exp Med 225: 71–76.

424. Bate P, Matyas T (1992) Negative transfer of training following brief practice of elbow tracking movements with electromyographic feedback from spastic antagonists. Arch Phys Med Rehabil 73: 1050–1058.

425. Crow J, Lincoln N, Nouri F, De Weerdt W (1989) The effectiveness of EMG biofeedback in the treatment of arm function after stroke. Int Disabil Stud 11: 155–160.

426. Armagan O, Tascioglu F, Oner C (2003) Electromyographic biofeedback in the treatment of the hemiplegic hand: a placebo-controlled study. Am J Phys Med Rehabil 82: 856–861.

427. Smith K (1979) Biofeedback in strokes. Aust J Physiother 25: 155–161.

428. Greenberg S, Fowler Jr R (1980) Kinesthetic biofeedback: a treatment modality for elbow range of motion in hemiplegia. Am J Occup Ther 34: 738–743.

429. Basmajian J, Gowland C, Brandstater M, Swanson L, Trotter J (1982) EMG feedback treatment of upper limb in hemiplegic stroke patients: a pilot study. Arch Phys Med Rehabil 63: 613–616.

430. Williams J (1982) Use of electromyographic biofeedback for pain reduction in the spastic hemiplegic shoulder: a pilot study. Physiother Can 34: 327–333.

431. Inglis J, Donald M, Monga T, Sproule M, Young M (1984) Electromyographic biofeedback and physical therapy of the hemiplegic upper limb. Arch Phys Med Rehabil 65: 755–759.

432. Basmajian J, Gowland C, Finlayson M, Hall A, Swanson L, et al. (1987) Stroke treatment: comparison of integrated behavioral-physical therapy vs traditional physical therapy programs. Arch Phys Med Rehabil 68: 267–272.

433. Dogan-Aslan M, Nakipoglu-Yuzer G, Dogan A, Karabay I, Ozgirgin N (2010) The effect of electromyographic biofeedback treatment in improving upper extremity functioning of patients with hemiplegic stroke. J Stroke Cerebrovasc Dis 21: 187–192.

434. Michaelsen S, Levin M (2004) Short-term effects of practice with trunk restraint on reaching movements in patients with chronic stroke: a controlled trial. Stroke 35: 1914–1919.

435. Thielman G (2010) Rehabilitation of reaching poststroke: a randomized pilot investigation of tactile versus auditory feedback for trunk control. J Neurol Phys Ther 34: 138–144.

436. Michaelsen S, Dannenbaum R, Levin M (2006) Task-specific training with trunk restraint on arm recovery in stroke: randomized control trial. Stroke 37: 186–192.

437. Carey L, Macdonell R, Matyas T (2011) SENSe: Study of the Effectiveness of Neurorehabilitation on Sensation: a randomized controlled trial. Neurorehabil Neural Repair 25: 304–313.

438. Heldmann B, Kerkhoff G, Struppler A, Havel P, Jahn T (2000) Repetitive peripheral magnetic stimulation alleviates tactile extinction. Neuroreport 11: 3193–3198.

439. Byl N, Roderick J, Mohamed O, Hanny M, Kotler J, et al. (2003) Effectiveness of sensory and motor rehabilitation of the upper limb following the principles of neuroplasticity: patients stable poststroke. Neurorehabil Neural Repair 17: 176–191.

440. Chen J, Liang C, Shaw F (2005) Facilitation of sensory and motor recovery by thermal intervention for the hemiplegic upper limb in acute stroke patients: a single-blind randomized clinical trial. Stroke 36: 2665–2669.

441. Byl N, Pitsch E, Abrams G (2008) Functional outcomes can vary by dose: learning-based sensorimotor training for patients stable poststroke. Neurorehabil Neural Repair 22: 494–504.

442. Wolny T, Saulicz E, Gnat R, Kokosz M (2010) Butler's neuromobilizations combined with proprioceptive neuromuscular facilitation are effective in reducing of upper limb sensory in late-stage stroke subjects: a three-group randomized trial. Clin Rehabil 24: 810–821.

443. Hunter S, Hammett L, Ball S, Smith N, Anderson C, et al. (2011) Dose-response study of mobilisation and tactile stimulation therapy for the upper extremity early after stroke: a phase I trial. Neurorehabil Neural Repair 25: 314–322.

444. Gordon N, Gulanick M, Costa F, Fletcher G, Franklin B, et al. (2004) Physical activity and exercise recommendations for stroke survivors: an American Heart Association scientific statement from the Council on Clinical Cardiology, Subcommittee on Exercise, Cardiac Rehabilitation, and Prevention; the Council on Cardiovascular Nursing; the Council on Nutrition, Physical Activity, and Metabolism; and the Stroke Council. Stroke 35: 1230–1240.

445. Brazzelli M, Saunders D, Greig C, Mead G (2011) Physical fitness training for stroke patients. Cochrane Database Syst Rev: CD003316.

446. Carr M, Jones J (2003) Physiological effects of exercise on stroke survivors. Top Stroke Rehabil 9: 57–64.

447. Lee M, Kilbreath S, Singh M, Zeman B, Lord S, et al. (2008) Comparison of effect of aerobic cycle training and progressive resistance training on walking ability after stroke: a randomized sham exercise-controlled study. J Am Geriatr Soc 56: 976–985.

448. Inaba M, Edberg E, Montgomery J, Gillis MK (1973) Effectiveness of functional training, active exercise, and resistive exercise for patients with hemiplegia. PhysTher 53: 28–35.

449. Glasser L (1986) Effects of isokinetic training on the rate of movement during ambulation in hemiparetic patients. Phys Ther 66: 673–676.

450. Kim C, Eng J, MacIntyre D, Dawson A (2001) Effects of isokinetic strength training on walking in persons with stroke: a double-blind controlled pilot study. J Stroke Cerebrovasc Dis 10: 265–273.

451. Bourbonnais D, Bilodeau S, Lepage Y, Beaudoin N, Gravel D, et al. (2002) Effect of force-feedback treatments in patients with chronic motor deficits after a stroke. Am J Phys Med Rehabil 81: 890–897.

452. Moreland J, Goldsmith C, Huijbregts M, Anderson R, Prentice D, et al. (2003) Progressive resistance strengthening exercises after stroke: a single-blind randomized controlled trial. Arch Phys Med Rehabil 84: 1433–1440.

453. Ouellette M, LeBrasseur N, Bean J, Phillips E, Stein J, et al. (2004) High-intensity resistance training improves muscle strength, self-reported function, and disability in long-term stroke survivors. Stroke 35: 1404–1409.

454. De Boissezon X, Burlot S, Glezes S, Roques C, Marque P (2005) A randomized controlled trial to compare isokinetic and conventional muscular strengthening in poststroke patients. Isokinet Exerc Sci: 91–92.

455. Akbari A, Karimi H (2006) The effect of strengthening exercises in exaggerated muscle tonicity in chronic hemiparesis following stroke. J Med Sci 6: 382–388.

456. Tihanyi T, Horvath M, Fazekas G, Hortobagyi T, Tihanyi J (2007) One session of whole body vibration increases voluntary muscle strength transiently in patients with stroke. Clin Rehabil 21: 782–793.

457. Bale M, Strand L (2008) Does functional strength training of the leg in subacute stroke improve physical performance? A pilot randomized controlled trial. Clin Rehabil 22: 911–921.

458. Flansbjer U, Miller M, Downham D, Lexell J (2008) Progressive resistance training after stroke: effects on muscle strength, muscle tone, gait performance and perceived participation. J Rehabil Med 40: 42–48.

459. Lee M, Kilbreath S, Singh M, Zeman B, Davis G (2010) Effect of progressive resistance training on muscle performance after chronic stroke. Med Sci Sports Exerc 42: 23–34.

460. Page S, Levine P, Teepen J, Hartman E (2008) Resistance-based, reciprocal upper and lower limb locomotor training in chronic stroke: a randomized, controlled crossover study. Clin Rehabil 22: 610–617.

461. Singh S (2008) Closed versus open kinematic chain exercises on gait performance in subacute stroke patients. Physiother Occup Ther J 1: 73–89.

462. Sims J, Galea M, Taylor N, Dodd K, Jespersen S, et al. (2009) Regenerate: assessing the feasibility of a strength-training program to enhance the physical and mental health of chronic post stroke patients with depression. Int J Geriatr Psychiatry 24: 76–83.

463. Cooke E, Tallis R, Clark A, Pomeroy V (2010) Efficacy of functional strength training on restoration of lower-limb motor function early after stroke: phase I randomized controlled trial. Neurorehabil Neural Repair 24: 88–96.

464. Tihanyi J, Di Giminiani R, Tihanyi T, Gyulai G, Trzaskoma L, et al. (2010) Low resonance frequency vibration affects strength of paretic and non-paretic leg differently in patients with stroke. Acta Physiol Hung 97: 172–182.

465. Lippert-Grüner M, Grüner M (1999) Muskelkrafttraining in der Rehabilitation des zentral paretischen Armes. Neurol Rehabil 5: 275–279.

466. Donaldson C, Tallis R, Miller S, Sunderland A, Lemon R, et al. (2009) Effects of conventional physical therapy and functional strength training on upper limb motor recovery after stroke: a randomized phase II study. Neurorehabil Neural Repair 23: 389–397.

467. Thielman G, Dean C, Gentile A (2004) Rehabilitation of reaching after stroke: task-related training versus progressive resistive exercise. Arch Phys Med Rehabil 85: 1613–1618.

468. Winstein C, Rose D, Tan S, Lewthwaite R, Chui H, et al. (2004) A randomized controlled comparison of upper-extremity rehabilitation strategies in acute stroke: A pilot study of immediate and long-term outcomes. Arch Phys Med Rehabil 85: 620–628.

469. Thielman G, Kaminski T, Gentile A (2008) Rehabilitation of reaching after stroke: comparing 2 training protocols utilizing trunk restraint. Neurorehabil Neural Repair 22: 697–705.

470. Potempa K, Lopez M, Braun L, Szidon J, Fogg L, et al. (1995) Physiological outcomes of aerobic exercise training in hemiparetic stroke patients. Stroke 26: 101–105.

471. Kamps A, Schüle K (2005) Cyclic movement training of the lower limb in stroke rehabilitation. Neurol Rehabil 11: S1–S12.

472. Katz-Leurer M, Carmeli E, Shochina M (2003) The effect of early aerobic training on independence six months post stroke. Clin Rehabil 17: 735–741.

473. Katz-Leurer M, Shochina M (2007) The influence of autonomic impairment on aerobic exercise outcome in stroke patients. NeuroRehabilitation 22: 267–272.

474. Lennon O, Carey A, Gaffney N, Stephenson J, Blake C (2008) A pilot randomized controlled trial to evaluate the benefit of the cardiac rehabilitation paradigm for the non-acute ischaemic stroke population. Clin Rehabil 22: 125–133.

475. Quaney B, Boyd L, McDowd J, Zahner L, He J, et al. (2009) Aerobic exercise improves cognition and motor function poststroke. Neurorehabil Neural Repair 23: 879–885.

476. Dobke B, Schüle K, Diehl W, Kaiser T (2010) Apparativ-assistive Bewegungstherapie in der Schlaganfallrehabilitation. Neurol Rehabil 16: 173–185.

477. Toledano-Zarhi A, Tanne D, Carmeli E, Katz-Leurer M (2011) Feasibility, safety and efficacy of an early aerobic rehabilitation program for patients after minor ischemic stroke: A pilot randomized controlled trial. NeuroRehabilitation 28: 85–90.

478. Teixeira-Salmela L, Olney S, Nadeau S, Brouwer B (1999) Muscle strengthening and physical conditioning to reduce impairment and disability in chronic stroke survivors. Arch Phys Med Rehabil 80: 1211–1218.

479. Duncan P, Studenski S, Richards L, Gollub S, Lai S, et al. (2003) Randomized clinical trial of therapeutic exercise in subacute stroke. Stroke 34: 2173–2180.

480. Richards C, Malouin F, Wood-Dauphinee S, Williams J, Bouchard J, et al. (1993) Task-specific physical therapy for optimization of gait recovery in acute stroke patients. Arch Phys Med Rehabil 74: 612–620.

481. Duncan P, Richards L, Wallace D, Stoker-Yates J, Pohl P, et al. (1998) A randomized, controlled pilot study of a home-based exercise program for individuals with mild and moderate stroke. Stroke 29: 2055–2060.

482. Rimmer J, Riley B, Creviston T, Nicola T (2000) Exercise training in a predominantly African-American group of stroke survivors. Med Sci Sports Exerc 32: 1990–1996.

483. Studenski S, Duncan P, Perera S, Reker D, Lai S, et al. (2005) Daily functioning and quality of life in a randomized controlled trial of therapeutic exercise for subacute stroke survivors. Stroke 36: 1764–1770.

484. Lai S, Studenski S, Richards L, Perera S, Reker D, et al. (2006) Therapeutic exercise and depressive symptoms after stroke. J Am Geriatr Soc 54: 240–247.

485. Olney S, Nymark J, Brouwer B, Culham E, Day A, et al. (2006) A randomized controlled trial of supervised versus unsupervised exercise programs for ambulatory stroke survivors. Stroke 37: 476–481.

486. Letombe A, Cornille C, Delahaye H, Khaled A, Morice O, et al. (2010) Early post-stroke physical conditioning in hemiplegic patients: a preliminary study. Ann Phys Rehabil Med 53: 632–642.

487. Outermans J, Van Peppen R, Wittink H, Takken T, Kwakkel G (2010) Effects of a high-intensity task-oriented training on gait performance early after stroke: a pilot study. Clin Rehabil 24: 979–987.

488. Donkervoort M, Dekker J, Stehmann-Saris F, Deelman B (2001) Efficacy of strategy training in left hemisphere stroke patients with apraxia: a randomised clinical trial. Neuropsychol Rehabil 11: 549–566.

489. Smania N, Girardi F, Domenicali C, Lora E, Aglioti S (2000) The rehabilitation of limb apraxia: a study in left-brain-damaged patients. Arch Phys Med Rehabil 81: 379–388.

490. Smania N, Aglioti SM, Girardi F, Tinazzi M, Fiaschi A, et al. (2006) Rehabilitation of limb apraxia improves daily life activities in patients with stroke. Neurology 67: 2050–2052.

491. Jongbloed L, Morgan D (1991) An investigation of involvement in leisure activities after a stroke. Am J Occup Ther 45: 420–427.

492. Drummond A, Walker M (1995) A randomized controlled trial of leisure rehabilitation after stroke. Clin Rehabil 9: 283–290.

493. Drummond A, Walker M (1996) Generalisation of the effects of leisure rehabilitation for stroke patients. Br J Occup Ther 59: 330–334.

494. Parker C, Gladman J, Drummond A, Dewey M, Lincoln N, et al. (2001) A multicentre randomized controlled trial of leisure therapy and conventional occupational therapy after stroke. TOTAL Study Group. Trial of Occupational Therapy and Leisure. Clin Rehabil 15: 42–52.

495. Nour K, Desrosiers J, Gauthier P, Carbonneau H (2002) Impact of a home leisure educadtional program for older adults who have had a stroke (Home Leisure Educational Program). Ther Recr J 36: 48–64.

496. Desrosiers J, Noreau L, Rochette A, Carbonneau H, Fontaine L, et al. (2007) Effect of a home leisure education program after stroke: a randomized controlled trial. Arch Phys Med Rehabil 88: 1095–1100.

497. Britto R, Rezende N, Marinho K, Torres J, Parreira V, et al. (2011) Inspiratory muscular training in chronic stroke survivors: a randomized controlled trial. Arch Phys Med Rehabil 92: 184–190.

498. Sütbeyaz S, Koseoglu F, Inan L, Coskun O (2010) Respiratory muscle training improves cardiopulmonary function and exercise tolerance in subjects with subacute stroke: a randomized controlled trial. Clin Rehabil 24: 240–250.

499. Young J, Forster A (1991) The Bradford community stroke trial: eight week results. Clin Rehabil 5: 283–292.

500. Young J, Forster A (1992) The Bradford community stroke trial: results at six months. BMJ 304: 1085–1089.

501. Baskett J, Broad J, Reekie G, Hocking C, Green G (1999) Shared responsibility for ongoing rehabilitation: a new approach to home-based therapy after stroke. Clin Rehabil 13: 23–33.

502. Gilbertson L, Langhorne P, Walker A, Allen A, Murray G (2000) Domiciliary occupational therapy for patients with stroke discharged from hospital: randomised controlled trial. BMJ 320: 603–606.

503. Rodgers H, Mackintosh J, Price C, Wood R, McNamee P, et al. (2003) Does an early increased-intensity interdisciplinary upper limb therapy programme following acute stroke improve outcome? Clin Rehabil 17: 579–589.

504. Glasgow Augmented Physiotherapy Study (GAPS) (2004) Can augmented physiotherapy input enhance recovery of mobility after stroke? A randomized controlled trial. Clin Rehabil 18: 529–537.

505. Platz T, Eickhof C, Van Kaick S, Engel U, Pinkowski C, et al. (2005) Impairment-oriented training or Bobath therapy for severe arm paresis after stroke: a single-blind, multicentre randomized controlled trial. Clin Rehabil 19: 714–724.

506. Davidson I, Hillier V, Waters K, Walton T, Booth J (2005) A study to assess the effect of nursing interventions at the weekend for people with stroke. Clin Rehabil 19: 126–137.

507. Harris J, Eng J, Miller W, Dawson A (2009) A self-administered Graded Repetitive Arm Supplementary Program (GRASP) improves arm function during inpatient stroke rehabilitation: a multi-site randomized controlled trial. Stroke 40: 2123–2128.

508. Harrington R, Taylor G, Hollinghurst S, Reed M, Kay H, et al. (2010) A community-based exercise and education scheme for stroke survivors: a randomized controlled trial and economic evaluation. Clin Rehabil 24: 3–15.

509. Hesse S, Welz A, Werner C, Quentin B, Wissel J (2011) Comparison of an intermittent high-intensity vs continuous low-intensity physiotherapy service over 12 months in community-dwelling people with stroke: a randomized trial. Clin Rehabil 25: 146–156.

510. Stern P, McDowell F, Miller J, Robinson M (1970) Effects of facilitation exercise techniques in stroke rehabilitation. Ann Phys Rehabil Med 51: 526–531.

511. Smith D, Goldenberg E, Ashburn A, Kinsella G, Sheikh K, et al. (1981) Remedial therapy after stroke: a randomised controlled trial. Br Med J (Clin Res Ed) 282: 517–520.

512. Sivenius S, Pyrorala K, Heinonen O, Salonen J, Riekkinen P (1985) The significance of intensity of rehabilitation of stroke–a controlled trial. Stroke 16: 928–931.

513. Sunderland A, Tinson D, Bradley E, Fletcher D, Langton Hewer R, et al. (1992) Enhanced physical therapy improves recovery of arm function after stroke. A randomised controlled trial. J Neurol Neurosurg Psychiatry 55: 530–535.

514. Werner R, Kessler S (1996) Effectiveness of an intensive outpatient rehabilitation program for postacute stroke patients. Am J Phys Med Rehabil 75: 114–120.

515. Logan P, Ahern J, Gladman J, Lincoln N (1997) A randomized controlled trial of enhanced Social Service occupational therapy for stroke patients. Clin Rehabil 11: 107–113.

516. Kwakkel G, Wagenaar R, Twisk J, Lankhorst G, Koetsier J (1999) Intensity of leg and arm training after primary middle-cerebral-artery stroke: a randomised trial. Lancet 354: 191–196.

517. Lincoln N, Parry R, Vass C (1999) Randomized, controlled trial to evaluate increased intensity of physiotherapy treatment of arm function after stroke. Stroke 30: 573–579.

518. Walker M, Gladman J, Lincoln N, Siemonsma P, Whiteley T (1999) Occupational therapy for stroke patients not admitted to hospital: a randomised controlled trial. Lancet 354: 278–280.

519. Partridge C, Mackenzie M, Edwards S, Reid A, Jayawardena S, et al. (2000) Is dosage of physiotherapy a critical factor in deciding patterns of recovery from stroke: a pragmatic randomized controlled trial. Physiother Res Int 5: 230–240.

520. Andersen H, Eriksen K, Brown A, Schultz-Larsen K, Forchhammer B (2002) Follow-up services for stroke survivors after hospital discharge–a randomized control study. Clin Rehabil 16: 593–603.

521. Slade A, Tennant A, Chamerlain M (2002) A randomised controlled trial to determine the effect of intensity of therapy upon length of stay in a neurological rehabilitation setting. J Rehabil Med 34: 260–266.

522. Di Lauro A, Pellegrino L, Savastano G, Ferraro C, Fusco M, et al. (2003) A randomized trial on the efficacy of intensive rehabilitation in the acute phase of ischemic stroke. J Neurol 250: 1206–1208.

523. Fang Y, Chen X, Lin H, Lin J, Huang R, et al. (2003) A study on additional early physiotherapy after stroke and factors affecting functional recovery. Clin Rehabil 17: 608–617.

524. Katz-Leurer M, Sender I, Keren O, Dvir Z (2006) The influence of early cycling training on balance in stroke patients at the subacute stage. Results of a preliminary trial. Clin Rehabil 20: 398–405.

525. Langhammer B, Lindmark B, Stanghelle J (2007) Stroke patients and long-term training: is it worthwhile? A randomized comparison of two different training strategies after rehabilitation. Clin Rehabil 21: 495–510.

526. Huijgen B, Vollenbroek-Hutten M, Zampolini M, Opisso E, Bernabeu M, et al. (2008) Feasibility of a home-based telerehabilitation system compared to usual care: arm/hand function in patients with stroke, traumatic brain injury and multiple sclerosis. J Telemed Telecare 14: 249–256.

527. Gelber D, Josefczyk P, Herman D, Good D, Verhulst S (1995) Comparison of two therapy approaches in the rehabilitation of the pure motor hemiparetic stroke patient. Neurorehabil Neural Repair 9: 191–196.

528. Langhammer B, Stanghelle J (2000) Bobath or motor relearning programme? A comparison of two different approaches of physiotherapy in stroke rehabilitation: a randomized controlled study. Clin Rehabil 14: 361–369.

529. Langhammer B, Stanghelle J (2003) Bobath or motor relearning programme? A follow-up one and four years post stroke. Clin Rehabil 17: 731–734.

530. Richards C, Malouin F, Bravo G, Dumas F, Wood-Dauphinee S (2004) The role of technology in task-oriented training in persons with subacute stroke: a randomized controlled trial. Neurorehabil Neural Repair 18: 199–211.

531. Tang Q, Yang Q, Wu Y, Wang G, Huang Z, et al. (2005) Effects of problem-oriented willed-movement therapy on motor abilities for people with poststroke cognitive deficits. Phys Ther 85: 1020–1033.

532. Van Vliet P, Lincoln N, Foxall A (2005) Comparison of Bobath based and movement science based treatment for stroke: a randomised controlled trial. J Neurol Neurosurg Psychiatry 76: 503–508.

533. Wang R, Chen H, Chen C, Yang Y (2005) Efficacy of Bobath versus orthopaedic approach on impairment and function at different motor recovery stages after stroke: a randomized controlled study. Clin Rehabil 19: 155–164.

534. Brock K, Haase G, Rothacher G, Cotton S (2011) Does physiotherapy based on the Bobath concept, in conjunction with a task practice, achieve greater improvement in walking ability in people with stroke compared to physiotherapy focused on structured task practice alone?: a pilot randomized controlled trial. Clin Rehabil 25: 903–912.

535. Bütefisch C, Hummelsheim H, Denzler P, Mauritz K (1995) Repetitive training of isolated movements improves the outcome of motor rehabilitation of the centrally paretic hand. J Neurol Sci 130: 59–68.

536. Dechaumont-Palacin S, Marque P, De Boissezon X, Castel-Lacanal E, Carel C, et al. (2008) Neural correlates of proprioceptive integration in the contralesional hemisphere of very impaired patients shortly after a subcortical stroke: an FMRI study. Neurorehabil Neural Repair 22: 154–165.

537. Chow D, Hauptman J, Wong T, Gonzalez N, Martin N, et al. (2012) Changes in stroke research productivity: a global perspective. Surg Neurol Int 3: 27.

538. Kennisnetwerk CVA Nederland (2012) Zorgstandaard CVA/TIA. Maastricht.

539. Otterman N, Van der Wees P, Bernhardt J, Kwakkel G (2012) Physical therapists' guideline adherence on early mobilization and intensity of practice at dutch acute stroke units: a country-wide survey. Stroke 43: 2395–2401.

540. Royal College of Physicians Clinical Effectiveness and Evaluation Unit on behalf of the Intercollegiate Stroke Working Party (2013) Sentinel Stroke Natinoal Audit Programme (SSNAP) – Clinical audit second pilot public report.

541. Kollen B, Lennon S, Lyons B, Wheatley-Smith L, Scheper M, et al. (2009) The effectiveness of the Bobath concept in stroke rehabilitation: what is the evidence? Stroke 40: e89–97.

542. Hebb D (1949) Organization of behavior: a neuropsychological theory. New York: John Wiley.

543. French B, Thomas L, Leathley M, Sutton C, McAdam J, et al. (2007) Repetitive task training for improving functional ability after stroke. Cochrane Database Syst Rev: CD006073.

544. Lee T, Swanson L, Hall A (1991) What is repeated in a repetition? Effects of practice conditions on motor skill acquisition. Phys Ther 71: 150–156.

545. Kwakkel G, Kollen B (2013) Predicting activities after stroke: what is clinically relevant? Int J Stroke 8: 25–32.

546. Dobkin B (2007) Confounders in rehabilitation trials of task-oriented training: lessons from the designs of the EXCITE and SCILT multicenter trials. Neurorehabil Neural Repair 21: 3–13.
547. Van Delden A, Peper C, Beek P, Kwakkel G (2013) Match and mismatch between objective and subjective improvements in upper limb function after stroke. Disabil Rehabil 35: 1961–1967.
548. O'Connor R, Cano S, Thompson A, Hobart J (2004) Exploring rating scale responsiveness: does the total score reflect the sum of its parts? Neurology 62: 1842–1844.
549. Ali M, English C, Bernhardt J, Sunnerhagen K, Brady M (2013) More outcomes than trials: a call for consistent data collection across stroke rehabilitation trials. Int J Stroke 8: 18–24.
550. Weaver C, Leonardi-Bee J, Bath-Hextall F, Bath P (2004) Sample size calculations in acute stroke trials: a systematic review of their reporting, characteristics, and relationship with outcome. Stroke 35: 1216–1224.
551. Dwan K, Gamble C, Williamson P, Kirkham J (2013) Systematic review of the empirical evidence of study publication bias and outcome reporting bias - an updated review. PLoS One 8: e66844.
552. Dobkin B, Duncan P (2012) Should body weight-supported treadmill training and robotic-assistive steppers for locomotor training trot back to the starting gate? Neurorehabil Neural Repair 26: 308–317.
553. Muir K (2002) Heterogeneity of stroke pathophysiology and neuroprotective clinical trial design. Stroke 33: 1545–1550.
554. Gabler N, Duan N, Liao D, Elmore J, Ganiats T, et al. (2009) Dealing with heterogeneity of treatment effects: is the literature up to the challenge? Trials 10: 43.
555. Kent D, Rothwell P, Ioannidis J, Altman D, Hayward R (2010) Assessing and reporting heterogeneity in treatment effects in clinical trials: a proposal. Trials 11: 85.
556. Altman D, Furberg C, Grimshaw J, Rothwell P (2006) Lead editorial: trials - using the opportunities of electronic publishing to improve the reporting of randomised trials. Trials 7: 6.
557. Schulz K, Altman D, Moher D (2010) CONSORT 2010 Statement: Updated guidelines for reporting parallel group randomised trials. J Clin Epidemiol 63: 834–840.
558. Hirst A, Altman D (2012) Are peer reviewers encouraged to use reporting guidelines? A survey of 116 health research journals. PLoS One 7: e35621.
559. Turner L, Shamseer L, Altman D, Weeks L, Peters J, et al. (2012) Consolidated standards of reporting trials (CONSORT) and the completeness of reporting of randomised controlled trials (RCTs) published in medical journals. Cochrane Database Syst Rev: MR000030.
560. Bernhardt J, Dewey H, Thrift A, Donnan G (2004) Inactive and alone: physical activity within the first 14 days of acute stroke unit care. Stroke 35: 1005–1009.
561. Murphy T, Corbett D (2009) Plasticity during stroke recovery: from synapse to behaviour. Nat Rev Neurosci 10: 861–872.
562. Keith R (1996) Rehabilitation after stroke: cost-effectiveness analyses. J R Soc Med 89: 631–633.
563. French B, Leathley M, Sutton C, McAdam J, Thomas L, et al. (2008) A systematic review of repetitive functional task practice with modelling of resource use, costs and effectiveness. Health Technol Assess 12: iii, ix-iii,117.
564. Sangvatanakul P, Hillege S, Lalor E, Levi C, Hill K, et al. (2010) Setting stroke research priorities: The consumer perspective. J Vasc Nurs 28: 121–131.
565. Pollock A, St George B, Fenton M, Firkins L (2012) Top ten research priorities relating to life after stroke. Lancet Neurol 11: 209.
566. Cooke E, Mares K, Clark A, Tallis R, Pomeroy V (2010) The effects of increased dose of exercise-based therapies to enhance motor recovery after stroke: a systematic review and meta-analysis. BMC Med 8: 60.
567. Johansson T, Wild C (2011) Telerehabilitation in stroke care–a systematic review. J Telemed Telecare 17: 1–6.
568. Levin M, Kleim J, Wolf S (2009) What do motor "recovery" and "compensation" mean in patients following stroke? Neurorehabil Neural Repair 23: 313–319.
569. Buma F, Kwakkel G, Ramsey N (2013) Understanding upper limb recovery after stroke. Restor Neurol Neurosci 31: 707–722.
570. Williams J, Pascual-Leone A, Fregni F (2010) Interhemispheric modulation induced by cortical stimulation and motor training. Phys Ther 90: 398–410.
571. Elsner B, Kugler J, Pohl M, Merholz J (2012) Transcranial direct current stimulation (tDCS) for improving function and activities of daily living in patients after stroke. Cochrane Database Syst Rev: CD009645.
572. Hsu W, Cheng C, Liao K, Lee I, Lin Y (2012) Effects of repetitive transcranial magnetic stimulation on motor functions in patients with stroke: a meta-analysis. Stroke 43: 1849–1857.
573. Chollet F, Tardy J, Albucher J, Thalamas C, Berard E, et al. (2011) Fluoxetine for motor recovery after acute ischaemic stroke (FLAME): a randomised placebo-controlled trial. Lancet Neurol 10: 123–130.
574. Vickrey B, Brott T, Koroshetz W (2013) Research priority setting: a summary of the 2012 NINDS Stroke Planning Meeting Report. Stroke 44: 2338–2342.
575. Craig L, Smith L (2008) The interaction between policy and education using stroke as an example. Nurse Educ Today 28: 77–84.
576. Smith L, Craig L, Weir C, McAlpine C (2008) Stroke education for healthcare professionals: making it fit for purpose. Nurse Educ Today 28: 337–347.
577. Kirkham J, Dwan K, Altman D, Gamble C, Dodd S, et al. (2010) The impact of outcome reporting bias in randomised controlled trials on a cohort of systematic reviews. BMJ 340: c365.
578. Riley R, Lambert P, Abo-Zaid G (2010) Meta-analysis of individual participant data: rationale, conduct, and reporting. BMJ 340: c221.
579. Hedges L, Pigott T (2004) The power of statistical tests for moderators in meta-analysis. Psychol Methods 9: 426–445.
580. Borenstein M, Higgins J (2013) Meta-analysis and subgroups. Prev Sci 14: 134–143.

6

Opinions of Youngsters with Congenital Below-Elbow Deficiency, and Those of Their Parents and Professionals Concerning Prosthetic Use and Rehabilitation Treatment

Ecaterina Vasluian[1]*, **Ingrid G. M. de Jong**[1], **Wim G. M. Janssen**[2], **Margriet J. Poelma**[3], **Iris van Wijk**[4], **Heleen A. Reinders-Messelink**[1], **Corry K. van der Sluis**[1]

1 Department of Rehabilitation Medicine, University Medical Center Groningen, University of Groningen, Groningen, The Netherlands, **2** Department of Rehabilitation Medicine, Erasmus Medical Center Rotterdam, Rotterdam, The Netherlands, **3** Rehabilitation Center De Sint Maartenskliniek, Nijmegen, The Netherlands, **4** Rehabilitation Center De Hoogstraat, Utrecht, The Netherlands

Abstract

Background: Youngsters with unilateral congenital below-elbow deficiency (UCBED) seem to function well with or without a prosthesis. Reasons for rejecting prostheses have been reported earlier, but unfortunately not those of the children themselves. Furthermore, reasons for acceptance are underexplored in the literature.

Objectives: To investigate opinions of children and early and late adolescents with UCBED, and those of their parents and healthcare professionals, concerning (1) reasons to wear or not to wear prostheses and (2) about rehabilitation care.

Methods: During one week of online focus group interviews, 42 children of 8–12 y/o, early and late adolescents of 13–16 and 17–20 y/o, 17 parents, and 19 healthcare professionals provided their opinions on various topics. This study addresses prosthetic use or non-use of prosthetics and rehabilitation care. Data were analyzed using the framework approach.

Results: Cosmesis was considered to be the prime factor for choosing and wearing a prosthesis, since this was deemed especially useful in avoiding stares from others. Although participants functioned well without prostheses, they agreed that it was an adjuvant in daily-life activities and sports. Weight and limited functionality constituted rejection reasons for a prosthesis. Children and adolescents who had accepted that they were different no longer needed the prosthesis to avoid being stared at. The majority of participants highly valued the peer-to-peer contact provided by the healthcare professionals.

Conclusions: For children and adolescents with UCBED, prostheses appeared particularly important for social integration, but much less so for functionality. Peer-to-peer contact seemed to provide support during the process of achieving social integration and should be embedded in the healthcare process.

Editor: Nicholas Jenkins, Edinburgh University, United Kingdom

Funding: This study was financed by grants from national foundations: the OIM Foundation, Beatrixoord Foundation, Orthopedietechniek De Hoogstraat Foundation and the Gratama Foundation. The funders had no role in study design, data collection and analysis, decision to publish, or preparation of the manuscript. The authors have no further financial relationships relevant to this article to disclose.

Competing Interests: The authors have declared that no competing interests exist.

* E-mail: e.golea.vasluian@umcg.nl

Introduction

Congenital upper limb defects affect between 19.5 and 21.5 births per 10,000 [1,2]. A considerable group of congenital upper limb anomalies result in reduction deficiencies (5.56 births per 10,000) [3]. Children with such impairments often receive prosthetic treatment in order to improve their functionality and to avoid developmental problems [4]. It is doubtful that prostheses fulfill these aims, since the rejection rate is high 35–45% [5], while no difference in functionality is seen between prostheses wearers and non-wearers [6,7]. Furthermore, prosthesis use seems to reduce manipulation, exploration, variation, and adaptation in the daily-life activities of young children with unilateral congenital below-elbow deficiency (UCBED) [8]. By developing compensa-

tory strategies and auxiliary movements using other body parts (e.g., head, legs, and trunk) to perform a task [9], children also tend to be more independent without prostheses [4]. Thus it is still unclear why some continue wearing prostheses.

Prostheses are typically accepted when people with upper limb impairment face a great deal of difficulty in daily-life activities, have a higher level of amputation (above the elbow), when the abilities of the prostheses are considered to be "fair," and when wearers are satisfied, in general, with their healthcare [10–12]. Advantages of early fitting with a prosthesis in children with UCBED are inconclusive in the literature [13–15] and are not associated with satisfaction with the prosthesis, functional use of the prosthesis, or motor skills [16].

Prostheses are often rejected when people do not experience many challenges in daily-life activities, have lower levels of amputation, are unsatisfied with certain features of the prostheses (sweating, cosmesis, or interface discomfort), or are unsatisfied with all healthcare areas (i.e., fitting, follow-up, repair, training, and information provision) [10–12]. Abnormal truncal movements that usually accompany the performance of activities in prosthetic users may also determine the rejection of prostheses [17]. Parents also play a role in the rejection of prostheses mostly because of disappointment with the limited benefits of prostheses, insufficient involvement in the treatment, and disappointment regarding socio-emotional guidance [13].

The literature is generally concerned with the reasons for rejection of prostheses in adults and provides abundant information as to quantitative outcomes. Information on self-reported reasons that elucidate why children and early and late adolescents choose or continue to wear a prosthesis is scarce. Knowing how psychosocial factors, vis-à-vis the more technical aspects, contribute to the rejection or acceptance of the prosthesis would be of great interest. Children's and adolescents' ideas about what aspects could be improved in a prosthesis have yet to be investigated. The rationale or role of the parents in choosing a prosthesis or in the decision to wear one is also unclear. The approach healthcare professionals take toward improving children's quality of life, including prosthetic prescription, has been previously described [18–20]. Nevertheless, there is not much information about patients' feedback about rehabilitation care, especially the feedback from children. Therefore, the direction of the current study is aimed at elucidating these aspects of how youngsters with UCBED function; the means chosen is a qualitative study design.

The aims of this study are (1) to investigate the opinions of children and early and late adolescents with UCBED, and that of their parents and professionals as to the reasons to wear or not to wear prostheses, and their opinions about (2) rehabilitation care, and to compare the differences in opinions and perspectives among children, early and late adolescents, parents, and healthcare professionals.

Methods

The current study is a part of a larger study which focused on the aspects of functioning of children and adolescents with UCBED: activities, participation, prosthetic use or non-use, psychosocial functioning, and rehabilitation care. The results concerning activities and participation, and those concerning psychosocial functioning have been published by De Jong and colleagues [21,22]. The aim of this published first study was to assess whether youngsters with UCBED encounter activity or participation limitations and, if so, what are their coping strategies for those limitations. The published second study investigated the psychosocial functioning of youngsters with UCBED, with a focus on their feelings about their deficiency and what their coping strategies are in terms of those feelings. The larger study as a whole was designed as a qualitative research study, using online focus group interviews for the data collection.

1 Study Design

Qualitative studies offer the possibility of gaining insight into underexplored research topics. Online focus group interviews are useful for exploring opinions, for obtaining a range of views from different age categories, and for observing interactions among a wide range of participants. Compared to classic face-to-face focus groups, the online version offers anonymous participation which minimizes the influence of social pressure and favors a more open

interaction; it provides a comfortable environment, and by avoiding the transcription process is inexpensive and time-efficient [23–25]. Online focus group interviews were considered appropriate for this study, because they are specifically suitable when rare diseases are the subject of interest and participants live in a widespread area. A group of 8 to 15 participants is believed to work successfully in asynchronous focus groups [26–28], and even 19 participants have been used in online settings [29].

2 Ethics Statement

Ethical approval was obtained from the Medical Ethical Committee of the University Medical Center Groningen, the Netherlands (number M09.079327). Each participant or child's parent/guardian provided an informed consent, and completed a demographic questionnaire prior to the beginning of the study. For the participation of the youngsters in the study, informed consent was obtained from the parents/guardians of those participants aged 8–11 y/o, from the participants aged 12–17 y/o and also from their parents/guardians, and it was obtained from the participants only, when aged 18–20 y/o. Regardless of whether their child actually participated, parents/guardians signed a separate informed consent allowing their own participation in the focus group interviews.

The participants were informed that they could contact an independent physician for any distress they experienced and that they could withdraw from the study at any time without any consequences. The confidentiality of the participant was also ensured by assigning a codename (for example, children were given names of types of fruit) to every participant. These codenames were used by the participants during the study and for the purpose of analysis. The credentials of the participants were accessible only to the researchers and to no one else.

3 Population

Five categories of participants were considered: children, early and late adolescents, parents, and healthcare professionals who had worked with the UCBED population.

3.1 Inclusion criteria for children and early and late adolescents. Purposive sampling was used [30], meaning that both prosthetic wearers and non-wearers with particular characteristics were selected: (1) aged between 8 and 20 years old, and (2) UCBED at a transradial level with a non-syndromic cause. Three categories were defined in concordance with school age: children aged 8–12 years old (primary school), early adolescents aged 13–16 years old (secondary school), and late adolescents aged 17–20 years old (secondary or higher education). By grouping participants in age categories, we aimed to detect specific age-related opinions on the research topics.

3.2 Inclusion criteria for parents and healthcare professionals. Eligible parents were those whose children met the criteria of inclusion for children and early and late adolescents. Eligible healthcare professionals were those with work experience with the UCBED pediatric group.

3.3 Exclusion criteria. Individuals with insufficient proficiency in the Dutch language and limited mental capacity were excluded.

3.4 Recruitment. Participants (except for healthcare professionals) were recruited through national rehabilitation centers and patient organizations. Patient organizations advertized the study on their websites and in newsletters. Twenty-five random people per group were approached, taking into account age, gender, prosthetic wearing/non-wearing, and referral center. Participants received a package with detailed information, a form for informed consent, and a letter approved by the attending rehabilitation physician stating that the physician supports the study and inviting the child or the parent to participate. Professionals were approached through rehabilitation centers and orthopedic workshops in the Netherlands.

4 Procedure

An expert provided methodological recommendations for designing and conducting the online focus group interviews. A website with five forums, one forum per group, was designed to facilitate the online focus group interviews. Participants were able to log in anonymously and post messages at any time of the day they preferred and from the location they preferred, within the timeframe of one week. Participants were instructed to omit names of people or rehabilitation centers.

A question about a specific topic was posted every morning during the first five days. The last two days were assigned to open discussions between group participants. The participants who did not access the website on a particular day would receive a reminder the following day asking them to answer not only the current day's question but also the question from the previous day. The participants were required to post at least one message as an answer to each of the five questions.

This study addressed aspects of the prosthetic use or non-use (day 3) and rehabilitation care (day 5), formulating queries as follows: "Tell us why you wear or do not wear a prosthesis," "Tell us how you evaluate the rehabilitation team and technicians," and "Do you have suggestions for improvement for them?" The rest of the topics were covered on other days: activities (day 1), participation (day 2), and psychosocial functioning (day 4).To ensure the correct understanding of the questions, the authors formulated them according to the participant's age. The study questions and the website with its five forums were pilot-tested on a group of non-impaired children and independent adults. Minor difficulties with understanding the questions and with using the forums were encountered during the pilot test. The website and the questions were improved based on participants' suggestions. To enable the comparison of perspectives between groups, parents and professionals were asked to express their feedback from the child's perspective. Multiple perspectives are important for gaining a richer and broader understanding of the studied population [27], and to help clinicians find suitable solutions for the barriers experienced by the parties dealing with UCBED, that is, children, early and late adolescents, parents, and healthcare professionals.

In order to cover a broad area of interest, the questions were based on the World Health Organization's International Classification of Functioning, Disability and Health for Children and Youth (ICF-CY). ICF-CY addresses issues on two levels: functioning and disability (body functions, body structures, activities, and participation), and contextual factors (environmental and personal factors) [31].

In order to address a possible bias induced by the lack of nonverbal communication, emoticons were made available. This enabled participants to express their feelings. Two moderators were online every day of the study from 8 a.m. to 11 p.m. to ensure that the online focus group interviews were conducted properly. They (IdJ and HRM) followed the moderator's principles [32] to allay some of the moderator's influences. The two moderators facilitated an interactive discussion between participants, but avoided influencing or dominating the discussions. Moderators refrained from rephrasing and evaluating statements; instead, they repeated comments using the participant's words, and provided positive reinforcement by using neutral comments and probing. Both moderators were experienced in the field of child and hand rehabilitation, in addition to a background in human movement sciences, and were not involved in the treatment of the participants. HRM had experience with qualitative data collection methods in pediatric populations. Moderators were in contact, during the study period, with a very experienced rehabilitation physician working with this type of patient. Whenever clarifications of an answer were needed or new information/issues appeared, moderators posted additional questions to individual or all participants until no other new information appeared. This is similar to reaching data saturation [30]. All the data is available in the Dutch language or, if requested, a translation in English can be provided as well.

5 Data Analysis

The most common methods in healthcare research used to analyze qualitative data are thematic analysis, grounded theory, and the framework approach [33]. The framework approach enables, as does thematic analysis, the corroboration of predefined research questions with the themes that emerge in the study. The advantage, however, is that it starts deductively from the clearly predefined objectives of the study, and is systematic and transparent, allowing easy access to the analytical process for the researcher as well as for other people [34]. The framework approach was used to analyze the data from this study. The approach contains five steps in which data is screened, condensed, and mapped into a thematic framework:

5.1 Familiarization. The data generated on the days allocated to prosthetic use and rehabilitation care were read by three authors (EV, HRM, and CvdS). The rest of the data was also read to extract remarks about prosthetic use and rehabilitation care. Key ideas and themes were identified in a meeting with the three authors. The themes were derived from subjects frequently mentioned by the participants.

5.2 Identifying a thematic framework. A coding framework was developed by EV to structure the collected information around key issues and themes (Table S1). Based on the aims of the study, the themes were grouped into main categories such as "reasons to wear a prosthesis," "reasons not to wear a prosthesis," or "tips for making a prosthesis better, adaptive devices, and other creative solutions." In addition, for each main category a "general" theme category was created for data not matching the other themes. The data in the "general" theme category (e.g., frequency, time and place for wearing the prosthesis) when considered appropriate were made available in the Results section to provide detailed information for the themes.

5.3 Indexing. EV and HRM tested the coding framework on ten percent of the data. After discussing minor differences in the manner of coding, agreement was reached upon the final version of the coding framework. EV correlated text pieces from the entire dataset with the appropriate code.

5.4 Charting. EV displayed the pieces of text corresponding to the matched code and affiliation group in the form of a matrix. The columns contained the framework themes, while the lines contained each participant's quotes on the theme. The quotes of wearers or non-wearers were thus easily identifiable from the matrix. The data accessibility of the matrix facilitated the analysis of the perspectives of the different groups, and of wearers and non-wearers.

5.5 Mapping and interpretation. The resulting matrix was verified for the correct code by HRM and CvdS. In order to draw conclusions, EV, HRM, and CvdS analyzed the matrix separately. All three discussed the similarities and differences that occurred. Consensus was found on interpretations and conclusions.

Results

From the total of 125 eligible participants, 77 (62%) participated in the study. Forty-two were either children, early adolescents, or late adolescents; 16 were parents; and 19 were healthcare professionals. No differences in age, gender, and provenance center were found between participants and non-participants. Non-wearers were represented by participants who had experience with prostheses (children 47%, early adolescents 54%, late adolescents 58%, and children of parents 63%), and participants without previous prosthetic experience (Table 1). Myoelectric prostheses were the most popular among wearers (Table 1). The healthcare professionals group consisted of five physiatrists, six occupational and physical therapists, six certified prosthetists, and two psychologists.

The participants were active in interacting with each other and with moderators. Each participant posted at least one message as an answer to each study question. Parents and healthcare professionals provided the most extensive answers.

1 Reasons to Choose and Wear Prostheses

1.1 Cosmetic, social, emotional, and identity reasons. Prostheses were chosen and worn primarily to provide cosmesis. Cosmesis helped participants of all age categories to manage relationships with the people in their environment. A frequently mentioned reason was to prevent adverse reactions like teasing and staring. For children, the prosthesis also offered a normal body appearance, while for early and late adolescents wearing a prosthesis allowed them to establish a good first impression and gave them a feeling of self-confidence.

"For walking on the street I found it [the prosthesis] enjoyable; everyone finds you normal then, because you then have two hands." (10 y/o girl, non-wearer with prosthesis experience)

The prostheses were worn every day, yet limited to being worn in public. In a safe home environment, the prosthesis had nothing to add and was therefore removed. The cosmesis also became more important during transitional periods such as puberty.

"At puberty, I noticed that they ask for it [the prosthesis] from a cosmetic point of view... They especially want a prosthesis, for example, when they go to secondary school." (Healthcare professional)

Professionals noticed that rejection of prosthesis use occurred in some children as soon as they became accustomed to a new environment.

Table 1. Characteristics of participants (n = 77).

Characteristics	Children	Early Adolescents	Late Adolescents	Parents
	No.(%) or Minimum-Maximum	No.(%) or Minimum-Maximum	No.(%) or Minimum-Maximum	No.(%) or Minimum-Maximum
Participants (approached, recruited, participated)	25, 17, 17	25, 15, 13	25, 13, 12	25, 19, 16
Distribution[a]	3, 3, 4, 4, 3	2, 3, 3, 5, 0	2, 3, 4, 3, 0	3, 3, 4, 6, 3
Gender (Male/Female)	9/8 (53/47)	3/10 (23/77)	4/8 (33/67)	10/6 (62.5/37.5)[b]
Age	8–12	13–16	17–20	12[b]
Age of fitting first prosthesis	9 mos.-8 y/o	6 mos.-8 y/o	6 mos.-9 y/o	6 mos.-6 y/o
User status				
Wearer	2 (12)	6 (46)	5 (42)	1 (6)[b]
Wearing frequency of current prosthesis (hours per day)	7.5, 4[c]	1–14	1.5–12	12[c]
Non-wearer	15 (88)	7 (54)	7 (58)	15 (94)[b]
Never wore prosthesis	7 (41)	–	–	5 (31)[b]
Type of current prosthesis	2 (12)	6 (46)	5 (42)	1 (6)[b]
Without grip function	–	1 (8)	2 (17)	–
With grip function	2 (12)	6 (46)	5 (42)	1 (6)[b]
Body powered	–	2 (15)	–	1 (6)[b]
Myoelectric	2 (12)	3 (23)	3 (25)	–
Type of prosthesis at first fitting	10 (59)	13 (100)	12 (100)	11 (69)[b]
Without grip function	5 (29)	12 (92)	9 (75)	6 (38)[b]
With grip function				
Body powered	1 (6)	–	1 (8)	3 (19)[b]
Myoelectric	4 (24)	–	1 (8)	2 (13)[b]
Unknown	–	1 (8)	1 (8)	–

Notations: mos. = months, y/o = years old.
[a]Number of participants distributed per participating rehabilitation center; the last number represents the number of participants recruited through other centers/organizations.
[b]Characteristics of children of participating parents.
[c]The values represent the actual number of hours per day (two wearers in children group and one wearer in parents' group).

1.2 Functionality, manipulation, dexterity reasons. Along with cosmesis, functionality was important for children and adolescents in the process of choosing and wearing prostheses. Being able to experience activities of daily life in a normal way, to grip with the impaired upper limb, and curiosity about whether the prosthesis offered more dexterity also led participants to opt for prostheses.

> "A cosmetic prosthesis often has to be practical too; that's why children/adolescents often want a myo [myoelectric prosthesis] then." (Healthcare professional)
> "I wanted to know if it would be handy or not to wear a prosthesis. I wanted to try and become handier so that everything might be a bit easier. " (13 y/o girl, non-wearer with prosthetic experience)

Wearers and non-wearers regarded the prosthesis as a "useful help accessory" for activities like managing school tasks, cutting, grasping, holding, and lifting.

Activity-specific use was noticed in early and late adolescents for activities such as cycling and driving more safely, or for leisure purposes such as playing sports like volleyball, hockey, and football.

At other times, participants managed to function perfectly well without prostheses. However, activities such as lifting heavy objects, playing sports like volleyball or hockey, or doing some jobs such as delivering newspapers were not performed without prostheses by several early adolescents.

1.3 Physical reasons. Some prosthetic wearers in every group considered wearing a prosthesis as something beneficial for muscle development, locomotion, posture, and balance.

> "When I play soccer, I have my prosthesis on… I have the feeling that I have better balance with it [the prosthesis] on and that I can manage better if I fall." (16 y/o girl, wearer)

1.4 Parents and prosthesis choice. Wearers in children's and late adolescent groups specified that they had been too young to make the choice on their own when the choice was initially made. Parents had therefore played an important role in the process of acquisition and wearing of prostheses.

Some parents had based their choice on the information and instructions about the benefits of early fitting that they had received from healthcare professionals. Other parents had followed their personal beliefs. They wanted to give the child the opportunity to experience a prosthesis so as to provide him/her with the knowledge to be able to make an informed choice later in life. Another reason for parents to choose a prosthesis for their child was that they had wanted to overcome the emotional stress of having a child with an upper-limb impairment.

> "When she was little, we allowed our daughter to use a prosthesis in the morning and go without the prosthesis in the afternoon. This way she could discover herself what was most suitable for her." (Parent of a 13 y/o girl, non-wearer with prosthetic experience)
> "There are parents that want a prosthesis per se, because that way they see their child as more complete, and they find it less difficult for themselves and the family." (Healthcare professional)

2 Reasons not to Choose and Wear Prostheses

2.1 Cosmetic, social, emotional, and identity reasons. Child non-wearers confronted the staring issue head on. They wanted acceptance and respect from the environment without having to wear a prosthesis. Early adolescents experienced self-confidence and self-identity without a prosthesis. Professionals explained this self-confidence on the part of adolescents as a result of realizing that they were able to perform everything just as well without the prosthesis.

Late adolescents, non-wearers, had negative feelings regarding the prosthesis. For them, the prosthesis was a statement about being disabled by highlighting the upper limb defect.

> "I felt myself disabled with that thing [the prosthesis] on… When I was wearing it, I had the feeling that it even made me stand out more [than without the prosthesis]." (20 y/o girl, non-wearer with prosthetic experience)

Non-wearers with or without prosthetic experience reached the stage of accepting their situation. The prosthesis could not substitute for a real hand; it was "a dead thing" or "a doll's hand," and it did not belong to the child. In that sense, the cosmesis of a prosthesis lost its value.

> "I did not want it [the prosthesis] anymore and I thought, 'I am how I am,' and that worked just as well." (9 y/o girl, non-wearer with prosthetic experience)
> "I never wanted it [the prosthesis] before, because I considered it a fake hand… I'm also not ashamed about it [the affected hand] [smiley face]." (11 y/o boy, non-wearer without prosthetic experience)

2.2 Functionality, manipulation, dexterity reasons. Children and adolescents felt more functional, more dexterous, or faster without prostheses. The majority of non-wearers were able to perform "everything and more" without the prosthesis. Parents and professionals noticed that children and adolescents saw little or no functional value in wearing prostheses.

> "Meanwhile he [parent's child] is at an age now (8 y/o), at which he has become very dexterous with his arm … He doesn't see his [affected] arm as a limitation and I think for him walking around with a prosthesis the whole day has no added value." (Parent of an 8y/o boy, non-wearer with prosthetic experience)

Wearers, on the other hand, specified that they did not use their prostheses for activities like eating, playing, tying shoelaces, manual work at school, or working with a computer, because they were more dexterous or had better grip without them.

> "I've been able to tie my shoelaces with and without a prosthesis since I was 3! I find it easier without the prosthesis, because then I have more grip on the lace." (15 y/o girl, wearer)

2.3 Technical and interface reasons. The most often mentioned complaint and reason for not wearing the prosthesis was a prosthesis's weight. The myoelectric prosthesis often required extra support with the sound hand to counterbalance the weight. Discomfort caused by the interface contact with the stump or the technical limitations of the prosthesis itself were also discussed. The interface caused stump irritations, sweating, bad odor, and difficulties fixing the stump in the socket.

"I found it annoying that the prosthesis was just stuck on my arm, and it [the arm] was sweating, and that's why it [the prosthesis] was difficult at first to put on and off." (10 y/o girl, non-wearer with prosthetic experience)

The prosthesis had a limited number of movements and grip functions. Other complaints of non-wearers include the presence of liners, frequent technical failure, and damaged or dirty gloves. Putting on and taking off were perceived as a difficult and laborious process. Manufacturing times were considered long, and learning to use a prosthesis was energy- and time-consuming.

Technical issues were not considered by the wearers to be reason enough not to wear prostheses, but rather as aspects that needed improvement.

2.4 Physical reasons.   Non-wearers were very disturbed by the lack of sensorial feedback from the stump, along with arm and shoulder fatigue, and pain from using prostheses.

"My arm was really tired after a day wearing a prosthesis and without [the prosthesis] not at all. With the prosthesis on, my shoulder used to start hurting easily. *Were these reasons, a tired arm and pain in the shoulder, the most important reasons to stop wearing the prosthesis?* Yes, actually they were." (16 y/o girl, non-wearer with prosthetic experience)

2.5 Parents and the prosthesis choice.   Parents who did not opt for a prosthesis for their child made this choice because they "first wanted to see his [child's] functionality without a prosthesis." Other parents considered a prosthesis to be useless, based on users' stories about daily-life experiences with prostheses.

3 Tips for Improving Prostheses

Late adolescents, parents, and professionals suggested lowering the costs of prostheses. Furthermore, they desired prostheses that were lighter, more attractive, easier to manipulate, and that had more hand positions and separate finger movements, sensorial feedback, and better glove quality. The harnesses on body-powered prostheses seemed to be very annoying, especially for boys:

"Harnesses can indeed be a problem, particularly among boys that want to get rid of the 'bra' [...]." (Healthcare professional)

Alternatives for prosthetic wearing.   The participants were creative in developing alternatives to wearing prostheses. The children or their relatives developed special techniques using body parts such as stump, head, trunk, mouth, or knees, and creative strategies such as bandages or tape to tie an object around the stump or to tie a magnet to it for holding objects.

Adaptive devices for the arm or prosthesis received a lot of attention among participants, especially for non-wearers with or without prosthetic experience, and were described as helpful tools for performing specific activities such as cycling, eating, playing sports, and playing a musical instrument. Professionals and parents suggested developing more adaptive devices, although it appeared to be difficult to get the costs of adaptive devices reimbursed.

4 Rehabilitation Care

4.1 General opinions.   The participants generally experienced good rehabilitation care. Many late adolescents were neutral, perceived the care as appropriate, or could not recall how they had felt about it. The participants had received proper guidance in choosing a prosthesis and had been adequately informed about functioning with a short arm and with a prosthesis.

4.2 Peer contact.   A recurrent theme in all groups was peer-to-peer contact. Parents with young children were eager to know what the possibilities and limitations were for their child in terms of normal functioning and development. Parents received answers to these questions during meetings with peer parents. Emotional support from experienced parents diminished the anxiety of less-experienced parents.

"We saw children in the peer-group meetings who were older [than their child] and they told us how they had found a solution for all the little problems. We benefited a lot from this and we still really enjoy going to these meetings... I think it can be very comforting for 'new' parents to have contact right away with 'experienced' parents so that a lot of the anxiety is taken away." (Parent of a 13 y/o boy, wearer)

Children and early adolescents also benefitted from peer-to-peer contact. Children referred to those meetings as "fun-time." Emotional support was offered even during the course of the online focus group to one child who was going through a difficult time.

"Right now I don't want to be around other children." (9 y/o boy, non-wearer with prosthetic experience)
Reaction from a participant: "I think it's sad that 'codename' [referring to the previous participant] is so sad; you've got to remember that you're perfect the way you are. [sad face]" (11 y/o boy, non-wearer without prosthetic experience)

Early adolescents added that the meetings were informative and emotionally helpful for them. They found out more about novel prostheses and solutions for performing difficult activities.

"I go about once a year to the meetings. I am the oldest one there, and so many people ask me things. I like this and also learn things, because they [other participants] help you with new things and improvements." (14 y/o girl, wearer)

The online focus group was seen by the children and early adolescents as an opportunity to share information about ways to perform certain activities like playing a musical instrument, playing sports, or tying shoelaces.

4.3 Psychosocial assistance.   Some children regarded the psychologist as vague and found the psychological tests unpleasant, or they simply did not want to talk and answer the question, "How are you doing?" However, early adolescents and parents mentioned that emotional and psychosocial help from the rehabilitation team was useful when they encountered difficult moments.

"I always enjoyed an hour with the social worker the most, always nice talks, and she helped me at the same time with things that were difficult for me at that time, such as bullying and other things." (16 y/o girl, non-wearer with prosthetic experience)

Professionals all agreed that psychosocial disciplines are an important and valuable part of the rehabilitation treatment.

4.4 Themes discussed by professionals. Professionals recognized that the clients' expectations were often too high. Children or their parents believed that a prosthesis could solve their problems with the short arm, but the outcome was not always the one they had aimed for.

Although professionals admitted that the current tendency of healthcare providers was to prescribe prostheses, and that more practice was needed until the child performed automatically with the prosthesis, some professionals had different ideas.

"I think that if you consider providing a prosthesis, then you should at least ensure that the child is not clumsier with a prosthesis than without it; so practicing is needed until his prosthesis can be pretty automatically manipulated." (Healthcare professional)

They stated that the team should not strive for bilateral handling of UCBED children, but that the child should grow up with a positive self-image and should be able to fulfill his wishes with or without a prosthesis. These professionals realized that they should listen carefully to the client's needs and to the strategies they had already found on their own, and should avoid imposing their own knowledge excessively.

Discussion

The children and adolescents with UCBED interviewed in our study seemed to choose and wear prostheses mostly for cosmetic reasons in order to avoid people staring at them. In adults with upper limb amputation, similar [35–37] and opposite outcomes were found (i.e., cosmesis was less important) [38]. On the other hand, our findings acknowledged that poor prosthetic cosmesis influenced the non-choice and rejection of the prosthesis [10,13]. The authors of a systematic review noticed a trend in qualitative studies in terms of reporting about the importance of cosmesis [39]. This being the case, the cosmetic aspects of prostheses in youngsters with UCBED deserve the full attention of manufacturers and of those recommending or prescribing them.

In terms of the World Health Organization's ICF classification, children and adolescents with UCBED have a body structure impairment [31]. Therefore, one might expect their functionality to be affected as well. However, the results of our study suggest that the functionality of children and adolescents is good, since many were able to perform activities with or without prostheses; this idea is supported in the literature as well [6,7]. The use of creative strategies (using sweatbands and/or other body parts for grasping and holding objects in place, choosing easier activities) to facilitate activities and participation in daily living may be an alternative to the use of prostheses [22].

In contrast to people with acquired arm amputations, children and adolescents with UCBED have no "sense of loss" regarding the short arm [40]. If children and adolescents with UCBED argue that they do not experience activity limitations and participation restrictions and have no "sense of loss," then there is no reason for them to believe they have an impairment and to feel disabled. However, there are mechanisms that make these youngsters aware of the impairment. Along with body structures and functions, activities and participation, the ICF considers the environmental

and the personal factors [31]. Environmental and the personal factors (gender, educational level, ability to adjust) may influence participation of people with amputations [41] and our findings support this.

When the children and adolescents with UCBED in our study did start to use prostheses, people from their close environment (parents, healthcare professionals) or from their external environment (strangers) exerted a great influence in this regard. Providing the child with a prosthesis in order to improve functionality or to disguise the impairment may be considered as strategies on the part of the parents to cope with their child being disabled. These strategies have been previously described [19,42]. Later on, when children and early and late adolescents become aware of the impact exerted by the short arm on their life, they find solutions to the problems they encounter. In addition to dealing with staring and hostile reactions from people, people with impairment of the upper limb have to deal with their own identity and values concerning body image, sexuality, and career [40]. This is the moment when cosmesis becomes more important and influences the choice of a prosthesis.

In the context of prosthetic use for cosmetic purposes, the concept of normality becomes a matter for discussion. One way to achieve normality for people with disabilities is to adjust and to fit into society [43]. In the research we conducted, participants of all ages experienced a need for normality, especially during transitional periods (a new school or applying for a job), which has been reported in previous studies as stressful events [40,44,45]. Therefore, more psychological attention and information about cosmetic options is needed from healthcare providers, especially in critical transitional phases like puberty.

For many children and adolescents in the study, the way to adjust to the environment and to ensure normality was to wear prostheses so as to appear bodily complete. Being able to perform daily, leisure, and school activities in the same way as their non-disabled peers may also be considered a form of normality. In these circumstances, the prosthesis seems to represent a source of empowerment that facilitates integration into society [43]. For a balanced relationship between youngsters with UCBED and their environment, it would also be appropriate for those people in their environment to adjust their way of thinking, perceiving, and approaching youngsters with UCBED.

Another way of achieving normality is to accept and acknowledge the impairment [43]. This was the case with the non-wearers in our current study. The non-wearers' wish for inclusion in society was based on being valued and accepted as they were. This might well mean that the psychosocial contribution of the prosthesis in combating others' staring at them is unnecessary after all. By not wearing an unnatural-looking prosthesis, children and adolescents believed they were not altering their appearance. This helped them reinforce their self-esteem and improve their self-identity. In addition, if prostheses are seen as having no functional gain [8,13,46], as being technically unsatisfactory and physically uncomfortable [47–49], and sometimes actually hampering effective performance [8] – issues we also found in the present research – the added value of the prosthesis disappears and rejection of it occurs. Interestingly, some of the participants succeeded in embracing acceptance and in using the prosthesis for some daily-life activities and in playing sports, a phenomenon also described in the literature [7,12]. These observations question prosthetic functionality and necessity: "Are prostheses the best solution for children's and adolescent's needs?" Our study also highlighted the perceived value children and adolescents expressed regarding the use of adaptive devices. These devices are lightweight, designed for specific activities, easy to manipulate and to put on [50]. Therefore, considering adaptive devices as an option for rehabilitating children and adolescents with UCBED may be of great value.

Participants' Perspectives about Prosthetic Use

Study participants, whether wearers or non-wearers, seemed to have the same expectations from a prosthesis when they decided to choose for one (i.e., nicer appearance and better functionality). After wearing and testing it, these expectations were not met for non-wearers, and only partially met for wearers. This discrepancy between a person's wishes and the outcomes of prosthetic use, detected by healthcare professionals in the present study, has also been reported in the literature by parents of these children [13] and by adults [51]. Providing information and clarifying the real possibilities and limitations of prosthetic use for consumers would serve to balance expectations versus real-life possibilities. More opportunities for trying and using prostheses before purchasing them would allow children and early and late adolescents to make a more informed choice. Providing these opportunities could be organized in the form of banks with prosthetic simulators that could be rented. A prosthetic simulator is a prosthesis which is adapted with fastening systems and can be attached on any type of arm (amputated, normal) [52].

Rehabilitation Care

The current research results were in line with the findings of other studies that stated that peer-to-peer contact provided emotional assistance for parents and children, as well as understanding, interaction, and identification with people in the same situation [9,40,53]. Incorporating regular peer-to-peer meetings into healthcare would address important aspects of the harmonious development of children and early and late adolescents with UCBED.

Patient-centered care was supported by healthcare professionals in our study. Patient-centered care considers three assumptions that would improve rehabilitation care: the patient (1) is the customer, (2) is the "owner of his body, mind, and soul," and (3) has requested a service in a health matter, so the service provided should focus on the patient's desires [54].

Study Strengths and Limitations

A subject of novelty in the literature and a strength of this study is the fact that children, early adolescents and late adolescents themselves were interviewed, and not only people in the immediate environment (e.g., parents), as in the majority of studies. Along with reasons for rejection – preferentially treated in the literature – the current study also explored the determinants for wearing prostheses in children and early and late adolescents with UCBED. Their opinions about prosthetic use and rehabilitation care allowed for a better understanding of the needs that a young person with UCBED experiences at a certain stage of life. The use of online focus group interviews proved to be an efficient method for collecting a large amount of data in a short period of time. For youngsters with UCBED, the online interaction was easy-going and convenient, since it offered anonymity and flexible participation hours [24,25,29].

This study also has some limitations. Opinions about prosthetic wear in the children and parents groups may have been underexplored due to the low number of wearers in these two groups. However, in all groups, the majority of the current non-wearers had previously worn prostheses. As such, opinions of non-wearers were also valuable for determining reasons for wearing prostheses. There were more females than males in the early adolescent, late adolescent, and parent groups. They might have influenced the results by highlighting the importance of cosmesis, but studies with a majority of males found the cosmetic aspect very important as well [35,51,55]. One may argue that the age of fitting the first prosthesis varies between the groups and might have had an influence on reporting reasons for prosthetic use. No clear proof exists in the literature regarding possible relationships between age of fitting and prosthetic use in later life [15,16].

The findings of this study should be interpreted in the context of qualitative studies and focus groups. Future studies in larger populations, designed as interviews or questionnaires, might explore in detail the reasons why children and early and late adolescents with UCBED either wear prostheses or do not do so.

Conclusions

Children and early and late adolescents with UCBED seem to choose and wear prostheses mainly for cosmetic reasons, in order to achieve social integration and not because of limited functionality. Peer-to-peer contact, organized by the rehabilitation teams in conjunction with other institutions, appeared to be an important informational and emotional support for children, early adolescents, and parents. When working with UCBED youngsters there should also be a focus on the importance of the cosmetic possibilities offered by a prosthesis. Extending the treatment options beyond prostheses to other solutions – such as, for example, the use of adaptive devices – would ease some daily-life activities for these children and adolescents. Further research should also focus on the psychosocial events and experiences in this young group.

Acknowledgments

The authors wish to thank Kiek Tates for methodological advice regarding the online focus group interviews. Esar van Hal is acknowledged for designing the website used in the study. We also thank Pieter U. Dijkstra for his assistance with the results presentation. We are grateful to all participants in the study and participants in the pilot study.

Author Contributions

Conceived and designed the experiments: IdJ WJ MP IvW HRM CvdS. Performed the experiments: IdJ HRM. Analyzed the data: EV HRM CvdS. Contributed reagents/materials/analysis tools: EV IdJ WJ MP IvW HRM CvdS. Wrote the paper: EV. Critical revision of manuscript for important intellectual content: IdJ WJ MP IvW HRM CvdS.

References

1. Giele H, Giele C, Bower C, Allison M (2001) The incidence and epidemiology of congenital upper limb anomalies: A total population study. J Hand Surg Am 26: 628–634.
2. Ekblom AG, Laurell T, Arner M (2010) Epidemiology of congenital upper limb anomalies in 562 children born in 1997 to 2007: A total population study from Stockholm, Sweden. J Hand Surg 35: 1742–1754.
3. Koskimies E, Lindfors N, Gissler M, Peltonen J, Nietosvaara Y (2011) Congenital upper limb deficiencies and associated malformations in Finland: A population-based study. J Hand Surg 36: 1058–1065.
4. Curran B, Hambrey R (1991) The prosthetic treatment of upper limb deficiency. Prosthet Orthot Int 15: 82–87.
5. Biddiss EA, Chau TT (2007) Upper limb prosthesis use and abandonment: A survey of the last 25 years. Prosthet Orthot Int 31: 236–257.

6. James MA, Bagley AM, Brasington K, Lutz C, McConnell S, et al. (2006) Impact of prostheses on function and quality of life for children with unilateral congenital below-the-elbow deficiency. J Bone Joint Surg Am 88: 2356–2365.

7. Buffart LM, Roebroeck ME, van Heijningen VG, Pesch-Batenburg JM, Stam HJ (2007) Evaluation of arm and prosthetic functioning in children with a congenital transverse reduction deficiency of the upper limb. J Rehabil Med 39: 379–386.

8. Hadders-Algra M, Reinders-Messelink HA, Huizing K, van den Berg R, van der Sluis CK, et al. (2012) Use and functioning of the affected limb in children with unilateral congenital below-elbow deficiency during infancy and preschool age: A longitudinal observational multiple case study. Early Hum Dev 89: 49–54.

9. Mundhenke L, Hermansson L, Sjoqvist Natterlund B (2010) Experiences of Swedish children with disabilities: Activities and social support in daily life. Scand J Occup Ther 17: 130–139.

10. Biddiss E, Chau T (2007) Upper-limb prosthetics: Critical factors in device abandonment. Am J Phys Med Rehabil 86: 977–987.

11. Biddiss EA, Chau TT (2008) Multivariate prediction of upper limb prosthesis acceptance or rejection. Disabil Rehabil Assist Technol 3: 181–192.

12. Davidson J (2002) A survey of the satisfaction of upper limb amputees with their prostheses, their lifestyles, and their abilities. J Hand Ther 15: 62–70.

13. Postema K, van der Donk V, van Limbeek J, Rijken RA, Poelma MJ (1999) Prosthesis rejection in children with a unilateral congenital arm defect. Clin Rehabil 13: 243–249.

14. Davids JR, Wagner LV, Meyer LC, Blackhurst DW (2006) Prosthetic management of children with unilateral congenital below-elbow deficiency. J Bone Joint Surg Am 88: 1294–1300.

15. Meurs M, Maathuis CG, Lucas C, Hadders-Algra M, van der Sluis CK (2006) Prescription of the first prosthesis and later use in children with congenital unilateral upper limb deficiency: A systematic review. Prosthet Orthot Int 30: 165–173.

16. Huizing K, Reinders-Messelink H, Maathuis C, Hadders-Algra M, van der Sluis CK (2010) Age at first prosthetic fitting and later functional outcome in children and young adults with unilateral congenital below-elbow deficiency: A cross-sectional study. Prosthet Orthot Int 34: 166–174.

17. Metzger AJ, Dromerick AW, Holley RJ, Lum PS (2012) Characterization of compensatory trunk movements during prosthetic upper limb reaching tasks. Arch Phys Med Rehabil 93: 2029–2034.

18. Nelson VS, Flood KM, Bryant PR, Huang ME, Pasquina PF, et al. (2006) Limb deficiency and prosthetic management. 1. Decision making in prosthetic prescription and management. Arch Phys Med Rehabil 87: S3–S9.

19. Krebs DE, Edelstein JE, Thornby MA (1991) Prosthetic management of children with limb deficiencies. Phys Ther 71: 920–934.

20. Kuyper MA, Breedijk M, Mulders AH, Post MW, Prevo AJ (2001) Prosthetic management of children in the Netherlands with upper limb deficiencies. Prosthet Orthot Int 25: 228–234.

21. de Jong IG, Reinders-Messelink HA, Janssen WG, Poelma MJ, van Wijk I, et al. (2012) Mixed feelings of children and adolescents with unilateral congenital below elbow deficiency: An online focus group study. PLoS One 7: e37099.

22. de Jong IG, Reinders-Messelink HA, Tates K, Janssen WG, Poelma MJ, et al. (2012) Activity and participation of children and adolescents with unilateral congenital below elbow deficiency: An online focus group study. J Rehabil Med 44: 885–892.

23. Rhodes SD, Bowie DA, Hergenrather KC (2003) Collecting behavioural data using the world wide web: Considerations for researchers. J Epidemiol Community Health 57: 68–73.

24. Tates K, Zwaanswijk M, Otten R, van Dulmen S, Hoogerbrugge PM, et al. (2009) Online focus groups as a tool to collect data in hard-to-include populations: Examples from paediatric oncology. BMC Med Res Methodol 9: 15.

25. Zwaanswijk M, Tates K, van Dulmen S, Hoogerbrugge PM, Kamps WA, et al. (2007) Young patients', parents', and survivors' communication preferences in paediatric oncology: Results of online focus groups. BMC Pediatr 7: 35.

26. Gaiser TJ (1997) Conducting on-line focus groups. Social Science Computer Review 15: 135–144.

27. Montoya-Weiss MM, Massey AP, Clapper DL (1998) On-line focus groups: Conceptual issues and a research tool. European Journal of Marketing 32: 713–723.

28. Zinchiak M (2001) Online focus group FAQs. Quirk's marketing research media. Available: http://www.quirks.com/articles/a2001/20010712.aspx?searchID=7987494. Accessed 16 August 2012.

29. Cher Ping L, Seng Chee T (2001) Online discussion boards for focus group interviews: An exploratory study. Journal of Educational Enquiry 2: 50–60.

30. Endacott R, Botti M (2007) Clinical research 3: Sample selection. Accid Emerg Nurs 15: 234–238.

31. World Health Organization (2007) International Classification of Functioning, Disability and Health: Children & Youth version: ICF-CY. Geneva: WHO.

32. Gill P, Stewart K, Treasure E, Chadwick B (2008) Methods of data collection in qualitative research: Interviews and focus groups. Br Dent J 204: 291–295.

33. Pope C, Mays N (2006) Qualitative research in health care. London: BMJ books: Blackwell Publishing. 153.

34. Pope C, Ziebland S, Mays N (2000) Qualitative research in health care. Analysing qualitative data. BMJ 320: 114–116.

35. Datta D, Selvarajah K, Davey N (2004) Functional outcome of patients with proximal upper limb deficiency–acquired and congenital. Clin Rehabil 18: 172–177.

36. Burger H, Marincek C (1994) Upper limb prosthetic use in Slovenia. Prosthet Orthot Int 18: 25–33.

37. Jang CH, Yang HS, Yang HE, Lee SY, Kwon JW, et al. (2011) A survey on activities of daily living and occupations of upper extremity amputees. Ann Rehabil Med 35: 907–921.

38. Atkins DJ, Heard DCY, Donovan WH (1996) Epidemiologic overview of individuals with upper-limb loss and their reported research priorities. JPO 8: 2–11.

39. Ritchie S, Wiggins S, Sanford A (2011) Perceptions of cosmesis and function in adults with upper limb prostheses: A systematic literature review. Prosthet Orthot Int 35: 332–341.

40. Jain S (1996) Rehabilitation in limb deficiency. 2. The pediatric amputee. Arch Phys Med Rehabil 77: S9–S13.

41. Ephraim PL, MacKenzie EJ, Wegener ST, Dillingham TR, Pezzin LE (2006) Environmental barriers experienced by amputees: The Craig hospital inventory of environmental factors-short form. Arch Phys Med Rehabil 87: 328–333.

42. Sheffler LC, Hanley C, Bagley A, Molitor F, James MA (2009) Comparison of self-reports and parent proxy-reports of function and quality of life of children with below-the-elbow deficiency. J Bone Joint Surg Am 91: 2852–2859.

43. Murray CD (2009) Being like everybody else: The personal meanings of being a prosthesis user. Disabil Rehabil 31: 573–581.

44. Schor EL (1986) Use of health care services by children and diagnoses received during presumably stressful life transitions. Pediatrics 77: 834–841.

45. Donkervoort M, Wiegerink DJ, van Meeteren J, Stam HJ, Roebroeck ME, et al. (2009) Transition to adulthood: Validation of the Rotterdam transition profile for young adults with cerebral palsy and normal intelligence. Dev Med Child Neurol 51: 53–62.

46. Wagner L, Bagley A, James M (2007) Reasons for prosthetic rejection by children with unilateral congenital transverse forearm total deficiency. Journal of Prosthetics & Orthotics, JPO 19: 51–54.

47. Biddiss E, Chau T (2007) The roles of predisposing characteristics, established need, and enabling resources on upper extremity prosthesis use and abandonment. Disabil Rehabil Assist Technol 2: 71–84.

48. Kejlaa GH (1993) Consumer concerns and the functional value of prostheses to upper limb amputees. Prosthet Orthot Int 17: 157–163.

49. Silcox DH,3rd, Rooks MD, Vogel RR, Fleming LL (1993) Myoelectric prostheses. A long-term follow-up and a study of the use of alternate prostheses. J Bone Joint Surg Am 75: 1781–1789.

50. Kanas JL, Holowka M (2009) Adaptive upper extremity prostheses for recreation and play. J Pediatr Rehabil Med 2: 181–187.

51. Saradjian A, Thompson AR, Datta D (2008) The experience of men using an upper limb prosthesis following amputation: Positive coping and minimizing feeling different. Disabil Rehabil 30: 871–883.

52. Romkema S, Bongers RM, van der Sluis CK (2012) Intermanual transfer in training with an upper-limb myoelectric prosthesis simulator. Phys Ther 93: 22–31.

53. Mathiesen AM, Frost CJ, Dent KM, Feldkamp ML (2012) Parental needs among children with birth defects: Defining a parent-to-parent support network. J Genet Couns 21: 862–872.

54. Kreitner C, Hartz AJ, Pflum RD (1994) Patient-centered care. Designing and delivering quality rehab services means placing patient needs over those of providers. Rehab Manag 7: 25–26, 29–30, 119.

55. Fraser CM (1998) An evaluation of the use made of cosmetic and functional prostheses by unilateral upper limb amputees. Prosthet Orthot Int 22: 216–223.

7

Final Disposition and Quality Auditing of the Rehabilitation Process in Wild Raptors Admitted to a Wildlife Rehabilitation Centre in Catalonia, Spain, during a Twelve Year Period (1995–2007)

Rafael A. Molina-López[1,2]*, **Jordi Casal[2,3]**, **Laila Darwich[2,3]**

1 Centre de Fauna Salvatge de Torreferrussa, Catalan Wildlife-Service-Forestal Catalana, Santa Perpètua de la Mogoda, Barcelona, Spain, 2 Departament de Sanitat i Anatomia Animals, Facultat de Veterinària, Universitat Autònoma de Barcelona, Cerdanyola del Vallès, Barcelona, Spain, 3 Centre de Recerca en Sanitat Animal (CReSA), UAB-IRTA, Campus Universitat Autònoma de Barcelona, Cerdanyola del Vallès, Barcelona, Spain

Abstract

Background: Variability in reporting and classification methods in previous published data of the final dispositions in the rehabilitation of wild raptors makes use of this data limited in trying to audit the quality of the rehabilitation process. Crude as well as stratified disposition rates are needed if quality auditing of the rehabilitation process is to be adequately performed.

Methodology: Final dispositions of 6221 hospitalized wild raptors admitted at a wildlife rehabilitation centre (WRC) of Catalonia during 1995–2007 were analyzed. These dispositions were calculated as the euthanasia (Er), unassisted mortality (Mr), release (Rr) and captivity rates (Cr)., time to death (Td) for dead and euthanized raptors, and length of stay for released (Tr) raptors was estimated. Stratified analyses by main causes of admission and clinical signs were performed.

Results: The disposition for the total population were: Er = 30.6%, Mr = 19.1%, Rr = 47.2%, and Cr = 3%. By main causes of admission, Er was higher in the trauma category (34.2%), whereas Mr was found similar between trauma (37.4%) and non-trauma categories (34.8%). The highest Rr was observed for the orphaned group (77.9%). Furthermore, Cr was low in all the categories (<4%). By clinical signs, the highest Er was found in animals suffering musculoskeletal (37.9%) or skin (32.3%) lesions; Mr was high in infectious/parasitic diseases (66.7%) and in case of neurological symptoms (64.5%). The euthanized birds had a median Td = 1 day (P_{10} = 0-P_{90} = 59) for both trauma and non-trauma categories, and Td = 36 days for the orphaned young group (P_{10} = 0; P_{90} = 596). The median Td in the unassisted dead birds was 2 days for all the categories (P_{10} = 0-P_{90} = 31). Finally, the median Tr in the centre was variable among categories.

Conclusions/Significance: Reporting of final dispositions in wildlife rehabilitation should include the crude and stratified rates (Er, Mr, Rr, and Cr), by causes and clinical presentation, as well as Td and Tr, to allow meaningful auditing of the rehabilitation process quality.

Editor: Justin David Brown, University of Georgia, United States of America

Funding: The study has been supported by the Catalan Wildlife-Service and Forestal Catalana. The funders had no role in study design, data collection and analysis, decision to publish, or preparation of the manuscript.

Competing Interests: The authors have declared that no competing interests exist.

* E-mail: rafael.molina@gencat.cat

Introduction

Rehabilitation of wild raptors is a complex process that includes both veterinary care of the injured bird and physical recovery and reconditioning of this animal for subsequent release in the wild [1]. The direct benefits derived from the recovery of wild birds could be summarized in several aspects: the improvement of the welfare of the individual animal, the reinforcement of the natural population after the release, especially in endangered species or long-lived birds, the identification of the causes of morbidity and mortality, and the regulatory changes implemented as a consequence of determining human influences and causes of admission [2,3].

Data published from wildlife rehabilitation centres (WRC) have been mainly focused on the causes of admission [4–7], on the investigation of some specific infectious or parasitic diseases and toxicoses [8–10] or on the establishment of bio-pathological reference values [11]. On the other hand, the final dispositions of the rehabilitation cases are commonly summarized or briefly described [12–14], but a stratified analysis by causes of the final disposition is rarely reported. This kind of analysis is crucial for building an evidence base for wildlife rehabilitation medicine and management.

Quality assessment is one of the strategic elements for the improvement and transformation of the modern human health system [15]. Outcomes research is an essential part of the quality control process, and quality indicators of medical performance have been defined by consensus in order to determine the quality of care in a measurable way [16,17]. In wildlife medicine, some clinical practice guidelines have been published which deal with welfare rehabilitation standards [18] and pre-release health screening protocols [19] but no quality indicators of the rehabilitation process have been defined.

The main objective of the present study was to analyze the outcomes of the rehabilitation of wild raptors in a WRC, adopting the four categories of the final disposition, the time until death and the length of stay as indicators of the quality audit of the rehabilitation process before release back to the wild.

Materials and Methods

Study design and animals

A retrospective study was performed using the original medical records of birds of prey admitted at the Wildlife Rehabilitation Centre (WRC) of Torreferrussa from 1995 to 2007. The centre is under the direction of the governmental Catalan Wildlife-Service. Samples were collected in compliance with the Ethical Principles in animal research guidelines in wildlife rehabilitation centres. The rehabilitation centres directly depend on the individual regional government wildlife services in Spain. Management and protocols were established according to the guidelines approved by each regional government according to legislation [20]. Animals that had to be euthanized for animal welfare reasons were administrated barbiturates by intravenous injection.

Definition of variables

Overall data about species, gender, age, date of admission, date of death or release, and primary cause of admission were included in the analyses. Classification of primary morbidity causes, criteria for sexing and ageing, as well as the geographical and demographical characteristics of the population were the same as those reported in a previous study [7].

The final disposition was divided into four categories adapted from Cooper (1987) [21]: euthanized animals (based on poor quality of life, or poor prognosis for survival on return to the wild), dead animals (with no human intervention), animals returned to the wild and permanently captive non-releasable animals (due to their poor prognosis of survivability in wilderness). The final dispositions were calculated by dividing the number of cases of each category by the total number of admissions in a given period of time; as a result, all four categories were expressed as rates: euthanasia rate (E_r), unassisted mortality rate (M_r), release rate (R_r), and captivity rate (C_r). In addition, R_r was analysed taking into account the season of admission and the season of release.

The final disposition was first analyzed based on the primary cause of admission grouped as trauma, non-trauma and orphaned young categories. It was then analyzed according to the main clinical signs of the animals at the time of the admission. This clinical presentation was based on the International Statistical Classification of Diseases and Related Health Problems-ICD-10 (WHO, 2004) [22] but adapting the categories to wildlife medicine. We have adopted a single-condition morbidity analysis in which the main condition was defined as the primary condition responsible for the patient's need for treatment or investigation. If there was more than one such condition, the one held most responsible for the greatest use of resources was selected. If no diagnosis was made, the main symptom, abnormal finding or problem was selected as the main condition. In this line, the initial signs were divided into the following categories: apparently healthy animals, infectious/parasitic diseases, endocrine/nutritional/met-

abolic diseases, behavioural abnormalities (imprinted or tame), eye and adnexa problems, skin and subcutaneous conditions, alterations in the different systems (nervous, respiratory, digestive and musculoskeletal), traumatic signs not classified in any of the previous categories, and others which included birds with different clinical signs not classified in the above categories. In order to minimize overlapping between diagnostic categories, the infectious/parasitic diseases category included all those diseases generally recognized as communicable or transmissible, despite the affected system.

Additional parameters such as time until death $(T_d$; difference between the date of admission and the date of the death) for euthanized and for dead animals, and length of stay in the centre for the released raptors $(T_r$; difference between the date of admission and the release date) were also evaluated. In order to study the cases with longest T_d, the percentiles 10 (P_{10}), 75 (P_{75}) and 90 (P_{90}) of this variable were selected as a cut-off point.

Quality indicators of the rehabilitation process conducted at the centre were evaluated based on different outcome variables following guidelines used in human medicine [23,24]. The main indicators adopted in our work were the four categories of the final disposition, the time until death (T_d) and the length of stay at the centre for the released raptors (T_r).

Statistical analysis

Descriptive statistics, normality test and inferential analyses were done at 95% confidence levels with SPSS Advanced Models ™ 15.0 (SPSS Inc. 233 South Wacker Drive, 11th Floor Chicago, IL 60606-6412). Median (P_{50}). Percentiles 10, 75 and 90 $(P_{10}; P_{75}; P_{90})$ were provided for the descriptive analysis of the dispositions T_d and T_r. Comparisons of the median were evaluated using the U-Mann-Whitney and Kruskal-Wallis test. Chi-square (χ^2) or Fisher exact tests were used for comparisons between the E_r, M_r, R_r and C_r and sex, age and order co-variables.

In order to compare the differences along the period of study of the final disposition categories, a ratio between the number of dispositions and the total number of cases per year was estimated. A linear regression model was used to estimate the trend of the dispositions during the period of study according to the main cause of admission categories and the order.

Results

Descriptive analyses of the total population

During a period of twelve years (from 1995 to 2007), a total of 7553 raptor admissions were reported at the WRC. After a critical review of all the admissions, 1332 cases were excluded for not fulfilling the inclusion criteria (739 cases were admitted dead and 593 cases included captive birds, captive-borne or falconry birds). Thus, the final population of this study was 6221 individuals distributed in the following orders: 3241 Strigiformes and 2980 Falconiformes.

The age distribution demonstrated that 46.3% (2884/6221) of birds were within their first year of age, 32.3% (2009/6221) were >1 calendar year and 21.3% (1328/6221) were of unknown age. Most of the animals, 59.4% (n = 3695), were classified as undetermined gender, 21.9% (n = 1363) of raptors were sexed as female and 18.7% (n = 1163) as males.

A crude analysis of the final disposition of the total raptor population showed the following rates: $E_r = 30.6\%$ (1903/6221), $M_r = 19.1\%$ (1191/6221), $R_r = 47.2\%$ (2939/6221), $C_r = 3\%$ (188/6221) (Fig. 1).

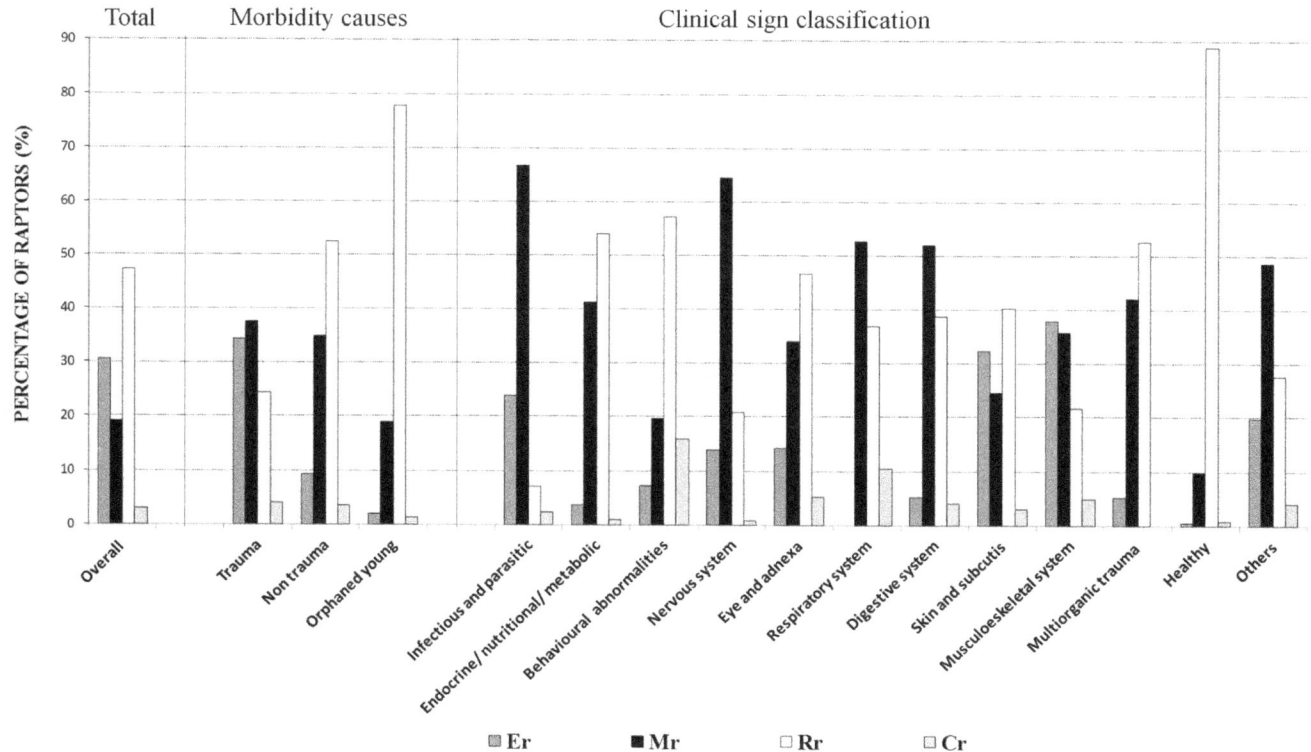

Figure 1. Resolution rates of euthanized (Er), dead (Mr), released (Rr) and captive (Cr) raptors relative to the overall population, the principal cause of the admission and the clinical signs.

Rehabilitation final dispositions by causes of admission

Stratifying by the primary cause of admission, 49.7% (3092/6221) of birds were classified into the trauma category, 15.7% (976/6221) in the non-trauma and 34.6% (2152/6221) in the orphaned young category. The euthanasia rate was notably higher in the trauma category (34.2%) compared to the non-trauma (9.2%) or orphaned young (2%) (Fig. 1), and mainly due to those cases related to electrocution and collisions with power lines (Table 1). The unassisted mortality rate was similar in both trauma (37.4%) and non-trauma (34.8%) categories but lower in the orphaned young (18.9%). Within the traumatic causes, animals found in traps (52.6%), and collisions with vehicles (46.5%) or fences (47.8%) presented the highest unassisted mortality rate. In the non-traumatic causes, infectious/parasitic diseases had the highest rate of mortality (70%). The release rate was significantly higher in the orphaned young (77.9%) and in non-trauma (52.5%) categories compared to the trauma category (24.3%). In the last category, birds who suffered collision with buildings had the best rates of release compared to the other traumatic causes. Finally, low rates of captivity were found in the three categories (4.1% trauma, 3.5% non-trauma) and particularly in the orphaned young birds (1.3%) (Table 1).

In the subgroup of animals with known sex and age, the unassisted mortality rate was higher in males than in females, in both non-trauma ($\chi^2 = 6.6$; $p = 0.0098$) and orphaned young ($\chi^2 = 15.8$; $p = 0.003$) categories.

Rehabilitation final dispositions by clinical signs

The euthanasia rate (E_r) was higher in those animals suffering lesions at the skin level (32.3%), mostly affected by extensive wounds and electric burns, or at the musculoskeletal system,

basically due to fractures and luxations (37.9%) (Fig. 1). By contrast, E_r was very low in adults presenting endocrine/nutritional/metabolic disorders (3.7%) and digestive disorders (5.3%). The unassisted mortality rate (Mr) was elevated in raptors with infectious/parasitic diseases (66.7%), mainly trichomoniasis, or with neurological symptoms like depression, ataxia and paralysis (64.5%). The highest rate of release was observed in the apparently healthy animals (88.9%), mostly represented by young orphaned birds and birds belonging to the fortuity category, including birds found inside buildings or other human structures. The R_r was also high for animals with behavioural abnormalities (57.3%) and in animals in the endocrine/nutritional/metabolic (54.1%) category when this comprised birds with low body condition and weakness as main general symptoms. Finally, the captivity rate was elevated in those animals with behavioural abnormalities (15.9%) and respiratory distress (10.5%) (Table 2).

Additional parameters: time until death and length of stay at the centre

The group of euthanized birds had a median $T_{d} = 1$ day ($P_{10} = 0$; $P_{90} = 59$) for the trauma ($P_{10} = 0$; $P_{90} = 41$) and non-trauma ($P_{10} = 0$; $P_{90} = 171$) categories, and $T_{d} = 36$ days for the orphaned young group ($P_{10} = 0$; $P_{90} = 596$) (Table 3). Interestingly, the median T_d in the dead birds was 2 days for all the categories ($P_{10} = 0$; $P_{90} = 31$). On the other hand, the median time of stay in the centre was highly variable among categories, presenting the trauma the longest times ($T_r = 115$) compared to non-trauma ($T_r = 58$) and orphaned young ($T_r = 59$) groups (Table 3).

Taking into account the season of the admission because it is of relevance for the decision of approving the release of rehabilitated animals, the median T_r was statistically different among seasons

Table 1. Description of the number and percentage of raptor cases according to their final disposition and the cause of admission at the wildlife rehabilitation centre.

Primary cause	Total	Euthanasia		Mortality		Release		Captivity	
Categories	N	n	Rate (%)	N	Rate (%)	n	Rate (%)	n	Rate (%)
Trauma	**3092**	**1058**	**34.2**	**1157**	**37.4**	**750**	**24.3**	**127**	**4.1**
Unknown trauma	1691	560	33.1	658	38.9	385	22.8	88	5.2
Gunshot	627	183	29.2	210	33.5	207	33.0	27	4.3
Vehicles	471	136	28.9	219	46.5	108	22.9	8	1.7
Electrocution	197	162	82.2	30	15.2	2	1.0	3	1.5
Building	52	3	5.8	17	32.7	32	61.5	0	0.0
Fences	23	9	39.1	11	47.8	3	13.0	0	0.0
Power lines	9	5	55.6	2	22.2	2	22.2	0	0.0
Trap	19	0	0.0	10	52.6	8	42.1	1	5.3
Predation	3	0	0.0	0	0.0	3	100.0	0	0.0
Non-trauma	**976**	**90**	**9.2**	**340**	**34.8**	**512**	**52.5**	**34**	**3.5**
Fortuity*	346	8	2.3	99	28.6	235	67.9	4	1.2
Undetermined	165	27	16.4	71	43.0	63	38.2	4	2.4
Metabolic/nutritional	223	27	12.1	95	42.6	94	42.2	7	3.1
Captivity	156	13	8.3	27	17.3	100	64.1	16	10.3
Infectious parasitic	84	15	17.9	46	54.8	20	23.8	3	3.6
Toxicoses	2	0	0.0	2	100.0	0	0.0	0	0.0
Orphaned young	**2153**	**43**	**2.0**	**406**	**18.9**	**1677**	**77.9**	**27**	**1.3**

*Fortuity includes all raptors found in manure heaps, bad weather conditions, etc, as previously defined by Molina-Lopez et al. (2011).

Table 2. Description of the number and percentage of raptor cases according to the final disposition and clinical signs presented at the admission at the wildlife rehabilitation centre.

Primary clinical signs	Total	Euthanasia		Mortality		Release		Captivity	
	N	n	Rate (%)	n	Rate (%)	n	Rate (%)	n	Rate (%)
Infectious and parasitic	42	10	23.8	28	66.7	3	7.1	1	2.4
Endocrine/nutritional/metabolic	862	32	3.7	355	41.2	466	54.1	9	1.0
Behavioural abnormalities	82	6	7.3	16	19.5	47	57.3	13	15.9
Nervous system	324	45	13.9	209	64.5	67	20.7	3	0.9
Eye and adnexa	206	29	14.1	70	34.0	96	46.6	11	5.3
Respiratory system	19	0	0.0	10	52.6	7	36.8	2	10.5
Digestive system	75	4	5.3	39	52.0	29	38.7	3	4.0
Skin and subcutis	679	219	32.3	166	24.4	273	40.2	21	3.1
Musculoeskeletal system	2110	799	37.9	751	35.6	456	21.6	104	4.9
Multi-organic trauma	19	1	5.3	8	42.1	10	52.6	0	0.0
Healthy	1610	8	0.5	157	9.8	1432	88.9	13	0.8
Others*	193	38	19.7	94	48.7	53	27.5	8	4.1

*Included all cases with other clinical signs not classified in any of the described categories.

($\chi^2 = 269.933$; p<0,001), with raptors admitted in spring presenting stays of 85 days ($P_{10} = 12$; $P_{90} = 296$), 53 days ($P_{10} = 16$; $P_{90} = 212$) if admitted in summer, 113 days ($P_{10} = 10$; $P_{90} = 386$) if admitted in autumn and 130.5 days ($P_{10} = 23$; $P_{90} = 418$) if admitted in winter.

Time evolution of dispositions along the study period

No statistically significant differences were observed among the final dispositions during the 12 years of the study in the overall group. However, in the traumatic category, a significant decrease in the unassisted mortality rate was observed (B = −0.12; p = 0.035).

Discussion

Historically, wildlife programs were developed as a consequence of the concern of modern society with both animal welfare and the negative impact of human activities in wildlife population. Rehabilitation of birds of prey and owls has led to the development

Table 3. Statistical descriptive of time that animals were keep in the rehabilitation centre until the final disposition.

	Time (days) from admission to final disposition											
	Euthanasia rate				Unassisted Mortality rate				Release rate			
Admission Causes	P_{10}	P_{50}	P_{75}	P_{90}	P_{10}	P_{50}	P_{75}	P_{90}	P_{10}	P_{50}	P_{75}	P_{90}
Trauma	0	1	7	41	0	2	5	26	24	115	265	443
Unknown trauma	0	1	7	57	0	2	5	27	24	94	240	416
Gunshot	0	2	22	82	0	3	7	74	66	207	320	621
Vehicles	0	1	10	28	0	2	5	15	14	95	239	485
Electrocution	0	0	1	4	0	2	4	7	N/A	N/A		N/A
Building	0	0	0	0	1	2	6	18	1	45	133	241
Fences	0	1	3	0	1	2	7	477	1	22	Na	N/A
Trap	0	N/A	N/A	N/A	N/A	8	11	15	5	15	148	N/A
Non-trauma	0	1	25	171	0	2	5	16	2	58	163	372
Fortuity	0	0	3	298	0	2	4	25	1	37	116	311
Undetermined	0	0	2	156	0	1	3	8	7	51	128	393
Metabolic/nutritional	0	1	25	96	0	2	5	18	11	63	110	280
Captivity	0	16	119	399	0	2	13	68	21	158	320	516
Infectious/parasitic	0	8	19	138	0	2	6	13	30	60	108	372
Orphaned young	0	36	187	596	0	2	14	51	18	59	87	179

P_{10}, P_{50}, P_{75}, P_{90}: percentiles 10, 50 (or median), 75 and 90; N/A, not applicable (just one case).

of many of these programs due to the sensitivity of wild birds to human threats, the unfavourable status of many species and the public interest in these predators [25].

A detailed description of primary causes of admission has been thoroughly reported [26] and welfare and general guidelines for rehabilitation of wild raptors are available [18]. However, the approach to the quality of audit in wildlife rehabilitation is poorly reported. In human medicine, quality indicators of the dispositions are employed to assess and improve the quality of care in many healthcare settings [27]. The data presented in the current study report the crude and stratified dispositions rates by cause and clinical entities, but also the time until death and the length of stay. All six parameters have been considered as quality indicators as a baseline for a quality audit.

From the data it is evident that less than half of raptors admitted to rehabilitation in Catalonia were successfully released. 52.8% of raptor admissions resulted in euthanasia, mortality or permanent captivity. Only 47.2% of birds were successfully returned to the wild. Nevertheless, an estimation of the final dispositions based on the main causes of admission or the clinical entities is essential in order to compare the results. The most simplistic and realistic classification is that consisting of two groups: 1) healthy young birds requiring rearing, 2) injured and ill birds, including those that have been kept illegally in captivity. Orphaned young birds represent an important part of the admissions to the WRC [28], usually concentrated in a short period of time and resulting in filling of rehabilitation facilities to maximum capacity and needing labour intensive care. Moreover, many of the birds are likely not true orphans, but because they are easily found by humans are brought to the WRC [29] and are apparently in good overall health. The proportion of releases in this group is high, and this influences the overall dispositions and results.

Literature on the dispositions of bird of prey rehabilitation is variable, making comparison between studies difficult. Most studies emphasise the release rate [30] as the main outcome, but overall causes are also frequently estimated [13,31]. In fact, two basic dispositions could be considered: releases and non-releases, including death, euthanasia and captivity of non-releasable birds. In the authors' opinion, the four categories (release, unassisted death, euthanasia and permanent captivity) should be analysed individually as a basic assessment of the quality indicators of the rehabilitation process, due to their different biological and management implications.

Euthanasia is an essential option in all wildlife rehabilitation, based on both animal welfare and optimization of economical resources [1,32]. However, beyond the situations in which the rehabilitation of the bird is not a viable option and euthanasia is the most appropriate disposition, legal policies preclude the final disposition of a bird of prey in some countries [33]. In our study, the overall rate of euthanasia was 30.6%, and the highest values were found in the trauma category (34.2%) mainly due to electrocutions and collisions with power lines. In our experience these animals frequently cannot be rehabilitated for release due to the severity of their injuries.

Mortality rate has been used as a quality indicator parameter in human medicine [34]. Unfortunately, in wildlife rehabilitation this parameter has been variably reported in most studies without defining criteria, making the comparison of results difficult. In some studies the mortality rate includes the proportion of deaths as well as the proportion of euthanized animals while others do not [13,35]. This approach may lead to overestimations of the actual rate of non-human intervention results. In our opinion, unassisted mortality rate and proportion of euthanized should be estimated separately and included in the general disposition report.

Our data demonstrated a similar rate of mortality for trauma (37.4%) and non-trauma (34.8%) cases. In the non-traumatic group, the higher M_r was due to infectious diseases, particularly trichomoniasis. It has previously been reported that the majority of cases demonstrating lesions produced by *Trichomonas spp* affecting the oral cavity and choanal slit, have a poor prognosis [36], and our findings confirmed this. In this study, the unassisted mortality rate due to gunshot was 33.5%, greater than that reported by Richards et al, 2005 (14%) [37] or Ress and Guyer, 2004 (<20%) [38]. This is due to regional differences in firearms availability, hunting and legislation. In our work M_r had an approximate 30% value in the three most prevalent causes of trauma. Most of those cases suffered severe trauma with multiple body systems affected. Finally, the unassisted mortality rate found in our young orphaned group (18.9%) was similar to other reports (16.1%) [39].

According to the classification of clinical signs, M_r was over 50% when the nervous, respiratory or digestive systems were primarily affected or in cases of general systemic infectious or parasitic disease. The M_r was higher in birds with integument and musculoskeletal conditions. On the other hand, the higher M_r in animals apparently healthy on admission or with nutritional and metabolic conditions is suggestive of captivity-related complications and requires further investigation. In the authors' opinion, the present classification focusing on clinical signs allows a more accurate assessment of the rehabilitation protocols than those based on the primary cause of admission. Both classifications are useful; clinical classification allows a veterinary perspective, while the primary cause of admission allows an assessment of environmental causes and problems, and should be included in the analysis of dispositions of the rehabilitation of wild birds of prey.

The release rate in our study was higher in the orphaned young group, followed by fortuity and captive birds that were mainly affected by minor health conditions. The overall release rate of trauma cases was 24.3% (ranging from 1% of electrocution cases to 61.5% of birds suffering impacts with buildings). The release rates of gunshot, collision with vehicles and unknown trauma were very similar to those previously reported [14,37,38], being under 35% in all cases. On the other hand, the permanent captivity rate differs and needs special consideration. The final disposition of a non-releasable bird depends on the welfare and legal policies of the country or of the centre. Therefore, comparison of this rate could be useless if the rehabilitation criteria and policies are not specified. In our centre, euthanasia decision-making is based on welfare and economical criteria; thus the rate of permanently captive birds is relatively low.

Length of stay is a quality indicator parameter frequently used in human medicine [40]. In rehabilitation of wild raptors the decision of when to release an animal is based on the criteria related with the rehabilitation process (health status, fitness and behaviour), but also on external/ecological factors [41]. In fact, the longest periods of stay observed in birds admitted in winter and autumn were explained by the dates of the hunting season in the area of the study, as well as adverse weather conditions. Some migratory species such as *Circaetus gallicus*, *Pernis apivorus* and *Otus scops* were maintained at the centre until the next spring migration. As a general rule, the length of stay must be as short as possible in order to reduce the risk of captive-related complications, infectious and parasitic disease, and behavioural abnormalities [42]. The length of stay is thus a critical parameter in assessing the quality of rehabilitation protocols.

The parameter time to death provides direct insight into the initial assessment and prognostication, the overall rehabilitation process, as well as the validity of veterinary protocols. This complements understanding of the mortality and euthanasia rates. In all time dependent variables we have included the extreme values because they highlight the real daily work of the rehabilitation centre, with birds remaining in captivity for unknown reasons. Interestingly, the median time to euthanasia was 1 day. That means that the decision is taken at the moment of the admission, resulting in optimization of welfare and financial resources. On the other hand, the median time of death was 2 days even for the young orphaned group. This fact suggests that special care and a complete clinical evaluation should be performed on all young birds, despite their apparently healthy appearance.

In our work, we paid attention into the M_r and E_r over the P_{90} of the T_d, as an indicator of undesirable or unexpected dispositions. The decision of euthanasia over 59 days was mostly taken due to complications related to trauma or musculoskeletal conditions. In our protocols, at 59 days most birds are in outside enclosures undergoing active flight conditioning. At this stage the decision to euthanize is taken in birds with musculoskeletal problems as well as those demonstrating abnormal behaviour incompatible with release to the wild.

Finally, a significant decrease in the unassisted mortality rate was observed in the traumatic category. This finding could be consequence of the improvement of both diagnostic and therapeutic protocols applied in the last years. The optimization of protocols for identifying specimens that are non-viable, has permitted the early euthanasia of these animals, avoiding unnecessary animal suffering and improving the management efficiency of resources.

In conclusion, the basic outcome research of the rehabilitation process of wild birds of prey and owls should include the four final disposition rates (Mr, Er, Rr and Cr), but also the parameters time until death (Td) and length of stay at the centre (Tr). The reports should also include the overall rates and the stratified analysis according to the cause of admission and the clinical entities. Moreover, both Td and Tr should be estimated by the overall group, but also stratifying by final decision and cause of admission and clinical entities. These six parameters are measurable items that should be considered as a baseline indicators for quality audits. Our results could represent a reference of a large amount of parameters related with the outcomes of the wildlife rehabilitation process that could be adapted by other centres as a start-point for further comparison. Finally, consensus of the professionals involved in rehabilitation of wild birds of prey is essential in order to develop evidence-based clinical guidelines and recommendations that will lead to an improvement of the rehabilitation procedure.

Acknowledgments

We are grateful to Sonia Almeria for the technical advice and review of the manuscript. We thank all the staff of the Torreferrussa Rehabilitation Centre (Catalan Wildlife-Service, Forestal Catalana).

Author Contributions

Conceived and designed the experiments: RAML JC LD. Performed the experiments: RAML JC LD. Analyzed the data: RAML JC LD. Contributed reagents/materials/analysis tools: RAML JC LD. Wrote the paper: RAML JC LD.

References

1. Redig PT, Arent L, Lopez H, Cruz L (2007) Rehabilitation. In: Bird DM, Bildstein KL, editors. Raptor Research and Management Techniques. Surrey: Hancock House Publishers LTD. 411–422.
2. Redig PT, Duke GE (1995) The effect and value of raptor rehabilitation in North America. Wildlife Management Institute. Transactions of the Sixtieth North American Wildlife and Natural Resources Conference. 24-29 March, 1995. Minneapolis, Minnesota. 163–172.
3. Sleeman JM and Clark EE (2003) Clinical Wildlife Medicine: A new paradigm for a new century. J Avian Med. Surg. 17: 33–37.
4. Martínez JA, Izquierdo A, Zuberogoitia I (2001) Causes of admission of raptors in rescue centres of the East of Spain and proximate causes of mortality. Biota 2: 163–169.
5. Brown JD, Sleeman JM (2002) Morbidity and mortality of reptiles admitted to the Wildlife Centre of Virginia, 1991 to 2000. J Wildl. Dis. 38: 699–705.
6. Kelly TR, Sleeman JM (2003) Morbidity and Mortality of Red Foxes (*Vulpes vulpes*) and Gray Foxes (*Urocyon cinereoargenteus*) Admitted to the Wildlife Centre of Virginia, 1993–2001. J Wildl. Dis. 39: 467–469.
7. Molina-López RA, Casal J, Darwich L (2011) Causes of Morbidity in Wild Raptor Populations Admitted at a Wildlife Rehabilitation Centre in Spain from 1995–2007: a Long Term Retrospective Study. PLoSOne 6 (9): e24603.
8. Kramer JL, Redig PT (1997) Sixteen years of lead poisoning in eagles, 1980–95: An epizootiologic view. J Raptor Res. 31: 327–332.
9. Smith WA, Mazet JAK, Hirsh DC (2002) Salmonella in California wildlife species: prevalence in rehabilitation centres and characterization of isolates. J Zoo Wildl. Med. 33: 228–235.
10. Cabezón O, García-Bocanegra I, Molina-López R, Marco I, Blanco JM, et al. Seropositivity and Risk Factors Associated with Toxoplasma gondii Infection in Wild Birds from Spain. PLoS ONE 6(12): e29549.
11. Black PA, McRuer DL, Horne LA (2011) Hematologic parameters in raptor species in a rehabilitation setting before release. J Avian Med. Surg. 25: 192–198.
12. Hartup BK (1996) Rehabilitation of native reptiles and amphibians in DuPage County, Illinois. J Wildl. Dis. 32: 109–112.
13. Deem SL, Terrell SP, Forrester DJ (1998) A retrospective study of morbidity and mortality of raptors in Florida: 1988–1994. J Zoo Wildl. Med. 29: 160–164.
14. Rodríguez B, Rodríguez A, Siverio F, Siverio M (2010) Causes of raptor admissions to a wildlife rehabilitation Center in Tenerife (Canary Islands). J Raptor Res. 44: 30–39.
15. García RE (2001) El concepto de calidad y su aplicación en Medicina. Rev Méd Chile 129: 825–26. [The concept of quality and its application in Medicine].
16. Soto J (2007) Implicación de la investigación de resultados en salud en la mejora continua de la calidad asistencial del Sistema Nacional de Salud. An Med.

Interna 24: 517–519. [Implication of results research on health in continual improvement in the National Health System social welfare quality].
17. Romero M, Soria V, Ruiz P, Rodríguez E, Aguayo JL (2010) Guidelines and clinical pathways. Is there really a difference? Cir. Esp. 88: 81–84.
18. Miller EA (2012) Minimum standards for wildlife rehabilitation. Fourth Edition. St. Cloud: NWRA & IWRC. 116.
19. Woodford MH (2000) Quarantine and Health Screening Protocols for Wildlife prior to Translocation and Release into the Wild. In: Woodford MH, editors. Gland: IUCN Species Survival Commission's Veterinary Specialist Group. 87.
20. R.D.1201/2005 of the Ministry of Presidency of Spain (10th October 2005). BOE 21st October 2005. Available: www.boe.es/boe/dias/2005/10/21/pdfs/A34367-34391.pdf. Accessed 2013 Feb 27.
21. Cooper JE (1987) Raptor care and rehabilitation: precedents, progress and potential. J Raptor Res 21: 21–26.
22. World Health Organization (2004) ICD-10: International Statistical Classification of Diseases and related Health problems: Tenth revision. Volume 2. Second Edition. Geneva: World Health Organization. 125.
23. Braun JP, Mende H, Bause H, Bloos F, Geldner G, et al (2010) Quality indicators in intensive care medicine: why? Use or burden for the intensivist. Germ Med. Sci. 8: Doc 22. doi:10.3205/000111.
24. Weiner BJ, Alexander JA, Shortell SM, Baker LC, Becker M, et al (2006) Quality Improvement Implementation and Hospital Performance on Quality Indicators. HSR: Health Services Research 41: 307–333.
25. Lawrence J (1997) A study of the benefits of raptor rehabilitation to the public. Senior Thesis Projects, 1993–2002. The University of Tennessee. Available: http://trace.tennessee.edu/utk_interstp2/17. Accessed 2013 Feb 27.
26. Morishita TY, Fullerton AT, Lownestine L, Gardner IA, Brooks DL (1998) Morbidity and mortality of free-living raptorial birds of Northern California: a retrospective study, 1983–1994. J Avian Med. Surg. 12: 78–90.
27. Kötter T, Blozik E, Scherer M (2012) Methods for the guideline-based development of quality indicators. A systematic review. Implementation Science 7: 21. Available: http://www.implementationscience.com/content/7/1/21. Accessed 2013 Feb 27.
28. Kirkwood JK (2003) Introduction: wildlife casualties and the veterinary surgeon. In: Mullineaux E, Best D, Cooper JE, editors. BSAVA Manual of Wildlife Casualties. Gloucester: British Small Animal Veterinary Association. 1–5.
29. Stocker L (2005) Birds of Prey. In: Stocker L, editor. Practical Wildlife Care. Second Edition. Oxford: Blackwell Publishing. 159–170.
30. Duke GE, Redig PT, Jones W (1981) Recoveries and resightings of released rehabilitated raptors. J Raptor Res. 15: 97–107.
31. Fix AS, Barrows SZ (1990) Raptors rehabilitated in Iowa during 1986 and 1987: A retrospective study. J Wildl. Dis. 26: 18–21.

32. Sleeman JM (2008) Use of Wildlife Rehabilitation Centres as monitors of ecosystem health. In: Fowler ME, Miller RE, editors. Zoo and Wild Animal Medicine. Saint Louis: Elsevier-Saunders. 97–104.

33. Millsap BA, Cooper MA, Holroyd G (2007) Legal Considerations. In: Bird DM, Bildstein KL, editors. Raptor Research and Management Techniques. Surrey: Hancock House Publishers LTD. 437–449.

34. Jiménez RE (2004) Indicadores de calidad y eficiencia de los servicios hospitalarios. Una mirada actual. Rev Cubana Salud Pública 30:17–36.

35. Punch P (2001) A retrospective study of the success of medical and surgical treatment of wild Australian raptors. Aust. Vet. J. 79: 747–752.

36. Samour JH, Naldo JL (2003) Diagnosis and therapeutic management of trichomoniasis in Falcons in Saudi Arabia. J Avian Med. Surg. 17: 136–143.

37. Richards J, Lickey A, Sleeman JM (2005) Decreasing Prevalence and Seasonal Variation of Gunshot Trauma in Raptors Admitted to the Wildlife Centre of Virginia: 1993–2002. J Zoo Wildl. Med. 36: 485–488.

38. Ress S, Guyer C (2004) A retrospective study of mortality and rehabilitation of raptors in the south-eastern region of the United States. J Raptor Res 38: 77–81.

39. Komnenou AT, Georgopoulou I, Savvas I, Dessiris A (2005) A retrospective study of presentation, treatment, and outcome of free-ranging raptors in Greece (1997–2000). J Zoo Wildl. Med. 36: 222–228.

40. OECD (2011) Average length of stay in hospitals. Health at a Glance 2011: OECD Indicators, OECD Publishing. Available: http://dx.doi.org/10.1787/health_glance-2011-33-en. Accessed 2013 Feb 27.

41. Arent L (2001) Reconditioning raptors: a training manual for the creance technique. Minneapolis: The Raptor Centre, College of Veterinary Medicine, University of Minnesota. 32–39.

42. Cooper JE, Cooper ME (2006) Ethical and legal implications of treating casualty wild animals. In Practice 28: 2–6.

8

Substantial Generalization of Sensorimotor Learning from Bilateral to Unilateral Movement Conditions

Jinsung Wang*, Yuming Lei, Khongchee Xiong, Katie Marek

Department of Kinesiology, The University of Wisconsin, Milwaukee, Wisconsin, United States of America

Abstract

Controversy exists regarding whether bimanual skill learning can generalize to unimanual performance. For example, some investigators showed that dynamic adaptation could only partially generalize between bilateral and unilateral movement conditions, while others demonstrated complete generalization of visuomotor adaptation. Here, we identified three potential factors that might have contributed to the discrepancy between the two sets of findings. In our first experiment, subjects performed reaching movements toward eight targets bilaterally with a novel force field applied to both arms, then unilaterally with the force field applied to one arm. Results showed that the dynamic adaptation generalized completely from bilateral to unilateral movements. In our second experiment, the same force field was only applied to one arm during both bilateral and unilateral movements. Results indicated complete transfer again. Finally, our subjects performed reaching movements toward a single target with the force field or a novel visuomotor rotation applied only to one arm during both bilateral and unilateral movements. The reduced breadth of experience obtained during bilateral movements resulted in incomplete transfer, which explains previous findings of limited generalization. These findings collectively suggest a substantial overlap between the neural processes underlying bilateral and unilateral movements, supporting the idea that bilateral training, often employed in stroke rehabilitation, is a valid method for improving unilateral performance. However, our findings also suggest that while the neural representations developed during bilateral training can generalize to facilitate unilateral performance, the extent of generalization may depend on the breadth of experience obtained during bilateral training.

Editor: Paul L. Gribble, The University of Western Ontario, Canada

Funding: This research was supported by the National Institutes of Health grant K01HD050245 (JW) and University of Wisconsin - Milwaukee SURF Awards (KX, KM). The funders had no role in study design, data collection and analysis, decision to publish, or preparation of the manuscript.

Competing Interests: The authors have declared that no competing interests exist.

* E-mail: wang34@uwm.edu

Introduction

Sensorimotor adaptation allows the nervous system a highly flexible control that can account for temporary, but predictable changes in response to varying constraints of a given task [1]. To understand the nature of sensorimotor adaptation, various types of generalization paradigms have been used, which include examining transfer of visuomotor or dynamic adaptation across different conditions within the same arm [2–4] or between the arms [5–7]. More recently, investigators started examining transfer of sensorimotor adaptation between bilateral and unilateral reaching conditions [8–11], which has major implications for stroke rehabilitation or athletic training. Bilateral arm training, for example, is used to improve motor function of the paretic arm post stroke and seems to have facilitative effects [12–14]. However, these claims are only valid if bilateral training can indeed generalize to unilateral performance.

Recently, the efficacy of bilateral arm training was questioned by Nozaki and colleagues, who showed that adaptation to a novel dynamic condition could generalize between bilateral and unilateral movement conditions, but only to a limited extent. Based on this finding, they suggested that only a partial overlap exists between the neural processes underlying the two types of movement. More recently, however, we demonstrated that adaptation to a novel visuomotor condition could generalize

completely from bilateral to unilateral conditions [10], [11], which contradicts Nozaki et al.'s argument.

To resolve this controversy, we identified three potential factors that might have contributed to the discrepancy between the two sets of findings. The first factor involves the nature of sensorimotor tasks: Nozaki and colleagues employed a dynamic adaptation task, whereas we employed a visuomotor adaptation task. In fact, it has been previously suggested that dynamic and visuomotor adaptation may involve distinct neural mechanisms [6], [15]. The second factor we identified concerns the fact that during bilateral adaptation, perturbations were simultaneously given to both arms in our studies, but only to one arm in Nozaki et al.'s study. The last factor concerns the breadth of experience obtained during sensorimotor adaptation. Subjects in our previous studies experienced eight target directions during reaching movements, whereas those in Nozaki et al.'s study experienced a single target. It seems plausible that a greater breadth of experience obtained during initial practice may lead to the development of a more complete sensorimotor transformation; and if so, multiple-target training during bilateral adaptation may lead to greater generalization as compared to single-target training.

In the present study, we examined the effects of these three factors on the extent of generalization of dynamic adaptation from bilateral to unilateral movement conditions in a series of three experiments. We investigated the pattern of generalization from bilateral to unilateral conditions, because generalization of motor learning in this direction would be more related to rehabilitation settings (e.g., bilateral training to improve paretic arm function post stroke), and thus more interesting to rehabilitation researchers and practitioners.

Experiment 1

This experiment served two purposes. The first, and main, purpose was to investigate generalization of dynamic adaptation from bilateral to unilateral conditions by employing an experimental paradigm used in our previous studies (i.e., a novel sensorimotor perturbation provided to both arms, reaching movements made toward multiple targets). If limited generalization were observed in this experiment, this would indicate that the discrepancy between Nozaki et al.'s findings and our previous findings was mainly due to the differences in the nature of sensorimotor tasks (i.e., dynamic vs. visuomotor). The second purpose was to determine whether the pattern of generalization from bilateral to unilateral conditions would depend on the consistency of movement directions between the arms (i.e., target directions extrinsically or intrinsically consistent between the arms).

Methods

Subjects. Subjects were 24 neurologically intact young adults (12 females and 12 males, aged between 21 and 26) who were right handed. The Edinburgh Handedness Inventory was used to determine handedness. They were recruited from the university community and paid for participation. The Institutional Review Board of the University of Wisconsin – Milwaukee approved this study; and every subject signed a written informed consent prior to his/her participation. Six subjects were tested in each of four subject groups. The number of subjects per group was determined based on a power analysis we performed using the data from our previous studies that employed similar tasks and performance measures [10], [11]. No subject participated in multiple experiments.

Apparatus. A bilateral robotic exoskeleton called KINARM (BKIN Technologies Ltd, Kingston, ON, Canada) was used to collect movement data. Subjects sat on the KINARM chair with their arms supported on the exoskeleton that provided gravitational support, and moved to bring their arms under a horizontal display (Fig. 1A). The KINARM was incorporated with a virtual reality system that projected visual targets on the display to make them appear in the same plane as the arms. Direct vision of the subjects' arm was blocked; and a cursor representing the tip of their index finger was provided to guide their reaching movements. The 2-D position data of the hand, elbow and shoulder were sampled at 1,000 Hz, low pass filtered at 15 Hz, and differentiated to yield resultant velocity and acceleration values. Computer algorithms for data processing and analysis were written in MATLAB.

Experimental design. Prior to movement, one of eight targets (2 cm in diameter; 10 cm away from the starting position), presented in a pseudorandom sequence within each cycle (eight consecutive trials including all target directions), was displayed on the horizontal tabletop (Fig. 1B). Subjects were instructed to move their index finger from the start circle (2 cm in diameter) to the target as straight and as fast as possible in response to the appearance of the target, and stop on it. The distance between the two start circles (one for each arm) was 50 cm for all subjects, which caused the joint angles to vary across the subjects.

The experiment consisted of three sessions: baseline, bilateral and unilateral sessions. The baseline session, provided to familiarize the subjects with the general bilateral reaching task, was followed by the bilateral session during which subjects performed bilateral reaching movements toward two targets that were either extrinsically or intrinsically consistent between the arms (Fig. 1B, top and bottom, respectively). Subjects were randomly assigned to the two consistency conditions. During the subsequent unilateral session, one half of the subjects in each of the two target conditions (extrinsic, intrinsic) performed unilateral reaching movements with their left arm, and the other half with their right arm (i.e., four subject groups total, six subjects per group). The three sessions (baseline, bilateral, unilateral) consisted of 96, 192 and 96 trials, respectively, which were organized into 12 (baseline, unilateral) or 24 (bilateral) cycles. Visual feedback of the cursor representing the index finger tip was available throughout the entire experiment.

To examine adaptation to a novel dynamic condition, a velocity-dependent endpoint force field (fx, fy) was mimicked using the torque motors of the robotic exoskeleton as follows:

$$\begin{pmatrix} Ts \\ Te \end{pmatrix} = \begin{pmatrix} -l2\sin\vartheta1 - l2\sin\vartheta2 & l1\cos\vartheta1 + l2\cos\vartheta2 \\ -l2\sin\vartheta2 & l2\cos\vartheta2 \end{pmatrix} \begin{pmatrix} fx \\ fy \end{pmatrix},$$

where Ts and Te are shoulder and elbow joint torques; l1 and l2 are upper arm and forearm lengths; $\varphi1$ and $\varphi2$ are shoulder and elbow angles. The force fields were fx = −15vy (−fx for left arm), fy = 15vx, where vy and vx are the y- and x-components of the endpoint velocity (m/s), respectively, and force is in Newtons. This force field was provided to both arms simultaneously during the bilateral session and to the moving arm during the unilateral session. During the bilateral session, the direction of the force fields applied to the arms was always extrinsically consistent (Fig. 1C). The force fields were only applied in the counter-clockwise direction throughout all experiments.

Data analysis. As our main performance measure, we calculated direction error at peak velocity (V_{max}), which was calculated as the angular difference between the vectors defined by the target and by the hand-path position at movement start and at V_{max}.

For statistical analysis, a repeated-measures ANOVA was conducted to examine the main effects of, and the interaction effects among, three variables: target consistency (extrinsically vs. intrinsically consistent; a between-subject factor), arm (left vs. right; a within-subject factor) and session (bilateral vs. unilateral; a within-subject factor). For the factor 'session', the mean direction error of the last two cycles (cycles 23 and 24) from the bilateral session and that of cycle 1 from the unilateral session were used. For the bilateral session, the mean direction error of the last two cycles was used because this mean error would reflect a more stable final adaptation level as compared to the direction error of the last cycle alone (e.g., performance in a single cycle near the end of a session could be influenced by certain factors such as boredom and fatigue). For the unilateral session, the direction error of only the first cycle was used because the performance at the very first cycle best reflects the extent of immediate transfer from the bilateral session. (Averaging the errors from cycles 1 and 2 is not ideal because a dramatic improvement typically occurs from cycle 1 to cycle 2.) The alpha level was set at .05 for statistical significance.

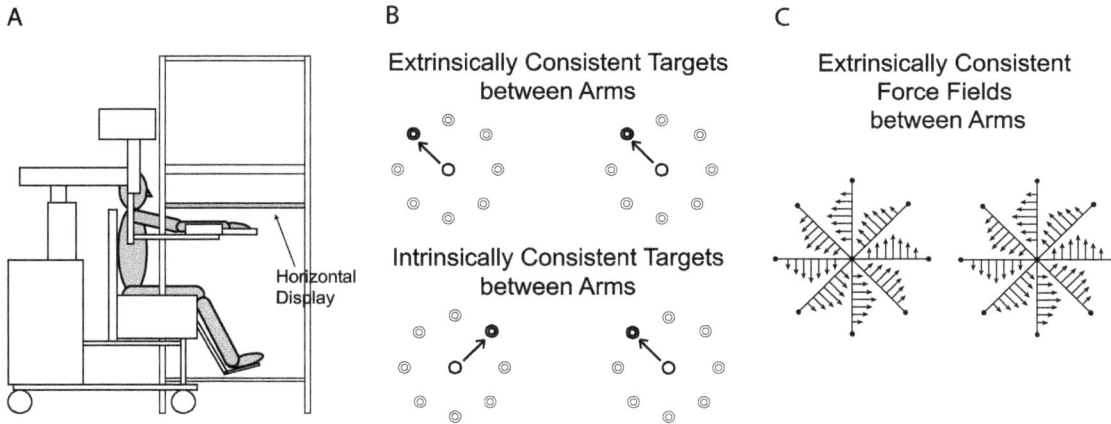

Figure 1. Experimental setup. A, Side view: subject sat on the KINARM chair with the arms placed under the horizontal display. B, Target was randomly displayed on one of eight target locations for each arm. Target directions were either extrinsically (top) or intrinsically (bottom) consistent between the arms during the bilateral session. C, Direction of a velocity-dependent force field applied to each arm during reaching movement. Longer arrows indicate greater forces. Force directions were always extrinsically consistent between the arms.

Results

Figure 2A illustrates typical hand-paths from a representative subject in one of the four subject groups (those who experienced the extrinsically consistent targets during the bilateral session and used the left arm during the unilateral session). Hand-paths shown in rows 1 and 2 represent the first and the last eight consecutive trials during the bilateral session, respectively; and those in row 3 represent the first eight consecutive trials during the unilateral session. Upon initial exposure to the force field during the bilateral session (row 1), the hand-paths obtained at the first cycle of both left and right arm performances were deviated substantially from a straight line between the start circle and the target. Following

adaptation to the force field, these paths became relatively straight and substantially more accurate (row 2). The hand-paths obtained during the unilateral session were relatively straight from the first cycle, indicating largely facilitative effects of bilateral training on subsequent unilateral performance. The facilitative effects of bilateral training, indicated by relatively straight and accurate hand-paths at the first cycle of the unilateral session, appeared to be similar across the four subject groups.

Figure 2B illustrates the mean values ($\pm$ SE) of direction error for two conditions: one in which the subjects performed the unilateral task with the left arm (top) and the other in which they performed the same task with the right arm (bottom). The repeated-measures ANOVA showed that none of the three factors

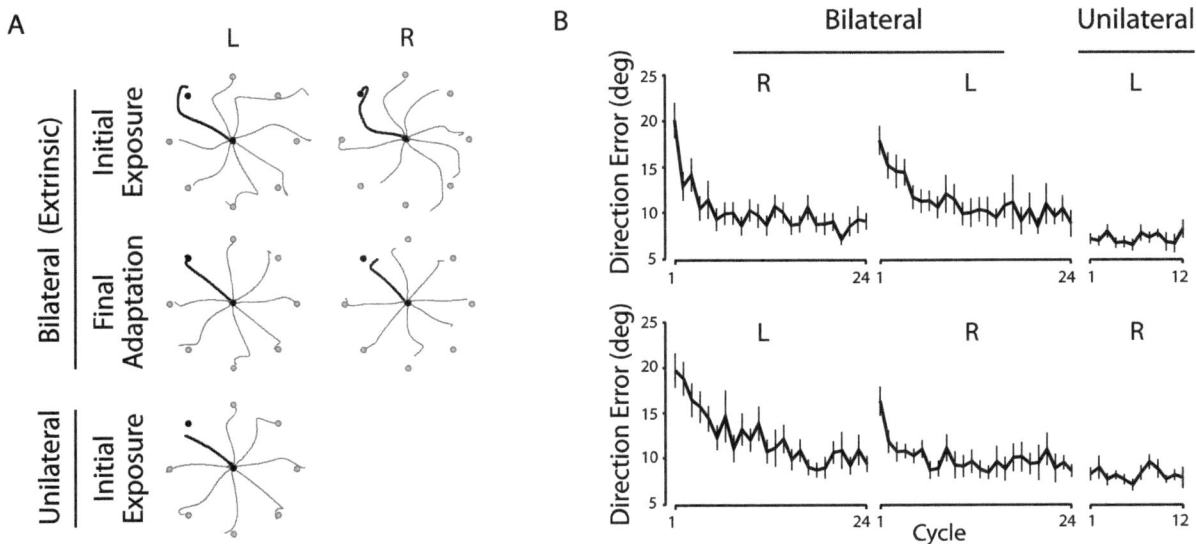

Figure 2. Reaching performance observed when the force field was provided to both arms during the bilateral session. A, Hand-paths obtained from a representative subject who reached toward extrinsically consistent targets during the bilateral session and used the left arm during the unilateral session. Hand-paths represent the first (rows 1, 3) or the last (row 2) eight consecutive trials in each session. Pairs (L and R) of black lines in the bilateral session indicate target directions presented simultaneously for bilateral performance. L above the hand-paths indicates left arm, R right arm. B, Mean direction errors. Every data point shown on X axis represents the average of 8 consecutive trials (cycle) across subjects (mean $\pm$ SE). Direction errors for the subjects who performed the unilateral task with the left (top) or the right (bottom) arm are shown separately (data collapsed across two target-consistency conditions due to lack of significant differences).

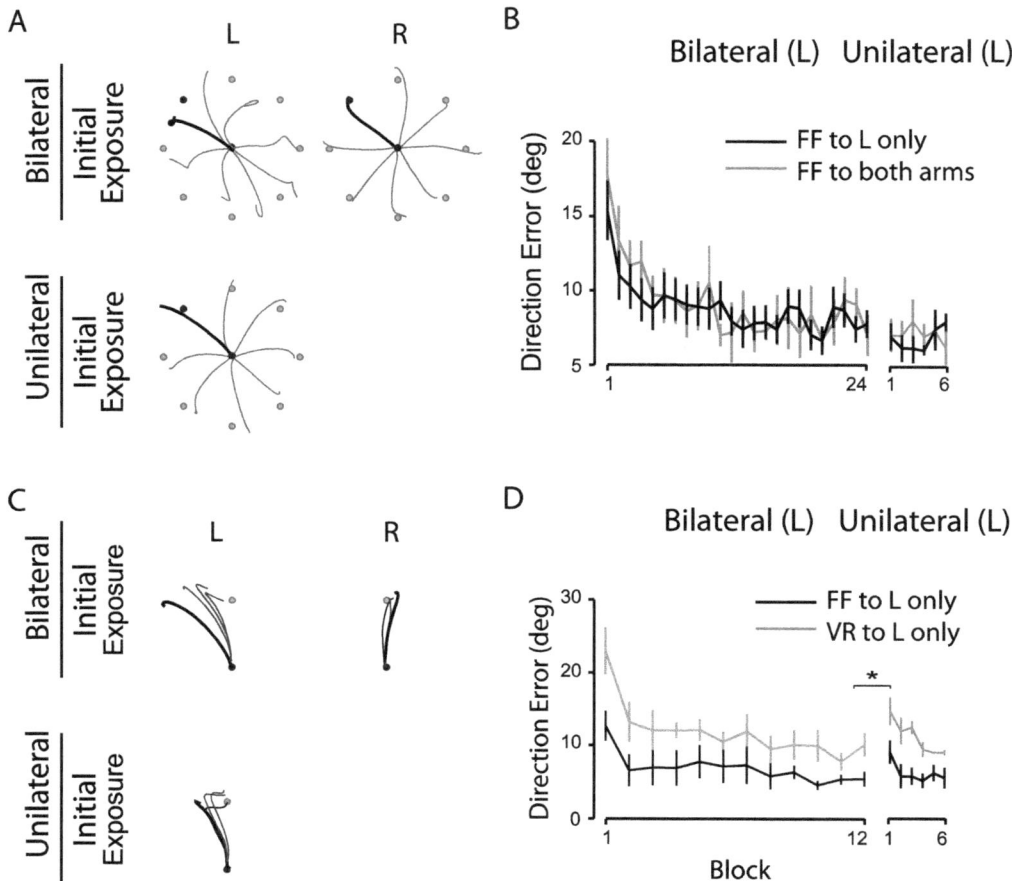

Figure 3. Reaching performance observed when the sensorimotor perturbation was only provided to the left arm. A, Hand-paths from a representative subject who experienced the force field provided only to the left arm during both the bilateral and unilateral sessions. B, Mean direction errors. Every data point shown on X axis represents the average of 8 consecutive trials (cycle) across subjects (mean ± SE) when the force field was provided only to the left arm (FF to L only, black lines) or to both arms (FF to both arms, grey lines). C, Hand-paths from a representative subject who experienced the force field provided only to the left arm during both the bilateral and unilateral sessions and reached toward a single target. D, Mean direction errors. Every data point shown on X axis represents the average of 8 consecutive trials (block) across subjects (mean ± SE) in the dynamic task condition (FF to L only, black lines) or in the visuomotor task condition (VR to L only, grey lines). * P<.05.

(target consistency, arm, session) had a significant main effect; and no interaction effect among those factors was significant. (Data shown in Figure 2B were collapsed across the two target-consistency conditions because no significant differences were observed between them.)

Additional post hoc analyses indicated that peak tangential velocity during reaching movements was not statistically different between bilateral and unilateral performances at the first and the last cycles.

Experiment 2

The results from experiment 1 indicated substantial generalization from the bilateral to unilateral sessions when the force field was provided to both arms. The purpose of experiment 2 was to investigate the generalization pattern from a bilateral to a unilateral session when the force field was only applied to one arm in both sessions.

Methods

Subjects. Subjects were 5 neurologically intact young adults (3 females and 2 males, aged between 21 and 25) who were right handed. No subject participated in the other experiments.

Experimental design. This experiment employed the same reaching tasks described above, and also consisted of the three sessions (baseline, bilateral, unilateral). During the bilateral session, however, all subjects experienced extrinsically consistent target directions between the arms. Extrinsically consistent target directions were used, because moving the two arms in extrinsically consistent directions was thought to be rather unnatural as compared with moving them in intrinsically consistent directions [16–19]; and we reasoned that if substantial generalization were observed in this condition, a good amount of generalization would be observed in the other (more natural) condition as well. During the unilateral session, all subjects performed the reaching task with their left arm. The left arm was tested, because the subjects in Nozaki et al.'s study also used the left arm during the unilateral session. The force field was only provided to the left arm during both the bilateral and unilateral sessions. The three sessions (baseline, bilateral, unilateral) consisted of 96, 192 and 48 trials (i.e., 12, 24 and 6 cycles), respectively.

Data analysis. For statistical analysis, direction errors from the aforementioned condition (i.e., the force field applied only to the left arm) were compared with those from one of the four conditions included in experiment 1 (i.e., the force field applied to both arms, target directions extrinsically consistent between the arms, the left arm tested during the unilateral session). A repeated-measures ANOVA was conducted to examine the main effects of, and the interaction effect between, two variables: force field (applied to both arms vs. one arm; a between-subject factor) and session (bilateral vs. unilateral; a within-subject factor). For the factor 'session', the mean direction error of the last two cycles (cycles 23 and 24) from the bilateral session and that of cycle 1 from the unilateral session were used. The alpha level was set at .05 for statistical significance.

Results

As observed in experiment 1, the hand-paths of a representative subject at the first cycle of the unilateral session (Fig. 3A, bottom) were substantially straighter than those observed at the first cycle of the bilateral session (top, left). The left arm performance, indicated by the mean direction errors (+ SE), improved substantially throughout the bilateral session in which the force field was provided only to the left arm (Fig. 3B, black s); and the level of performance observed at the end of the bilateral session appeared similar to that observed at the beginning of the subsequent unilateral session. The pattern of adaptation, as well as generalization, observed in this condition was similar to that observed in the other condition in which the force field was provided to both arms during the bilateral session (Fig. 3B, grey lines). The repeated-measures ANOVA indicated that neither force field nor session had a significant main effect; and the interaction effect between the two factors was not significant either, indicating substantial transfer of dynamic adaptation again.

Experiment 3

The results from experiments 1 and 2 indicated substantial generalization from the bilateral to unilateral sessions regardless of whether the force field was provided to both arms or only to one arm. The purpose of experiment 3 was to investigate the generalization pattern from a bilateral to a unilateral session when subjects reached only toward a single target in both sessions. In this experiment, we also included a comparable condition in which subjects adapted to a novel visuomotor rotation to determine the similarities between the pattern of generalization following dynamic and visuomotor adaptation.

Methods

Subjects. Subjects were 10 neurologically intact young adults (5 females and 5 males, aged between 22 and 25) who were right handed. No subject participated in the other experiments. Five subjects were tested in each subject group.

Experimental design. Two experimental conditions were employed: one in which the subjects adapted to a novel force field condition, and the other in which they adapted to a novel visuomotor rotation. The former condition was identical to the condition tested in experiment 2, except that the subjects only reached toward a single target ("12 o'clock" direction) with each arm during both the bilateral and unilateral sessions. In the latter condition, the cursor representing the index finger tip location was rotated 30 degrees counterclockwise about the start circle as it moved toward the same target during both the bilateral and unilateral sessions. A similar visuomotor adaptation task (i.e., 30 degree counterclockwise rotation, but reaching toward eight different targets) was employed in our previous studies [10], [11]. The three sessions (baseline, bilateral, unilateral) consisted of 48, 96 and 48 trials (6, 12 and 6 blocks, with each block representing the mean of eight consecutive trials), respectively.

Data analysis. A repeated-measures ANOVA was conducted to examine the main effects of, and the interaction effect between, two variables: task (dynamic vs. visuomotor; a between-subject factor) and session (bilateral vs. unilateral; a within-subject factor). For the factor 'session', the mean direction error of the last two cycles (blocks 11 and 12) from the bilateral session and that of block 1 from the unilateral session were used. The alpha level was set at .05 for statistical significance.

Results

Figure 3C illustrates the hand-paths of a representative subject from the dynamic adaptation condition. The hand-paths at the first four trials of the unilateral session (Fig. 3C, bottom) were straighter than those observed at the first four trials of the bilateral session (top, left), although they still deviated substantially from a straight line between the start circle and the target. The hand-paths of the subjects tested in the visuomotor adaptation condition were almost the same as those described above, except that the deviations from a straight line between the start circle and the target were somewhat greater in the visuomotor condition.

The left arm performance, indicated by the mean direction errors (+ SE), improved substantially throughout the bilateral session in both task conditions (Fig. 3D). However, the level of performance observed at the beginning of the unilateral session was poorer than that observed at the end of the bilateral session regardless of the task condition. The repeated-measures ANOVA indicated that the task main effect was not significant, but the session main effect was (p = .002). The interaction effect between the two factors was not significant. This indicates limited generalization of both dynamic and visuomotor adaptation from the bilateral to the unilateral session.

Discussion

We previously demonstrated that visuomotor adaptation could generalize completely from bilateral to unilateral movement conditions, regardless of the consistency between the arms in terms of target directions or visual rotation directions [10], [11]. In the present study, we demonstrated that dynamic adaptation could also generalize substantially from bilateral to unilateral conditions. Complete generalization was observed regardless of whether the force field was provided to both arms (experiment 1) or only to one arm (experiment 2). These findings indicate that the learning that occurred in the two bilateral conditions had similar effects, which is in line with the finding that learning of a force field in one arm was the same regardless of whether the other arm made movements in a null field or in a force field [20]. Our findings also indicate that the effect of bilateral training on subsequent unilateral performance is quite robust and not overly sensitive to the context of bilateral training. It has been suggested that bilateral movements in different contexts may engage distinct representations of the limb dynamics and kinematics [21]. Considering that, bilateral movements performed in our two conditions in experiment 1, one in which the movement directions were the same between the arms and the other in which the directions were opposite, might have engaged two distinct neural representations. Our results, however, were similar (statistically not different) between the two conditions, indicating that substantial generalization can occur from bilateral to unilateral conditions regardless of the contexts of bilateral training. These findings are in agreement with a recent finding that adapting to a novel disturbance torque during a bimanual tracking task facilitated performing the same task unilaterally regardless of whether the torque was applied symmetrically or asymmetrically to the two arms [22].

In experiment 3, we observed limited generalization of dynamic adaptation from the bilateral to the unilateral session when the subjects reached only toward a single target during initial training. The extent of transfer observed in this experiment is comparable to that observed in Nozaki et al.'s study (~60% transfer observed in their study, Fig. 1f). The mean (± SE) direction errors at block 1 and blocks 11~12 of the bilateral session and at block 1 of the unilateral session in experiment 3 were 12. 38 (±4.78), 5.45 (±1.59) and 8.53 (±2.95) degrees, respectively. This indicates that approximately 56% transfer occurred from the bilateral to the unilateral session when the subjects only experienced a single target during reaching movements. It should be noted here that the number of trials in the bilateral session was smaller in experiment 3 as compared with the number of trials in the same session in experiments 1 and 2 (96 vs 192 trials, respectively). We used a smaller number of trials because reaching toward a single target for too many trials could have a negative effect on the initial adaptation due to certain factors such as the loss of motivation and boredom. One may argue that the limited generalization observed in this experiment was influenced by the reduced number of trials. However, the number of trials for the given target direction (12 o'clock direction) was four times more in this experiment than in experiments 1 and 2 (96 vs. 24 trials, respectively). In addition, the learning curve observed in experiment 3 was very similar to that observed in the other experiments. Thus, it is unlikely that the smaller number of trials in this experiment had a substantial influence on the observed extent of generalization.

We also investigated generalization of visuomotor adaptation from the bilateral to the unilateral session in experiment 3. Our results showed limited generalization, indicated by a significant difference between the direction errors at the last blocks of the bilateral performance and those at the first block of the unilateral performance, when the subjects only experienced a single target direction. This finding is very different from the findings from our previous studies [10], [11], in which complete generalization of visuomotor adaptation occurred from the bilateral to the unilateral session when the subjects experienced eight different target directions (as our subjects did in the current study, experiment 1). This is in line with the well-known variability of practice principle of motor learning, which posits that experiences with task variations are crucial to the development of motor memories that are responsible for motor control and learning [23], [24]. It is, thus, speculated that experiencing a broader range of movement (target directions in our case) during bilateral adaptation may lead to the development of a neural representation associated with a novel sensorimotor transform (whether it is visuomotor or dynamic in nature) that is less task-specific or less context-dependent, thus resulting in greater generalization across different types of movements. This idea is also in agreement with the finding

reported by Seidler [25] that experiencing a variety of motor learning paradigms can facilitate the acquisition of general, transferable knowledge about skill learning processes, regardless of similarities among the experienced paradigms (e.g., visual rotations, gain change, sequence learning).

Our current findings have an implication for rehabilitation. Whether generalization of sensorimotor adaptation investigated in our study is indeed a good model of what happens during stroke rehabilitation is an open question. Nonetheless, our findings clearly indicate that the neural mechanisms underlying this type of motor learning overlap substantially between bilateral and unilateral training, which provides support to the idea that bilateral arm training employed in stroke rehabilitation can facilitate functional recovery of the paretic arm in stroke patients with hemiparesis [12–14]. In stroke rehabilitation, different types of bilateral arm training are employed, such as bilateral isokinematic training, machine-assisted bilateral training, bilateral mirror therapy and bilateral priming (see [13] for review). When investigating the effects of these training methods, investigators typically employ symmetrical, as compared with asymmetrical, movements between the arms because symmetrical movements may involve the generation of similar neural commands to control the two arms, which is thought to be more beneficial for improving motor function of the paretic arm. Studies that investigated bilateral coordination in healthy young adults suggest that bilateral coordination is more stable, in terms of both temporal and spatial domains, when the arms perform symmetrical, as compared to asymmetrical, movements (e.g., [16–19]). Symmetrical bilateral movements have also been shown to involve similar neural processes in both hemispheres (e.g., [26–28]). However, our current findings, along with our previous findings [11], indicate that complete generalization of both dynamic and visuomotor learning can occur regardless of whether the arms move symmetrically or asymmetrically. A small number of investigators employed both symmetrical and asymmetrical bilateral arm training in their stroke intervention studies. However, a systematic comparison between the two types of training was not done in those studies because they had the same stroke patients experience both types of movement during bilateral training (e.g., [29]) and/or because they did not have a sufficient number of patients in the two movement conditions (e.g., [30]). Further research is necessary to determine whether symmetrical and asymmetrical bilateral training are equally effective for improving motor function of the paretic arm post stroke as well.

Author Contributions

Assisted with writing the manuscript: YL KX KM. Conceived and designed the experiments: JW. Performed the experiments: YL KX KM. Analyzed the data: JW YL KX KM. Contributed reagents/materials/analysis tools: JW YL. Wrote the paper: JW.

References

1. Bastian AJ (2008) Understanding sensorimotor adaptation and learning for rehabilitation. Curr Opin Neurol 21: 628–633.
2. Shadmehr R, Moussavi ZM (2000) Spatial generalization from learning dynamics of reaching movements. J Neurosci 20: 7807–7815.
3. Baraduc P, Wolpert DM (2002) Adaptation to a visuomotor shift depends on the starting posture. J Neurosci 88: 973–981.
4. Wang J, Sainburg RL (2005) Adaptation to visuomotor rotations remaps movement vectors, not final positions. J Neurosci 25: 4024–4030.
5. Sainburg RL, Wang J (2002) Interlimb transfer of visuomotor rotations: independence of direction and final position information. Experimental Brain Research 145: 437–447.
6. Wang J, Sainburg RL (2004) Interlimb transfer of novel inertial dynamics is asymmetrical. J Neurophysiol 92: 349–360.
7. Galea JM, Miall RC, Woolley DG (2007) Asymmetric interlimb transfer of concurrent adaptation to opposing dynamic forces. Exp Brain Res 182: 267–273.
8. Nozaki D, Kurtzer I, Scott SH (2006) Limited transfer of learning between unimanual and bimanual skills within the same limb. Nature Neurosci 9: 1364–1366.
9. Burgess JK, Bareither R, Patton JL (2007) Single limb performance following contralateral bimanual limb training. IEEE Trans Neural Syst Rehabil Eng 15: 347–355.
10. Wang J, Sainburg RL (2009) Generalization of visuomotor learning between bilateral and unilateral conditions. J Neurophysiol 102: 2090–2099.
11. Wang J, Mordkoff JT, Sainburg RL (2010) Visuomotor learning generalizes between bilateral and unilateral conditions despite varying degrees of bilateral interference. J Neurophysiol 104: 2913–2921.

12. Stewart KC, Cauraugh JH, Summers JJ (2006) Bilateral movement training and stroke rehabilitation: a systematic review and meta-analysis. J Neurol Sci 244: 89–95.

13. Stoykov ME, Corcos DM (2009) A review of bilateral training for upper extremity hemiparesis. Occup Ther Int 16: 190–203.

14. Cauraugh JH, Lodha N, Naik SK, Summers JJ (2010) Bilateral movement training and stroke motor recovery progress: a structured review and meta-analysis. Hum Mov Sci 29: 853–870.

15. Krakauer JW, Ghilardi MF, Ghez C (1999) Independent learning of internal models for kinematic and dynamic control of reaching. Nat Neurosci 2: 1026–1031.

16. Franz EA, Zelaznik HN, McCabe G (1991) Evidence of common timing processes in the control of manual, orofacial, and speech movements. J Mot Behav 24: 281–287.

17. Heuer H (1996) Coordination. In: Handbook of Perception and Action: Motor Skills, edited by Heuer H, Keele SW. San Diego, CA: Academic Press. 2: 121–180.

18. Swinnen SP (2002) Intermanual coordination: from behavioural principles to neural-network interactions. Nat Rev Neurosci 3: 348–359.

19. Carson RG (2005) Neural pathways mediating bilateral interactions between the upper limbs. Brain Res Brain Res Rev 49: 641–662.

20. Tcheang L, Bays PM, Ingram JN, Wolpert DM (2007) Simultaneous bimanual dynamics are leant without interference. Exp Brain Res 127: 182–192.

21. Howard IS, Ingram JN, Wolpert DM (2010) Context-dependent partitioning of motor learning in bimanual movements. J Neurophysiol 104: 2082–2091.

22. Trlep M, Mihelj M, Munih M (2012) Skill transfer from symmetric and asymmetric bimanual training using a robotic system to single limb performance. J Neuroeng Rehabil 9: 43.

23. Shea CH, Kohl RM (1990) Specificity and variability of practice. Res Q Exerc Sport 61: 169–177.

24. Schmidt RA, Bjork RA (1992) New conceptualizations of practice: Common principles in three paradigms suggest new concepts for training. Psychol Sci 3: 207–217.

25. Seidler RD (2004) Multiple motor learning experiences enhance motor adaptability. J Cogn Neurosci 16: 65–73.

26. Jancke L, Peters M, Himmelbach M, Nosselt T, Shah J, et al. (2000) FMRI study of bimanual coordination. Neuropsychologia 38: 164–174.

27. Swinnen SP, Wenderoth N (2004) Two hands, one brain: Cognitive neuroscience of bimanual skill. Trends Cogn Sci 8: 18–25.

28. Nachev P, Kennard C, Husain M (2008) Functional role of the supplementary and pre-supplementary motor areas. Nat Rev Neurosci 9: 856–869.

29. McCombe Waller S, Whitall J (2004) Fine motor control in adults with and without chronic hemiparesis: Baseline comparison to nondisabled adults and effects of bilateral arm training. Arch Phys Med Rehabil 85: 1076–1083.

30. Stinear JW, Byblow WD (2004) Rhythmic bilateral movement training modulates corticomotor excitability and enhances upper limb motricity poststroke: A pilot study. J Clin Neurophysiol 21: 124–131.

9

Cardiopulmonary Fitness Correlates with Regional Cerebral Grey Matter Perfusion and Density in Men with Coronary Artery Disease

Bradley J. MacIntosh[1,2,4]*, Walter Swardfager[1,3], David E. Crane[1], Nipuni Ranepura[3], Mahwesh Saleem[3], Paul I. Oh[5,7], Bojana Stefanovic[1,2,3], Nathan Herrmann[3,6], Krista L. Lanctôt[1,3,6]

1 Heart and Stroke Foundation Canadian Partnership for Stroke Recovery, Sunnybrook Research Institute, Toronto, Ontario, Canada, 2 Physical Sciences, Sunnybrook Research Institute, Toronto, Ontario, Canada, 3 Neuropsychopharmacology Research Group, Sunnybrook Research Institute, Toronto, Ontario, Canada, 4 Department of Medical Biophysics, University of Toronto, Toronto, Ontario, Canada, 5 Department of Clinical Pharmacology, University of Toronto, Toronto, Ontario, Canada, 6 Department of Psychiatry, University of Toronto, Toronto, Ontario, Canada, 7 Toronto Rehabilitation Institute, Toronto, Ontario, Canada

Abstract

Purpose: Physical activity is associated with positive effects on the brain but there is a paucity of clinical neuroimaging data in patients with coronary artery disease (CAD), a cardiovascular condition associated with grey matter loss. The purpose of this study was to determine which brain regions are impacted by cardiopulmonary fitness and with the change in fitness after 6 months of exercise-based cardiac rehabilitation.

Methods: CAD patients underwent magnetic resonance imaging at baseline, and peak volume of oxygen uptake during exercise testing (VO_{2Peak}) was measured at baseline and after 6 months of training. T1-weighted structural images were used to perform grey matter (GM) voxel-based morphometry (VBM). Pseudo-continuous arterial spin labeling (pcASL) was used to produce cerebral blood flow (CBF) images. VBM and CBF data were tested voxel-wise using VO_{2Peak} and age as explanatory variables.

Results: In 30 men with CAD (mean age 65 ± 7 years), VBM and CBF identified 7 and 5 respective regions positively associated with baseline VO_{2Peak}. These included the pre- and post-central, paracingulate, caudate, hippocampal regions and converging findings in the putamen. VO_{2Peak} increased by 20% at follow-up in 29 patients (t = 9.6, df = 28, p<0.0001). Baseline CBF in the left post-central gyrus and baseline GM density in the right putamen predicted greater change in VO_{2Peak}.

Conclusion: Perfusion and GM density were associated with fitness at baseline and with greater fitness gains with exercise. This study identifies new neurobiological correlates of fitness and demonstrates the utility of multi-modal MRI to evaluate the effects of exercise in CAD patients.

Editor: Francisco J. Esteban, University of Jaén, Spain

Funding: Funding support was provided by: Canadian Institutes of Health Research (Lanctot MOP-114913) and the Heart and Stroke Foundation Centre for Stroke Recovery. The funders had no role in study design, data collection and analysis, decision to publish, or preparation of the manuscript.

Competing Interests: The authors have read the journal's policy and have the following conflicts to disclose (initials denote the coauthor): BJM has received funding from Philips Healthcare. NH has received honoraria and support from Lundbeck, Pfizer, Janssen Ortho, Sanofi Aventis, AbbVie and Roche. KL has received honoraria and support from AbbVie, Lundbeck, MedImmune, Pfizer, Janssen Ortho, Sanofi Aventis and Roche.

* E-mail: bmac@sri.utoronto.ca

Introduction

Aerobic exercise not only reduces cardiovascular risk but also affects the brain by increasing angiogenesis, neurogenesis and synaptogenesis [1]. Animal studies have identified brain regions that respond to exercise, including angiogenesis-related processes in motor circuits in rats [2,3], mature aged monkeys [4], as well as the mouse hippocampus [5]. Replication of these findings in human studies has been limited to date, and performed primarily in healthy cohorts. For example, healthy older adults participated in a 12 month walking intervention and this contributed to increasing the volume of the hippocampus [6]. Cross-sectionally,

highly active older adults have increased perfusion in the precuneus region compared to age-matched sedentary adults [7]. Peak volume of oxygen uptake (VO_{2Peak}), a measure of the capacity to transport and use oxygen during exercise, is associated with increased grey matter volume in multiple brain regions among older healthy adults. The regions include the anterior cingulate, inferior frontal gyrus and superior temporal gyrus, as reported by others [8]. Aside from the hippocampus, subcortical grey matter regions are typically not reported in human exercise neuroimaging literature, despite evidence from the animal studies that exercise impacts the basal ganglia [9,10]. These studies and compelling reports on Alzheimer's patients [11,12] provide the impetus to further characterize exercise-related effects on the brain in older clinical populations at risk for cognitive decline [13]. Cardiovascular and/or cerebrovascular patients are likely to garner significant benefits [14] and they are therefore the focus of the current study.

Coronary artery disease (CAD) involves intraluminal narrowing of the arteries that supply blood to the heart and it is associated with a cluster of vascular risk factors such as hypertension, dyslipidemia, history of smoking, increased central adiposity and sedentary behaviour. These factors have been variably linked with grey matter loss [15–17] and posited to contribute to brain hypoperfusion [18]. Importantly, VO_{2Peak} is a strong predictor of cardiac and all-cause mortality in CAD patients [19]. Exercise-based cardiac rehabilitation is thus indicated for the secondary prevention of cardiovascular events. The cardiopulmonary exercise test (CPET) is used to quantify VO_{2Peak}, a highly reproducible objective measure of cardiopulmonary fitness. Clinically, the VO_{2Peak} is used to assess the efficacy of exercise interventions. Although increasing VO_{2Peak} is linearly related to a decreased risk of cardiovascular mortality [20], individual responses to exercise interventions can vary considerably.

In the current study, VO_{2Peak} is used to explain within-cohort variance seen on two magnetic resonance imaging (MRI) techniques: 1) cortical and subcortical grey matter (GM) density using voxel based morphometry (VBM) and 2) cerebral blood flow (CBF) using whole brain pseudocontinuous arterial spin labeling (pcASL). VBM is an ideal structural analysis technique to study both cortical and subcortical grey matter. Previous neuroimaging studies in healthy adults have found GM density in both cortical [8] and subcortical [6] regions to be correlated with exercise. pcASL is a sensitive technique that can provide blood flow measures that complement structural imaging [21]. In the present study, it is hypothesized that VO_{2Peak} will be correlated with increased perfusion and grey matter density in distinct brain regions in patients with CAD. In addition, it is hypothesized that baseline grey matter perfusion and density in these regions will predict changes in VO_{2Peak} over the course of an exercise intervention.

Methods

Participants

This study was approved by Sunnybrook and University Health Network research ethics boards. Participants entering a cardiac rehabilitation program were approached to participate in this study. Seventy participants were screened, 58 showed evidence of CAD, 42 were willing to be contacted by study personnel of which 10 were excluded (see below) and 32 provided written informed consent. Two participants were excluded due to poor quality MRI resulting in 30 patients for analysis in study. Due to the 4.5 to 1 bias of men CAD patients entering cardiac rehabilitation compared to women CAD patients [22] and established sex differences in cerebral blood flow [23],[24], male sex was an inclusion criteria for this study. Other inclusion criteria included age 55–80 years, a documented history of CAD: myocardial infarction (MI), narrowing of at least one major coronary artery, percutaneous coronary intervention (PCI), or coronary artery bypass graft surgery (CABG). Patients were excluded if they had contraindications to an MRI or any neurodegenerative disorder. In addition to cardiac history, demographic information, concomitant medications, body mass index (BMI), and histories of hyperlipidemia, diabetes mellitus, hypertension and smoking were ascertained.

Cardiopulmonary exercise test

Cardiopulmonary fitness was assessed using a cycle ergometer (Ergoselect 200P, Ergoline, Bitz, Germany) symptom-limited graded exercise test at baseline and after 6 months of exercise. Workload was increased by 16.7 W every minute. Breath-by-breath gas samples were collected and averaged over a 20-second period using a calibrated metabolic cart (Vmax Encore, Sensor-Medics, Yorba Linda, CA) [25]. The peak volume of oxygen uptake per minute (VO_{2Peak}) was calculated after dividing by the patient's mass to obtain VO_{2Peak} in units of mL/kg/min. MRI was performed within 1 month of CPET and within 2 weeks of beginning exercise.

Cardiac rehabilitation exercise program

Cardiac rehabilitation consisted of aerobic and resistance training in a group setting under the supervision of exercise and medical specialists. Patients attended supervised exercise visits that included an aerobic walk or walk/jog once per week for 24 weeks. The 6-month cardiac rehabilitation program was at no cost to the participants due to national healthcare coverage and they received no remuneration to participate in the study. Patients were also expected to exercise five out of seven days of the week at home and document the duration, intensity and frequency of the exercise in weekly exercise diaries, which were monitored every week for compliance by an assigned exercise supervisor. Previously, we have reported on the efficacy of this program [26], and established that compliance is high in this population [27]. Patients were provided with nutrition documentation at the start of the program during education classes, but no formal diet was recommended/undertaken. Initial exercise prescription was a walking distance of approximately 1.6 km at an intensity equivalent to 60% of VO_{2Peak}. Prescriptions progressed every 2 weeks to a maximum of 6.4 km and then to a maximum intensity of 80% of VO_{2Peak} as estimated from maximum heart rate measurements. Prescriptions did not exceed a maximum daily duration of 60 minutes.

Magnetic resonance imaging

Neuroimaging was performed on a 3 Tesla MRI system (Discovery MR750, General Electric Healthcare) and using a body radio frequency (RF) coil for transmission and an 8 channel phased array RF head coil for signal detection. Structural imaging included: 1) high resolution T1-weighted data using 3D spoiled gradient recalled echo (TR/TE/TI = 8.1/3.2/650 ms, flip angle = 8deg, acquisition matrix 256×192×186, nominal spatial resolution 0.9×0.9×1 mm), 2) fluid attenuated inversion recovery (FLAIR) sequence (TR/TE/TI = 9700/141/2200 ms, flip angle = 90deg, acquisition matrix 256×192×48, nominal spatial resolution 0.9×0.9×3 mm) and 3) dual proton density, T2-weighted images (TR/TE1/TE2 = 2500/11/90 ms, flip angle = 90deg, acquisition matrix 256×192×48, nominal spatial resolution 0.9×0.9×3 mm). FLAIR images were used to enable automatic identification and masking of white matter hyperintensity (WMH) voxels that would otherwise influence GM density estimates on the VBM analysis. Proton density images were used to extract the brain from head. These latter two considerations are part of Lesion Explorer software, described elsewhere [28].

Perfusion weighted images were acquired using a pseudo-continuous arterial spin labeling (pcASL) sequence that was developed in the laboratory [29], performed with a labeling duration of 1500 ms and a post label delay of 1700 ms [30]. The labeling plane was prescribed with the help of time-of-flight angiography images at the level of or just superior to the carotid bifurcation. Labeling was typically done at the level of the 2nd cervical vertebrae where internal carotids and vertebral arteries

Change in VO2-Peak

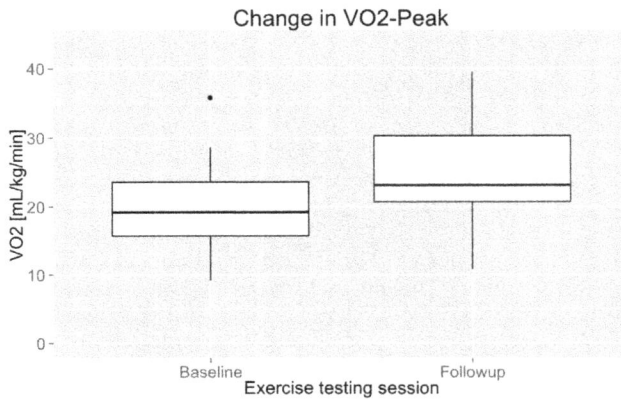

Figure 1. Mean cardiopulmonary fitness at baseline (N = 30) and after 6 months of exercise intervention (n = 29). The paired comparison shows a significant session effect (t = 9.6, df = 28, p<0.0001).

run parallel to one another. Twenty-five control and tag images were acquired sequentially in the axial plane using TR/TE/Flip angle = 4000 ms/17 ms/90deg and single shot echo planar imaging (EPI) readout. Seventeen slices were collected with gap of 1.4 mm, slice thickness of 4.2 mm and nominal voxel dimensions of 3.4 by 3.4 by 5.6 mm^3. The pcASL volume was planned based on maximum coverage of cerebrum. In practise this meant that the cerebellum and superior portion of the cerebrum were not covered consistently.

Post processing

Voxel based morphometry (VBM) was performed in FMRIB Software Library (FSL), with additional customized steps to account for white matter changes: 1) non-brain regions on T1 images were identified using brain extraction tool (BET), 2) FLAIR images were co-registered to the T1, 3) WMH masks were warped to T1, 4) voxels within WMH regions were replaced with intensity values equivalent to mean healthy WM along with Gaussian noise, thereby creating a flat intensity profile over the WMH region to ensure proper GM segmentation, and 5) grey matter estimates were generated in standard space using the standard FSL-VBM processing pipeline with a 4.6 mm full-width half-max Gaussian smoothing kernel [31].

ASL images were processed using FMRIB Software Library (FSL) tools. Post processing of ASL data included: perfusion-weighted difference images, motion correction and spatial smoothing by a Gaussian kernel of 5 mm full width at half

Table 1. Participant Demographics (BMI = body mass index, DBP = diastolic blood pressure, SBP = systolic blood pressure, CABG = coronary artery bypass graft, MI = myocardial infarction, ASA = acetylsalicylic acid, ACE = angiotensin-converting-enzyme).

Demographics		Mean±SD or %
Age [years]		65.0±7.0
Education [years]		16.9±3.1
Marital status [partnered]		90%
Ethnicity [number, %]		
	Caucasian	27 (87%)
	South Asian	2 (6.5%)
	African American/Afro-Caribbean	2 (6.5%)
Employment status [number, %]		
	Employed	14 (45%)
	Not working/retired	17 (55%)
Vascular risk factors		
	BMI [kg/m^2]	27.9±3.8
	Body Fat [%]	25.7±5.7
	DBP [mmHg]	73.4±7.9
	SBP [mmHg]	124.3±15.2
	Hypertension	40%
	History of smoking	53%
Cardiac history		
	Stent	47%
	CABG	47%
	MI	37%
Concomitant medications		
	ASA use	100%
	Statin	97%
	Beta-blocker	73%
	ACE inhibitor	57%

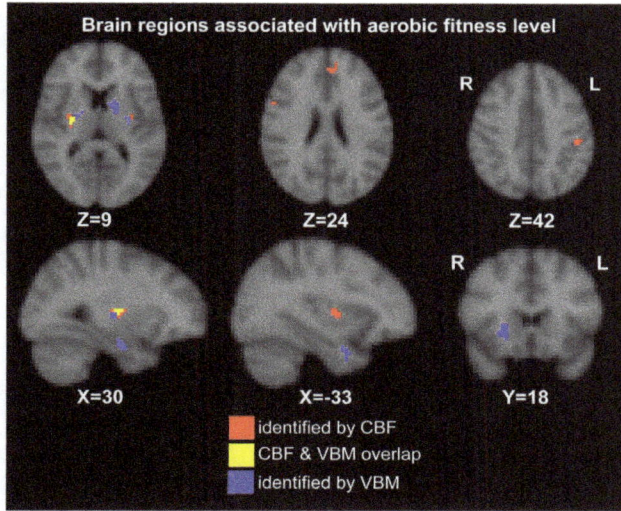

Figure 2. Voxel-wise analyses for CBF and GM density. Brain regions shown in color are significantly correlated with baseline VO_{2Peak} after controlling for age and correcting for multiple comparisons. CBF voxels are shown in red; VBM voxels are shown in blue; the region in yellow is the right putamen and found to be overlapping for CBF and GM data.

maximum using "asl_preproc" available in FSL. CBF images were intensity normalized to a global level of 40 ml/100 g/min [32] and co-registered to a standard space atlas using affine registration. The CBF intensity normalization was done to reduce the between subject variance and thereby increase the sensitivity to the VO_{2Peak} effect of interest. Others report an increase in sensitivity from this normalization in clinical pcASL cohort studies [33].

Statistics

VO_{2Peak} data were tested for normality in R (www.R-project. org) using the Shapiro test. Voxel-wise group analyses were performed using a general linear model whereby VO_{2Peak} was the explanatory variable of interest and age was included as a covariate. Statistical maps were calculated to determine voxels with a positive association of VO_{2Peak} on the MRI data. Images were reformatted to 3 mm isotropic voxels in standard space to ensure consistency between the two modalities. Randomise in FSL was used with 5000 permutations to characterize the null distribution of the data empirically [34]. Correction for multiple comparisons was performed using a two step procedure: 1) an evaluation of the false discovery rate (FDR) using the FSL program called FDR with a one way q = 0.05 followed by 2) a cluster level threshold of contiguous voxels with a minimum volume of 8 voxels (.22 mL) using the program 3dclust in AFNI. A secondary group analysis was performed on the baseline ASL and VBM data using the change in VO_{2Peak} (i.e. VO_{2Peak} at follow-up minus VO_{2Peak} at baseline). The same multiple comparison corrections were used in this case for the CBF and GM data. Finally, linear regression analyses were performed in R using change in VO_{2Peak} and age as independent variables of the baseline MRI data. These analyses were restricted to the areas identified by the cross-sectional findings.

Results

Baseline and change in VO_{2Peak}

Table 1 shows baseline participant demographics. The time since most recent hospitalization for an acute coronary syndrome or intervention was 11.1 weeks (range 6.86–13.43). Twenty-nine out of 30 participants completed 6 months of cardiac rehabilitation and returned for follow-up CPET VO_{2Peak} testing. All 29 patients were compliant with cardiac rehabilitation protocols as assessed by their case manager based on exercise logs, attendance and fitness assessments. At baseline, the mean VO_{2Peak} was 20.5±5.9 mL/kg/min, which is 16% below the age-adjusted norm [35]. At

Table 2. Brain regions identified by the voxel-wise CBF and grey matter density analyses.

	Brain Region	MNI Coordinates				Baseline VO_{2Peak} model				Change in VO_{2Peak} model			
		# Voxels	X	Y	Z	adj R^2	t-stat	p-value	sig	adj R^2	t-stat	p-value	sig
CBF													
1	Putamen, left	23	−30	9	3	0.30	3.37	0.0023	**	−0.01	0.26	0.3999	
2	Putamen, right	16	30	−9	9	0.24	3.14	0.0041	**	−0.05	−0.26	0.4004	
3	Anterior cingulate, left	12	−3	42	24	0.34	3.65	0.0011	**	0.02	−0.35	0.3659	
4	Premotor cortex, right	9	51	9	27	0.24	2.78	0.0097	**	0.03	0.61	0.2751	
5	Postcentral gyrus, left	8	−48	−27	42	0.42	3.42	0.0020	**	0.30	1.78	0.0430	*
VBM													
1	Planum temporale, right	46	42	−15	−9	0.62	6.64	0.0000	**	0.00	0.00	0.5000	
2	Temporal pole, left	26	−33	3	−36	0.51	5.47	0.0000	**	0.00	0.66	0.2580	
3	Hippocampus, right	22	21	−21	−12	0.54	3.99	0.0005	**	0.26	−0.10	0.4599	
4	Caudate, left	20	−15	−3	6	0.64	4.31	0.0002	**	0.40	0.94	0.1778	
5	Putamen, right	18	21	18	−9	0.42	3.82	0.0007	**	0.26	2.24	0.0170	*
6	Hippocampus, right	12	33	−9	−24	0.60	4.35	0.0002	**	0.32	−0.63	0.2664	
7	Putamen, left	12	−30	−15	6	0.42	4.42	0.0001	**	0.00	−0.12	0.4541	

The number of voxels and MNI coordinates are listed. These regions were then used in a linear regression model to assess the effect of VO_{2Peak} and change in VO_{2Peak} with age as a covariate. * denotes significant at P = 0.05 on a 1-tailed test and ** denotes 2-tailed test.

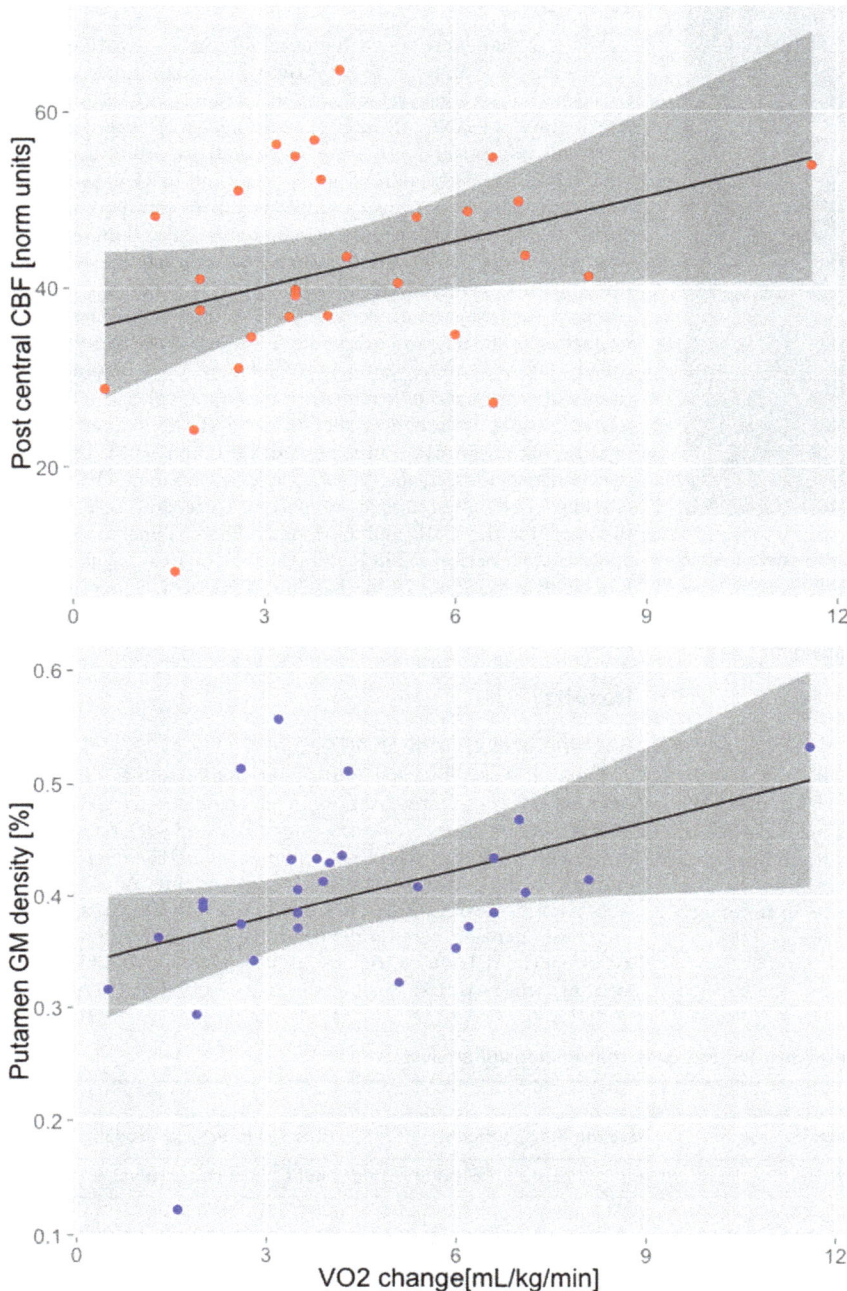

Figure 3. Scatter plots show MRI findings at baseline versus the change in VO$_{2Peak}$. The linear regression analyses for these two regions / measures were significant (P<0.01). The line of best fit is shown with the grey shaded region showing the 95% confidence interval.

follow-up, the mean VO$_{2Peak}$ was 24.7±6.7 mL/kg/min among the 29 completers, 4% above the norm and significantly higher than baseline (t = 9.6, df = 28, p<0.0001; Figure 1).

Effect of VO$_{2Peak}$ and baseline grey matter perfusion and density

Figure 2 shows the brain regions that were identified voxel-wise as significantly positively correlated with VO$_{2Peak}$ after accounting for age as a covariate. Significant voxels for the CBF data are shown in red and included bilateral putamen, left anterior

cingulate, right premotor cortex and the left postcentral gyrus regions. Significant voxels for the VBM are shown in blue and included bilateral putamen, left caudate, right hippocampus, left temporal pole and right planum temporale. Voxels in the left and right bilateral putamen were detected by both VBM and CBF modalities (Figure 2; shown in yellow). Significant voxel volumes, i.e. cluster sizes, and Montreal Neurological Institute coordinates are listed in Table 2.

Voxel-wise analysis on the change in VO$_{2Peak}$ data did not produce any significant voxels after multiple comparison correction. Linear regression analyses however found two significant brain regions from Figure 2 that were significantly related to the change in VO_{2Peak} (i.e. follow-up minus baseline) for a 1-tailed test at $P = 0.05$ (see Table 2). Scatter plots for CBF in the left post-central gyrus and the GM density in the right putamen versus change in VO_{2Peak} are shown in Figure 3.

Discussion

This study demonstrates that cardiopulmonary fitness (VO_{2Peak}) is positively associated with regional cerebral blood flow and grey matter hypertrophy in specific regions among adults with CAD. One striking finding was the localization of an exercise effect in the putamen, with converging evidence provided by both CBF and VBM analyses. The present multi-modal approach provides complementary structural and perfusion findings, illustrating that CBF was uniquely associated with cardiopulmonary fitness in cortical structures like the sensorimotor and premotor cortices, as well as the anterior cingulate. By contrast, cardiopulmonary fitness was associated with increased GM density in subcortical structures, the hippocampus, caudate and temporal regions, which are brain regions previously identified in studies of healthy adults[6–8].

Within the striatum, the results of the current study identified the putamen in both the ASL and VBM datasets, and the caudate in the VBM dataset as being positively associated with VO_{2Peak}. These results are not altogether unexpected as they parallel the animal exercise literature For instance, McCloskey et al. used an optical method to show increased cytochrome oxidase metabolism in hindlimb and forelimb motor cortices and striatum due to chronic exercise [9]_ENREF_22. In another study, rats that underwent treadmill training showed a similar pattern of regional changes as seen by functional activation, namely basal ganglia, cerebellum, thalamus, and sensorimotor cortex [10].The putamen is known to receive motor pathway connections and is implicated in motor learning, while the caudate receives dorsolateral prefrontal pathway connections and is implicated in learning, feedback and reward [36].

The current study provides new evidence that brain measures prior to starting an exercise intervention can predict the change in fitness. As reflected in Table 2, it was putamen grey matter density and sensorimotor CBF at baseline predicted greater increases in VO_{2Peak} over the course of this exercise interventions. While much emphasis has been placed on understanding the effects of exercise on the brain, less has been done to establish neurobiological markers that predict who will benefit from an exercise program. These data add to limited and emerging literature suggesting that brain function can predict the effectiveness of exercise interventions [37,38] and the current study suggests that these phenomena

may have a quantifiable neurobiological basis. Further efforts will be needed to translate these preliminary findings into strategies to predict and improve outcomes.

This study has limitations, such as a relatively small sample size. In addition a non-CAD control group would have helped to establish whether the observed brain associations would generalize to a non-clinical cohort. Having said this the imaging methodologies were sensitive enough to detect associations with adequate power. Only men were considered for this study due to the preponderance of male participants in cardiac rehabilitation and the possibility that including a relatively small proportion of women might introduce heterogeneity in a small sample; therefore, the results cannot be generalized to women. Moreover, apart from gender, although the demographics of the included participants are characteristic of those who undertake cardiac rehabilitation, the study may have been subject to bias based on patterns of referral and intake into cardiac rehabilitation, further reducing generalizability. Although the study identifies a temporal relationship between VO_{2Peak} and grey matter measures, follow-up MRI was not performed, precluding our ability to establish a direct causation. Finally, the present study does not elucidate relationships between perfusion at rest and perfusion during exercise [39], which remains an important area for further exploration.

The association between putamen volume and VO_{2Peak} in this study of older men with CAD concurs with that reported recently in adolescents [40], identifying a consistent correlate of fitness throughout the human lifespan. Moreover, in the present study, larger right putamen volumes were associated with larger changes in VO_{2Peak} associated with the exercise intervention. The findings would be consistent with the involvement of the putamen in mediating changes to the dopaminergic reward system in response to exercise [41] and with a role of the putamen in initiating physical activity behaviours based on a history of reward [42]. These findings, taken together with the putamen's pivotal position in the striatal circuitry controlling motor function, implicate the putamen as a critical node in the relationship between brain and behaviour. Sensorimotor CBF was associated with baseline VO_{2Peak} and change in VO_{2Peak}, which to our knowledge is a unique clinical finding to date and aligns with primate work showing exercise increases motor cortex vascular density [4].

Author Contributions

Conceived and designed the experiments: BJM WS DEC PO NH KLL. Performed the experiments: WS NR MS PO BS. Analyzed the data: BJM WS DEC NH KLL. Contributed reagents/materials/analysis tools: BJM WS DEC PO BS KLL. Wrote the paper: BJM WS DEC PO BS NH KLL.

References

1. Thomas AG, Dennis A, Bandettini PA, Johansen-Berg H (2012) The effects of aerobic activity on brain structure. Front Psychol 3: 86.
2. Kleim JA, Cooper NR, VandenBerg PM (2002) Exercise induces angiogenesis but does not alter movement representations within rat motor cortex. Brain Res 934: 1–6.
3. Holschneider DP, Maarek JM, Yang J, Harimoto J, Scremin OU (2003) Functional brain mapping in freely moving rats during treadmill walking. J Cereb Blood Flow Metab 23: 925–932.
4. Rhyu IJ, Bytheway JA, Kohler SJ, Lange H, Lee KJ, et al. (2010) Effects of aerobic exercise training on cognitive function and cortical vascularity in monkeys. Neuroscience 167: 1239–1248.
5. Pereira AC, Huddleston DE, Brickman AM, Sosunov AA, Hen R, et al. (2007) An in vivo correlate of exercise-induced neurogenesis in the adult dentate gyrus. Proc Natl Acad Sci U S A 104: 5638–5643.
6. Erickson KI, Voss MW, Prakash RS, Basak C, Szabo A, et al. (2011) Exercise training increases size of hippocampus and improves memory. Proc Natl Acad Sci U S A 108: 3017–3022.
7. Thomas BP, Yezhuvath US, Tseng BY, Liu P, Levine BD, et al. (2013) Life-long aerobic exercise preserved baseline cerebral blood flow but reduced vascular reactivity to CO. J Magn Reson Imaging.
8. Colcombe SJ, Erickson KI, Scalf PE, Kim JS, Prakash R, et al. (2006) Aerobic exercise training increases brain volume in aging humans. J Gerontol A Biol Sci Med Sci 61: 1166–1170.
9. McCloskey DP, Adamo DS, Anderson BJ (2001) Exercise increases metabolic capacity in the motor cortex and striatum, but not in the hippocampus. Brain Res 891: 168–175.
10. Holschneider DP, Yang J, Guo Y, Maarek JM (2007) Reorganization of functional brain maps after exercise training: Importance of cerebellar-thalamic-cortical pathway. Brain Res 1184: 96–107.
11. Honea RA, Thomas GP, Harsha A, Anderson HS, Donnelly JE, et al. (2009) Cardiorespiratory fitness and preserved medial temporal lobe volume in Alzheimer disease. Alzheimer Dis Assoc Disord 23: 188–197.
12. Burns JM, Cronk BB, Anderson HS, Donnelly JE, Thomas GP, et al. (2008) Cardiorespiratory fitness and brain atrophy in early Alzheimer disease. Neurology 71: 210–216.

13. Ahlskog JE, Geda YE, Graff-Radford NR, Petersen RC (2011) Physical exercise as a preventive or disease-modifying treatment of dementia and brain aging. Mayo Clin Proc 86: 876–884.

14. Lee CD, Folsom AR, Blair SN (2003) Physical activity and stroke risk: a meta-analysis. Stroke 34: 2475–2481.

15. Gianaros PJ, Greer PJ, Ryan CM, Jennings JR (2006) Higher blood pressure predicts lower regional grey matter volume: Consequences on short-term information processing. Neuroimage 31: 754–765.

16. Jagust W, Harvey D, Mungas D, Haan M (2005) Central obesity and the aging brain. Arch Neurol 62: 1545–1548.

17. Chen X, Wen W, Anstey KJ, Sachdev PS (2006) Effects of cerebrovascular risk factors on gray matter volume in adults aged 60-64 years: a voxel-based morphometric study. Psychiatry Res 147: 105–114.

18. Adachi T, Kobayashi S, Yamaguchi S (2002) Frequency and pathogenesis of silent subcortical brain infarction in acute first-ever ischemic stroke. Intern Med 41: 103–108.

19. Kavanagh T, Mertens DJ, Hamm LF, Beyene J, Kennedy J, et al. (2002) Prediction of long-term prognosis in 12 169 men referred for cardiac rehabilitation. Circulation 106: 666–671.

20. Vanhees L, Fagard R, Thijs L, Amery A (1995) Prognostic value of training-induced change in peak exercise capacity in patients with myocardial infarcts and patients with coronary bypass surgery. Am J Cardiol 76: 1014–1019.

21. Kuller LH, Longstreth WT Jr, Arnold AM, Bernick C, Bryan RN, et al. (2004) White matter hyperintensity on cranial magnetic resonance imaging: a predictor of stroke. Stroke 35: 1821–1825.

22. Marzolini S, Brooks D, Oh PI (2008) Sex differences in completion of a 12-month cardiac rehabilitation programme: an analysis of 5922 women and men. Eur J Cardiovasc Prev Rehabil 15: 698–703.

23. MacIntosh BJ, Filippini N, Chappell MA, Woolrich MW, Mackay CE, et al. (2010) Assessment of arterial arrival times derived from multiple inversion time pulsed arterial spin labeling MRI. Magn Reson Med 63: 641–647.

24. Parkes LM, Rashid W, Chard DT, Tofts PS (2004) Normal cerebral perfusion measurements using arterial spin labeling: reproducibility, stability, and age and gender effects. Magn Reson Med 51: 736–743.

25. Hamm LF, Kavanagh T (2000) The Toronto Cardiac Rehabilitation and Secondary Prevention Program: 1968 into the new millennium. J Cardiopulm Rehabil 20: 16–22.

26. Marzolini S, Oh PI, Thomas SG, Goodman JM (2008) Aerobic and resistance training in coronary disease: single versus multiple sets. Med Sci Sports Exerc 40: 1557–1564.

27. Marzolini S, Mertens DJ, Oh PI, Plyley MJ (2010) Self-reported compliance to home-based resistance training in cardiac patients. Eur J Cardiovasc Prev Rehabil 17: 35–41, quiz 42–39.

28. Longstreth WT Jr, Bernick C, Manolio TA, Bryan N, Jungreis CA, et al. (1998) Lacunar infarcts defined by magnetic resonance imaging of 3660 elderly people: the Cardiovascular Health Study. Arch Neurol 55: 1217–1225.

29. Kamijo K, Nishihira Y, Hatta A, Kaneda T, Wasaka T, et al. (2004) Differential influences of exercise intensity on information processing in the central nervous system. Eur J Appl Physiol 92: 305–311.

30. van Osch MJ, Teeuwisse WM, Walderveen MAA, Hendrikse J, Kies DA, et al. (2009) Can Arterial Spin Labeling Detect White Matter Perfusion Signal? Magn Reson Med 62: 165–173.

31. Douaud G, Smith S, Jenkinson M, Behrens T, Johansen-Berg H, et al. (2007) Anatomically related grey and white matter abnormalities in adolescent-onset schizophrenia. Brain 130: 2375–2386.

32. Last D, Alsop DC, Abduljalil AM, Marquis RP, de Bazelaire C, et al. (2007) Global and regional effects of type 2 diabetes on brain tissue volumes and cerebral vasoreactivity. Diabetes Care 30: 1193–1199.

33. Benar CG, Gross DW, Wang Y, Petre V, Pike B, et al. (2002) The BOLD response to interictal epileptiform discharges. Neuroimage 17: 1182–1192.

34. Nichols TE, Holmes AP (2002) Nonparametric permutation tests for functional neuroimaging: a primer with examples. Hum Brain Mapp 15: 1–25.

35. Jones NL, Campbell EJM (1982) Clinical exercise testing: Philadelphia: W. B. Saunders.

36. Alexander GE, Crutcher MD, DeLong MR (1990) Basal ganglia-thalamocortical circuits: parallel substrates for motor, oculomotor, "prefrontal" and "limbic" functions. Prog Brain Res 85: 119–146.

37. Kakos LS, Szabo AJ, Gunstad J, Stanek KM, Waechter D, et al. (2010) Reduced executive functioning is associated with poorer outcome in cardiac rehabilitation. Prev Cardiol 13: 100–103.

38. Swardfager W, Herrmann N, Marzolini S, Oh PI, Saleem M, et al. (2011) Verbal memory performance and completion of cardiac rehabilitation in patients with coronary artery disease. Psychosom Med 73: 580–587.

39. Macintosh BJ, Crane DE, Sage MD, Rajab AS, Donahue MJ, et al. (2014) Impact of a single bout of aerobic exercise on regional brain perfusion and activation responses in healthy young adults. PLoS One 9: e85163.

40. Chaddock L, Hillman CH, Pontifex MB, Johnson CR, Raine LB, et al. (2012) Childhood aerobic fitness predicts cognitive performance one year later. J Sports Sci 30: 421–430.

41. Evero N, Hackett LC, Clark RD, Phelan S, Hagobian TA (2012) Aerobic exercise reduces neuronal responses in food reward brain regions. J Appl Physiol 112: 1612–1619.

42. Muranishi M, Inokawa H, Yamada H, Ueda Y, Matsumoto N, et al. (2011) Inactivation of the putamen selectively impairs reward history-based action selection. Exp Brain Res 209: 235–246.

10

Postoperative Admission to a Dedicated Geriatric Unit Decreases Mortality in Elderly Patients with Hip Fracture

Jacques Boddaert[1,2*¶], Judith Cohen-Bittan[1], Frédéric Khiami[3], Yannick Le Manach[4], Mathieu Raux[1,5,8], Jean-Yves Beinis[6], Marc Verny[1,2], Bruno Riou[1,7,8]

1 Université Pierre et Marie Curie (UMRS 956, UMRS 1158), Paris, France, 2 Department of Geriatrics, Groupe hospitalier (GH) Pitié-Salpêtrière, Assistance Publique Hôpitaux de Paris (APHP), Paris, France, 3 Department of Orthopedic Surgery and Trauma, GH Pitié-Salpêtrière, APHP, Paris, France, 4 Departments of Anesthesia & Clinical Epidemiology and Biostatistics, Michael DeGroote School of Medicine, Faculty of Health Sciences, McMaster University, Hamilton, Ontario, Canada, 5 Department of Anesthesiology and Critical Care, GH Pitié-Salpêtrière, APHP, Paris, France, 6 Department of Rehabilitation, Groupe Hospitalier Charles Foix, APHP, Ivry-sur-Seine, France, 7 Department of Emergency Medicine and Surgery, GH Pitié-Salpêtrière, APHP, Paris, France, 8 Institut national de la santé et de la recherche médicale (UMRS 956, UMRS 1158, UMR 689), Paris, France

Abstract

Background: Elderly patients with hip fracture have a 5 to 8 fold increased risk of death during the months following surgery. We tested the hypothesis that early geriatric management of these patients focused on co-morbidities and rehabilitation improved long term mortality.

Methods and Findings: In a cohort study over a 6 year period, we compared patients aged >70 years with hip fracture admitted to orthopedic versus geriatric departments in a time series analysis corresponding to the creation of a dedicated geriatric unit. Co-morbidities were assessed using the Cumulative Illness Rating Scale (CIRS). Each cohort was compared to matched cohorts extracted from a national registry (n = 51,275) to validate the observed results. Main outcome measure was 6-month mortality. We included 131 patients in the orthopedic cohort and 203 in the geriatric cohort. Co-morbidities were more frequent in the geriatric cohort (median CIRS: 8 vs 5, $P<0.001$). In the geriatric cohort, the proportion of patients who never walked again decreased (6% versus 22%, $P<0.001$). At 6 months, re-admission (14% versus 29%, P = 0.007) and mortality (15% versus 24%, P = 0.04) were decreased. When co-morbidities were taken into account, the risk ratio of death at 6 months was reduced (0·43, 95%CI 0·25 to 0·73, P = 0.002). Using matched cohorts, the average treatment effects on the treated associated to early geriatric management indicated a reduction in hospital mortality (−63%; 95% CI: −92% to −6%, P = 0.006).

Conclusions: Early admission to a dedicated geriatric unit improved 6-month mortality and morbidity in elderly patients with hip fracture.

Editor: Darwin Ang, University of South Florida, United States of America

Funding: All authors declare that no authors have support from any company for the submitted work; no authors have relationships with any company that might have an interest in the submitted work in the previous 3 years; their spouses, partners, or children have do not have any financial relationships that may be relevant to the submitted work; and no authors have any-financial interests that may be relevant to the submitted work.

Competing Interests: The authors have declared that no competing interests exist.

* E-mail: jacques.boddaert@psl.aphp.fr

¶ Pr J. Boddaert is the designated author signing on behalf of all co-authors of the contribution.

Introduction

Worldwide 1.6 million patients suffer a hip fracture each year [1] and as the population continues to age this figure has increased by 25% each decade [2]. In the elderly patient hip fracture has devastating consequences. The hospital mortality of the condition ranges from 2.3% to 13.9% [3–7], with patients discharged home having a 5 to 8 fold increased risk of death in the months immediately following surgery [8]. This risk persists well beyond the immediate surgical period with 6 month mortality rates ranging from 12 to 23 % [7,9–12], and it is estimated that hip fractures account for more than 1.5% of all deaths in patients aged 50 years or more [13].

When compared to elective total hip replacements, patients presenting with hip fracture have a 6 to 15 fold mortality risk [14].

This can largely be explained by the high prevalence of pre-existing medical conditions seen in this population: 75% of patients are older than 70 years [1], and 95% of them present with at least one major preoperative comorbidity [15]. However studies suggest that only 1 in 4 of hip fracture associated deaths may be causally related to the fracture itself rather than due to pre-existing medical conditions [13]. This suggests that the insult of the hip fracture destabilizes an elderly population with a high burden of pre-existing morbidities thereby resulting in excess mortality.

Despite the magnitude of this problem there are no established effective strategies to prevent mortality after hip fracture. Approaches that combine both orthopedic and geriatric management have been studied but these have provided conflicting results

[16–20] and few studies report an improvement in short and long term clinical outcomes [21].

To address this significant public health problem, we formed a multi-disciplinary management team and created a dedicated care unit with the aim of providing integrated postoperative orthopedic and geriatric care for elderly patients with hip fracture. We hypothesized that the provision of early care with specific management of these patients focused on co-morbidity management and rehabilitation would significantly impact long term mortality. To evaluate the impact of this strategy we conducted an interrupted time series study. In addition, we used a national registry to provide external validation of our results.

Methods

Ethics statement

Our hospital ethics committee (CPP Ile de France VI, Paris, France) approved this study and authorized waived informed consent since the study was observational. The database was declared to the French National Commission on Computing and Liberty (CNIL, Paris, France).

Patients

From September 2005 to March 2012 all consecutive patients admitted to our Emergency Department (ED) were evaluated for eligibility. Patients were included if their primary presentation was due to hip fracture and if they were ≥70 years of age. Patients were excluded if they presented with multiple fractures, a metastatic fracture, a fracture complicated by a previous hip prosthesis or osteosynthesis, if they had been transferred to another hospital before surgery, or were already hospitalized at the time of diagnosis.

Intervention

In June 2009, we created a new geriatric unit (Unit for Post-Operative Geriatric Care, UPOG) devoted to the post-operative care of elderly patients with hip fracture. Before its opening, the medical staff from the emergency, anesthesiology and critical care, geriatric, orthopedic surgery, and rehabilitation departments met to define priorities for patients who would be admitted. Four key factors were identified: (1) early alert from the ED; (2) consideration of hip fracture as an emergency case requiring emergency surgery as soon as feasible (i.e. 24 hours a day); (3) rapid transfer to the UPOG after surgery (<48 h); and (4) rapid transfer of stable patients to a dedicated rehabilitation unit. Management strategy focused on early mobilization -with the aim of chair-sitting and walking (first steps) within 24 and 48 hours after arrival respectively, pain management -using acetaminophen and morphine, the provision of air-filled mattresses for patients with pressure ulcers or a high risk of pressure ulcers as evaluated by the Braden scale [22], swallowing disorders detected using a systematic medical survey, detection of stool impaction and urinary retention using ultrasound, the presence of anemia and liberal transfusion of packed red blood cells (usually when the hemoglobin level was <10 g.L^{-1}), detection of delirium using the Confusion Assessment Method [23], and malnutrition detection and management in conjunction with a nutritionist. All skills are regrouped in the same ward, allowing a common plan of care for all patients, implicating physicians, nurses, physiotherapists, speech therapist and nutritionist.

Data collection

Data were collected from computerized ED medical charts (instituted September 1st, 2005) and from hand-written medical charts of other departments. Since the opening of the UPOG in June 2009, data were prospectively entered in the database. The following variables were collected: age, sex, home or nursing home living conditions, walking ability, previous medical history, type of fracture and surgical treatment, delay and duration of surgery. Co-morbidity severity was assessed using the Cumulative Illness Rating Scale (CIRS) in which co-occurring medical conditions are weighted from 0 to 4 in 13 main systems [24]. We recorded the preoperative hemoglobin level and its lowest value during the acute care period. Anemia was defined following WHO guidelines [25]. We measured serum creatinine and estimated creatinine clearance [26]. All complications during the acute care period were recorded including delirium, need for physical restraints, stool impaction, urinary retention requiring drainage, morphine administration, pressure ulcer, infection, thromboembolic event, need for blood transfusion, aspiration related to swallowing disorders, cardiac insufficiency (i.e. acute cardiac failure or acute pulmonary edema), and admission into an intensive care unit (ICU).

Patients were followed until death or 6 months after admission. Surviving patients or their family were contacted and interviewed by telephone. Missing patients were tracked through health care providers, particularly general practitioners, or any identified acquaintances.

Study cohort

We compared the intervention cohort of patients admitted to the UPOG (geriatric cohort) to a control cohort of patients admitted to the orthopedic surgery department (orthopedic cohort). All patients transferred >48 h after surgery to the UPOG were assigned to the orthopedic cohort. After the opening of the UPOG, the proportion of patients admitted to the orthopedic department rapidly decreased as did the proportion of transfers to other hospitals (Figure 1), providing a nearly perfect time series analysis [27]. There was no selection of the patients admitted into the UPOG. Nevertheless, before the opening of the UPOG, a selection of patients admitted to the orthopedic department (versus transfer) was very likely. Thus it was expected that the co-morbidities of the cohorts may differ, the patients in the orthopedic cohort being expected to be less severe.

External validation cohort

We identified all patients admitted to French private or public health institutions in 2010 (n = 7,051,113) (See Table S1 in File S1). To create a hip fracture validation cohort we identified all patients undergoing surgery for hip/femur fracture related to a recent trauma, and then excluded patients <70 years of age and those from our institution. We then extracted patient age, sex, length of acute care stay and presence of pre-existing medical conditions (See Table S2 in File S1) and in-hospital mortality.

End points

The primary end point was 6-month mortality. The main secondary endpoints were re-hospitalization, re-fracture, new admission into a nursing home, and ability to walk 6 months after admission. We also considered length of stay and mortality while in acute care and rehabilitation facilities, admission into an ICU, delay to first sitting and first walking, and the ability to walk after the acute care and/or rehabilitation period. For the comparison with the external national validation cohort, only hospital mortality was available and this was used as the primary endpoint.

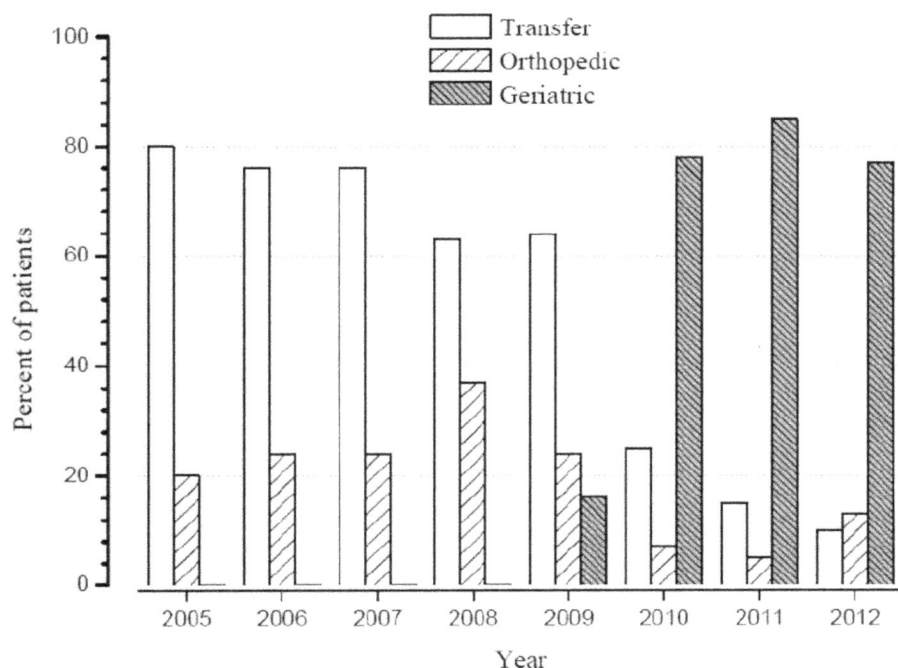

Figure 1. Transfers and allocation of patients. Evolution of transfers out of the hospital (n = 392) and allocation to the orthopedic (n = 131) and geriatric (n = 203) cohorts during the study period. There were only 4 months (September to December) in 2005 and 3 months (January to March) in 2012.

Sample size calculation

Assuming a baseline 6 month mortality rate of 20% [7] and a mortality reduction of 40% (*i.e.* from 20% to 12%) in the geriatric cohort, we estimated that we would require 298 patients to obtain a 80% power with a two-tailed *P* value of 0·05. This estimation hypothesized a weak relationship between the predictors of the primary endpoint and the strategy tested, which was sustained by the design of the study and by the absence of major change in the recruitment of these patients. A study period of at least 30 months after the opening of the UPOG was planned.

Statistical analysis

Data are presented as mean ± SD, median [25–75 inter-quartile] for non-Gaussian variables, or number (percentages). Comparison between cohorts was performed using the unpaired Student t test, Mann-Whitney test, Fisher's exact method, and multivariate analysis of variance when appropriate. Survival was estimated by the Kaplan-Meier method and differences were assessed by the log-rank test. In a preliminary analysis (n = 100) using a multivariate Cox proportional-hazards model we determined that three variables (age, sex, CIRS) were associated with 6-month mortality. We tested the impact of the intervention by calculating the hazard ratio and its 95 percent confidence interval (CI) in association with these prognostic variables.

To provide external validation all patients in the geriatric and orthopedic cohorts were matched with patients drawn from the external national validation cohort. Logistic models using all variables specified in Table S2 in File S1 were developed to determine the probabilities to be in the geriatric or in the orthopedic cohorts. These probabilities (*i.e.* propensity scores) were used to match the patients of the geriatric cohort and those of the orthopedic cohort to patients from the national cohort. Matching was performed using a nearest neighbor matching method with a

caliper of 20% of the *logit* of these probabilities. Each patient from the geriatric and orthopedic cohorts was matched to 3 patients from the national cohort using this probability [28]. The absolute standardized difference (ASD) was used to assess balance between the groups. An ASD above 10 to 15% is considered to represent meaningful imbalance [29]. The average treatment effect on the treated (ATT) was estimated in these two cohorts, which represents the average impact of the care program among those who have been exposed to it, was estimated in these two cohorts. We also conducted a sensitivity analysis without caliper use.

All P values were two-sided and P<0.05 was considered significant. R 2.14 software (www.cran.r-project.org last date accessed February 2, 2013) was used for statistical analyses.

Results

Among the 726 elderly patients with hip fracture admitted to the ED, 334 were selected, 131 in the orthopedic cohort and 203 in the geriatric cohort (Figure 2). Only 3 patients were transferred to UPOG more than 48 hours after surgery and so were assigned to the orthopedic cohort.

Patients from the two cohorts differed slightly in the prevalence of co-morbidities and the proportion who received gamma nail and dynamic screw fixation (Table 1). Patients in the geriatric cohort underwent surgery 1 hour before the orthopedic cohort, a clinically insignificant difference but the proportion of patients delayed for >48 h did not. Surgery duration was shorter in the geriatric cohort, probably as a result of the higher proportion of gamma nails (effect of surgical treatment: F = 11.92, P<0·001; effect of cohort: F = 0·09, P = 0·78) (Table 1). The observed difference in surgery duration (10 min) was not considered to be clinically relevant.

During the acute care period, patients in the geriatric cohort received more morphine, less physical restraint, were transfused

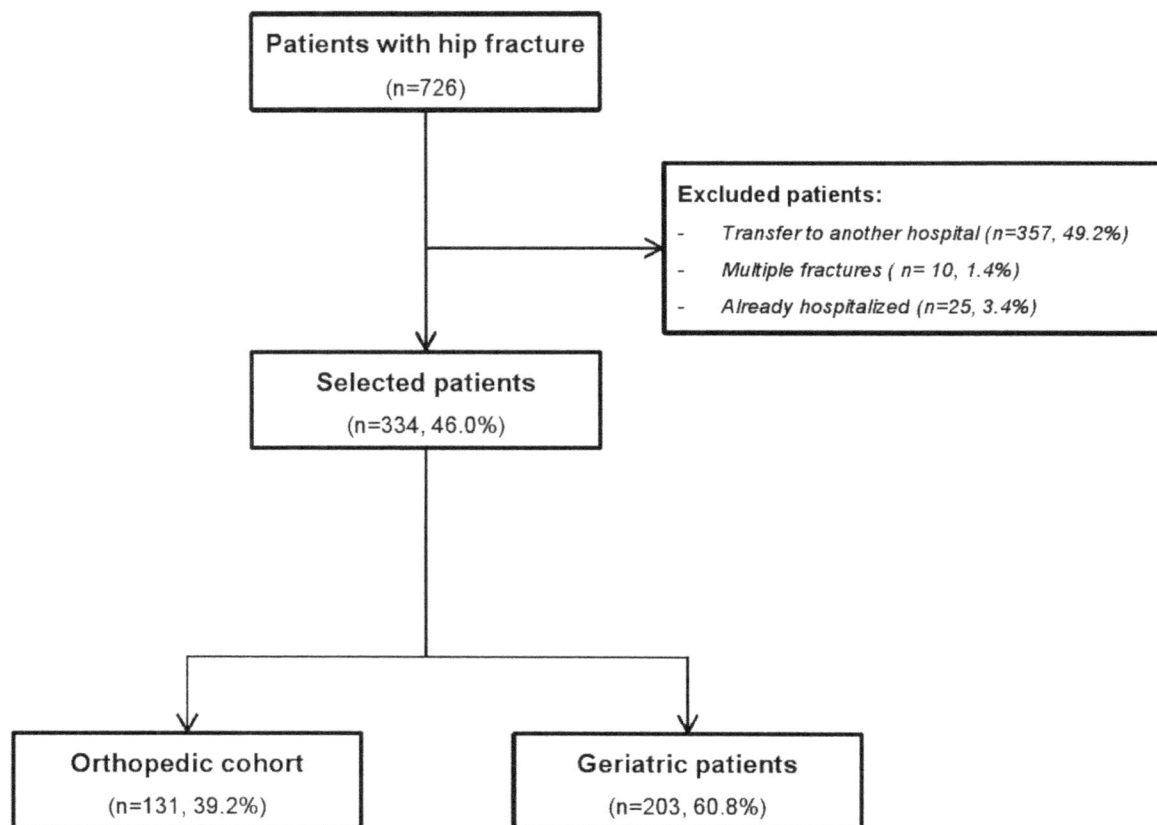

Figure 2. Study flow chart.

more frequently, and were diagnosed with stool impaction and swallowing disorders more frequently. They were less frequently admitted into an ICU and suffered fewer pressure ulcers. However episodes of cardiac insufficiency occurred more frequently. Patients in the geriatric cohort had a markedly reduced time to first sitting and first walking, a much shorter stay in acute care, and a greater proportion of walking patients at the end of the intervention period (Table 2).

Only 3 (0.9%) patients were lost to follow-up, 2 in the geriatric cohort and 1 in the orthopedic cohort (all due to transfer to foreign countries). During the follow up period, both mortality and re-hospitalization risks were significantly reduced in the geriatric cohort (Figure 3). When taking into account age, sex, and co-morbidities (using the CIRS), patients in the geriatric cohort showed a profound reduction in both risks of mortality and re-hospitalization. No significant difference was observed for the risk of re-fracture or new admission to a nursing home (Table 3).

In the unmatched cohorts, hospital mortality was 7.6 % in the orthopedic cohort (n = 131), 3·0 % in the geriatric cohort (n = 203), and 3.9 % in the external national validation cohort (n = 51,275) but large imbalances were observed between these cohorts (See Table S2 in File S1). After matching, the highest ASD was 9.8% in the geriatric cohort (23 discarded patients) and 13.5% in the orthopedic cohort (18 discarded patients). In the matched populations, hospital mortality was significantly lower in the geriatric cohort compared to the external national validation cohort (2.5% versus 5.4%, log rank test P = 0·04), but not significantly different in the orthopedic cohort (6.3% versus 5.4%, log rank test P = 0.72) (Figure 4). The relative ATT associated to

the geriatric cohort indicated a significant reduction in mortality (−63%; 95% CI: −92% to −6%; P = 0.006) whereas the relative ATT associated with the orthopedic cohort was not significantly different from zero (32%; 95% CI: −2 to +67%; P = 0.57).

In the matching procedure conducted without calipers (i.e., no discarded patients in geriatric and orthopedic cohorts) the population characteristics were not similar with most variables showing an AST>15%. However the relative ATT was −70% (95%CI: −98% to −3%; P<0.001) in the matched geriatric cohort and 51% (95%CI: −12% to 111%; P = 0.83) in the matched orthopedic cohort.

Lastly, we compared the key management factors previously identified (*vide supra*) between patients who were alive at 6 month and those who died. There was no significant difference between groups swallowing disorders (19 vs 26%, P = 0.20), physical restraint (5 vs 10%, P = 0.12), stool impaction (31 vs 39%, P = 0.28), morphine administration (59 vs 62%, P = 0.65), blood transfusion (62 vs 74 %, P = 0.08), and delay for surgery (22 [13–34] vs 23 [15–44] hours, P = 0.23). In contrast, we observed significant differences in pressure ulcers (16 vs 28 %, P = 0.037), delirium (33 vs 61 %, P<0.001), urinary retention (23 vs 37 %, P = 0.04), delay to first sitting (2 [1–3] vs 2 [1–5] days, P = 0.015), delay to first walking (3 [1–5] vs 5 [2–8] days, P<0.001), and proportion of patients who never walked (3 vs 52 %, P<0.001).

Discussion

In this study, we observed that elderly patients with hip fracture, admitted early into a dedicated geriatric unit and managed with a

Table 1. Comparison of the main characteristics of the two study cohorts.

	Orthopedic cohort (n = 131)	Geriatric cohort (n = 203)	All patients (n = 334)
Age (years)	85±6	86±6	86±6
Male	44 (34)	50 (25)	94 (28)
Medical history			
Obesity[a]	3 (2)	20 (10)	23 (7)
Dementia	32 (24)	78 (38)*	110 (33)
Diabetes	16 (12)	27 (13)	43 (13)
Hypertension	74 (56)	138 (68)*	212 (63)
Cardiac failure	18 (14)	33 (16)	51 (15)
Coronary artery disease	22 (17)	27 (13)	49 (15)
Heart valve disease	9 (7)	17 (8)	26 (8)
Atrial fibrillation	28 (21)	47 (23)	75 (22)
Peripheral vascular disease	5 (4)	12 (6)	17(5)
Stroke	17 (13)	33 (16)	50 (15)
Hemiplegia/paraglegia	1 (1)	8 (4)	9 (3)
Cancer	24 (18)	37 (18)	61 (18)
COPD	10 (8)	15 (7)	25 (7)
Pulmonary hypertension	0 (0)	2 (1)	2(1)
Alcohol abuse	2 (2)	10 (5)	12 (4)
Chronic renal insufficiency	16 (12)	31 (15)	47 (14)
Creatinine clearance (ml.min^{-1})[b]	53±25	53±22	53±23
CIRS 52	5 [3–8]	8 [6–11]	7[4–10]
Hemoglobin (g.dL^{-1})	12.0±1.8	12.1±1.4	12.1±1.5
Anemia	70 (53)	98 (48)	168 (50)
Living status			
Living at home	117 (89)	182 (90)	299 (90)
Living in institution	14 (11)	21 (10)	35 (10)
Unknown	0	0	0
Live alone	42 (37)	28 (14)*	70 (21)
Unknown	19	0	19
Walking ability			
No walking disability	118 (90)	187 (92)	305 (91)
Moderate walking disability	11 (8)	14 (7)	25 (7)
Does not walk	2 (2)	2 (1)	4 (1)
Unknown	0	0	0
Fracture			
Femoral neck fracture	59 (45)	112 (55)	171 (51)
Intertrochanteric fracture	72 (55)	91 (45)	163 (49)
Surgery			
Delay to surgery (h)	23 [15–40]	22 [12–34]	22 [14–35]
Delay to surgery >48 h	25 (19)	26 (13)	51 (15)
Duration of surgery (min)	150 [120–175]	140 [110–160]*	140 [120–170]
Gamma nail	33 (25)	102 (50)*	135 (40)
Dynamic hip screw	39 (30)	24 (12)*	63 (19)
Unipolar prosthesis	52 (40)	70 (34)	122 (36)
Bipolar prosthesis	7 (5)	7 (3)	14 (4)

Data are mean ± SD, median [25–75 interquartile], or number (percentage). COPD: chronic obstructive pulmonary disease; CIRS: cumulative illness rating scale;
[a]: defined as body mass index >30 kg.m^{-2};
[b]: creatinine clearance could be calculated in 99 (76%) and 200 (98%) patients in the orthopedic and geriatric cohorts respectively.
*: P<0.05 vs Orthopedic cohort.

Table 2. Acute care, rehabilitation, and walking ability.

	Orthopedic cohort (n = 131)	Geriatric cohort (n = 203)	P value
Delay to first sitting (days)	3 [2–4]	1 [1–2]	<0.001
Delay to first walking (days)	5 [3–9]	2 [1–4]	<0.001
Walking initially contra-indicated	8 (6)	9 (4)	0.61
Acute care complications			
Delirium	49/118 (41)	72/203 (35)	0.29
Physical restraint	18/121 (15)	1/203 (0.5)	<0.001
Morphine administration	37/116 (32)	152/203 (75)	<0.001
Swallowing disorders	8/120 (7)	56/203 (28)	<0.001
Lowest hemoglobin (g.dL^{-1})	9.3±1.7	9.2±1.3	0.54
Blood transfusion	72/131 (55)	141/203 (69)	0.008
Stool impaction	23/120 (19)	83/203 (41)	<0.001
Urinary retention	26/120 (22)	57/203 (28)	0.24
Pressure ulcer	40/121 (33)	18/203 (9)	<0.001
Acute heart failure	6/120 (5)	33/203 (16)	0.002
Infection	31/123 (25)	40/203 (20)	0.27
Venous thromboembolism	1/122 (1)	10/203 (5)	0.06
Fall	9/120 (7)	9/203 (4)	0.32
Admission into ICU	17/131 (13)	8/203 (4)	0.005
LOS acute care (days)	13 [10–20]	11 [8–16]	0.001
Admission to rehabilitation care[a]	91/121 (75)	167/197 (85)	0.04
LOS rehabilitation care (days)	41 [25–71]	42 [30–62]	0.78
Total LOS (acute and rehabilitation care) (days)	43 [22–70]	49 [30–68]	0.41
Death during acute care	10/131 (8)	6/203 (3)	0.07
Death during rehabilitation	10/91 (11)	14/166 (8)	0.51
Death during acute care and/or rehabilitation	20/130 (15)	20/202 (10)	0.17
Return to home[b]	92/129 (71)	149/202 (74)	0.70
New admission into nursing home[c]	14/97 (14)	25/163 (15)	1.00
Unknown	2	1	
Readmission within 30 days[d]	19/111 (17)	10/183 (5)	0.002
Redo surgery within 30 days	6/130 (5)	3/201 (1)	0.16
Unknown	2	1	
Walking ability			
After acute care/rehabilitation			
No walking disability	41/111 (37)	88/182 (48)	0.07
Moderate walking disability	55/111 (50)	88/182 (48)	0.90
Does not walk	15/111 (14)	6/182 (3)	0.002
Missing data	0	1	
After 6 months			
No walking disability	33/99 (33)	57/172 (33)	1.00
Moderate walking disability	56/99 (57)	107/172 (62)	0.37
Does not walk	10/99 (10)	8/172 (5)	0.13
Missing data	1	2	
Never walked	29/131 (22)	12/203 (6)	<0.001

Data are mean ± SD, median [25–75 interquartile], or number (percentage). LOS: length of stay; ICU: intensive care unit;
[a]: excluding death during acute care;
[b]: institution was considered as "home" in patients previously living in an institution;
[c]: excluding patients previously living in an institution;
[d]: excluding patients who died in acute care and/or rehabilitation.

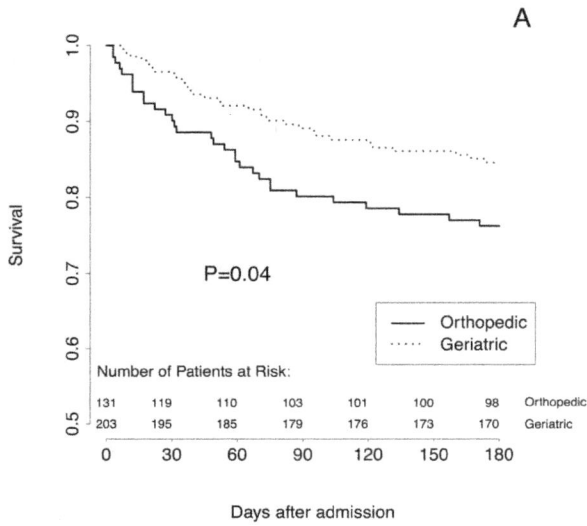

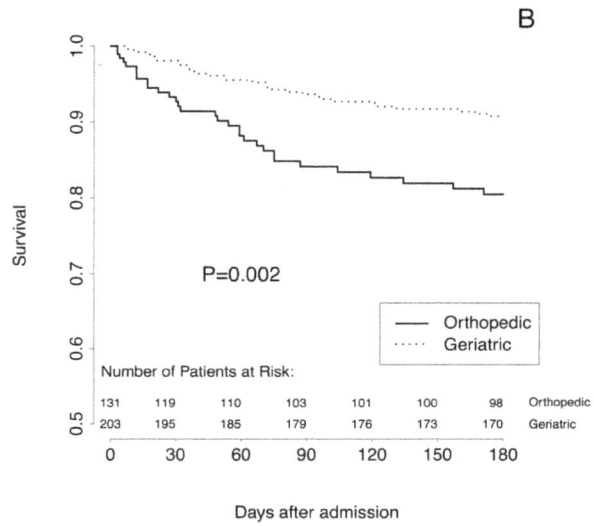

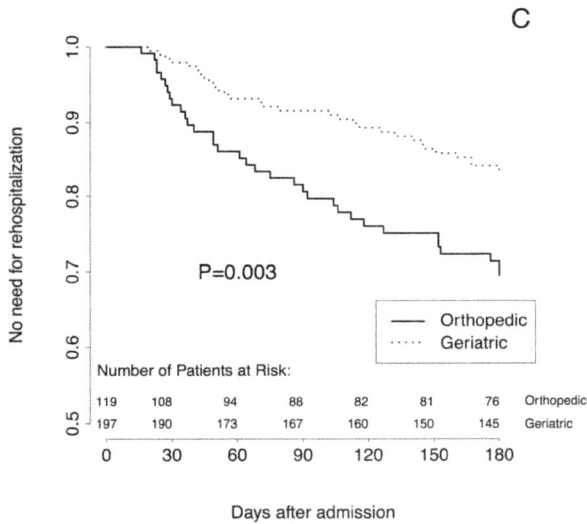

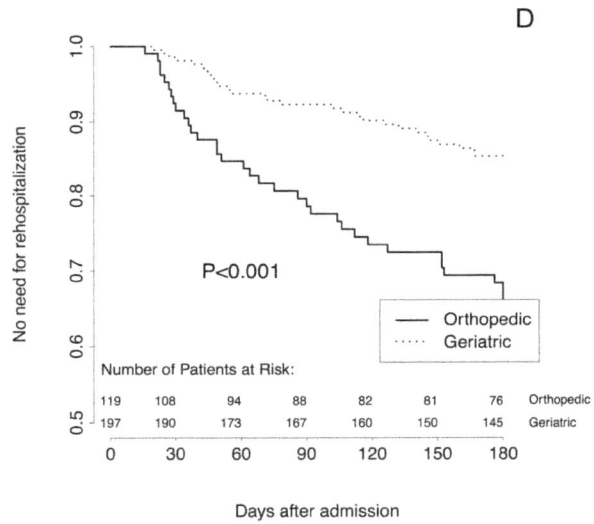

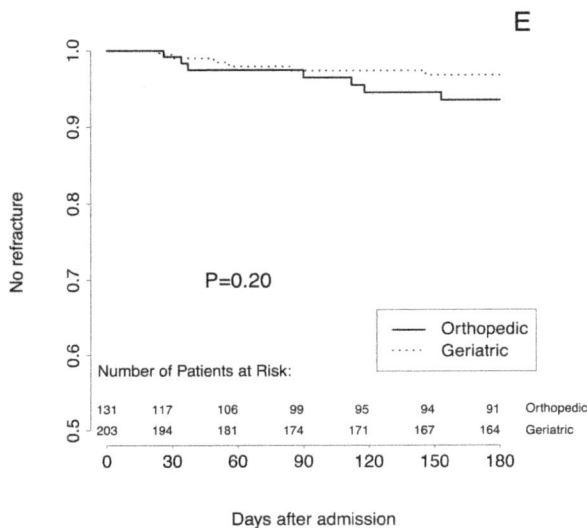

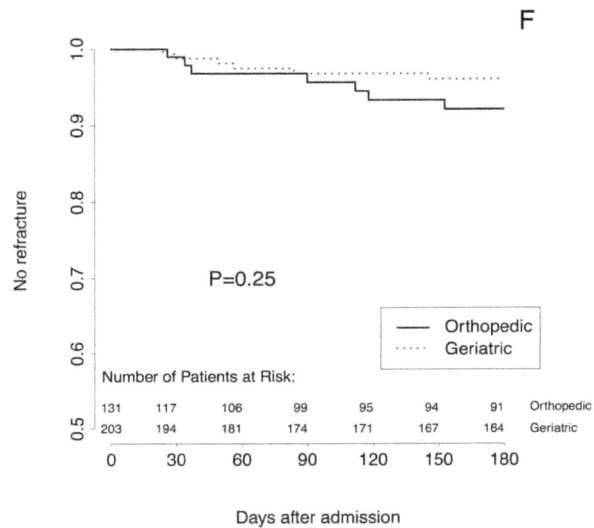

Figure 3. Survival curves for mortality, re-hospitalization, and re-fracture. Survival curves for mortality, re-hospitalization, and re-fracture for patients in the orthopedic (solid lines) and geriatric (dotted line) cohorts. Survival is non-adjusted (panels A, C, and E) and adjusted (panels B, D, and F) for age, sex and Cumulative Illness Rating Scale (CIRS) calculated with a Cox regression analysis. For re-hospitalization and re-fracture, death was considered as a censored observation. *P* values refer to log-rank test.

multidisciplinary approach, had reduced long term mortality and improved walking ability. These observations were externally validated against a matched cohorts derived from a national hospital database.

Various approaches have been taken to integrate orthopedic and geriatric care, also known collectively as orthogeriatrics, for hip fracture patients. As in our study, some of these measures have included admission into a geriatric ward under the specialist care of an orthopedic consultant [16,17]. However, no previous studies have demonstrated a clear mortality benefit with this approach. Alternative approaches have included using an orthopedic ward with geriatric consultation [30], or an orthopedic ward with daily geriatric management [31–33]. When these approaches have shown mortality reduction, it was transient or without reduction in detailed patient morbidity. To our knowledge, this is the first orthogeriatric study that has shown sustained mortality reduction, together with improved walking ability and less morbidity.

We observed a marked reduction (risk ratio 0.43) in the risk of death at 6 months (Table 3). This treatment effect is approximately twice that observed in randomized trials conducted to demonstrate the benefit of early surgery in hip fracture patients [34]. In the geriatric cohort we observed a significant reduction in the length of stay in acute care facilities, but this was not observed when taking into account the rehabilitation period. We believe that some patients in the orthopedic cohort may have been discharged prematurely and that this may at least partially explain the higher proportion of readmitted patients. However, we cannot rule out the possibility that these differences may be due to the lower number of co-morbidities in the orthopedic cohort. When comparing patients who survived at 6 months and those who did not, it seems that early sitting and walking, prevention of pressure ulcer, early identification of urinary retention and delirium, may be the most important management factors associated with survival improvement. Irrespective of the reasons behind this difference our results emphasize the role played by the rehabilitation facilities as well as the importance of the cooperation between acute care and rehabilitation facilities.

Despite considering geriatric hip fracture as an emergency requiring surgery as soon as feasible (i.e. 24 hours a day) [34,35], we were unable to observe any significant reductions in the time delay until surgery (Table 1). However, in both cohorts, the proportion of patients with delayed surgery was lower than that reported in previous studies [19,30,35], suggesting that this goal had already been appropriately implemented in our hospital. Moreover, surgery must sometimes be postponed in some patients due to their pre-existing conditions, including drugs that interfere with hemostasis. The delays to surgery reported in previous orthogeriatric studies were usually longer [19,30,35].

Some events in the geriatric cohort such as stool impaction, swallowing disorders, venous thromboembolism, and acute heart failure were more frequently reported. Although these differences may be due to the retrospective recording of data in the orthopedic cohort, we believe that they were detected more frequently in the UPOG due to improved surveillance. Swallowing disorders are a strong risk factor for the development of aspiration pneumonia, and their detection has led to food consistency being thickened and heightened pneumonia surveillance. Despite this we did not observe a significant difference in infection rates. Stool impaction

represents a source of discomfort for patients, with increased risk of urinary retention, which may delay rehabilitation and result in life-threatening complications [35]. We cannot rule out the hypothesis that increased morphine consumption in the geriatric cohort may have lead to higher rates of stool impaction. Improved surveillance probably explains the increased venous thromboembolism detection while the increased incidence of acute heart failure could be related either to better clinical detection or intolerance to blood transfusion. However, these differences probably had a limited influence on outcome.

Patients in the geriatric cohort received more blood transfusions and this is explained by our strict adherence to French national transfusion guidelines [36]. These recommend maintaining a hemoglobin >10 g/dL in geriatric patients who are unable to tolerate anemia. This goal was modified in 2011 after Carson et al. [37] showed no benefit of a liberal transfusion regimen as compared to a restrictive one.

Our study has several limitations. First, it was an observational study and the orthopedic cohort data were collected retrospectively. However, we validated our results externally against matched cohorts derived from a national hospital database, used mortality as our primary endpoint, and successfully followed-up

Table 3. Multivariate cox proportional-hazards analysis predicting death, re-fracture, and re-hospitalization.

Variables	Risk Ratio[95% CI]	P value
Prediction of death (n = 334)		
Age	1.04 [1.00–1.08]	0.047
Male sex	1.88 [1.11–3.18]	0.02
CIRS	1.17 [1.10–1.25]	<0.001
Geriatric cohort	0.43 [0.25–0.73]	0.002
Prediction of re-fracture (n = 334)		
Age	0.98 [0.90–1.06]	0.58
Male sex	0.22 [0.03–1.76]	0.16
CIRS	1.00 [0.85–1.17]	0.97
Geriatric cohort	0.50 [0.15–1.65]	0.26
Prediction of re-hospitalization (n = 294)[a]		
Age	0.99 [0.95–1.03]	0.68
Male sex	0.76 [0.41–1.41]	0.39
CIRS	1.08 [1.00–1.16]	0.04
Geriatric cohort	0.40 [0.23–0.70]	0.001
Prediction of admission into a new institution (n = 296)[b]		
Age	1.08 [1.03–1.14]	0.003
Male sex	1.71 [0.86–3.41]	0.13
CIRS	1.06 [0.97–1.15]	0.21
Geriatric cohort	0.98 [0.47–2.00]	0.95

CI: confidence interval; CIRS: cumulative illness rating scale;
[a]: only patients who survived to acute care and rehabilitation were considered;
[b]: only patients who were not previously living in an institution were considered. For re-hospitalization and re-fracture, death was considered as a censored observation.

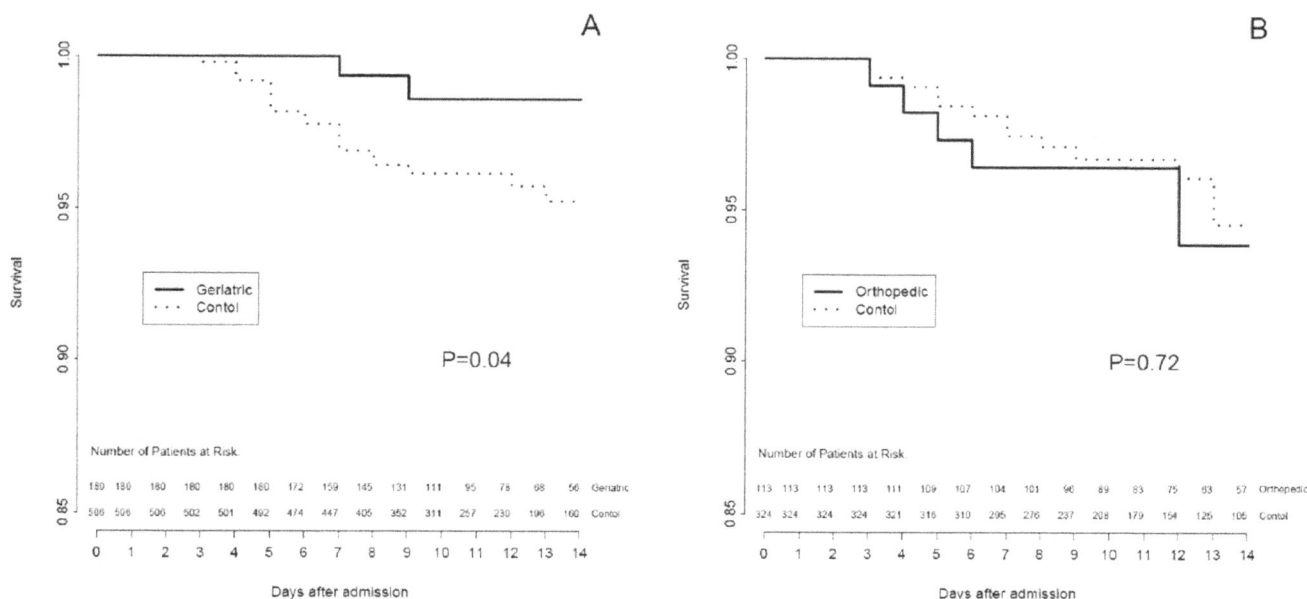

Figure 4. Survival curves for in-hospital mortality. Survival curves for in-hospital mortality in the geriatric (Panel A) and orthopedic (Panel B) cohorts, and their respective matched cohorts from the national registry. *P* values refer to log-rank test.

99% of enrolled patients. When comparing complex health procedures, randomized trials are difficult to conduct and interrupted time series analysis are often used. A multicenter cluster randomized study may also be an appropriate methodology. Second, we were unable to compare our results to other models of orthogeriatric reported in the literature [15–19]. Comparisons of this nature are difficult due to differences between health care systems and/or local hospital organization, varying study end points, and a lack of reported long term outcomes [30–33]. However, our results suggest that an alignment of multidisciplinary hospital teams (physicians and nurses) and hospital care paths (from ED admission to rehabilitation care) toward optimal care of the geriatric hip fracture patient is key factor in successful patient management. Lastly, our results may in part be attributable to certain characteristics of the French health care system and may not be appropriate in countries with different health systems.

Conclusion

We observed that elderly patients with hip fracture, admitted early into a dedicated geriatric unit and managed with a multidisciplinary approach, had reduced long term mortality and an improved walking ability.

References

1. Johnell O, Kanis JA (2006) An estimate of the worldwide prevalence and disability associated with osteoporotic fractures. Osteoporosis Int 17: 1726–33.
2. Johnell O, Kanis JA (2004) An estimate of the worldwide prevalence, mortality and disability associated with hip fracture. Osteoporosis Int 15: 897–902.
3. Rapp K, Becker C, Lamb SE, Icks A, Klenk J (2008) Hip fractures in institutionalized elderly people: incidence rates and excess mortality. J Bone Mineral Res 23: 1825–31.
4. Jiang HX, Majumdar SR, Dick DA, Moreau M, Raso J, et al. (2005) Development and initial validation of a risk score for predicting in-hospital and 1-year mortality in patients with hip fractures. J Bone Mineral Res 20: 494–500.
5. Myers AH, Robinson EG, Van Natta ML, Michelson JD, Collins K, et al. (1991) Hip fractures among the elderly: factors associated with in-hospital mortality. Am J Epidemiol 134: 1128–37.

Acknowledgments

We thank Dr. David Baker, DM, FRCA, (Department of Anesthesiology and Critical Care, Hôpital Necker-Enfants Malades, Paris) and Dr. Reitze Rodseth, MB ChB, FRCA (Lecturer, Perioperative Research Group, Department of Anaesthetics, University of KwaZulu-Natal, Durban, South Africa & Research Fellow, Population Health Research Institute, Hamilton, Canada) for reviewing the manuscript.

Author Contributions

Conceived and designed the experiments: JB BR YLM. Performed the experiments: JB JCB FK MR JYB. Analyzed the data: JB BR YLM. Contributed reagents/materials/analysis tools: YLM BR. Wrote the paper: JB YLM BR. Critical revision of the manuscript for important intellectual content: JB JCB FK MR JYB MV BR.

6. Endo Y, Aharonoff GB, Zuckerman JD, Egol KA, Koval KJ (2005) Gender differences in patients with hip fracture: a greater risk of morbidity and mortality in men. J Orthop Trauma 19: 29–35.
7. Abrahamsen B, van Staa T, Ariely R, Olson M, Cooper C (2009) Excess mortality following hip fracture: a systematic epidemiological review. Osteoporosis Int 20: 1633–50.
8. Haentjens P, Magaziner J, Colón-Emeric CS, Vanderschueren D, Milisen K, et al. (2010) Meta-analysis: excess mortality after hip fracture among older women and men. Ann Intern Med 152: 380–90.
9. Penrod JD, Litke A, Hawkes WG, Magaziner J, Doucette JT, et al. (2008) The association of race, gender, and comorbidity with mortality and function after hip fracture. J Gerontol A Biol Sci Med Sci 63: 867–72.

10. Bentler SE, Liu L, Obrizan M, Cook EA, Wright KB, et al. (2009) The aftermath of hip fracture: discharge placement, functional status change, and mortality. Am J Epidemiol 170: 1290–9.
11. Hannan EL, Magaziner J, Wang JJ, Eastwood EA, Silberzweig SB, et al. (2001) Mortality and locomotion 6 months after hospitalization for hip fracture: risk factors and risk-adjusted hospital outcomes. JAMA 285: 2736–42.
12. Bass E, French DD, Bradham DD, Rubenstein LZ (2007) Risk-adjusted mortality rates of elderly veterans with hip fractures. Ann Epidemiol 17: 514–9.
13. Kanis JA, Oden A, Johnell O, De Laet C, Jonsson B, et al. (2003) The components of excess mortality after hip fracture. Bone 32: 468–73.
14. Cram P, Lu X, Kaboli PJ, Vaughan-Sarrazin MS, Cai X, et al. (2011) Clinical characteristics and outcomes of Medicare patients undergoing total hip arthroplasty, 1991–2008. JAMA 305: 1560–7.
15. Nikkel LE, Fox EJ, Black KP, Davis C, Andersen L, et al. (2012) Impact of comorbidities on hospitalization costs following hip fracture. J Bone Joint Surg Am 94: 9–17.
16. Gilchrist WJ, Newman RJ, Hamblen DL, Williams BO (1988) Prospective randomised study of an orthopaedic geriatric inpatient service. BMJ 297: 1116–8.
17. Adunsky A, Lusky A, Arad M, Heruti RJ (2003) A comparative study of rehabilitation outcomes of elderly hip fracture patients: the advantage of a comprehensive orthogeriatric approach. J Gerontol A Biol Sci Med Sci 58: 542–7.
18. Kennie DC, Reid J, Richardson IR, Kiamari AA, Kelt C (1988) Effectiveness of geriatric rehabilitative care after fractures of the proximal femur in elderly women: a randomised clinical trial. BMJ 297: 1083–6.
19. Naglie G, Tansey C, Kirkland JL, Ogilvie-Harris DJ, Detsky AS, et al. (2002) Interdisciplinary inpatient care for elderly people with hip fracture: a randomized controlled trial. CMAJ 167: 25–32.
20. Friedman SM, Mendelson DA, Bingham KW, Kates SL (2009) Impact of a comanaged geriatric fracture center on short-term hip fracture outcomes. Arch Intern Med 169: 1712–7.
21. Kammerlander C, Roth T, Friedman SM, Suhm N, Luger TJ, et al. (2010) Ortho-geriatric service–a literature review comparing different models. Osteoporosis Int 21: S637–46.
22. Bergstrom N, Demuth PJ, Braden BJ (1987) A clinical trial of the Braden Scale for predicting pressure sore risk. Nurs Clin North Am 22: 417–28.
23. Inouye SK, van Dyck CH, Alessi CA, Balkin S, Siegal AP, et al. (1990) Clarifying confusion: the confusion assessment method. A new method for detection of delirium. Ann Intern Med 113: 941–8.
24. Linn BS, Linn MW, Gurel L (1968) Cumulative illness rating scale. J Am Geriatr Soc 16: 622–6.
25. McLean E, Cogswell M, Egli I, Wojdyla D, de Benoist B (2009) Worldwide prevalence of anaemia, WHO Vitamin and Mineral Nutrition Information System, 1993–2005. Public Health Nutr 12: 444–54.
26. Cockcroft DW, Gault MH (1976) Prediction of creatinine clearance from serum creatinine. Nephron 16:31–41.
27. Ramsay CR, Matowe L, Grilli R, Grimshaw JM, Thomas RE (2003) Interrupted time series designs in health technology assessment: lessons from two systematic reviews of behavior change strategies. Int J Technol Assess Health Care 19: 613–23.
28. Austin PC (2011) Optimal caliper widths for propensity-score matching when estimating differences in means and differences in proportions in observational studies. Pharm Stat 10: 150–61.
29. Austin PC (2009) Balance diagnostics for comparing the distribution of baseline covariates between treatment groups in propensity-score matched samples. Stat Med 28: 3083–107.
30. Leung AH, Lam TP, Cheung WH, Chan T, Sze PC, et al. (2011) An orthogeriatric collaborative intervention program for fragility fractures: a retrospective cohort study. J Trauma 71: 1390–4.
31. Fisher AA, Davis MW, Rubenach SE, Sivakumaran S, Smith PN, et al. (2006) Outcomes for older patients with hip fractures: the impact of orthopedic and geriatric medicine cocare. J Orthop Trauma 20: 172–8.
32. Koval KJ, Chen AL, Aharonoff GB, Egol KA, Zuckerman JD (2004) Clinical pathway for hip fractures in the elderly: the Hospital for Joint Diseases experience. Clin Orthop Relat Res 425: 72–81.
33. Vidan M, Serra JA, Moreno C, Riquelme G, Ortiz J (2005) Efficacy of a comprehensive geriatric intervention in older patients hospitalized for hip fracture: a randomized, controlled trial. J Am Geriatr Soc 53: 1476–82.
34. Simunovic N, Devereaux PJ, Sprague S, Guyatt GH, Schemitsch E, et al. (2010) Effect of early surgery after hip fracture on mortality and complications: systematic review and meta-analysis. CMAJ 182: 1609–16.
35. Vidan MT, Sanchez E, Gracia Y, Maranon E, Vaquero J, et al. (2011) Causes and effects of surgical delay in patients with hip fracture: a cohort study. Ann Intern Med 155:226–33.
36. Agence Nationale de Sécurité du Médicament (ANSM) (2002) Recommandations pour la transfusion de globules rouges homologues: produits, indications, alternatives. http://ansm.sante.fr/var/ansm_site/storage/original/application/3a08e904ce75401d27f52e600d53a0cc.pdf (last access March 21, 2013).
37. Carson JL, Terrin ML, Noveck H, Sanders DW, Chaitman BR, et al. (2011) Liberal or restrictive transfusion in high-risk patients after hip surgery. N Engl J Med 365: 2453–62.

11

The NHV Rehabilitation Services Program Improves Long-Term Physical Functioning in Survivors of the 2008 Sichuan Earthquake: A Longitudinal Quasi Experiment

Xia Zhang[1,2⑨], **Jan D. Reinhardt**[2,3,4⑨], **James E. Gosney**[2], **Jianan Li**[1,2]*

1 The First Affiliated Hospital of Nanjing Medical University, Nanjing, People's Republic of China, **2** World Health Organization Liaison Sub–Committee on Rehabilitation Disaster Relief of the International Society of Physical and Rehabilitation Medicine, Geneva, Switzerland, **3** Swiss Paraplegic Research, Nottwil, Switzerland, **4** Department of Health Sciences and Health Policy, University of Lucerne, Lucerne, Switzerland

Abstract

Background: Long-term disability following natural disasters significantly burdens survivors and the impacted society. Nevertheless, medical rehabilitation programming has been historically neglected in disaster relief planning. 'NHV' is a rehabilitation services program comprised of non–governmental organizations (NGOs) (N), local health departments (H), and professional rehabilitation volunteers (V) which aims to improve long-term physical functioning in survivors of the 2008 Sichuan earthquake. We aimed to evaluate the effectiveness of the NHV program.

Methods/Findings: 510 of 591 enrolled earthquake survivors participated in this longitudinal quasi-experimental study (86.3%). The early intervention group (NHV–E) consisted of 298 survivors who received institutional-based rehabilitation (IBR) followed by community-based rehabilitation (CBR); the late intervention group (NHV–L) was comprised of 101 survivors who began rehabilitation one year later. The control group of 111 earthquake survivors did not receive IBR/CBR. Physical functioning was assessed using the Barthel Index (BI). Data were analyzed with a mixed-effects Tobit regression model. Physical functioning was significantly increased in the NHV–E and NHV–L groups at follow-up but not in the control group after adjustment for gender, age, type of injury, and time to measurement. We found significant effects of both NHV (11.14, 95% CI 9.0–13.3) and sponaneaous recovery (5.03; 95% CI 1.73–8.34). The effect of NHV-E (11.3, 95% CI 9.0–13.7) was marginally greater than that of NHV-L (10.7, 95% CI 7.9–13.6). It could, however, not be determined whether specific IBR or CBR program components were effective since individual component exposures were not evaluated.

Conclusion: Our analysis shows that the NHV improved the long-term physical functioning of Sichuan earthquake survivors with disabling injuries. The comprehensive rehabilitation program benefitted the individual and society, rehabilitation services in China, and international rehabilitation disaster relief planning. Similar IBR/CBR programs should therefore be considered for future large-scale rehabilitation disaster relief efforts.

Editor: Anthony E. Kline, University of Pittsburgh, United States of America

Funding: This study was funded by the Hong Kong Caring for Children Foundation. The funders had no role in study design, data collection and analysis, decision to publish, or preparation of the manuscript.

Competing Interests: The authors have declared that no competing interests exist.

* E-mail: lijianan@carm.org.cn

⑨ These authors contributed equally to this work.

Introduction

Long-term physical disability following natural disasters significantly burdens the impacted society, even more so than immediate medical needs [1,2,3]. Nevertheless, medical rehabilitation programming has been historically neglected in disaster relief planning [4,5,6,7,8,9]. Robust scientific evidence on effectiveness of medical rehabilitation in victims of earthquakes has not been previously reported in the medical literature [4]. The Sichuan earthquake of May 12, 2008 affected 46 million people, resulting in 87,476 deaths and over 350,000 persons injured, more than 10,000 of them severely [10,11]. Many of these had disabling injuries, including fractures, amputation, spinal cord injury (SCI), and traumatic brain injury (TBI), all of which require physical rehabilitation to optimize long-term physical functioning and prevent medical complications [12,13,14,15,16].

The large volume of traumatic injuries overwhelmed the severely damaged local medical infrastructure of Sichuan province, resulting in mass evacuation of medically stable patients to hospitals across China [17,18]. Anticipating the significant surgical and physical rehabilitation needs of the returning victims [19,20], the Chinese Association of Rehabilitation Medicine (CARM) partnered with local health ministries as well as non-governmental organizations (NGOs) (N), local health departments (H), and rehabilitation volunteers (V) to form NHV, the medical relief strategy's rehabilitation services component. Local health department resources were capacitated by volunteer rehabilitation professional expertise and NGO funding and other resources in

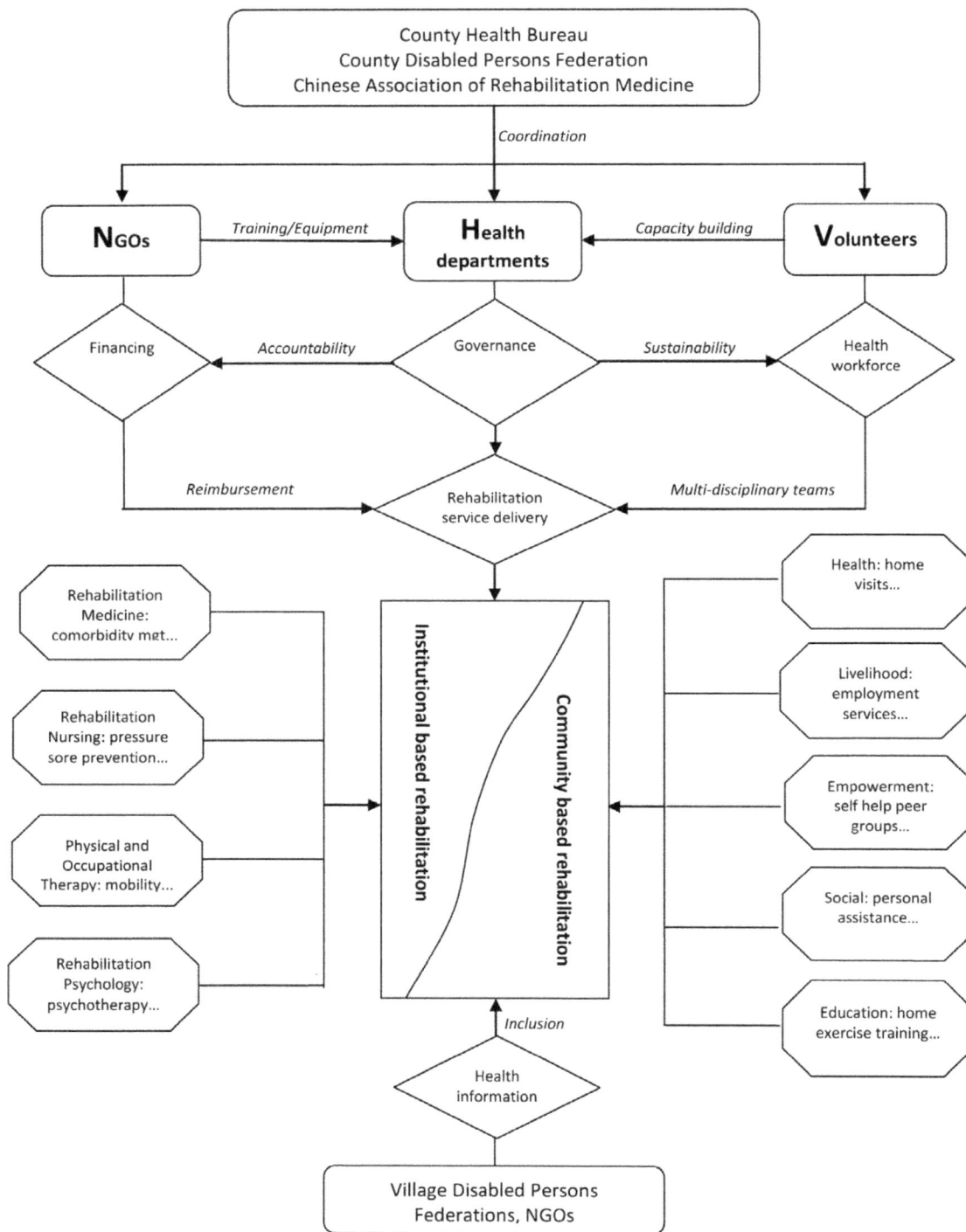

Figure 1. NHV program components and rehabilitation services.

providing a comprehensive continuum of institutional and community–based rehabilitation (IBR, CBR) services designed to improve the long-term physical functioning and quality of life of injured survivors [7].

IBR was administered in county hospital rehabilitation departments where patients participated in individualized physical rehabilitation programs. Rehabilitation interventions included muscle strengthening and range of motion exercises, training in self care and mobility activities, education in bladder, bowel and skin care management, and provision of assistive devices. Traditional Chinese therapies including acupuncture and massage were also provided. Following discharge to the community, CBR health sector services including medical care, rehabilitation, assistive devices, health prevention, and health promotion were provided [21]. Other CBR sectors comprising livelihood, social support, and empowerment were addressed via employment services, personal assistants, and patient self-help peer groups, respectively, among other interventions [21]. NHV focused initially on IBR and shifted to CBR as most earthquake victims were discharged into the community. Figure 1 shows the NHV program components and rehabilitation services.

Currently, NHV operates in two counties which accounted for more than 20% of the earthquake casualties [22]. A comprehensive prospective evaluation of NHV effectiveness attributing program causal effects has not been performed. Cumulative evidence on effectiveness of health service delivery following natural disasters is sparse due to compromised record keeping and lack of systematic planning [4,6,23,24,25]. Our study aims to quantify the effectiveness of the NHV rehabilitation program as measured by improvement in long-term physical functioning of Sichuan earthquake survivors with disabling injuries as assessed by the Barthel Index (BI).

Methods

Ethical Statement

This research has been approved by the ethical review board of the Medical Faculty of the Nanjing Medical University. Informed consent has been obtained from all study participants. All clinical investigations have been conducted according to the principles expressed in the Declaration of Helsinki.

Design

We use a longitudinal quasi–experimental design with two points of measurement and two intervention groups and a control group.

Setting

NHV IBR was implemented initially in a hospital in County A (NHV-E) which provided specialized rehabilitation care in its newly established rehabilitation department as part of comprehensive medical management of victims. CBR services were concurrently implemented in the community for patients' benefit following discharge by an international rehabilitation services NGO. Due to the urgent need to rehabilitate additional victims and given NHV's operational efficiency the program was implemented in neighbouring County B after one year (NHV-L). Due to resource and political constraints NHV was not implemented in neighbouring county C which served as the control group. Earthquake impact and victim demographics were comparable in the neighboring counties evaluated.

Participants

Five hundred and ninety-one earthquake survivors were originally identified and enrolled. Eligibility criteria for this study

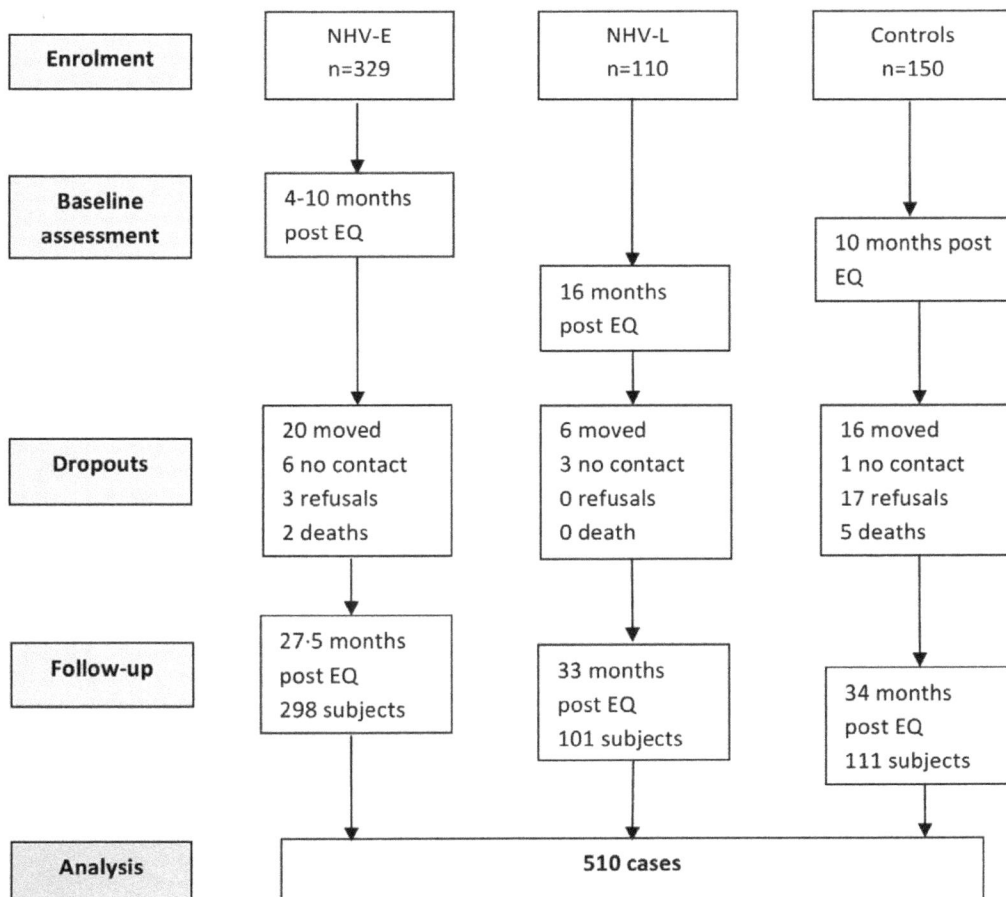

Figure 2. Subject flow in the NHV effectiveness study.

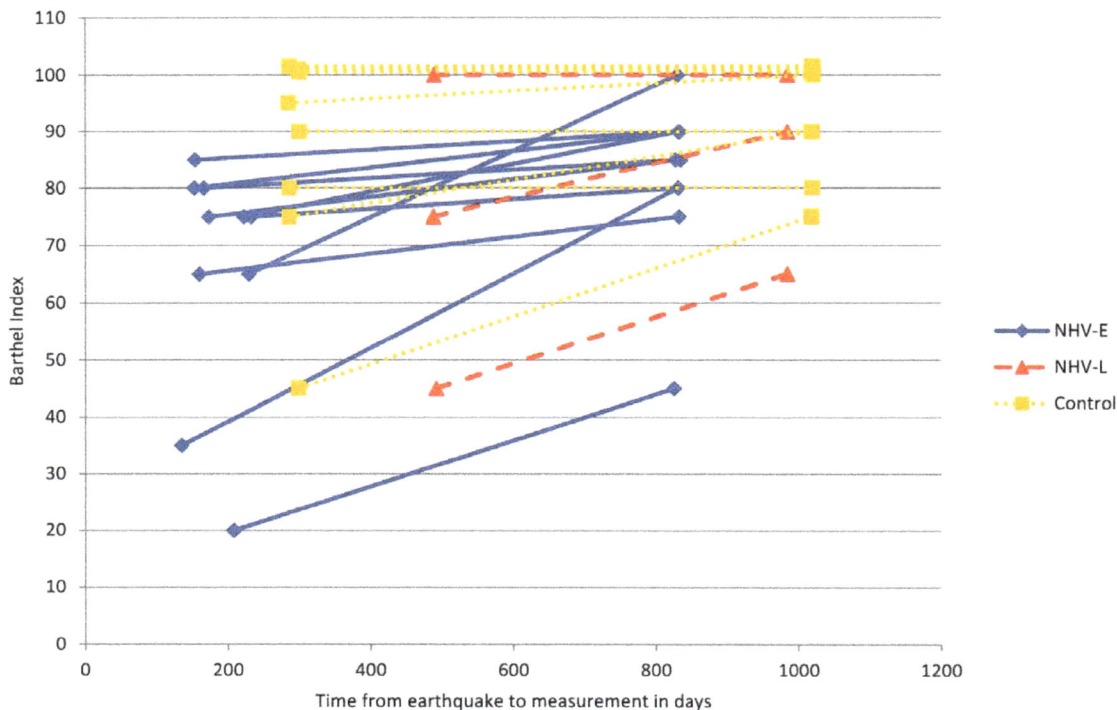

Figure 3. Ceiling effect of the Barthel Index in amputees (three patients from the control group and one from NHV-L begin with a censored score at baseline). Observations for one patient at different time points are connected by lines.

were: 1) age of 18 years and older; 2) diagnosis of a disabling injury requiring physical rehabilitation caused by the earthquake, and 3) no complicating internal injury. Based on these criteria, two patients were excluded due to complicating internal injuries. Written informed consent was obtained from participants in the intervention groups. Verbal telephonic consent was obtained from

patients in the control group due primarily to limited volunteer availability. Identical consent forms were used. Five hundred and ten subjects completed the study of which 298 subjects were assigned to NHV–E, 101 participants to NHV-L, and 111 to the control group (Figure 2).

Table 1. Baseline characteristics of the NHV study groups.

Characteristics	NHV–E (n = 298)	NHV–L(n = 101)	Control Group (n = 111)	P[‡]
Age, mean (SD)	55.2(16.6)	53.4(15.7)	51.8 (16.2)	0.156
Gender, % male	34.9	30.7	39.6	0.392
Injury classification, % (n)				
-Fracture	83.2% (248)	85.1% (86)	80.2% (89)	0.618
-Spinal cord injury	8.7% (26)	3.0% (3)	3.6% (4)	0.048
-Traumatic brain injury	1.7% (5)	1.0% (1)	6.3% (7)	0.017
-Amputation	3.7% (11)	3.0% (3)	7.2% (8)	0.226
-Other injury	2.7% (8)	7.9% (8)	2.7% (3)	0.045
BI at baseline, mean (SD)	77.5 (18.1)	80.1 (18.0)	82.4 (15.1)	0.032*
Time earthquake to baseline in days, mean (SD)	190.3 (32.5)	290.8 (9.1)	490.3 (1.5)	<0.001
Time earthquake to follow up in days, mean (SD)	829.5 (2.8)	984.4 (0.5)	1019.4 (1.1)	<0.001
Duration of Rehabilitation in days, mean (SD)	52.6 (19.1)	51.5 (19.0)	Not applicable	0.641†

SD = Standard Deviation; BI = Barthel Index. [‡]F–test for metric; Chi–square for categorical variables. *Significant difference between NHV-E and Controls only, according to post hoc tests (Scheffé), [†]T-test.

Measures

Physical functioning was assessed with the Chinese version of the Barthel Index (BI), a measure of performance of ADLs, comprised of personal hygiene, bathing, eating, toileting, ambulation, dressing, bladder and bowel control, transfers, and mobility [26]. BI scores range from zero to 100 with higher scores indicating greater independence [26]. The BI was used since it enhances comparability with other Chinese data on rehabilitation of disabled persons as it is the most widely used non-injury specific assessment measure of functioning in China; Chinese versions of comparable measures used in international research have not yet been validated.

Diagnostic data on injury type were retrieved from patient hospital charts. Demographic information including gender and age as well as date of assessment were also recorded. Baseline intervention group data were obtained prior to the onset of IBR; NHV-E data were obtained at 4–10 months post-earthquake and data for the NHV-L group at 16 months. Baseline control group data were collected at 10 months post-earthquake. Follow-up data for the three groups were collected at 27.5 to 34 months (Figure 2). Measurement points were largely determined by the availability of volunteers for data collection, requiring mathematical adjustment for time to measurement (see below).

Effect of NHV on daily physical functioning

Due to a ceiling effect of the BI (Figure 3) we computed a longitudinal Tobit model to estimate the effectiveness of rehabilitation achieved through NHV-E and NHV-L [27,28]. The use of this model in longitudinal analysis of BI data has been recommended by Twisk and Rijmen [24].

A ceiling effect implies that variance of BI scores cannot be measured above the scale maximum score due to the scale design. Scores, however, can be mathematically estimated with the Tobit model which employs a latent dependent variable that can assume values above the scale maximum. Estimation of supramaximal values allows correction for the baseline imbalance of physical functioning across study groups as the NHV-L and control groups had higher baseline values (see Table 1), leaving less margin for improvement up to the scale ceiling. The estimation of values above the scale maximum and the modelling of both an effect of time to measurement and of rehabilitation makes it possible to appropriately differentiate between influences of the rehabilitation program and the natural course of healing. Without correction for the BI's ceiling effect improvement in NHV-L and control group due to spontaneous recovery may have been underestimated.

Since observations i $(1,..,n_i)$ at different time points (level 1) were nested in individuals j $(1,...,n_j)$ (level 2) who in turn were nested in different intervention groups (level 3) or counties k (1,2,3), random intercepts δ_j and ϕ_k were introduced on the individual and county level, respectively. To model individual responsiveness to recovery over time, a random slope γ_j for the time from the earthquake to the respective measurement points in days (TimeEQMP) was considered. In the fixed part of the model, BI values Y^* (latent) were estimated using patients' age, TimeEQMP, and receipt of NHV rehabilitation services at follow up in the early (NHV_E_fu) or late intervention group (NHV_L_fu) as time-varying covariates. Gender (male = 1), injury type (dummies were introduced for fractures, amputation, SCI, and TB; other injuries was the reference group), and presence in an intervention (NHV_E_base vs. NHV_L_base) or control county (reference) were time-constant covariates. Random effects and residuals ε were assumed to be normally distributed with a mean of zero and variance of σ^2.

The formula of the resulting three-level Tobit model is:

$$
\begin{aligned}
Y*k_{ji} = {} & \beta_0 + \beta_1 age_{kji} + \beta_2 male_{kj} + \beta_3 fracture_{kj} + \beta_4 SCI_{kj} \\
& + \beta_5 TBI_{kj} + \beta_6 amputation_{kj} + \beta_7 TimeEQMP_{kji} \\
& + \beta_8 NHV\_E\_base_{kj} + \beta_9 NHV\_L\_base_{kj} \\
& + \beta_{10} NHV\_E\_fu_{kji} + \beta_{11} NHV\_L\_fu_{kji} \\
& + \delta_j + \gamma_j TimeEQMP + \vartheta_k + \varepsilon_{ijk}
\end{aligned}
$$

With

$$
\varepsilon_{ijk} \sim N\left(0, \sigma^2\right); \delta_j \sim N\left(0, \sigma^2\right)
$$

$$
\gamma_j \sim N\left(0, \sigma^2\right); \phi_k \sim N\left(0, \sigma^2\right)
$$

$$
Y_{ijk} = Y*_{kji} \text{ if } Y*_{kji} < 100
$$

$$
Y_{ijk} = 100 \text{ if } Y*_{kji} \geq 100
$$

Based on the fixed parameter estimates of this model we predicted BI values for the study groups at baseline and follow-up while adjusting for other model covariates. Bonferroni correction was applied to adjust confidence intervals (CIs) for multiple testing.

Counterfactual analysis

To differentiate the effect of IBR/CBR from the effect of recovery over time attributable to other factors, counterfactual predictions [29] were calculated by factoring out the rehabilitation effect in the model equation. Comparison of the slopes of change in BI from baseline to follow-up for the full and the counterfactual predictions indicates the difference between the NHV causal effect and the effect of recovery over time.

Sensitivity Analysis

To determine the possible degree to which study dropouts may have resulted in estimation bias, the model was re-estimated by imputing BI dropout data for three scenarios: a) BI remained constant over time; b) BI decreased by ten points; c) BI remained constant in dropouts from the intervention groups while increasing by ten points in controls (censored observation stayed at 100). Fatalities were excluded.

All data were analysed with Stata 12. The three-level Tobit model was implemented with the gllamm command [27,30]. All codes, estimates, analyses of residuals, and details of model development are available from the authors on request.

Results

Table 1 shows baseline characteristics of the study groups. In terms of injury classification prevalence, significantly more patients are diagnosed with SCI in NHV–E, more patients with TBI are among controls, and more patients with other injuries can be found in NHV-L. Baseline BI scores and times from the earthquake to measurements vary significantly across groups, requiring statistical adjustment. Dropout characteristics are addressed with the related sensitivity analysis below. Without further adjustment, differences between baseline and follow up BI are significant in all groups (NHV-E: 13.6, 95%CI 11.3 to 16.0; NHV-L: 9.3, 95% CI 7.5 to 12.0; controls: 6.1, 95% CI 3.8 to 8.4).

Parameter estimates of the multi-level Tobit model (Table 2) show baseline physical functioning to be approximately 12 points lower in the NHV-E and 6 points lower in the NHV-L group than in controls. While NHV-E improved BI scores by about eleven points at follow up (11.3, 95% CI 9.0 to 13.7), the effect of NHV-L was marginally smaller (10.7, 95% CI 7.9 to 13.6). An effect of recovery over time is also noted as BI improved by almost one point over 100 days (0.0083*100). On the individual level, random intercept and random slope were strongly negatively correlated; the higher the baseline BI scores, the less the individual recovery over time.

Marginal predictions show significant differences in baseline and follow-up BI scores in NHV-E (baseline: 73.8, 95% CI 72.5 to 75.2; follow up: 90.5, 95% CI 88.9 to 92.0) and NHV-L (baseline: 82.2, 95% CI 76.5 to 87.8; follow up: 96.9, 95% CI 92.4 to 101.4), while the difference is no longer significant in the control group (baseline: 86.8, 95% CI 83.6 to 90.1; follow up: 92.8, 95% CI 89.7 to 96.0) due to the absence of the NHV effect (Figure 4).

Figure 5 shows the overall effect of NHV IBR/CBR (11.14, 95% CI 9.0 to 13.3) compared to recovery over time (5.03; 95% CI 1.73–8.34) (Figure 5a) as well as separate NHV-E and NHV-L group effects (Table 2) compared to respective recovery over time (Figure 5b). The positive effect on physical functioning due to NHV is nearly twice that of recovery over time. The recovery over time effect is greater in NHV-E than in NHV-L (5.3; 95% CI 2.7 to 7.8 vs. 4.0, 95% CI −2.1 to 10.1).

Regarding dropouts and their potential impact on estimation of NHV effects, more males dropped from the study than females (63.3 vs. 36.8%, $X^2 = 22.9$, p<0.001). Dropouts were also significantly younger (38.2 vs. 54.1, T = 7.8; p<0.001) and had higher baseline BI scores in the intervention groups (94.3 vs. 78.1, T = 6.8, p<0.001). Sensitivity analysis showed the greatest relative decrease in NHV rehabilitation effects for imputation scenario B in which dropout BI scores were decreased by ten points (Figure 6). The NHV-E and NHV-L effects remained significant in all scenarios, however (p<0.01).

Discussion

The NHV rehabilitation services program improved long-term physical functioning of severely disabled survivors of the 2008 Sichuan earthquake. Our fully adjusted multi-level Tobit model estimated a statistically significant and clinically meaningful 11 point increase in BI in the intervention groups compared to controls; patients who received comprehensive IBR/CBR in two heavily-impacted, neighboring counties (sequenced implementation) benefitted. Statistically meaningful improvement in physical functioning was thus shown in both early and late intervention groups, demonstrating benefit from rehabilitation delivered nearly 1.5 years after injury.

To compare our results with findings from the literature, we performed a systematic review (May 2012) in PubMed, Embase, and CINAHL using the search terms "rehabilitation" AND "earthquake" AND ("outcome"* OR" effectiveness"). Four studies reporting quantitative data on functional outcomes of rehabilitation interventions on adult earthquake subjects were identified; all investigated populations from Sichuan. Two employed a cross-sectional design with a control group [14,31] and the other two used a pre-post intervention design [32]. A cross-sectional study on fracture victims of the Sichuan earthquakes revealed better outcomes in victims who received rehabilitation than controls at 27 months post-earthquake [14].

However, this study did not adequately adjust for baseline functioning. The other cross-sectional study was conducted in patients with tibial shaft fractures and performed a multivariate logistic regression to determine the effect of rehabilitation training on functional recovery. The odds of being in the two study groups which showed the greatest physical independence were five times higher for patients who received rehabilitation training [31]. However, this study is highly prone to bias since bivariate analysis was used to determine the multivariate model variables without correcting for multiple testing [33]. Li et al. [13] compared physical functioning at admission and discharge (institutional rehabilitation) in 51 Sichuan survivors with SCI and noted significant improvement. However, isolation of an effect of rehabilitation from spontaneous recovery was not possible since no control group was employed. Ning et. al [32] studied a team-based rehabilitation intervention and reported that the percentage of patients with complete functional dependence decreased from 89% at baseline to 38% at follow-up. However, it is unclear how functional dependence was measured, no control group was used, and no adjustment for other factors was performed.

Evidence on the effectiveness of medical rehabilitation in earthquake victims is scarce. Of the four relevant studies, two were of questionable methodological quality and none employed a pre-post intervention design using a control group. Our study is the first to employ a longitudinal design with a control group, allowing estimation of a causal effect of rehabilitation programming on physical functioning. The comparably large sample sizes allowed for appropriate adjustment for patient demographics and injury types. This study thereby contributes significantly to the evidence base on medical rehabilitation of earthquake victims.

Limitations of our research require that its results be viewed with caution, however. Counterfactual analysis allowed us to differentiate the effect of NHV IBR/CBR from that of recovery over time. However, although effectiveness of the NHV IBR/CBR program was demonstrated, it could not be determined whether specific IBR or CBR program components were effective since individual component exposures were not evaluated. IBR is believed to have made a significant contribution as has been found in other studies [13] since individualized therapy programs were designed to improve specific functional outcomes, including ADLs. However, BI was not administered at discharge, precluding isolation of an effect due to IBR. The effect of CBR would be more challenging to determine since discharged patients received various CBR health sector services, including rehabilitation (less structured and administered primarily by the patient or caregiver), in addition to other CBR sector services which likely positively affected functional outcomes. Future studies could be designed to distinguish between relative IBR and CBR effects as well as subcomponent effects on rehabilitation program effectiveness (the effect of specific IBR therapies or of CBR self-help peer groups, for example). CBR effects are expected to be further clarified by results of the third victim assessment performed in 2012 (data unavailable).

Although the BI ceiling effect was corrected using a Tobit model, actual improvement of patients who started IBR with censored scores was nonetheless not measured in this study. Future studies could employ other functional status measures which allow more precise evaluation of functional improvement, potentially based on WHO's International Classification of Functioning, Disability and Health (ICF) [34]. Measures of physical functioning that can be used for both clinical evaluation as well as population-based, survey assessment remain to be developed, however [4,35].

Increased dropouts in controls compared to intervention groups may have also biased results; nonetheless, the NHV effect

Table 2. Parameter estimates for Barthel Index (BI) based on the three-level Tobit model.

Predictors	Coefficient	SE	z	95% Confidence Interval	
Age	−0.0328	0.0256	−1.3	−0.0831	0.0174
Male	1.3257	0.8428	1.6	−0.3262	2.9776
Fracture	6.8478	2.0357	3.4***	2.8579	10.8377
SCI	5.6715	2.571	2.2*	0.6325	10.7105
TBI	7.5046	2.9879	2.5*	1.6484	13.3607
Amputation	2.7665	2.8281	1.0	−2.7764	8.3095
Time from EQ to MP in days	0.0083	0.0016	5.2***	0.0052	0.0115
NHV-E baseline	−12.0477	1.51	−8.0***	−15.0073	−9.0881
NHV-L baseline	−5.9792	2.4302	−2.5*	−10.7424	−1.216
NHV-E follow up	11.3622	1.1982	9.5***	9.0137	13.7107
NHV-L follow up	10.7119	1.4589	7.3***	7.8526	13.5712
Intercept	79.2396	2.5876	30.62***	74.168	84.3112
Variances/co-variances and SEs of random effects					
Level 1	35.6958	3.4261			
Level 2 (subject): intercept	501.4740	28.8731			
Level 2 (subject): slope	0.0002	<0.0001			
Level 2 (subject): cov (intercept, slope)	−0.2609	0.0270			
Level 3 (group) intercept	<0.0001	<0.0001			

Log Likelihood: −3415.094; Bayesian Information Criterion (BIC): 6947.956.
SE = standard error, z = standardized coefficient; EQ = earthquake; MP = point of measurement; cov = covariance *p<0.05, **p<0.01, *** p<0.001.

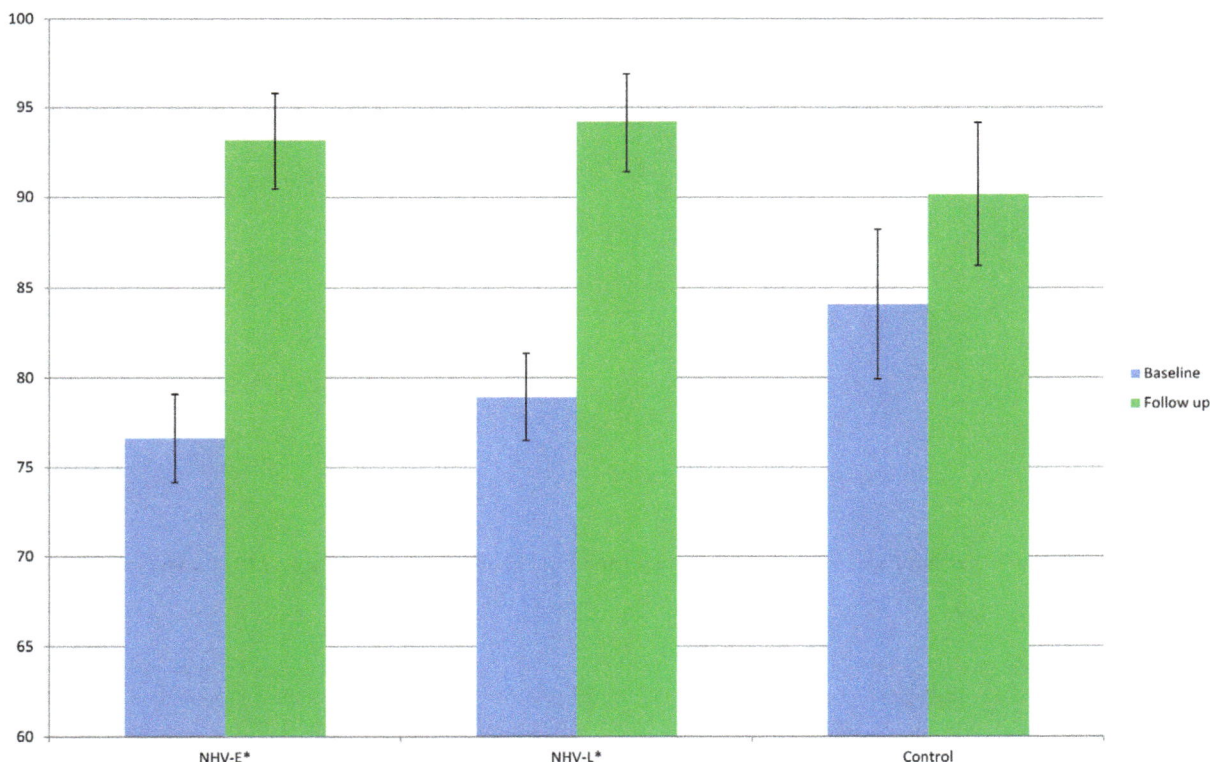

Figure 4. Marginal predictions of Barthel Index mean scores for the NHV study groups at time points based on the three-level Tobit model.

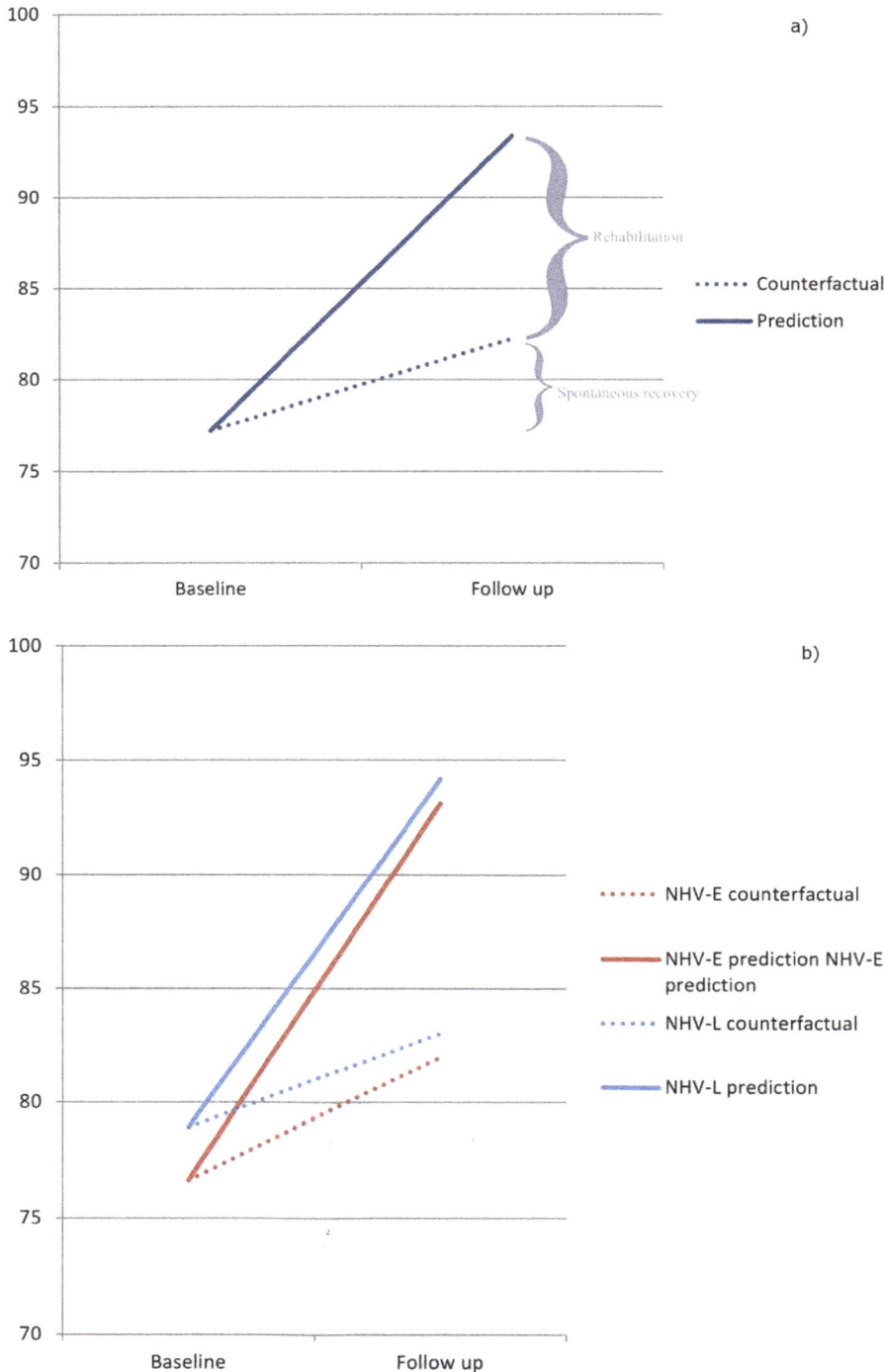

Figure 5. Relative combined effect of NHV and recovery over time (a) and individual effects of NHV-E and NHV-L and recovery over time (b).

remained significant in our sensitivity analysis. Younger persons with better functional status at baseline dropped from the study, presumably migrating to other counties for employment [36]. Overestimation of the effect of recovery over time (population level) may have resulted since patients starting with higher baseline functioning are more likely to show smaller recovery over time effect based on random effect analysis.

Our study has significant implications for rehabilitation disaster-related research, for the study population, for the impacted area, and for rehabilitation disaster relief within China and internationally. Regarding disaster-related research, this analysis reinforces the significance of systematic needs and functional assessment data collection in support of long-term outcomes

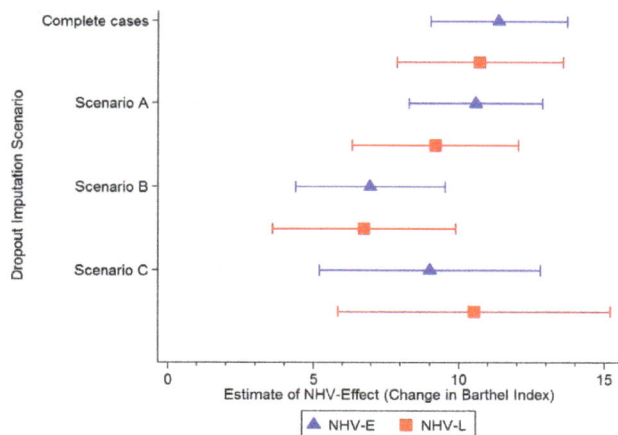

Figure 6. Sensitivity analysis: estimated change in NHV rehabilitation effect based on different dropout imputation scenarios. Legend: Scenario A = no dropouts incurred any change in Barthel Index; Scenario B = all dropouts decreased by ten points in Barthel Index at follow up; Scenario C = dropouts from the intervention groups did not change between baseline and follow up, while dropouts from the control group increased by ten points in Barthel Index; Complete cases = model estimation with valid cases only (see Table 2). Error bars represent 95% confidence intervals.

follow up studies. Such studies are required to improve the scientific base of disaster relief planning [25].

Sichuan earthquake victims with improved physical functioning are able to perform daily activities more independently, requiring less assistance. Moreover, they can perform household domestic tasks and work outside the home, contributing to the overall recovery of post-disaster society with reduced demand on health and social services. Greater victim community integration also enhances personal empowerment and well-being. The NHV rehabilitation services programme has thereby reduced the potential long-term burden of the earthquake on individuals and the community in this resource-constrained area.

The significant development of rehabilitation infrastructure via NHV demonstrates how large-scale natural disasters, particularly earthquakes, present an opportunity to expand rehabilitation services in low-resource regions. When the international rehabilitation services NGO departs in 2013 at the end of its five-year commitment, significantly developed IBR and CBR services will remain in place. Rehabilitation departments of hospitals in County

A and B are now treating traumatic victims of motor vehicle accidents as well as other disabling injuries and rehabilitation diagnoses.

The rapid, close, and continued coordination between multiple rehabilitation stakeholders, including local authorities, national and international NGOs, and professional societies, serves as an example to guide future disaster responses in China and internationally. Capitalizing on the established operational mechanism and employing experienced program leadership, NHV was implemented in only half the time in County B (two weeks). The use of a professional volunteer recruitment database to hasten response underscores the recognized need within the international humanitarian response community for an international register of foreign medical team provider organizations [37]. NHV IBR/CBR also exemplifies the recognition within the international humanitarian community for close linkage of surgical and rehabilitation services as well as for a spectrum of required rehabilitation services following a large-scale disaster with significant disabling injuries [4,9,38].

In conclusion, our study provides evidence that the NHV program was effective in improving physical functioning of injured earthquake survivors of the 2008 Sichuan earthquake. The comprehensive rehabilitation program benefitted the individual and society, rehabilitation services in China, and international rehabilitation disaster relief planning. Similar IBR/CBR programs should therefore be considered for future large-scale rehabilitation disaster relief efforts.

Acknowledgments

We acknowledge the support of the Hong Kong Caring For Children Foundation, the Chinese Association of Rehabilitation Medicine, the Nanjing Medical University, Handicap International, the Sichuan Province and Mianzhu County Government, the Mianzhu County People's Hospital, the Anxian Traditional Chinese Medicine Hospital, and the Hong Kong Rehabilitation Society. We deeply thank the rehabilitation volunteers who participated in this study. The investigation would not have been possible without the significant contributions of Xiaorong Hu, Sijing Chen, and Shouguo Liu, who were intimately involved in NHV design and data collection. Carolina Ballert, Nandini Devi, Bernd Fellinghauer, Per von Groote, Andrew Pennycott, and Sheng Cai are kindly acknowledged as well for their technical contributions.

Author Contributions

Conceived and designed the experiments: XZ JL JR. Performed the experiments: XZ JL. Analyzed the data: JR. Contributed reagents/materials/analysis tools: JR. Wrote the paper: XZ JR JG JL.

References

1. Redmond AD, Li J (2011) The UK medical response to the Sichuan earthquake. Emerg Med J 28: 516–520.
2. Burns AS, O'Connell C, Rathore F (2012) Meeting the challenges of spinal cord injury care following sudden onset disaster: lessons learned. J Rehabil Med 44: 414–420.
3. Landry MD, O'Connell C, Tardif G, Burns A (2010) Post-earthquake Haiti: the critical role for rehabilitation services following a humanitarian crisis. Disabil Rehabil 32: 1616–1618.
4. Reinhardt JD, Li J, Gosney J, Rathore FA, Haig AJ, et al. (2011) Disability and health-related rehabilitation in international disaster relief. Glob Health Action 4: 7191.
5. Kett M, van Ommeren M (2009) Disability, conflict, and emergencies. Lancet 374: 1801–1803.
6. Gosney J, Reinhardt JD, Haig AJ, Li J (2011) Developing post-disaster physical rehabilitation: role of the World Health Organization Liaison Sub-Committee on Rehabilitation Disaster Relief of the International Society of Physical and Rehabilitation Medicine. J Rehabil Med 43: 965–968.
7. WHO (2005) Disasters, disability and rehabilitation. Available: http://www.who.int/violence_injury_prevention/other_injury/disaster_disability2.pdf. Accessed 2011 Nov 10.

8. Rathore FA, Gosney JE, Reinhardt JD, Haig AJ, Li J, et al. (2012) Medical rehabilitation after natural disasters: why, when, and how? Arch Phys Med Rehabil 93: 1875–1881.
9. Redmond AD, Mardel S, Taithe B, Calvot T, Gosney J, et al. (2011) A qualitative and quantitative study of the surgical and rehabilitation response to the earthquake in Haiti, January 2010. Prehosp Disaster Med 26: 449–456.
10. Centre for Research on the Epidemiology of Disasters – CRED (2012) EM-DAT. The international disaster database. Available: www.emdat.be. Accessed 2012 May 1.
11. You C, Chen X, Yao L (2009) How China responded to the May 2008 earthquake during the emergency and rescue period. J Public Health Policy 30: 379–393; discussion 393–374.
12. Dong ZH, Yang ZG, Chen TW, Feng YC, Wang QL, et al. (2009) Spinal injuries in the Sichuan earthquake. N Engl J Med 361: 636–637.
13. Li Y, Reinhardt JD, Gosney JE, Zhang X, Hu X, et al. (2012) Evaluation of functional outcomes of physical rehabilitation and medical complications in spinal cord injury victims of the Sichuan earthquake. J Rehabil Med 44: 534–540.

14. Zhang X, Hu XR, Reinhardt JD, Zhu HJ, Gosney JE, et al. (2012) Functional outcomes and health-related quality of life in fracture victims 27 months after the Sichuan earthquake. J Rehabil Med 44: 206–209.

15. Wong CN, Yu JM, Law SW, Lau HM, Chan CK (2010) Bilateral transtibial amputation with concomitant thoracolumbar vertebral collapse in a Sichuan earthquake survivor. J Orthop Surg Res 5: 43.

16. Gu J, Yang W, Cheng J, Yang T, Qu Y, et al. (2010) Temporal and spatial characteristics and treatment strategies of traumatic brain injury in Wenchuan earthquake. Emerg Med J 27: 216–219.

17. Zhang L, Liu X, Li Y, Liu Y, Liu Z, et al. (2012) Emergency medical rescue efforts after a major earthquake: lessons from the 2008 Wenchuan earthquake. Lancet 379: 853–861.

18. Chen J, Zhao W, Xian M, Lu J, Liang Z (2009) Trans-province transfer of 10,373 patients injured in Wenchuan earthquake. J Evid Based Med 2: 270–276.

19. Chan EY, Kim J (2011) Chronic health needs immediately after natural disasters in middle-income countries: the case of the 2008 Sichuan, China earthquake. Eur J Emerg Med 18: 111–114.

20. Li Y, Pan F (2009) Analysis of rehabilitation needs, measures taken, and their effectiveness for the wounded following the Wenchuan Earthquake. J Evid Based Med 2: 258–264.

21. WHO (2010) Community-based rehabilitation: CBR guidelines. Introductory booklet. Available: http://whqlibdoc.who.int/publications/2010/9789241548052_introductory_eng.pdf. Accessed 2010 May 1.

22. Zhang L, Liu Y, Liu X, Zhang Y (2011) Rescue efforts management and characteristics of casualties of the Wenchuan earthquake in China. Emerg Med J 28: 618–622.

23. Rathore FA, Gosney JE, Reinhardt JD, Haig AJ, Li J, et al. (2012) Medical Rehabilitation after natural disasters: Why, When and How? Arch Phys Med Rehabil.

24. Waeckerle JF (1991) Disaster planning and response. N Engl J Med 324: 815–821.

25. Roy N, Thakkar P, Shah H (2011) Developing-world disaster research: present evidence and future priorities. Disaster Med Public Health Prep 5: 112–116.

26. Leung SO, Chan CC, Shah S (2007) Development of a Chinese version of the Modified Barthel Index– validity and reliability. Clin Rehabil 21: 912–922.

27. Rabe-Hesketh S, Skrondal A (2005) Multilevel and longitudinal modeling using Stata. Lakeway Drive (Texas): Stata Press.

28. Twisk J, Rijmen F (2009) Longitudinal tobit regression: a new approach to analyze outcome variables with floor or ceiling effects. J Clin Epidemiol 62: 953–958.

29. Garnett GP, Cousens S, Hallett TB, Steketee R, Walker N (2011) Mathematical models in the evaluation of health programmes. Lancet 378: 515–525.

30. Rabe-Hesketh S (2004) Tobit with gllamm. statalist.Available: http://statalist.1588530.n2.nabble.com/Tobit-with-gllamm-td5377417.html. Accessed 2012 Feb 15.

31. Xiao M, Li J, Zhang X, Zhao Z (2011) Factors affecting functional outcome of Sichuan-earthquake survivors with tibial shaft fractures: a follow-up study. J Rehabil Med 43: 515–520.

32. Ning N, Liao D-B, He F-Q, Wang R-Z, Cheng Y-J (2008) Effect of a teamwork intervention in amputated patients following an earthquake [Chinese]. Chinese Journal of Evidence-Based Medicine 8: 496–498.

33. Babyak MA (2004) What you see may not be what you get: a brief, nontechnical introduction to overfitting in regression-type models. Psychosom Med 66: 411–421.

34. WHO (2001) International Classification of Functioning, Disability, and Health – ICF. Geneva: WHO Press.

35. WHO, World Bank (2011) World Report on Disability. Geneva: WHO Press.

36. Gong P, Liang S, Carlton EJ, Jiang Q, Wu J, et al. (2012) Urbanisation and health in China. Lancet 379: 843–852.

37. Redmond AD, O'Dempsey TJ, Taithe B (2011) Disasters and a register for foreign medical teams. Lancet 377: 1054–1055.

38. Knowlton LM, Gosney JE, Chackungal S, Altschuler E, Black L, et al. (2011) Consensus statements regarding the multidisciplinary care of limb amputation patients in disasters or humanitarian emergencies: report of the 2011 humanitarian action summit surgical working group on amputations following disasters or conflict. Prehosp Disaster Med 26: 438–448.

12

Are the 10 Meter and 6 Minute Walk Tests Redundant in Patients with Spinal Cord Injury?

Gail F. Forrest[1,2]*, Karen Hutchinson[3], Douglas J. Lorenz[4,5], Jeffrey J. Buehner[6], Leslie R. VanHiel[7], Sue Ann Sisto[8], D. Michele Basso[9]

1 Human Performance and Engineering Laboratory, Kessler Foundation Research Center, West Orange, New Jersey, United States of America, **2** Department of Physical Medicine and Rehabilitation, Rutgers, New Jersey Medical School, Newark, New Jersey, United States of America, **3** Department of Physical Therapy and Athletic Training, Boston University, Boston, Massachusetts, United States of America, **4** Department of Bioinformatics and Biostatistics, School of Public Health and Information Sciences, University of Louisville, Louisville, Kentucky, United States of America, **5** Kentucky Spinal Cord Research Center, University of Louisville, Louisville, Kentucky, United States of America, **6** Wexner Medical Center at the Ohio State University- Dodd Hall, Columbus, Ohio, United States of America, **7** Hulse Spinal Cord Injury Lab and Crawford Research Institute, Shepherd Center, Atlanta, Georgia, United States of America, **8** State University of New York at Stony Brook, School of Health Technology and Management, Research and Development Park, Rehabilitation Research and Movement Performance Laboratory, Stony Brook, New York, United States of America, **9** The Ohio State University, School of Allied Medical Professions, Center for Brain and Spinal Cord Repair, Columbus, Ohio, United States of America

Abstract

Objective: To evaluate the relationship and redundancy between gait speeds measured by the 10 Meter Walk Test (10MWT) and 6 Minute Walk Test (6MWT) after motor incomplete spinal cord injury (iSCI). To identify gait speed thresholds supporting functional ambulation as measured with the Spinal Cord Injury Functional Ambulation Inventory (SCI-FAI).

Design: Prospective observational cohort.

Setting: Seven outpatient rehabilitation centers from the Christopher and Dana Reeve Foundation NeuroRecovery Network (NRN).

Participants: 249 NRN patients with American Spinal Injury Association Impairment Scale (AIS) level C (n = 20), D (n = 179) and (n = 50) iSCI not AIS evaluated, from February 2008 through April 2011.

Interventions: Locomotor training using body weight support and walking on a treadmill, overground and home/community practice.

Main Outcome Measure(s): 10MWT and 6MWT collected at enrollment, approximately every 20 sessions, and upon discharge.

Results: The 10MWT and 6MWT speeds were highly correlated and the 10MWT speeds were generally faster. However, the predicted 6MWT gait speed from the 10MWT, revealed increasing error with increased gait speed. Regression lines remained significantly different from lines of agreement, when the group was divided into fast (≥0.44 m/s) and slow walkers (< 0.44 m/s). Significant differences between 6MWT and 10MWT gait speeds were observed across SCI-FAI walking mobility categories (Wilcoxon sign rank test p<.001), and mean speed thresholds for limited community ambulation differed for each measure. The smallest real difference for the 6MWT and 10MWT, as well as the minimally clinically important difference (MCID) values, were also distinct for the two tests.

Conclusions: While the speeds were correlated between the 6MWT and 10MWT, redundancy in the tests using predictive modeling was not observed. Different speed thresholds and separate MCIDs were defined for community ambulation for each test.

Editor: Michael Fehlings, University of Toronto, Canada

Funding: Funding for this work is from the Christopher and Dana Reeve Foundation; NRN-2008. THESE FUNDERS AIDED IN PAYMENT OF TREATMENT SESSIONS/ STAFF. The funders had no role in study design, data collection and analysis, decision to publish, or preparation of the manuscript.

Competing Interests: The authors have declared that no competing interests exist.

* E-mail: gforrest@kesslerfoundation.org

Introduction

In people with incomplete spinal cord injury (iSCI), walking capacity - comprised of walking speed and endurance - is an important construct in evaluating efficacy of gait training

rehabilitation[1]. Currently, the most accepted standardized timed tests used in studies of persons with iSCI are the 10 Meter Walk Test (10MWT) for speed and 6 Minute Walk Test (6MWT) for walking endurance[2]. These outcome measures are valid, reliable and responsive for acute to chronic iSCI[3]. The pragmatic characteristics of timed walking tests, such as ease and time burden to perform, often determine whether both will be used for clinical outcomes or research trials.

Recent studies advocate the use of only a single walking test, specifically the 10MWT, for clinical research in individuals with SCI[4;5] due to ease of administration. When compared to age-matched normative data[6] and data on stroke survivors after rehabilitation[7], the 10MWT and 6MWT showed little clinical differences for speed. Additionally, strong correlations between the 10MWT and the 6MWT exist at a single time point after recovery periods for individuals with iSCI[8;9]. However, each walking test appears to perform differently when measuring preferred vs. maximum walking speed. Higher speeds occurred most often with the 10MWT compared to the 6MWT when measuring maximum speeds, but during tests of preferred speed, the highest speeds occurred most often using the 6MWT[5;10]. Thus, measured walking speed appears to differ for the two walking tests according to walking speed demands. Indeed, Barbeau[4] found that people with iSCI produced similar walking speeds on the 15.2 Meter Walking Test (15.2 MWT) and the 6MWT when maximum speeds were below 0.9 m/s. However, when higher speeds were attained, the two walking tests produced significantly different values from each other. These differences were postulated to be *clinically* irrelevant, because subjects were all independent ambulators and considered to have sufficient capacity to perform unrestricted community walking, although the community ambulation scores were not reported. Thus, there is a need to determine whether different walking speeds on the two tests reflect true differences in function and community ambulation. Furthermore, although speed thresholds for community ambulation after iSCI been described for the 10MWT[11] they have yet to be identified for the 6MWT.

Support for the use of a single walking test may lie in the interpretation of the redundancy between walking tests. Barbeau et al. considered redundancy to be the degree of equivalency, or the comparison between the average gait speed during a short walking test and the 6MWT[4]. Another method for evaluating redundancy is to model the relationship between the 10MWT and the 6MWT and compare the predicted 6MWT walking speed (from the 10MWT data) to the actual 6MWT speed. The two walking tests would be considered redundant if the error between the predicted and actual values was small across all ranges of gait speed. Thus, knowledge of speed on one test could be used to accurately predict speed on the other, mitigating the need for conducting both tests. To our knowledge, predictive modeling has not been used to determine if the 10MWT and 6MWT provide unique measures of walking capacity across a range of speeds and over time after iSCI.

To delineate the unique or redundant contributions of the 10MWT and the 6MWT, a measure of functional capacity must be used. Recently gait speed from the 10MWT was validated as a predictor of community ambulation in a large European study[11]. A minimum gait speed of 0.44 m/s was the threshold for community ambulation as determined by partitioning components of the Spinal Cord Independence Measure (SCIM)[11]. By contrast, the mobility portion of the Spinal Cord Injury Functional Ambulation Inventory (SCI-FAI), which relies on patient self-report of gait parameters and frequency of walking in the home and community, has not been examined relative to gait speed. The SCI-FAI is a reliable, valid and sensitive measure of walking ability in individuals with SCI[12]. In the present study, we analyzed gait speed at each successive level of ambulatory capacity, as defined by the SCI-FAI mobility scale, to determine the validity of walking

speed measurements in discriminating household and community ambulation. We also separately analyzed the 6MWT and 10MWT data using the 0.44 m/s threshold for identifying slow (household) and fast (community) gait speeds[11].

The first purpose of this study was to evaluate the relationship and redundancy between gait speeds measured by the 10MWT and the 6MWT after motor iSCI. If redundancy exists then the scores should be highly correlated and one of the measures would predict performance of the other. Speeds collected before, during and after Locomotor Training rehabilitation will determine whether differences between the two walk tests depend on the extent of recovery. The second purpose was to examine if the variability between these gait speed measures was unique at fast or relatively slow gaits speeds. We propose that there are differences in walking test performance, not previously identified, for both slow walking speeds (less than 0.44 m/s) and fast walking speeds (those equal or greater than 0.44 m/s)[13]. The third purpose was to establish whether statistical and clinically relevant differences exist between the 10MWT and 6MWT. Measures of smallest real difference (SRD) and functional walking capacity (e.g. household vs. community ambulation with SCI-FAI) were examined. We propose that differences in the inter-evaluation variability between the walking tests may best signify whether both tests are clinically meaningful, or if only one test is needed.

Methods

Study Participants

Two hundred forty-nine patients, enrolled in the standardized Locomotor Training therapy program described in detail elsewhere[14–16]. Patients who were admitted between February 2008 through April 2011 were evaluated at seven out-patient clinical sites in the Christopher and Dana Reeve Foundation (CDRF) NeuroRecovery Network (NRN). Sites included Boston Medical Center, Boston, MA; Frazier Rehabilitation Institute, Louisville, KY; Kessler Institute for Rehabilitation, West Orange, NJ; Magee Rehabilitation Hospital, Philadelphia, PA; the Ohio State University Medical Center, Columbus, OH; Shepherd Center, Atlanta, GA; and The Institute for Rehabilitation and Research, Houston, TX. From each center an IRB-approved written statement of consent was obtained in writing prior to collecting clinical information and administering the outcome measures. Participants provided their written informed consent to participate in this study. The IRB institutions were as follows: Institutional Review Board of Boston University Medical Campus and Boston Medical Center, Boston, MA; Kentucky One Health Research Center, Institute of Review Board, Louisville, KY; Kessler Foundation Institutional Review Board, West Orange, NJ; Magee Rehabilitation Institutional Review Board, Philadelphia, PA; Biomedical Sciences Institutional Review Board, the Ohio State University, Columbus, OH; Research Review Committee at Shepherd Center, Atlanta, GA; University of Texas Health Science Center Houston, Texas. Patients were selected for participation in the NRN Locomotor Training program and outcome assessments based on 1) the presence of a non-progressive spinal cord lesion, 2) neurological level of injury above T11 as determined by the International Standards for Neurological Classification of Spinal Cord Injury (ISNCSCI), 3) completion of an in-patient rehabilitation program, 4) no use of Botox or other medications for chemodenervation for spasticity for the 3 months prior to enrollment, 5) some lower limb movement or visible voluntary contraction, 6) the capacity to generate a lower limb reciprocal alternating flexion/extension stepping pattern in the body-weight supported step training environment, and 7) medical referral by a physician for physical therapy. Patients on anti-spasticity medications were weaned during participation in the NRN program as directed by their NRN physicians. The patients underwent at least the baseline evaluation, a minimum of 20 training sessions and at least one additional evaluation of the functional outcome measures.

Outcome Measures

The 6MWT and the 10MWT were captured as part of a battery of measures at baseline in a single session or over two consecutive days, depending on the abilities of the participants to perform them. These measures were captured approximately every 20 treatment sessions thereafter, and at discharge from the Locomotor Training program. The standardized procedures for gait assessment within the NRN have been outlined in a previous manuscript[16]. For the 6MWT, the placement of turns, precise verbal feedback and location of the observer conformed to standardized methods[17]. The need for physical assistance or to sit ended the test. For the 10MWT, a 14-meter path with a flying start was used to avoid acceleration/deceleration effects associated with starting and stopping during this assessment. The middle 10 meters of this path were used for the measurement. Patients were instructed to "walk as fast as they can". Both tests included use of assistive devices when required; however, no lower limb bracing or physical assistance was allowed. When patients changed assistive devices over the course of treatment, each gait outcome measure was conducted twice – once with the device used at enrollment, termed the "initial device" and once with the device currently being used, termed the "current device". Five minutes of seated rest preceded each of the gait tests. Our data represent the fastest walking speed attained, irrespective of ambulation device. The walking mobility scale of the SCI-FAI was used to classify the individuals' self- reported level of home or community ambulation. The walking mobility portion of the SCI-FAI scale classifies individuals from 0 to 5. A score of 0 indicates self-reported non-ambulatory status or ambulation with physical assistance only; scores 1–3 indicate in-home but not community ambulation; and scores 4–5 indicate limited and independent community ambulation ability.

Data Analysis

Of 249 patients, 6MWT and 10 MWT data were available for 217 at enrollment, 249 at discharge and 249 at interim evaluations. Thirty-two (32) were unable to complete one or both of the walk tests at enrollment. One hundred seventy patients had enrollment and discharge measurements of the 10MWT, 6MWT and SCI-FAI mobility measure. On this sample, we calculated the SRDs and conducted the analysis of changes in the 10MWT and 6MWT. One hundred twenty-five patients had enrollment and discharge measurements of the 10MWT and 6MWT as well as an enrollment SCI-FAI score below 5. On this sample, we calculated minimum clinically important differences (MCIDs). The details of the calculation of SRD and MCID are provided below.

The relationship between the 10MWT and 6MWT was evaluated using correlation and regression methods for measurements taken at enrollment, discharge, and over the entire period of participation in the NRN. Simple linear regression models were fit and Pearson correlation coefficients calculated on the enrollment and discharge data using 10MWT speed as the predictor and 6MWT speed as the outcome. The regression models were fit with generalized least squares to permit the modeling of heterogeneous residual variance. The same models – 6MWT speeds predicted by 10MWT speeds – were fit for all of the data (i.e. enrollment, interim, and discharge measurements) using the linear mixed effects model. The 10MWT speed served as the only fixed and random effect, and variance functions to model heterogeneous variance patterns were included[18]. Pearson correlation coefficients calculated on the full data were calculated utilizing recently developed methods for clustered data[19]. We calculated these clustered data coefficients to account for dependence among repeated evaluations of NRN patients and control for the potential biasing effect of informative cluster size, in this case the varying number of observations contributed by NRN patients.

We compared 10MWT and 6MWT speeds over categories defined by the SCI-FAI mobility subscale using the Kruskal-Wallis test, with pairwise comparisons of SCI-FAI categories conducted using the Wilcoxon rank sum test with the Hochberg correction for multiple testing[20]. We compared the measurement properties of the 10MWT and 6MWT by calculating the SRD and the MCID. The SRD was calculated according to a modified version of a formula proposed by Beckerman[21]; a discussion of the modification to the SRD formula is in the Appendix (Appendix S1). The MCID was calculated through a receiver-operator characteristic (ROC) analysis utilized by Tilson, et al.[22] which we describe briefly. We selected a one-unit increase in the SCI-FAI mobility subscale to represent clinically relevant change in a patient's walking function and divided patients into responders and non-responders based on this criterion[12;22]. We constructed ROC curves for enrollment-to-discharge changes in the 10MWT and 6MWT, from which we calculated the area under the curve (AUC) with 95% confidence intervals. The walk tests were defined to be in significant correspondence with 1-unit increases in the SCI-FAI if the 95% confidence interval for the AUC did not contain 0.5. Each point on the ROC curve defines a threshold for the change in walking speed, above which a patient is classified as a responder and below a non-responder. At each of these speed thresholds on the ROC curve we calculated two quantities: (1) sensitivity, defined as the proportion of patients classified as responders among those experiencing clinically relevant improvement (a one-unit increase in SCI-FAI), and (2) specificity, defined as the proportion of patients classified as non-responders among those not experiencing clinically relevant improvement. We defined the MCID to be the threshold at which the sum of the sensitivity and specificity was maximized[23]. All analyses were conducted using the full data and for two subgroups of data – slow walks, defined as walk speeds less than 0.44 m/s, and fast walks were equal to or greater than 0.44 m/s per van Hedel, 2009[11;23]. Demographic and clinical characteristics at NRN enrollment were summarized using means and standard deviations for continuous, symmetric data, medians and extrema for continuous skewed data, and counts and percentages for categorical data. Hypothesis tests were conducted at the .05 significance level. Analyses were conducted using the open-source R software package[24].

Results

Demographic, Clinical, and Treatment Characteristics

The demographic and clinical characteristics of our sample of 249 patients (Table 1) corresponded with those of other samples of NRN data[8;13;25] and with the incomplete SCI population[26]. Patients were enrolled in the NRN for a median 3.4 months and received a median of 40 treatment sessions, with the highest enrollment time and number of completed treatment sessions being 52.5 months and 353 sessions, respectively. The number of evaluations ranged from 2–18 with a median of 4 evaluations per patient at which 6MWT and 10MWT were measured.

Table 1. Demographic, clinical, and treatment characteristics.

Demographics (N = 249)	
Sex	
F	59 (24)
M	190 (76)
Age	42±16
AIS	
C	20 (8)
D	179 (72)
Not evaluated	*50 (20)*
Time Since SCI (years)	0.7 [0.1, 21.6]
Mechanism of Injury	
MVA	83 (33)
Fall	54 (22)
Sporting	45 (18)
Med-Surg	25 (10)
Violence	17 (7)
Non-Trauma	15 (6)
Other	10 (5)
Treatment Characteristics	
Time in NRN (months)	3.4 [0.2, 52.5]
Treatment Sessions	40 [2, 353]
Evaluations	4 [2,18]

Values are counts (percentages), mean ± SD, or median [min, max].

Little Redundancy between 10MWT and 6MWT Gait Speeds

To examine redundancy, we reasoned that the scores for the 10MWT and the 6MWT should be highly correlated and one measure would predict the performance on the other. Speeds from the 10MWT and 6MWT were highly correlated (Table 2, Figure 1) at enrollment (0.93), at discharge (0.94) and for all evaluations (r = 0.94). Speeds from the 10MWT were generally faster than those from the 6MWT. However, it is noteworthy that for up to 23% of cases, gait speeds on 6MWT were faster than 10MWT. Corresponding to each plot, in Figure 1 we compared the regression line of best fit with the line of agreement, defined by an intercept of 0 and a slope of 1, as a measure of redundancy. The lines differed significantly at enrollment, at discharge and for all evaluations, indicating that speeds from the 10MWT and 6MWT were not equivalent (F-test, p<.001; Figure 1).

From the linear models, we predicted the 6MWT gait speed from 10MWT and examined the error in prediction across a range of speeds (Table 3, Figure 2). In fitting the linear mixed effects models, we modeled the residual variance as an increasing power function of 10MWT speed (see the Appendix S1, for technical specifications and details of modeling variance heterogeneity). At the enrollment evaluation, residual standard error increased from 0.05 m/s to 0.31 m/s as 6MWT speeds increased from 0.20 m/s to 2.0 m/s. Comparable increases were observed for discharge evaluations (error increased from 0.08 m/s to 0.21 m/s) and for all evaluations (0.07 m/s to 0.22 m/s).

Inequalities between 10MWT and 6MWT Occur for Fast and Slow Walkers

Given that Barbeau et al.[4] established differences at faster speeds and we established substantial error at slow speeds we repeated the analyses of the relationship between the 10MWT and 6MWT for two groups of patients – fast walkers, those with gait speeds meeting or exceeding 0.44 m/s, and slow walkers, with gait speeds less than 0.44 m/s. This cutoff was selected based on prior research identifying 0.44 m/s as a threshold for community ambulation[13;27]. Compared to the overall sample, correlations between the 10MWT and 6MWT were reduced within the fast group and, to a greater extent, the slow group (Table 2, Figure). Gait speeds from the 10MWT continued to exceed 6MWT speeds in the two groups, although to a lesser extent in the slow walk group (Figure 3). Sixty-six percent (55 of 83) of enrollment evaluations, 73% (46/63) of discharge evaluations and 70% (282/404) of all evaluations had 10MWT speeds greater than 6MWT speeds for slow walkers. Conversely, up to 34% of gait speeds were higher during the 6MWT for slow walkers. For fast walkers, 85% (80/94) of enrollment evaluations, 88% (152/172) of discharge evaluations and 86% (480/559) of all evaluations registered higher speeds on the 10MWT than the 6MWT. Conversely, up to 15% of gait speeds were higher during the 6MWT for fast walkers. The lines of best fit remained significantly different from the lines of agreement in both slow and fast walking groups (Figure 1, Table 2, p<.001), although disparity from the line of agreement was greater in the fast group. The slopes of the regression lines for fast walkers were substantially below the line of agreement for each plot while the slopes for slow walkers were modestly displaced.

Table 2. Assessment of linear relationship between 6MWT and 10MWT via correlation and regression.

Walk Type	Evaluations	Correlation	Intercept	Slope
All Walks	Enrollment (N = 217)	0.93 (0.91, 0.95)	0.01 (0.00, 0.02)	0.80 (0.76, 0.84)
	Discharge (N = 240)	0.94 (0.92, 0.95)	0.04 (0.01, 0.06)	0.77 (0.74, 0.80)
	All (N = 249, 1028 observations)	0.94 (0.92, 0.96)	0.05 (0.04, 0.07)	0.74 (0.71, 0.77)
Slow Walks	Enrollment (N = 123)	0.84 (0.76, 0.89)	0.01 (0.00, 0.01)	0.87 (0.79, 0.94)
	Discharge (N = 68)	0.73 (0.59, 0.83)	0.00 (−0.01, 0.02)	0.89 (0.79, 0.99)
	All (N = 143, 469 observations)	0.80 (0.73, 0.86)	0.03 (0.01, 0.04)	0.77 (0.71, 0.84)
Fast Walks	Enrollment (N = 94)	0.85 (0.78, 0.90)	0.17 (0.10, 0.24)	0.60 (0.52, 0.68)
	Discharge (N = 172)	0.90 (0.86, 0.92)	0.10 (0.04, 0.16)	0.71 (0.66, 0.76)
	All (N = 178, 559 observations)	0.89 (0.85, 0.92)	0.14 (0.10, 0.18)	0.66 (0.62, 0.70)

For enrollment, discharge, and all evaluations, nonparametric Spearman correlation coefficients and slopes and intercepts from lines of best fit are given with 95% confidence intervals. Results are presented for all walk evaluations, slow walk evaluations (<.44 m/s) and fast walk evaluations (≥.44 m/s).

Linear models fit to the two subgroups continued to exhibit increasing prediction errors with increased gait speed (Table 3, Figure 3), which was modeled with a power function as before.

Smallest Real Difference is Lower for 6MWT

To determine whether the differences in 6MWT and 10MWT surpassed the error of the measurement we calculated the SRD. Average improvement from enrollment to discharge in 10MWT and 6MWT speeds was 0.30 m/s and 0.26 m/s, respectively (Table 4, Figure 4), and slow walkers tended to show greater improvement than fast walkers. Previous reports[9;28] have estimated the test-retest intraclass correlation coefficient of both the 6MWT and 10MWT to be 0.98. Using this estimate and the estimated standard deviation of enrollment-to-discharge changes in the 6MWT and 10MWT, we calculated the SRD for the 6MWT and 10MWT to be 0.08 m/s and 0.10 m/s, respectively. The SRDs for walkers defined as slow (<0.44 m/s) and fast (≥ 0.44 m/s) at enrollment were nearly identical to the SRD for the overall sample (Table 4).

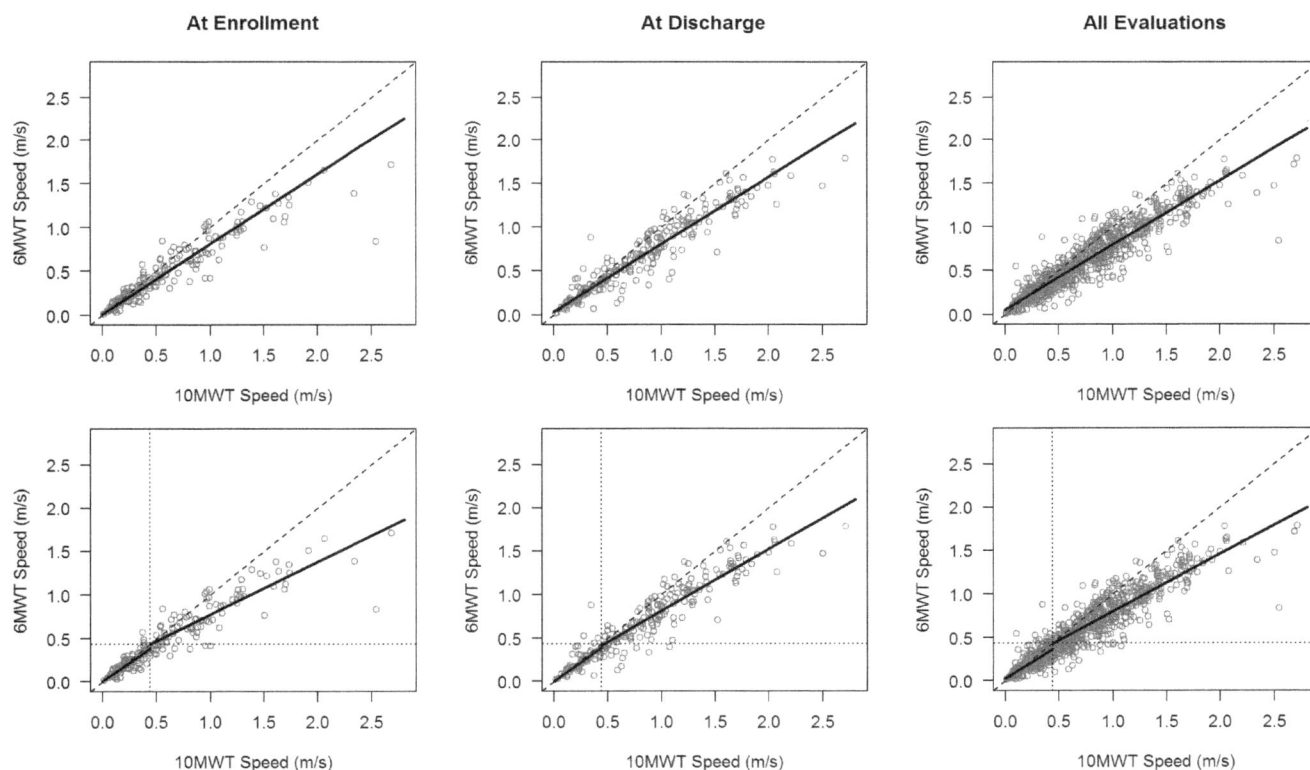

Figure 1. Lines of best fit from linear models predicting 6MWT speeds with 10MWT speeds at enrollment, discharge, and all evaluations. Top row: linear models fit to all observations. Bottom row: linear models fit to slow and fast walkers (separated by dotted line). Dashed line is 45-degree line of agreement.

Table 3. Residual standard errors for linear models using 10MWT speeds to predict 6MWT speeds at selected speeds.

10MWT Speed (m/s)	FULL MODEL			SLOW/FAST MODELS		
	Enrollment (N = 217)	Discharge (N = 240)	All (N = 249)	Enrollment (N = 217)	Discharge (N = 240)	All (N = 249)
0.2	0.05	0.08	0.07	0.05	0.06	0.07
0.4	0.08	0.11	0.10	0.09	0.11	0.10
0.6	0.12	0.13	0.12	0.12	0.15	0.14
0.8	0.15	0.15	0.14	0.14	0.16	0.15
1.0	0.18	0.16	0.15	0.16	0.16	0.16
1.25	0.21	0.18	0.17	0.19	0.17	0.17
1.5	0.25	0.19	0.19	0.21	0.17	0.17
2.0	0.31	0.21	0.22	0.25	0.18	0.18

Standard errors were modeled as a power function of the 10MWT speeds. Results presented for modeling all of the data and for modeling slow and fast walkers separately. Models including the heterogeneous variance function fit the data significantly better than models without (ANOVA F-test, p<.001), justifying their use in models of the 6MWT and 10MWT.

Gait Speeds and Functional Walking Capacity Classified by SCI-FAI

To understand whether clinical measures of gait speed align with functional walking, we partitioned patients with the SCI-FAI walking mobility scale into non-walkers (score 0), limited in-home ambulators (scores 1–3) and community ambulators (scores 4–5). A small number of patients (n = 19) who indicated a SCI-FAI score of 0 ambulated sufficiently at initial evaluation in the clinic to complete the 10MWT and 6MWT, albeit at gait speeds near 0 m/s (Table 5). Significantly higher speeds occurred with higher classifications for both the 6MWT and 10MWT (Kruskall-Wallis tests, p<.001, Table 5). Those classified as extensive community ambulators (SCI-FAI 5) had significantly faster gait speeds than all other classifications regardless of which walking test was used to measure gait speed (Wilcoxon test, Hochberg correction, p<.001). Gait speeds for adjacent SCI-FAI categories 1–4 were not significantly different (p>.06) whereas separations of more than one category resulted in significant differences using either walking measure (p<.04). For example, gait speeds in patients with SCI-FAI score of 2 did not significantly differ from gait speeds in patients with SCI-FAI scores 1 or 3, but were significantly lower than gait speeds of patients with SCI-FAI scores of 4 or 5.

10MWT and 6 MWT Differ from Each other across Functional Classifications

The 10MWT and 6MWT did not perform equally for each walking category on the SCI-FAI. For most SCI-FAI levels, mean gait speed on the 6MWT was slower than that on the 10MWT (Table 5). The differences between 10MWT and 6MWT gait speeds were significant for SCI-FAI categories 3, 4 and 5 (Wilcoxon sign rank test p<.001) (Table 5). The mean speed threshold for limited community ambulation (SCI-FAI 4) at initial evaluation was 0.39 m/s vs. 0.49 m/s for the 6MWT and 10MWT, respectively, and corresponded closely to the reported minimum speed for community ambulation of 0.44 m/s identified by van Hedel (2008)[11].

To determine if differences in gait speed between the two walk tests were functionally or clinically relevant, we calculated the MCID for all patients with enrollment and discharge measurements of the 10MWT, 6MWT, and SCI-FAI, and had SCI-FAI scores less than 5 at enrollment (n = 125). Of these patients, 78% (98/125) experienced at least a 1 unit improvement. The MCIDs were 0.11 m/s for the 6MWT and 0.15 m/s for the 10MWT (Table 4). ROC analyses showed that increases in the 6MWT and 10MWT corresponded well with 1-unit improvements in the SCI-FAI. The area under the ROC curve for the 6MWT was 0.85 (95% CI: 0.77, 0.94) and for the 10MWT was 0.83 (95% CI: 0.73, 0.92). The substantial overlap of these 95% confidence intervals

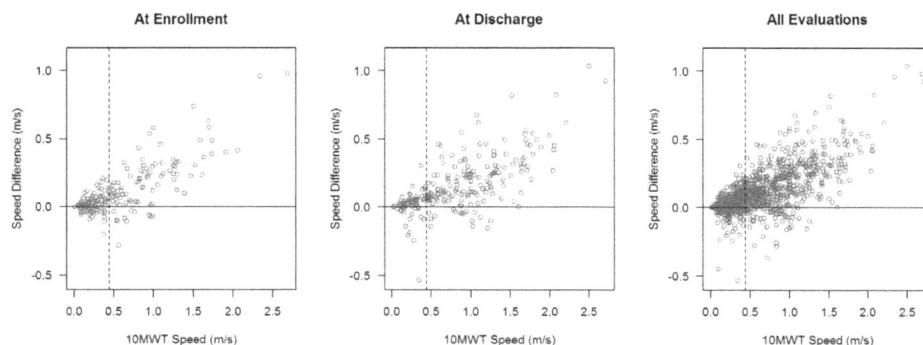

Figure 2. Difference in walk speeds (10MWT−6MWT) by speed on 10MWT for enrollment, discharge, and all evaluations. Vertical dashed line is at 0.44 m/s, separating slow and fast walkers. Negative values represent faster gait speeds on the 6MWT than the 10MWT.

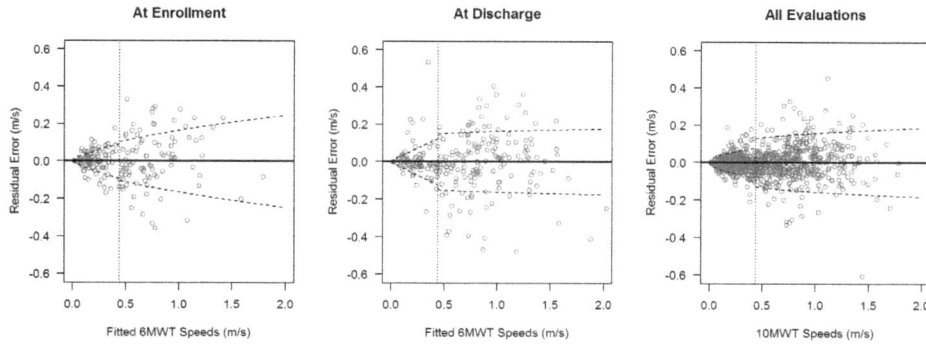

Figure 3. Residuals from linear models predicting 6MWT speeds with 10MWT speeds at enrollment, discharge, and all evaluations. Linear models fit to slow and fast walkers (separated by dotted line). Dashed lines are estimated residual standard errors from models.

indicated that the measures did not significantly differ in their correspondence with clinically relevant change. The sensitivity for each of the 6MWT and 10MWT at their respective MCID were 0.81 and 0.74 with a specificity of 0.81 for both tests.

When partitioned into slow and fast walkers, 73 slow walkers (77%) and 25 fast walkers (83%) had at least a 1 unit increase in the SCI-FAI. The MCID for slow walkers were 0.10 to 0.15; and in close correspondence with the MCID for all walkers. We did not calculate the MCID for fast walkers, because too few people were available to yield interpretable results (i.e. only 6 fast walkers failed to improve on SCI-FAI).

Discussion

This study examined whether two common walking tests detect both statistically and clinically significant changes in walking function for a large cohort of individuals with relatively chronic iSCI. The primary finding was that walking speeds collected from the 10MWT and the 6MWT differed from each other across a broad range of speeds and for people who were self-reported in-home or community ambulators. While the speeds were correlated between the two tests, we did not find redundancy in the tests using predictive modeling. Importantly, we defined different speed thresholds for community ambulation and separate MCIDs for each test.

The current view of timed walking tests for iSCI is that the 10MWT and 6MWT produce largely equivalent measures of gait speed[4;5]. While strong correlations between the measures suggest redundancy, especially at slow speeds, several findings

raise questions about whether outcomes measured by the 10MWT and the 6MWT are indeed equivalent. Significant differences in gait speeds collected with the 10MWT and the 6MWT have been identified in fast walkers[4]. Recent evidence also showed that the change in performance over time on these two measures for a given intervention was not strongly correlated[8]. Taken together, it appears that the 10MWT and the 6MWT may measure different aspects of walking function and is the foundation of the current study[4;29–31].

Little Redundancy of Walking Measures for Slow and Fast Walkers

In this study, strong correlations occurred between 6MWT and 10MWT speeds for all walkers and when classified as slow or fast walkers (Table 2), which is consistent with the literature and has previously been used as evidence for redundancy between measures[4;9]. However, we present three lines of evidence that the 6MWT and 10MWT appear to capture different aspects of walking performance which warrant using both tests.

First, individual walking performance differed significantly as measured by the 10MWT and the 6MWT (Figure 1). Using the line of equivalence as a measure of redundancy as described by Barbeau et al.[4], we found that the line of best fit differed significantly from this for enrollment, discharge and all evaluations collected during treatment (slope<1.0). These differences remained significant for both slow and fast walkers and indicates that most slow and fast walkers had higher gait speeds on the 10MWT than on the 6MWT (Table 2). While differences have been reported for fast walkers above 0.9 m/s previously[4], this may be

Table 4. Walking speeds at enrollment and discharge (m/s), smallest real difference (SRD), minimal clinically important difference (MCID), and area under the curve (AUC) calculated for 6MWT and 10MWT (in m/s), all and by speed group at enrollment.

Measure	6MWT			10MWT		
	All	Slow	Fast	All	Slow	Fast
Speed at Enrollment (m/s)	0.40±0.39	0.13±0.13	0.77±0.32	0.51±0.53	0.15±0.14	0.98±0.48
Speed at Discharge (m/s)	0.67±0.43	0.42±0.29	0.99±0.38	0.81±0.55	0.50±0.37	1.23±0.48
Change in Speed (m/s)	0.26±0.28	0.28±0.28	0.23±0.26	0.30±0.35	0.35±0.35	0.25±0.35
SRD	0.08	0.08	0.07	0.10	0.10	0.10
MCID	0.10	0.11	NA	0.15	0.15	NA
AUC	0.85(0.77, 0.94)	0.90(0.84, 0.96)	0.66(0.31, 1)	0.83(0.73, 0.92)	0.87(0.79, 0.94)	0.62(0.23, 1)

NA: among fast walkers, the 6MWT and 10MWT did not significantly correspond with clinically relevant change and reliable MCID could not be calculated.

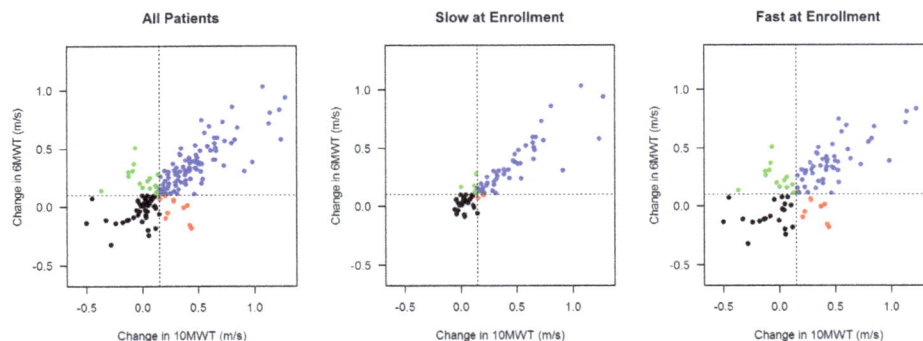

Figure 4. Enrollment-to-discharge improvements in 6MWT speed by enrollment-to-discharge improvements in 10MWT speed for all patients (n = 170), patients that walked slow (<0.44 m/s) at enrollment (n = 78), and patients that walked fast (≥0.44 m/s) at enrollment (n = 92). Plots restricted to patients that had enrollment and discharge evaluations of the 6MWT and 10MWT. Dotted lines are plotted at the MCID for the 6MWT (0.10 m/s) and 10MWT (0.15 m/s). Blue = improvements exceeded MCID for both 6MWT and 10MWT, red = improvements exceeded MCID for 10MWT only, green = improvements exceeded MCID for 6MWT only, black = improvements did not exceed MCID for either 6MWT or 10MWT.

the first report of statistically significant differences at much slower speeds <0.44m/s but its clinical importance remains to be determined. This implies that even in slow walkers or during early recovery when walking is slow, the two tests may not capture a change in walking capacity similarly.

Second, prediction error from linear regression models can serve as another marker of redundancy. If the results from one test can be predicted with minimal error from the results of a different test, then the two tests could be considered redundant – knowledge of the results of one test provide an accurate estimate of the results of another, mitigating the need for the test being performed. The smallest real differences we calculated for the 10MWT and 6MWT (0.10 and 0.08) provide reasonable thresholds for prediction error from a linear model. Based on these thresholds, we found substantial error in the estimates of 6MWT performance at gait speeds of 0.4 m/s and above for enrollment data and 0.2 m/s and above for discharge evaluations for the entire sample.

When partitioned into slow and fast walkers, the error surpassed the SRD at a gait speed of 0.4 m/s on the 10MWT. The magnitude of the error increased as 10MWT gait speed increased, suggesting that performance on one walking test is distinct from performance on the other walking test. Importantly, the error in predicting 6MWT speeds from 10MWT speeds surpassed even the 6MWT MCID at speeds as low as 0.6 m/s. Therefore, both

statistically (SRD) and clinically relevant (MCID) errors exist when predicting the performance of the 6MWT based on the 10MWT at slow, fast, and over all speeds. Therefore our data suggests that the 6MWT cannot be accurately predicted from the 10MWT via a linear regression model, in - contrast with the findings of van Hedel's group[5]. In their study of subacute iSCI, regression analysis showed no differences between walking speeds from 6MWT and 10MWT, collected at preferred and maximum walking speeds.

The differences between our study and previous work may be explained by sample size and chronicity of the injury. Our sample was 249 subjects with time since injury ranging from 8 months to 21 years post SCI, whereas van Hedel studied a smaller sample (n = 51) and 1–6 months post SCI. In addition, in the current study, data collection occurred without physical assistance provided during ambulation, whereas earlier studies allowed up to moderate physical assistance during ambulation testing [4]. Another distinction between the reported studies and our work is the instructions given for the walking tests, in our work the instruction for 6MWT was "walk as far as you can" whereas for another study the instructions were given to, "Walk as fast as you can safely walk"[4]. Also, while differences in rehabilitation interventions surely exist, it is doubtful that the LT intervention impacted our large residual errors, because we observed these

Table 5. Summary statistics for 6MWT and 10MWT at enrollment, discharge, and all evaluations by SCI-FAI Walking Mobility score.

Enrollment			Discharge		
SCI-FAI	6MWT (m/s)	10MWT(m/s)	SCI-FAI	6MWT(m/s)	10MWT(m/s)
0 (N = 18)	0.01±0.03	0.02±0.04	0 (N = 3)	0.18±0.21	0.15±0.13
1 (N = 20)	0.18±0.13	0.17±0.09	1 (N = 2)	0.16±0.08	0.17±0.07
2 (N = 19)	0.27±0.26	0.26±0.21	2 (N = 7)	0.18±0.10	0.29±0.17
3 (N = 21)	0.28±0.13*	0.37±0.19	3 (N = 16)	0.28±0.20*	0.30±0.20
4 (N = 38)	0.39±0.21*	0.49±0.32	4 (N = 30)	0.44±0.28*	0.58±0.34
5 (N = 61)	0.84±0.35*	1.07±0.54	5 (N = 118)	0.89±0.37*	1.08±0.50

Values are mean ± SD. SCI-FAI score 0 indicates non-ambulatory status or ambulation with physical assistance only, scores 1–3 indicate in-home but no community ambulation, and scores 4–5 indicate occasional or regular community ambulation. Table includes 177 patients with enrollment and discharge measurements of the SCI-FAI, 6MWT, and 10MWT. SCI-FAI categories 3, 4, and 5 exhibited significant 6MW–10MW differences.
*p<.04.

prediction errors in analyses restricted to enrollment data, before training began. The fact that residual error was similar at enrollment and discharge suggests that outcomes from the two tests reflect walking capacity more than type of intervention.

Third, differences between speeds derived from the two tests were also evident when the outcomes were classified according to function rather than a speed threshold (0.44 m/s). Using the SCI-FAI, we stratified our sample into 5 groups ranging from little or no ability to walk (SCI-FAI score 0) to some assisted or independent community ambulation (SCI-FAI score 4–5). We found statistically significant differences between 6MWT and 10MWT gait speeds for SCI-FAI classifications 3, 4 and 5 at enrollment and discharge. Our data suggest that each walking test captures walking capacity differently for slow and fast walkers and for individuals with greater capability (SCI-FAI, Table 5) and supports the use of both tests throughout recovery after an iSCI. However, if only a single test can be used, our data suggests that the 6MWT may be more responsive to walking ability. The 6MWT had a higher sensitivity than 10MWT (0.81 vs. 0.74, respectively) when measuring individuals that improved at least one category on the SCI-FAI, detecting more responders than the 10MWT. Additionally, the 6MWT had a smaller SRD than the 10MWT (Table 3). Given that SRD reflects the smallest difference needed to exceed measurement error of the test, the 6MWT appears to have less volatility than 10MWT and may be more responsive to walking recovery. Our sample is comprised of a wide range of functional abilities from walking a few steps to independent community ambulation which allows for good generalizability. In this paper, we calculated SRD with computation modifications that potentially improve the accuracy of threshold for SCI[28;32;33]. Further we calculated the value for a much larger population than has previously been reported[28;32;33]. Both of these criteria strengthen the assertion that the SRD threshold gait speed between the 6MWT and 10MWT, independent of error, is much lower than reported previously[28]. Given the lower threshold identified, previous studies might have under reported differences between these two walk tests. However SRD only peripherally relates to clinical significance since it is the value that represents change that cannot be attributed to error. Subsequently our calculated MCID values would provide much more accurate thresholds for the determination of real clinically relevant change.

Gait Speeds Associated with SCI-FAI Functional Classifications

The 10MWT and 6MWT are often used as surrogates for functional ambulation in which gait speed over short distances (10MWT) is thought to represent crossing the street, while longer distances (6MWT) likely reflect endurance required for community ambulation. Here we directly compare gait speeds over short and long distances to self-reported walking function on the SCI-FAI mobility scale. To our knowledge, this is the first time that gait speed thresholds for different walking capacities have been determined using the 6MWT. Previously, van Hedel et al.

generated 10MWT speed thresholds for 5 functional ambulation groups defined from the Spinal Cord Independence Measure (SCIM)[27]. These classifications were similar to those defined on the SCI-FAI. When considering limited community ambulation (category 4 for SCIM and SCI-FAI 4), we found that both the 6MWT and 10MWT speeds at initial and discharge aligned with van Hedel's minimum walking speed of 0.44 m/s. These data strongly supports his assertion that 0.44 m/s is a plausible threshold for limited community ambulation after iSCI. For independent community ambulation, van Hedel proposed an average 10MWT speed of 0.80 m/s which is consistent with our 6MWT SCI-FAI Category 5 walk speed at enrollment (0.84 m/s) and discharge (0.89 m/s). However, our average 10MWT speeds were much higher than reported by van Hedel[27].

Our SCI-FAI results are novel and in contrast to Barbeau et al., who assessed walking speeds from the 15.2MWT and 6MWT in 120 subjects with iSCI and found significant separation between the two tests at gait speeds greater than 0.9 m/s[4]. We, like van Hedel et al.[11], suggest that much lower speed thresholds for community ambulation exist for iSCI regardless of whether a short or long distance walking test is used.

Limitations

The SCI-FAI mobility subscale does have face validity, but it also demonstrates significant ceiling effects[34], as noted in the current study. Fifty-two percent of our patients identified themselves as a SCI-FAI category 5 level of mobility at enrollment which means that any improvement made during rehabilitation would not have been detected with the SCI-FAI mobility scale. These ceiling effects prevented us from calculating MCID for fast walkers. It appears that perhaps a category 6 might be warranted for the SCI-FAI, which could reflect a greater return to high-level pre-morbid ambulation activities than the current scale allows. In addition, the SCI-FAI was designed to assess functional ambulation, but walking speed is only included in the description of category 5, where speed is expected to be "at least 50% of normal". Convergent validity of the SCI-FAI instrument was established by finding that mobility scores correlated with walking speed (Pearson $r \sim = -0.742$) collected over a 3.8 meter distance, using a small sample of 22 people with incomplete SCI. The differences between our gait speed data per SCI-FAI category and the original SCI-FAI work warrants further investigation.

Author Contributions

Conceived and designed the experiments: GFF KH DJL JB LVH SAS DMB. Performed the experiments: GFF KH DJL JB LVH SAS DMB. Analyzed the data: GFF KH DJL JB LVH SAS DMB. Contributed reagents/materials/analysis tools: GFF KH DJL JB LVH SAS DMB. Wrote the paper: GFF KH DJL JB LVH SAS DMB.

References

1. Ditunno JF Jr, Burns AS, Marino RJ (2005) Neurological and functional capacity outcome measures: essential to spinal cord injury clinical trials, J Rehabil Res Dev. 42: 35–41.
2. Jackson AB, Carnel CT, Ditunno JF, Read MS, Boninger ML, et al. (2008) Outcome measures for gait and ambulation in the spinal cord injury population, J Spinal Cord Med 31: 487–499.
3. Tyson S, Connell L (2009) The psychometric properties and clinical utility of measures of walking and mobility in neurological conditions: a systematic review, Clin Rehabil 23: 1018–1033.
4. Barbeau H, Elashoff R, DeForge D, Ditunno J, Saulino M, et al. (2007) Comparison of speeds used for the 15.2-meter and 6-minute walks over the year after an incomplete spinal cord injury: the SCILT Trial, Neurorehabil Neural Repair 21: 302–306.
5. van Hedel HJ, Dietz V, Curt A (2007) Assessment of walking speed and distance in subjects with an incomplete spinal cord injury, Neurorehabil Neural Repair 21: 295–301.

6. Steffen TM, Hacker TA, Mollinger L (2002) Age- and gender-related test performance in community-dwelling elderly people: Six-Minute Walk Test, Berg Balance Scale, Timed Up & Go Test, and gait speeds, Phys Ther. 82: 128–137.

7. Dobkin BH (2006) Short-distance walking speed and timed walking distance: redundant measures for clinical trials?, Neurology 66: 584–586.

8. Forrest GF, Lorenz DJ, Hutchinson K, Vanhiel LR, Basso DM (2012) Ambulation and balance outcomes measure different aspects of recovery in individuals with chronic, incomplete spinal cord injury, Arch Phys Med Rehabil 93: 1553–1564.

9. van Hedel HJ, Wirz M, Dietz V (2005) Assessing walking ability in subjects with spinal cord injury: validity and reliability of 3 walking tests, Arch Phys Med Rehabil 86: 190–6.

10. van Hedel HJ, Wirth B, Dietz V (2005) Limits of locomotor ability in subjects with a spinal cord injury, Spinal Cord 43: 593–603.

11. van Hedel HJ (2009) Gait speed in relation to categories of functional ambulation after spinal cord injury, Neurorehabil Neural Repair: 23343–350.

12. Field-Fote EC, Fluet GG, Schafer SD, Schneider EM, Smith R, et al. (2001) The Spinal Cord Injury Functional Ambulation Inventory (SCI-FAI), J Rehabil Med 33: 177–81.

13. Buehner JJ, Forrest GF, Schmidt-Read M, White S, Tansey K (2012) Relationship Between ASIA Examination and Functional Outcomes in the NeuroRecovery Network Locomotor Training Program, Arch Phys Med Rehabil 93: 1530–1540.

14. Behrman AK, Lawless-Dixon AR, Davis SB, Bowden MG, Nair P, et al. (2005) Locomotor training progression and outcomes after incomplete spinal cord injury, Phys Ther 85: 1356–71.

15. Behrman AL, Harkema SJ (2000) Locomotor training after human spinal cord injury: a series of case studies, Phys Ther 80: 688–700.

16. Harkema SJ, Schmidt-Read M, Lorenz DJ, Edgerton VR, Behrman AL (2012) Balance and ambulation improvements in individuals with chronic incomplete spinal cord injury using locomotor training-based rehabilitation, Arch Phys Med Rehabil 93: 1508–1517.

17. Brooks D, Solway S, Gibbons WJ (2003) ATS statement on six-minute walk test, Am. J Respir. Crit Care Med 167: 1287.

18. Pinheiro JC, Bates DM (2000) Mixed Effects Models in S and S-Plus., Springer Verlag, New York.

19. Lorenz DJ, Datta S, Harkema SJ (2011) Marginal association measures for clustered data, Stat.Med 30: 3181–3191.

20. Hochberg Y (1988) A sharper Bonferroni procedure for multiple tests of significance. Biometrika 75: 800–8002.

21. Beckerman H, Roebroeck ME, Lankhorst GJ, Becher JG, Bezemer PD, et al. (2001) Smallest real difference, a link between reproducibility and responsiveness, Qual.Life Res 10: 571–578.

22. Tilson JK, Sullivan KJ, Cen SY, Rose DK, Koradia CH, et al. (2010) Meaningful gait speed improvement during the first 60 days poststroke: minimal clinically important difference, Phys Ther. 90: 196–208.

23. YOUDEN WJ (1950) Index for rating diagnostic tests, Cancer 3 32–35.

24. R Development Core Team (2011) A Language and Environment for Statistical Computing, Vienna, Austria. The R Foundation for Statistical Computing. 11-11-2011. Ref Type: Electronic Citation

25. Harkema SJ, Schmidt-Read M, Lorenz D, Edgerton VR, Behrman AL (2011) Balance and Ambulation Improvements in Individuals With Chronic Incomplete Spinal Cord Injury Using Locomotor Training-Based Rehabilitation, Arch Phys Med Rehabil Sep; 93(9): 1508–17.

26. DeVivo MJ (2012) Epidemiology of traumatic spinal cord injury: trends and future implications, Spinal Cord 50: 365–372.

27. van Hedel HJ, Dietz V (2009) Walking during daily life can be validly and responsively assessed in subjects with a spinal cord injury, Neurorehabil Neural Repair 23: 117–124.

28. Lam T, Noonan VK, Eng JJ (2008) A systematic review of functional ambulation outcome measures in spinal cord injury, Spinal Cord 46: 246–254.

29. Dixon RE, Ellaway PH, Hansen SM, Pascoe JE (1969) Regularizing of fusimotor discharges by a descending 5-hydroxy-tryptaminergic pathway, J Physiol 202: 68P–69P.

30. Wirz M, Zorner B, Rupp R, Dietz V (2010) Outcome after incomplete spinal cord injury: central cord versus Brown-Sequard syndrome, Spinal Cord 48: 407–414.

31. Kim CM, Eng JJ, Whittaker MW (2004) Level walking and ambulatory capacity in persons with incomplete spinal cord injury: relationship with muscle strength, Spinal Cord 42: 156–162.

32. Musselman KE, Yang JF (2007) Walking tasks encountered by urban-dwelling adults and persons with incomplete spinal cord injuries, J Rehabil Med 39: 567–574.

33. Musselman K (2007) Clinical Significance Testing In Rehabilitation Research: What, Why, And How?, Physical Therapy Reviews 12: 287–296.

34. Lemay JF, Nadeau S (2010) Standing balance assessment in ASIA D paraplegic and tetraplegic participants: concurrent validity of the Berg Balance Scale, Spinal Cord 48: 245–250.

13

The Effect of Telephone Support Interventions on Coronary Artery Disease (CAD) Patient Outcomes during Cardiac Rehabilitation

Ahmed Kotb[1,2]*, Shuching Hsieh[2], George A. Wells[1,2]

1 Department of Epidemiology and Community Medicine, University of Ottawa, Ottawa, Canada, **2** Cardiovascular Research Methods Centre, University of Ottawa Heart Institute, Ottawa, Canada

Abstract

Background: Cardiac rehabilitation is offered to individuals after cardiac events to aid recovery and reduce the likelihood of further cardiac illness. However, patient participation remains suboptimal and the provision of high quality care to an expanding population of patients with chronic heart conditions is becoming increasingly difficult. A systematic review and meta-analysis was conducted to determine the effect of telephone support interventions compared with standard post-discharge care on coronary artery disease patient outcomes.

Methods: The Cochrane Library, MEDLINE, EMBASE, and CINAHL were searched and randomized controlled trials that directly compared telephone interventions with standard post-discharge care in adults following a myocardial infarction or a revascularization procedure were included. Study selection, data extraction and quality assessment were completed independently by two reviewers. Where appropriate, outcome data were combined and analyzed using a random effects model. For each dichotomous outcome, odds ratios (OR) and 95% confidence intervals (CI) were derived for each outcome. For continuous outcomes, weighted mean differences (WMD) and standardized mean differences (SMD) and 95% CI were calculated.

Results: 26 studies met the inclusion criteria. No difference was observed in mortality between the telephone group and the group receiving standard care OR 1.12 (0.71, 1.77). The intervention was significantly associated with fewer hospitalizations than the comparison group OR 0.62 (0.40, 0.97). Significantly more participants in the telephone group stopped smoking OR 1.32 (1.07, 1.62); had lower systolic blood pressure WMD −0.22 (−0.40, −0.04); lower depression scores SMD −0.10 (−0.21, −0.00); and lower anxiety scores SMD −0.14 (−0.24, −0.04). However, no significant difference was observed for low-density lipoprotein levels WMD −0.10 (−0.23, 0.03).

Conclusions: Compared to standard post-discharge care, regular telephone support interventions may help reduce feelings of anxiety and depression as well as, improve systolic blood pressure control and the likelihood of smoking cessation.

Editor: Yiru Guo, University of Louisville, United States of America

Funding: This research was funded by an Ontario Graduate Scholarship. The funders had no role in study design, data collection and analysis, decision to publish, or the preparation of the manuscript.

Competing Interests: The authors have declared that no competing interests exist.

* E-mail: akotb@ottawaheart.ca

Introduction

Cardiac rehabilitation (CR) is offered to individuals after cardiac events to aid recovery and reduce the likelihood of further cardiac illness. They have been previously shown to improve physical health as well as decrease subsequent morbidity and mortality through exercise, education, behavior change, counseling and other strategies aimed at targeting traditional risk factors for cardiovascular disease [1–6]. Despite these benefits however, patient participation in these programs remains suboptimal [7].

Some evidence suggests that interventions involving motivational communications delivered through letters, telephone calls and home visits may increase the uptake of cardiac rehabilitation

[8]. This offers promise as the provision of high quality care to an expanding population of older patients with chronic heart conditions becomes increasingly difficult. On the other hand, patients may be unwilling or unable to make frequent clinic attendance due to financial, transport or disability constraints [9].

To date, much of the evidence available has been focused on examining the effect of complex and multifactorial telemedicine interventions on heart failure (HF) patients. HF is a complex debilitating syndrome that results from a cardiac dysfunction that impairs the ability of the ventricle to fill with or eject blood[10]. More recently however, more basic telephone support interventions have been adapted for use in coronary artery disease (CAD) patient populations CAD is one of the most common forms of heart disease that results from an impedance or blockage of one or more arteries that supply blood to the heart [11–12].

Previous reports have examined the impact of multifaceted interventions on chronic diseases in general. When multifaceted interventions are examined, it becomes difficult to determine specifically which method of telemedicine appears most effective for this particular patient population. The aim of this systematic review and meta-analysis is to examine the literature on the impact of receiving structured telephone support, during cardiac rehabilitation, on clinical events, cardiac risk factors and patient reported outcomes in individuals with CAD compared to receiving usual follow-up care alone. The research questions addressed were: (1) What impact does structured telephone support (STS) have on mortality and hospitalization? (2) What impact does STS have on controlling risk factors such as smoking, systolic blood pressure, and low-density lipoprotein? (3) What does STS have on patient reported outcomes such as anxiety and depression?

Methods

Data Sources and Searches

Relevant randomized controlled trials published before September 2012 were identified by searching the following databases: Cochrane Central Register of Controlled Trials (CENTRAL), Database of Abstracts of Reviews of Effects (DARE) and Health Technology Assessment Database (HTA) on The Cochrane Library, MEDLINE, EMBASE, CINAHL, AMED, and the Web of Knowledge. Language restrictions were not applied to any of the searches. Bibliographies of included trials were examined to identify other potentially relevant studies.

Study Selection

Randomized controlled trials were included if they directly compared the impact of telephone-delivered post-discharge interventions with standard care at discharge in adults (18 years or older) who had experienced a myocardial infarction (MI), a revascularization procedure (coronary artery bypass grafting (CABG) or percutaneous transluminal coronary angioplasty (PTCA)), and those with angina, or angiographically defined coronary heart disease. The primary outcome was all-cause hospitalization. Secondary outcomes included all-cause mortality, depression, anxiety as well as measures taken to reduce the risk of further cardiac illness such as smoking cessation, reducing systolic blood pressure, and low-density lipoprotein cholesterol levels.

In the first phase of screening, the titles and abstracts of all identified citations were screened by two independent reviewers (AK and SC). In the second phase of screening, full manuscripts were retrieved and screened by two independent reviewers on the basis of our predefined patient population, intervention, comparison, outcomes and study design of interest. Disagreements were resolved through discussion or through adjudication by a third reviewer (GW).

Data Extraction and Quality Assessment

For each included paper, one review author (AK) extracted data and a second author (SC) checked the extracted data and disagreements were resolved by discussion between the two review authors. If no agreement could be reached, a third author (GW) was required for adjudication.

The SIGN-50 checklist and the Cochrane Collaboration's tool for assessing risk of bias (ROB) were used to evaluate the methodological quality of included trials. Two independent reviewers conducted the quality assessments (AK and SC).

Disagreements between reviewers were resolved by discussion or through adjudication by a third reviewer (GW).

Data Synthesis and Analysis

The primary analysis was a comparison of telephone follow-up with usual care. Heterogeneity amongst included studies was explored qualitatively by comparing the characteristics of included studies, visual inspection of forest plots and quantitatively using Cochrane's Q test and I^2 statistic. For continuous data (using the same measuring instrument) the weighted mean difference (WMD) and 95% confidence intervals (CI) are reported. Where the studies have used different instruments to measure the same conceptual outcome, the standardized mean difference (SMD) is reported. In studies that report dichotomous data, the odds ratios (OR) or risk ratios (RR) and confidence intervals (CI) are reported. To account for heterogeneity and take a more conservative approach, the analyses were carried out using the random-effects model are presented. Sensitivity analyses using fixed effect models were conducted for comparison.

Results

Search results

The electronic search conducted yielded a total of 1,538 titles. The reference lists of studies later included were hand-searched and resulted in the selection of 53 studies for additional screening. After duplicates were removed, the titles and abstracts of 1,235 studies were screened. A total of 1,075 studies were excluded and 160 studies were retrieved for possible inclusion. After examining their full texts, 26 studies were included [13–38] and 134 were excluded. The study selection process and the reasons for exclusion are summarized in the PRISMA flow diagram shown in Figure 1.

Description of studies

All included randomized controlled trials (4,081 participants) compared a telephone intervention designed to improve cardiac patients' outcomes directly to standard post-discharge care. Nine of the included studies were conducted in Canada [13,16,20,30,31,32,33,34,35] 8 in Australia[17,25–29,37,38], 5 in the United States of America[14,21–23,38] 3 in Europe [18,19,24] and 1 in Iran [15]. Thirteen studies had longer than 6 months of follow-up [19,21,22,24,25,26,28,29,30,31–33,38]. Seven studies reported less than 6 months of follow-up [15–17,20,27,34,35] and 6 reported outcomes at 6 months [13,14,18,23,36,37]. Sample sizes varied considerably across studies (range: 59 to 792) as well as the number of calls made to participants (range: 3 to 24).

Of the 26 included studies, 8 studies recruited patients diagnosed with Acute Coronary Syndrome [14,21,23,25–29] 8 recruited patients who had undergone revascularization patients [13,15,16,20,31–33,37] 4 studies recruited patients diagnosed with a myocardial infarction [18,19,34,38] and 6 recruited any patients diagnosed with coronary artery disease [17,22,24,30,35,36]. Ten studies described their patient populations as having received some degree of cardiac rehabilitation [13,15,17,19,24,31–33,36,37]. Of those 10 studies, only 7 provided the proportion of patients who participated in CR (range: from 32% to 100%) [17,24,31–33,36,37]. Five studies described their patient populations as not accessing CR [25–29] and the remaining 11 studies did not provide detail regarding how much of their included participants also took part in cardiac rehabilitation [14,16,18,20–23,30,34,35,38].

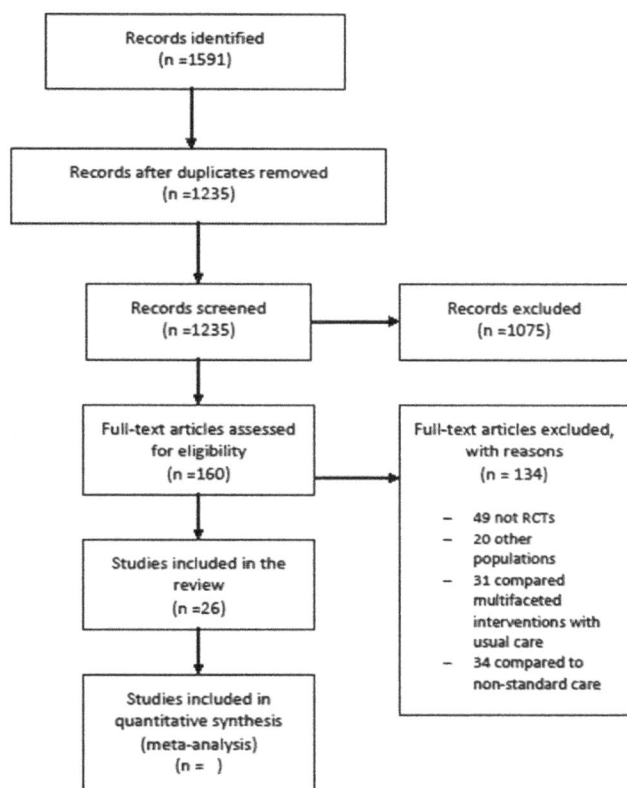

Figure 1. Modified PRISMA diagram.

The frequency of calls made varied between 3–6 times in fourteen studies and was greater than 6 calls in five studies. In 8 studies, the frequency of the intervention was not detailed [18,19,22,28,34,35,36,38]. In most studies, the telephone support intervention was delivered by a clinician with nurses being the most commonly reported delivery personnel. The second most common professional delivering the intervention was an exercise specialist. This occurred when the interventions' main component was exercise [13,31–33]. In one instance, when the intervention was focused primarily on lowering cholesterol levels, the intervention was delivered by a dietitian [37]. In one instance when the intervention was designed to address a multitude of risk factors, the intervention was delivered by a health educator. Further detail is available in Table 1 regarding the design of each included study, the type of patients included, and the interventions compared.

Risk of bias in included studies

Using the SIGN-50 quality assessment tool for randomized controlled trials, 14 studies were considered to be of high quality [13,20,26–37] 11 were considered to be of acceptable quality[14,16–19,21–25,38] and 1 was considered to be low [15] (see Table 1). A summary of the risk of bias of included studies is described in Figure 2. The risk of bias assessment of each study is detailed in Figure S1. Funnel plots were only considered for the outcome of mortality due to the fact that the number of studies was deemed sufficient to produce a reliable assessment (Figure S2). No considerable asymmetry was apparent.

Structured telephone support interventions versus usual care. Figure 3 provides a summary of the intervention's main effects compared to usual care for the following outcomes of

interest: all-cause mortality, all-cause hospitalization, smoking cessation, and depression. Further detail on the meta-analysis of the following outcomes: systolic blood pressure, low-density lipoprotein levels, and anxiety are available in Figures S3-S8.

Clinical events

Data on all-cause mortality was available and considered appropriate to be combined across 11 studies (Figure 3). Five studies were conducted in N. America, 4 in Australia and 2 in Europe. The quality was judged to be high for 5 studies and acceptable for 6. With the exception of one study, all included studies followed patients for at least 6 months. Four studies described their included patient population as having had an acute myocardial infarction, 4 as having acute coronary syndrome and 3 as having had a revascularization procedure. In 5 studies, a significant proportion of the included population participated in a cardiac rehabilitation program. In the remaining six studies, the participation of patients in a cardiac rehabilitation program was not described. In 7 of the studies the intervention was delivered by a nurse who offered support and education on topics that included risk factor control and improved symptom recognition. In the remaining 4 studies, the professionals delivering the intervention included health educators, pharmacists, dietitians, and exercise specialist. When the intervention was delivered by an exercise specialist the intervention focused more on physical activity in the period following an event. Where the intervention was delivered by a dietitian or pharmacist the focus shifted more towards lipid control. The $I^2 = 0\%$ and the overall effect estimate found showed no difference in the odds of mortality between the intervention and comparison group [OR 1.12 95% CI (0.71, 1.77)].

A total of 4 studies reported on hospitalization after discharge (Figure 3). Three of the four studies were conducted in Canada and one was conducted in Norway. Three of the four studies were considered to be of high quality and the fourth study was judged to be of acceptable quality. Heterogeneity was further examined according to the PICO statement of individual trials. In three out of the four studies, the majority of the CAD patient population had undergone a revascularization procedure. With the exception of the study by Smith (2011), three out of the four studies involved telephone follow-up carried out by a nurse that focused on the provision of support and education. Furthermore, only the study by Smith (2011) included a large portion of individuals who were participating in a cardiac rehabilitation program. The statistical measure of heterogeneity was low ($I^2 = 15\%$) and the overall effect estimate indicated significantly lower odds of hospitalization [OR 0.62 95% CI (0.40, 0.97)] in the telephone group. It is important to note however, that when a sensitivity analysis was conducted with and without the most outlying study, Beckie (1989), the significant effect was no longer found [OR 0.68 95% CI (0.45, 1.01)].

Modifiable risk factors. A total of 6 studies reported data on smoking cessation (Figure 3). Two studies were conducted in N. America, 2 in Europe and 2 in Australia. All six studies were considered to be of either acceptable or high quality. The follow-up period in all six studies was 6 or more months. In all six studies, the patient population was described as individuals recovering from either an AMI or CABG procedure. In all studies, the intervention was delivered by nurses who took part in coaching, supporting and educating participants. In only two studies, participants were described as having received cardiac rehabilitation. When combined together the overall effect estimate indicated significantly greater odds of smoking cessation in the group

Table 1. Characteristics of included studies.

Author/Year	Country	Population	Comparisons	Follow-up	Quality
1.Arthur 2002 [13]	Canada	CABG patients (N = 242). Participating in a Cardiac Rehabilitation program: Yes	Intervention: In addition to exercise, patients were telephoned every 2 weeks by the exercise specialist. Comparison: Hospital based exercise training	6 months	High quality
2.Bambauer 2005 [14]	USA	ACS patients (N = 100). Participating in a Cardiac Rehabilitation program: Not described	Intervention: Six 30 minute telephone counseling sessions. Comparison: Patients received a booklet on coping with chronic illness and were instructed to contact their primary care physician if they experienced any warning signs of more significant depression.	6 months	Acceptable
3.Bazargani 2011 [15]	Iran	CABG patients (N = 300). Participating in a Cardiac Rehabilitation program: Yes	Intervention: 6 sessions (150 min/week) of psycho-education. Comparison: Not described	3 months	Unacceptable
4.Beckie 1989 [16]	Canada	CABG patients (N = 74). Participating in a Cardiac Rehabilitation program: Not described	Intervention: 4 to 6 supportive-educative telephone calls with a cardiac rehabilitation nurse specialist. Comparison: Received routine in-hospital teaching available to all patients undergoing cardiac surgery.	1.5 months	Acceptable
5.Gallagher 2003 [17]	Australia	Women with CAD (N = 196). Participating in a Cardiac Rehabilitation program: 32% did	Intervention: 4 telephone calls to assist coping with recovery. Comparison: All inpatients received a Phase I education program, and all women were referred to local cardiac rehabilitation programs.	3 months	Acceptable
6.Hanssen 2007 [18]	Norway	AMI patients (N = 288). Participating in a Cardiac Rehabilitation program: Not described	Intervention: Nurse-initiated telephone calls after discharge. Comparison: All patients in the control group were managed in accordance with the current clinical practice, which encompassed one visit to a physician at the outpatient clinic 6–8 weeks after discharge, and subsequent visits to the patient's general practitioner.	6 months	Acceptable
7.Hanssen 2009 [19]	Norway	AMI patients (N = 288). Participating in a Cardiac Rehabilitation program: A very small proportion were referred	Intervention: Nurse-initiated telephone calls after discharge. Comparison: All patients in the control group were managed in accordance with the current clinical practice, which encompassed one visit to a physician at the outpatient clinic 6–8 weeks after discharge, and subsequent visits to the patient's general practitioner.	18 months	Acceptable
8.Hartford 2002 [20]	Canada	CABG patients (N = 166) who have a caregiver. Participating in a Cardiac Rehabilitation program: Not described	Intervention: 6 telephone calls to patients and partners. Comparison: The control group received usual care, which did not include systematic follow-up	2 months	High quality
9.Holmes-Rovner 2008 [21]	USA	ACS patients (N = 525). Participating in a Cardiac Rehabilitation program: Not described	Intervention: Six-session telephone counseling calls by a health educator. Comparison: Patients received a written discharge contract listing recommended outpatient medications, cardiac rehabilitation recommendations, and health behavior changes (smoking cessation, diet modification, and exercise), as well as numerical values for ejection fraction and cholesterol.	8 months	Acceptable

Table 1. Cont.

Author/Year	Country	Population	Comparisons	Follow-up	Quality
10.Ma 2010 [22]	USA	CAD patients (N = 689). Participating in a Cardiac Rehabilitation program: Not described	Intervention: Pharmacist-delivered telephone counseling calls. Comparison: consisted of normal clinical care as determined by the patient's provider.	12 months	Acceptable
11.Mclaughlin 2005 [23]	USA	ACS patients (N = 100) with symptoms of depressive illness or anxiety. Participating in a Cardiac Rehabilitation program: Not described	Intervention: 3–6 telephone counseling sessions of 30 minutes by clinicians. Comparison: Patients received a booklet on coping with cardiac illness typical of those given at hospital discharge and were instructed to contact their primary care physician if they experienced any warning signs of depression.	6 months	Acceptable
12.Mittag 2006 [24]	Germany	CAD patients (N = 343). Participating in a Cardiac Rehabilitation program: All received 3 weeks of inpatient Cardiac Rehabilitation	Intervention: Monthly nurse-initiated telephone contacts. Comparison: The control group received six flyers on general health topics (relaxation, sports and physical exercise, sleep disorders, low back pain, nutrition) by mail every second month as an attention placebo. Patients in the intervention group were given the same written information	12 months	Acceptable
13.Neubeck 2009 [25]	Australia	ACS patients (N = 208). Participating in a Cardiac Rehabilitation program: Not accessing CR	Intervention: A clinic visit plus 3 months of phone support. Comparison: ongoing conventional health care. Managing cardiovascular health in consultation with their GP and cardiologist.	48 months	Acceptable
14.Neubeck 2011 [26]	Australia	ACS patients (N = 208). Participating in a Cardiac Rehabilitation program: Not accessing CR	Intervention: 1-hour consultation and telephone calls over 3 months. Comparison: ongoing conventional health care. Managing cardiovascular health in consultation with their GP and cardiologist.	48 months	High quality
15.Redfern 2008 [27]	Australia	ACS patients (N = 208). Participating in a Cardiac Rehabilitation program: Not accessing CR	Intervention: 1-hour consultation and approximately four 10-minute follow-up calls. Comparison: Participants continued to manage their cardiovascular health as directed by their family physician often in consultation with their cardiologist.	3 months	High quality
16.Redfern 2009 [28]	Australia	ACS patients (N = 208). Participating in a Cardiac Rehabilitation program: Not accessing CR	Intervention: Clinic visit plus telephone support and tailored preferential risk modification. Comparison: continuing conventional care but no centrally coordinated secondary prevention	12 months	High quality
17.Redfern 2010 [29]	Australia	ACS patients (N = 208). Participating in a Cardiac Rehabilitation program: Not accessing CR	Intervention: One-hour initial consultation and four 10 minute follow-up phone calls over three months. Comparison: participated in ongoing conventional care, aimed at managing their cardiovascular health as directed by their General Practitioner, ideally in consultation with their Cardiologist.	12 months	High quality
18.Reid 2007 [30]	Canada	CAD patients (N = 100) who were also current smokers. Participating in a Cardiac Rehabilitation program: Not described	Intervention: Automatic telephone contact plus counseling by up to three 20-min telephone sessions. Comparison: All participants received advice to quit smoking; access to Nicotine Replacement Therapy during hospitalization (if necessary); brief bedside counseling with a nurse-specialist; a self-help guide; and the provision of information about the hospital's outpatient smoking cessation program and other community programs.	12 months	High quality

Table 1. Cont.

Author/Year	Country	Population	Comparisons	Follow-up	Quality
19.Smith 2004 [31]	Canada	CABG patients (N = 222). Participating in a Cardiac Rehabilitation program: All participated in CR (home vs. hospital-based)	Intervention: Exercise program and telephone follow-up every 2 weeks by an exercise specialist. Comparison: Patients assigned to the Hospital based exercise group were expected to attend supervised exercise sessions 3 times per week for 6 months.	12 months	High quality
20.Smith 2007 [32]	Canada	CABG patients (N = 196). Participating in a Cardiac Rehabilitation program: All participated in CR (home vs. hospital-based)	Intervention: Exercise program and telephone follow-up every 2 weeks by an exercise specialist. Comparison: Patients assigned to the Hospital based exercise group were expected to attend supervised exercise sessions 3 times per week for 6 months.	72 months	High quality
21.Smith 2011 [33]	Canada	CABG patients (N = 196). Participating in a Cardiac Rehabilitation program: All participated in CR (home vs. hospital-based)	Intervention: Exercise program and telephone follow-up every 2 weeks by an exercise specialist. Comparison: Patients assigned to the Hospital based exercise group were expected to attend supervised exercise sessions 3 times per week for 6 months.	72 months	High quality
22.Stevens 1985 [34]	Canada	MI patients (N = 59). Participating in a Cardiac Rehabilitation program: Not described	Intervention: Received telephone calls by 2 nurses and the investigator. Comparison: nurses educated MI patients prior to discharge and all got a booklet to take home. Upon discharge patients were returned to the care of the GP and received usual follow-up.	1.5–2 months	High quality
23.Tranmer 2004 [35]	Canada	CAD patients (N = 200). Participating in a Cardiac Rehabilitation program: Not described	Intervention: Follow-up via nurse-initiated telephone calls. Comparison: Usual care included preoperative and discharge preparation by the nurse, provision of an education booklet and home care follow-up, as necessary.	1.25 months	High quality
24.Vale 2003 [36]	Australia	CAD patients (N = 792). Participating in a Cardiac Rehabilitation program: 53% of patients in the intervention group and 57% of the patients in the control group attended a cardiac rehabilitation program.	Intervention: Patients received coaching sessions by telephone. Comparison: Patients received a hospital discharge summary, a one page chart of risk factor for CHD secondary prevention to them and their medical caregivers as well as contacted once after discharge at 24 weeks for follow-up assessment	6 months	High quality
25.Vale 2002 [37]	Australia	CABG or PCI patients (N = 245). Participating in a Cardiac Rehabilitation program: 53% of patients in the intervention group and 50% of the patients in the control group attended a cardiac rehabilitation program.	Intervention: Dietitian contacted patients 5 times by telephone regarding lipid levels. Comparison: All patients in the study (including patients in the coaching intervention group) were offered information about a cardiac rehabilitation program and were encouraged to attend. Patients in the usual care group were contacted at 24 weeks postrandomization to obtain a fasting serum lipid profile within the next 2 weeks.	6 months	High quality
26.Van Elderen 1994 [38]	USA	AMI patients (N = 60). Participating in a Cardiac Rehabilitation program: Not described	Intervention: Nurse contacted the patient by telephone. Comparison: Patients received standard medical care only; consisting primarily of medical care. A standard physical rehabilitation program was mplemented in the nursing ward.	12 months	Acceptable

Note: Studies underlined and in bold were included in the meta-analysis. The other studies were described qualitatively. CABG = Coronary artery bypass graft. ACS = Acute coronary syndrome. AMI = Acute myocardial infarction. CAD = Coronary artery disease. PCI = Percutaneous coronary intervention.

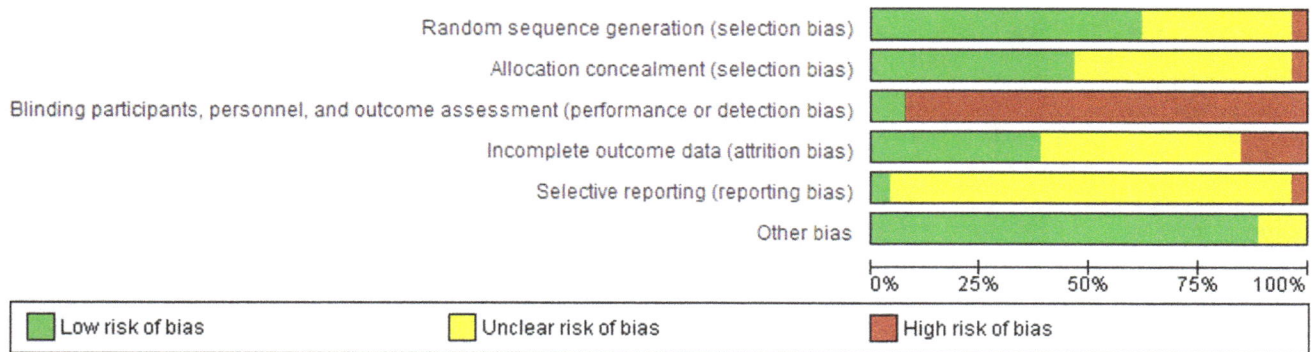

Figure 2. Risk of bias graph.

receiving the telephone intervention [Risk Ratio 1.32 95% CI (1.07, 1.62)].

Two studies reported data on SBP differences between treatment groups. The follow-up period in both studies was 12 or more months. The study by Mittag (2006) was conducted in Germany and the study by Neubeck (2011) was conducted in Australia. The quality of both studies was considered to be acceptable. Both studies included acute CAD patients and both telephone follow-up interventions were delivered by nurses and focused on risk factor reduction. The $I^2 = 0\%$ and the overall calculated WMD for SBP was significantly lower for the telephone group [WMD -4.22 95% CI (-7.58, -0.85)].

A total of 4 studies reported data regarding the change in LDL levels between treatment groups. In three out of the 4 studies the follow-up period was greater than or equal to 12 months. Two studies were conducted in N. America and two were conducted in Australia. The quality of the studies was considered high in 3 studies and acceptable in 1. Three studies described their patient population as acute coronary syndrome or recovering from a revascularization procedure while one study only broadly defined patients as having coronary heart disease (CHD). The telephone intervention was delivered by a different type of specialist in each study. This included a dietitian, an exercise specialist, a nurse, and a pharmacist. The I^2 statistic $= 71\%$ when these studies were analyzed together using a random effects model. When only studies of longer than 6 months follow-up were examined, the I^2 statistic was reduced to 16% and the overall WMD for LDL was not found to significantly differ between comparison groups (WMD -0.07 [-0.20, 0.05]).

Patient reported outcomes. In total 5 studies measured and reported on the outcome of depression (Figure 3). In 4 out of the 5 studies, the follow-up period was greater than or equal to 6 months. Two studies were conducted in the United States, two in Australia and one in Germany. The quality of the studies was judged to be acceptable in 4 studies and high in one. In three studies, the patient populations were described to have an acute myocardial infarction (AMI). The patient populations in the remaining two studies were described as having an acute coronary syndrome (ACS) and having undergone was revascularization. In 3 out of 5 studies, a significant portion of the patients received some cardiac rehabilitation services. In 4 out of 5 studies the intervention was delivered by a nurse. In the study that did not involve nurses in the delivery, the intervention was delivered by clinicians. The I^2 statistic $= 0\%$ and the overall calculated SMD showed a significantly lower (p $= 0.04$) depression score in the

telephone group than the comparison [SMD -0.10 95% CI (-0.21, -0.00)].

Six studies examined the impact of regular telephone follow-up on feelings of anxiety. In 4 out of the 6 studies the follow-up period was greater than or equal to 6 months. Three studies were conducted in N. America, 2 in Australia and 1 in Europe. The quality of the studies was judged to be acceptable in 5 studies and high in one. The patient population was described as having had an AMI or CABG in 5 studies and as ACS in one. In 3 out of 6 studies, a significant portion of the included population received some cardiac rehabilitation services. In 5 out of 6 studies, the nurses delivered the telephone support intervention and in one study the intervention was delivered by a clinician.

Even though the overall calculated SMD indicated that participants in the telephone group had significantly lower anxiety scores than those in the comparison group [SMD -0.29 95% CI (-0.56, -0.01)], the forest plot and I^2 ($I^2 = 81\%$) indicated that a considerable amount of heterogeneity was evident across studies. The most outlying study by Beckie (1989) had the shortest follow-up having only followed patients for a period of 6 weeks and included CAD patients who were less severe or acutely ill than the patients in other studies. This study was excluded from subsequent analyses that examined studies of longer than 6 weeks of follow-up.

When studies of at least 3 months of follow-up were examined, the analysis included 5 out of the 6 studies. The $I^2 = 29\%$ and the telephone group was found to have reduced feelings of anxiety than the control group [SMD -0.14 95% CI (-0.24, -0.04)]. This effect remained when studies of 6 or more months of follow-up were examined. This analysis included 4 out of 6 studies and demonstrated that the participants in the telephone intervention group had significantly lower anxiety scores [SMD -0.18 95% CI (-0.30, -0.07)].

Discussion

Many patients with CAD continue to face challenges maintaining their adherence to recommendations for risk reduction such as managing their blood pressure, lowering their low-density lipoprotein levels and abstaining from smoking. A wealth of available evidence also suggests a strong link between increased feelings of depression and anxiety in the period that follows having a coronary event. Together, these continued challenges place individuals with these diseases at an increased risk of further cardiac illness and death. The hypothesis in this review was that the availability of remote monitoring and support services for recovering patients may facilitate access to care and improve

A) All-cause mortality

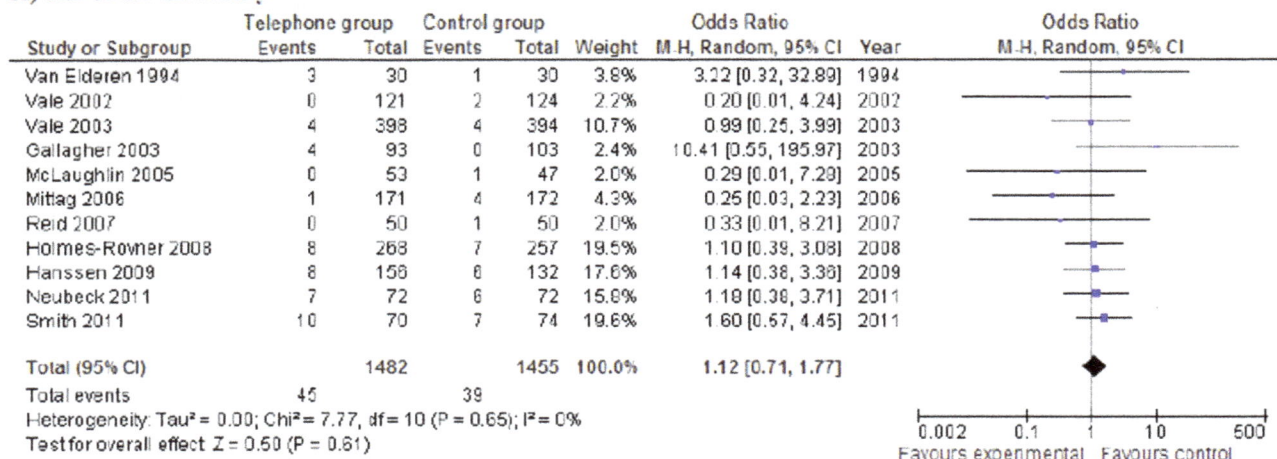

Study or Subgroup	Telephone group Events	Total	Control group Events	Total	Weight	Odds Ratio M-H, Random, 95% CI	Year	Odds Ratio M-H, Random, 95% CI
Van Elderen 1994	3	30	1	30	3.8%	3.22 [0.32, 32.89]	1994	
Vale 2002	0	121	2	124	2.2%	0.20 [0.01, 4.24]	2002	
Vale 2003	4	398	4	394	10.7%	0.99 [0.25, 3.99]	2003	
Gallagher 2003	4	93	0	103	2.4%	10.41 [0.55, 195.97]	2003	
McLaughlin 2005	0	53	1	47	2.0%	0.29 [0.01, 7.29]	2005	
Mittag 2006	1	171	4	172	4.3%	0.25 [0.03, 2.23]	2006	
Reid 2007	0	50	1	50	2.0%	0.33 [0.01, 8.21]	2007	
Holmes-Rovner 2008	8	268	7	257	19.5%	1.10 [0.39, 3.08]	2008	
Hanssen 2009	8	156	8	132	17.6%	1.14 [0.38, 3.38]	2009	
Neubeck 2011	7	72	6	72	15.8%	1.18 [0.38, 3.71]	2011	
Smith 2011	10	70	7	74	19.6%	1.60 [0.57, 4.45]	2011	
Total (95% CI)		1482		1455	100.0%	1.12 [0.71, 1.77]		
Total events	45		39					

Heterogeneity: Tau² = 0.00; Chi² = 7.77, df = 10 (P = 0.65); I² = 0%
Test for overall effect: Z = 0.50 (P = 0.61)

0.002   0.1   1   10   500
Favours experimental   Favours control

B) All-cause hospitalization

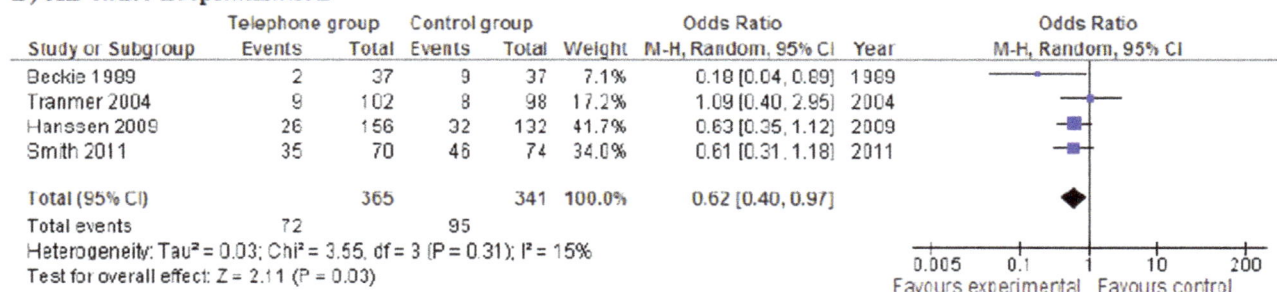

Study or Subgroup	Telephone group Events	Total	Control group Events	Total	Weight	Odds Ratio M-H, Random, 95% CI	Year	Odds Ratio M-H, Random, 95% CI
Beckie 1989	2	37	9	37	7.1%	0.18 [0.04, 0.89]	1989	
Tranmer 2004	9	102	8	98	17.2%	1.09 [0.40, 2.95]	2004	
Hanssen 2009	26	156	32	132	41.7%	0.63 [0.35, 1.12]	2009	
Smith 2011	35	70	46	74	34.0%	0.61 [0.31, 1.18]	2011	
Total (95% CI)		365		341	100.0%	0.62 [0.40, 0.97]		
Total events	72		95					

Heterogeneity: Tau² = 0.03; Chi² = 3.55, df = 3 (P = 0.31); I² = 15%
Test for overall effect: Z = 2.11 (P = 0.03)

0.005   0.1   1   10   200
Favours experimental   Favours control

C) Smoking cessation

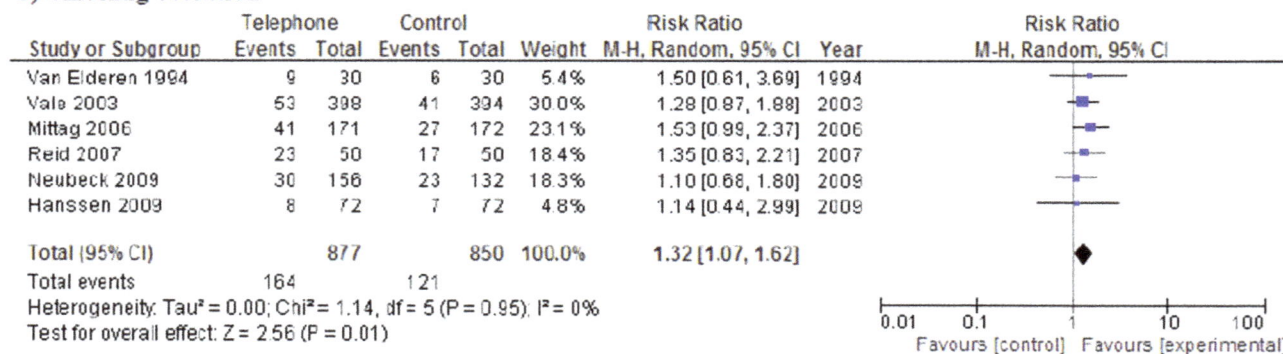

Study or Subgroup	Telephone Events	Total	Control Events	Total	Weight	Risk Ratio M-H, Random, 95% CI	Year	Risk Ratio M-H, Random, 95% CI
Van Elderen 1994	9	30	6	30	5.4%	1.50 [0.61, 3.69]	1994	
Vale 2003	53	398	41	394	30.0%	1.28 [0.87, 1.88]	2003	
Mittag 2006	41	171	27	172	23.1%	1.53 [0.99, 2.37]	2006	
Reid 2007	23	50	17	50	18.4%	1.35 [0.83, 2.21]	2007	
Neubeck 2009	30	156	23	132	18.3%	1.10 [0.68, 1.80]	2009	
Hanssen 2009	8	72	7	72	4.8%	1.14 [0.44, 2.99]	2009	
Total (95% CI)		877		850	100.0%	1.32 [1.07, 1.62]		
Total events	164		121					

Heterogeneity: Tau² = 0.00; Chi² = 1.14, df = 5 (P = 0.95); I² = 0%
Test for overall effect: Z = 2.56 (P = 0.01)

0.01   0.1   1   10   100
Favours [control]   Favours [experimental]

D) Depression

Study or Subgroup	Telephone group Mean	SD	Total	Control group Mean	SD	Total	Weight	Std. Mean Difference IV, Random, 95% CI	Year	Std. Mean Difference IV, Random, 95% CI
Van Elderen 1994	23.23	6.19	30	25.15	7.58	30	4.0%	-0.27 [-0.78, 0.23]	1994	
Gallagher 2003	4.3	4.6	93	4.1	4.2	103	13.1%	0.05 [-0.24, 0.33]	2003	
Vale 2003	-4.9	21.31	398	-2.8	19.18	394	53.2%	-0.10 [-0.24, 0.04]	2003	
McLaughlin 2005	5.7	3.6	53	6.6	3.9	47	6.7%	-0.24 [-0.63, 0.16]	2005	
Mittag 2006	11	8.6	171	12.1	8.9	172	23.0%	-0.13 [-0.34, 0.09]	2006	
Total (95% CI)			745			746	100.0%	-0.10 [-0.21, -0.00]		

Heterogeneity: Tau² = 0.00; Chi² = 2.00, df = 4 (P = 0.73); I² = 0%
Test for overall effect: Z = 2.02 (P = 0.04)

-2   -1   0   1   2
Favours experimental   Favours control

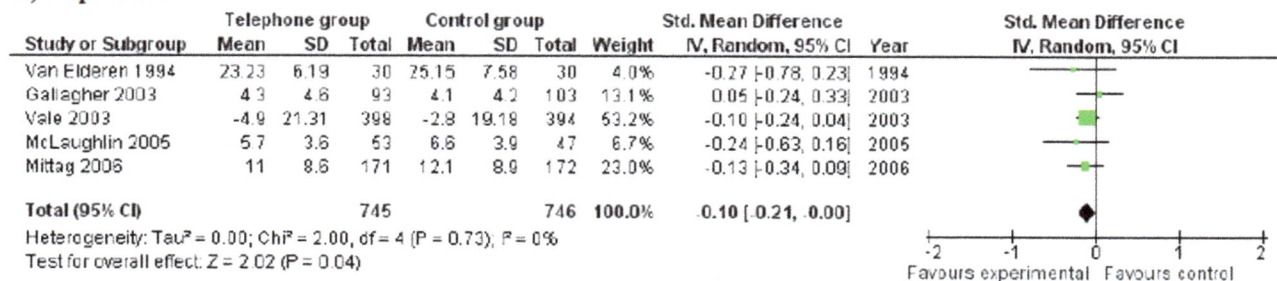

Figure 3. Comparing telephone support with usual care.

patients' outcomes through cardiac risk reduction and improved patient outcomes.

Study participants were mostly males, aged between of 50 and 70 years old, and diagnosed as acute CAD patients defined as having had an MI or a revascularization procedure. With the exception of one study that was conducted in the Middle East, all studies were conducted in either N. America, Europe or Australia. With the exception of one study, the quality of included studies was either high or acceptable and the follow-up period was typically six or more months. The telephone support intervention was typically delivered by a nurse who supported patients and educated them on matters that included cardiac risk reduction and improved symptom recognition. Outcomes considered included clinical events (all-cause mortality and hospitalization), modifiable risk factors (smoking cessation, low-density lipoprotein, and systolic blood pressure), and other patient outcomes (depression and anxiety).

No evidence was found to support any additional benefit as a result of the telephone intervention in terms of a reduction in mortality and level of low-density lipoprotein. These findings were consistent with findings by Neubeck (2009) and Whalley (2011) that showed no strong evidence for reductions in total deaths and the review by Taylor (2010) that found no difference between groups in terms of LDL levels [40,41].

In this review, participants receiving the telephone intervention did however have significantly fewer hospitalizations. They also experienced significant reductions in systolic blood pressure and were more likely to stop smoking. These findings were similar to those by Barth (2008) and by Neubeck (2009), where telephone support was found to significantly promote smoking cessation in patients with coronary heart disease [11,39]. Neubeck (2009) also demonstrated that participants in the telephone group had significantly lower systolic blood pressure.

Patients receiving the telephone intervention also had significantly lower depression and anxiety scores were observed in participants who received the telephone intervention. Symptoms of anxiety and depression are commonly experienced by patients with coronary artery diseases (CAD). Depression and anxiety have been previously associated the with increased severity of CAD, the number and length of cardiac-related hospitalizations and all-cause mortality, and can predict greater risk major adverse cardiac events in patients with stable CAD[42–44]. Evidence from this systematic review and meta-analysis is therefore in support of conducting a randomized controlled trial of sufficient power and at least 12 months of follow-up to compare the impact associated with the delivery of a regular telephone intervention alongside usual care for monitoring and supporting coronary artery disease patients following an acute cardiac event or revascularization procedure.

This review has several important limitations to consider. Like any systematic review, the strengths of the results depends primarily on the quality and completeness of the data currently available from included studies. Detailed descriptions around participants' attendance and compliance rates for cardiac rehabilitation programs were inadequately reported. This limited how thoroughly this issue can investigated in order to determine if the benefits associated with telephone support are perhaps due to an increased participation in cardiac rehabilitation programs. Furthermore, intensive monitoring can add to more contact with providers and in some instances, more tests. This can occur for an intervention of this sort. Almost all studies were conducted in what are considered to be high-income countries. This in turn limits the generalizability of the findings to settings outside of N. America, Europe and Australia. As is commonly expected, the patient populations varied slightly across included studies. Although only patients with an acute form of coronary artery disease patients who had not advanced to heart failure were considered for this review, included studies described their patients as having either had an acute myocardial infarction, diagnosis of acute coronary syndrome or had undergone a revascularization procedure. A randomized controlled trial that compares the effect of standard care and a telephone support intervention delivered by nurses to aid in the education and counseling of either one of the aforementioned patient groups therefore remains warranted. Even though such resource utilization implications may compromise the benefits associated with telephone support, there was no data available from included studies to address this concern. Further research is needed to examine the cost-effectiveness of this intervention as it compares to the current standard of post-discharge care.

Conclusions

The effectiveness of this simple telephone intervention is of relevance given that most cardiac rehabilitation programs involve one or more of the following: routine monitoring, counseling, and educating. Some of these benefits can be feasibly delivered remotely using telephone technology as a medium. Evidence from this review suggests that telephone support and monitoring appear more effective in reducing certain risk factors than others, physicians may identify, depending on each patient's rehabilitation goals, which patients would be most likely to benefit from the intervention. Through reducing feelings of anxiety and depression, improved control over cardiac risk reduction and fewer hospitalizations, structured telephone support and follow-up can aid in the delivery of specialist preventive care to patients who may otherwise not have access to them and may have the potential to reduce some of the burden on the healthcare system. If hospitalization, anxiety and depression are indeed reduced this would be extremely valuable and possibly cost effective. A larger definitive randomized controlled trial of this intervention targeted to a specific population likely to benefit most is therefore merited.

Acknowledgments

We gratefully acknowledge the help of Dr. Alaa Kotb for providing his expertise in the field of cardiology and Agnieszka Szczotka for her help in devising the search strategies needed for conducting this review.

Author Contributions

Conceived and designed the experiments: AK GW SH. Performed the experiments: AK GW SH. Analyzed the data: AK GW. Wrote the paper: AK. Wrote the first draft of the manuscript: AK. Contributed to the writing of the manuscript: AK GW SH.

References

1. Jolliffe JA, Rees K, Taylor RS, Thompson D, Oldridge N, et al. (2001) Exercise-based rehabilitation for coronary heart disease. Cochrane Database of Systematic Reviews, Issue 1. [DOI: 10.1002/14651858.CD001800].

2. Taylor RS, Brown A, Ebrahim S, Jolliffe J, Noorani H, et al. (2004) Exercise-based rehabilitation for patients with coronary heart disease: systematic review and meta-analysis of randomized controlled trials. American Journal of Medicine 116(10): 682–92.

3. Balady GJ, Williams MA, Ades PA, Bittner V, Comoss P, et al. (2007) Core components of cardiac rehabilitation/secondary prevention programs: 2007 update: a scientific statement from the American Heart Association Exercise, Cardiac Rehabilitation, and Prevention Committee, the Council on Clinical Cardiology; the Councils on Cardiovascular Nursing, Epidemiology and Prevention, and Nutrition, Physical Activity, and Metabolism; and the American Association of Cardiovascular and Pulmonary Rehabilitation. Circulation 115(20):2675–82.

4. Graham I, Atar D, Borch-Johnsen K, Boysen G, Burell G, et al. (2007) European guidelines on cardiovascular disease prevention in clinical practice: full text. Fourth Joint Task Force of the European Society of Cardiology and other societies on cardiovascular disease prevention in clinical practice (constituted by representatives of nine societies and by invited experts). European Journal of Cardiovascular Prevention and Rehabilitation (Suppl 2):S1–113.

5. National Institute for Health and Clinical Excellence (2007) MI: Secondary prevention. Secondary prevention in primary and secondary care for patients following a myocardial infarction. Available at http://www.nice.org.uk/CG48 [accessed 18 2 2008]. London, UK: National Institute for Health and Clinical Excellence.

6. Stone JA, Arthur HM (2005) Canadian guidelines for cardiac rehabilitation and cardiovascular disease prevention, second edition, 2004: executive summary. Canadian Journal of Cardiology;21 (Suppl D):3D–19D.

7. Beswick AD, Rees K, Griebsch I, Taylor FC, Burke M, et al. (2004) Provision, uptake and cost of cardiac rehabilitation programmes: improving services to under-represented groups. Health Technology Assessment 8(41):1–166.

8. Davies P, Taylor F, Beswick A, Wise F, Moxham T, et al. (2010) Promoting patient uptake and adherence in cardiac rehabilitation (Review). Cochrane Database of Systematic Reviews, Issue 7.

9. Inglis SC, Clark RA, McAlister FA, Ball J, Lewinter C, et al. (2010) Structured telephone support or telemonitoring programmes for patients with chronic heart failure. Cochrane Database of Systematic Reviews Issue 8. Art. No.: CD007228. DOI: 10.1002/14651858.CD007228.pub2.

10. Definition of Heart Failure. MedicineNet.com. MedicineNet.com, n.d. Web. 23 January 2013. http://www.medterms.com/script/main/art.asp?articlekey = 3672

11. Neubeck L, Redfern J, Fernandez R, Briffa T, Baumane A, et al. (2009) Telehealth interventions for the secondary prevention of coronary heart disease: a systematic review. European Journal of Cardiovascular Prevention & Rehabilitation 16: 281–289.

12. Definition of Coronary artery disease. MedicineNet.com. MedicineNet.com, n.d. Web. 25 June 2012. www.medterms.com/script/main/art.asp?articlekey = 10267

13. Arthur HM, Smith KM, Kodis J, McKelvie R (2002) A controlled trial of hospital versus home-based exercise in cardiac patients. Medicine and Science in Sports and Exercise. 34(10)15441550doi: 10.1249/01.MSS.0000030847.23854.CB

14. Bambauer KZ, Aupont O, Stone PH, Locke SE, Mullan MG, et al. (2005) "The effect of a telephone counseling intervention on self-rated health of cardiac patients." Psychosomatic Medicine 67(4): 539–545.

15. Bazargani RH, Besharat MA, Ehsan HB, Nejatian M, Hosseini K (2011) The efficacy of Chronic Disease Self Management Programs and Tele-health on psychosocial adjustment by increasing self-efficacy in patients with CABG. Procedia - Social and Behavioral Sciences, 30: 817–821.

16. Beckie T (1989) A supportive-educative telephone program: Impact on knowledge and anxiety after coronary artery bypass graft surgery. Heart and Lung: Journal of Critical Care 18(1): 46–55.

17. Gallagher R, McKinley S, Dracup K (2003) Effects of a telephone counseling intervention on psychosocial adjustment in women following a cardiac event. Heart and Lung: Journal of Acute and Critical Care 32(2): 79–87.

18. Hanssen TA, Nordrehaug JE, Eide GE, Rokne B (2007) Improving outcomes after myocardial infarction: A randomized controlled trial evaluating effects of a telephone follow-up intervention. European Journal of Cardiovascular Prevention and Rehabilitation 14 (3): 429–437.

19. Hanssen TA, Nordrehaug JE, Eide GE, Hanestad BR (2009) Does a telephone follow-up intervention for patients discharged with acute myocardial infarction have long-term effects on health-related quality of life? A randomised controlled trial. Journal of Clinical Nursing 18(9): 1334–1345.

20. Hartford K, Wong C, Zakaria D (2002) Randomized controlled trial of a telephone intervention by nurses to provide information and support to patients and their partners after elective coronary artery bypass graft surgery: Effects of anxiety. Heart and Lung: Journal of Acute and Critical Care, 31(3), 199–206.

21. Holmes-Rovner M, Stommel M, Corser WD, Olomu A, Holtrop JS, et al. (2008) Does outpatient telephone coaching add to hospital quality improvement following hospitalization for acute coronary syndrome? Journal of General Internal Medicine 23(9): 1464–70.

22. Ma Y, Ockene IS, Rosal MC, Merriam PA, Ockene JK, et al. (2010) Randomized trial of a pharmacist-delivered intervention for improving lipid-lowering medication adherence among patients with coronary heart disease. Cholesterol 2010:1–11.

23. McLaughlin TJ, Aupont O, Bambauer K, Stone P, Mullan MG, et al. (2005) Improving psychologic adjustment to chronic illness in cardiac patients: The role of depression and anxiety. Journal of General Internal Medicine 20(12): 1084–1090.

24. Mittag O, China C, Hoberg E, Juers E, Kolenda K, et al. (2006) Outcomes of cardiac rehabilitation with versus without a follow-up intervention rendered by telephone (Luebeck follow-up trial): overall and gender-specific effects International journal of rehabilitation research Internationale Zeitschrift fur Rehabilitationsforschung. Revue internationale de recherches de readaptation29(4): 295–302.

25. Neubeck L, Redfern J, Briffa T, Ascanio R, Freedman SB, et al. (2009) Cardiovascular risk benefits of the CHOICE (Choice of Health Options In prevention of Cardiovascular Events) program are maintained for four years: Randomised controlled trial. European Heart Journal Conference: European Society of Cardiology, ESC Congress 2009 Barcelona Spain. Conference Start: 20090829 Conference End: 20090902. Conference Publication: (var.pagings)30: 76.

26. Neubeck L, Freedman SB, Briffa T, Bauman A, Redfern J (2011) Four-year follow-up of the choice of health options in prevention of cardiovascular events randomized controlled trial. European Journal of Cardiovascular Prevention and Rehabilitation.18(2)278286

27. Redfern J, Briffa T, Ellis E, Freedman SB (2008) Patient-centered modular secondary prevention following acute coronary syndrome: A randomized controlled trial. Journal of Cardiopulmonary Rehabilitation and Prevention.28(2)107117

28. Redfern J, Briffa T, Ellis E, Freedman SB (2009) Choice of secondary prevention improves risk factors after acute coronary syndrome: 1-Year follow-up of the CHOICE (Choice of Health Options in prevention of Cardiovascular Events) randomised controlled trial. Heart 95 (6): 468–475.

29. Redfern J, Menzies M, Briffa T, Freedman SB (2010) Impact of medical consultation frequency on modifiable risk factors and medications at 12 months after acute coronary syndrome in the CHOICE randomised controlled trial. International Journal of Cardiology 145 (3): 481–486.

30. Reid RD, Pipe AL, Quinlan B, Oda J (2007) Interactive voice response telephony to promote smoking cessation in patients with heart disease: A pilot study. Patient Education and Counseling 66 (3): 319–326.

31. Smith KM, Arthur HM, McKelvie RS, Kodis J (2004) Differences in sustainability of exercise and health-related quality of life outcomes following home or hospital-based cardiac rehabilitation. European Journal of Cardiovascular Prevention and Rehabilitation 11(4): 313–319.

32. Smith KM (2007) Sustainability of exercise capacity and quality of life after home or hospital based exercise training in low-risk patients following coronary artery bypass graft surgery: a six-year follow-up of a randomized controlled trial, McMaster University (Canada): 176 p–176 p.

33. Smith KM, McKelvie RS, Thorpe KE, Arthur HM (2011) Six-year follow-up of a randomised controlled trial examining hospital versus home-based exercise training after coronary artery bypass graft surgery. Heart 97(14): 1169–1174.

34. Stevens B (1985) The effectiveness of patient education follow-up by telephone on knowledge of post-myocardial infarction patients. (M.Nus., University of Alberta (Canada)). ProQuest Dissertations and Theses (303461144).

35. Tranmer JE, Parry MJE (2004) Enhancing postoperative recovery of cardiac surgery patients - A randomized clinical trial of an advanced practice nursing intervention. Western Journal of Nursing Research 26(5): 515–532.

36. Vale MJ, Jelinek MV, Best JD, Dart AM, Grigg LE, et al. (2003) Coaching patients on achieving cardiovascular health (COACH): A multicenter randomized trial in patients with coronary heart disease. Archives of Internal Medicine–.163(22)27752783

37. Vale MJ, Jelinek MV, Best JD, Santamaria JD (2002) Coaching patients with coronary heart disease to achieve the target cholesterol: A method to bridge the gap between evidence-based medicine and the "real world" - randomized controlled trial. Journal of Clinical Epidemiology.55(3)245252

38. van Elderen-van Kemenade T, Maes S, van den Broek Y (1994) Effects of a health education programme with telephone follow-up during cardiac rehabilitation. British Journal of Clinical Psychology 33(3): 367–378.

39. Barth J, Critchley JA, Bengel J (2008) Psychosocial interventions for smoking cessation in patients with coronary heart disease. Cochrane Database of Systematic Reviews, Issue 1. Art. No.: CD006886. DOI: 10.1002/14651858.CD006886.

40. Taylor RS, Dalal H, Jolly K, Moxham T, Zawada A (2010) Home-based versus centre-based cardiac rehabilitation. Cochrane Database of Systematic Reviews, Issue 1. Art. No.: CD007130. DOI: 10.1002/14651858.CD007130.pub2.

41. Whalley B, Rees K, Davies P, Bennett P, Ebrahim S, et al. (2011) Psychological interventions for coronary heart disease. Cochrane Database of Systematic Reviews 2011, Issue 8. Art. No.: CD002902. DOI:10.1002/14651858.CD002902.pub3.

42. Versteeg H, Hoogwegt MT, Hansen TB, Pedersen SS, Zwisler AD, et al. (2013) Depression, not anxiety, is independently associated with 5-year hospitalizations and mortality in patients with ischemic heart disease. Journal of psychosomatic research 75(6): 518–25.

43. Ekici B, Ercan EA, Cehreli S, Tore HF (2014) The effect of emotional status and health-related quality of life on the severity of coronary artery disease." Kardiol Pol [Epub ahead of print].

44. Frasure-Smith N, Lesperance F (2008). Depression and anxiety as predictors of 2-year cardiac events in patients with stable coronary artery disease. Arch Gen Psychiatry 65(1): 62–71.

14

Virtual Reality Therapy for Adults Post-Stroke: A Systematic Review and Meta-Analysis Exploring Virtual Environments and Commercial Games in Therapy

Keith R. Lohse[1,2]*, Courtney G. E. Hilderman[3], Katharine L. Cheung[3], Sandy Tatla[4], H. F. Machiel Van der Loos[5]

1 School of Kinesiology, Auburn University, Auburn, Alabama, United States of America, 2 School of Kinesiology, University of British Columbia, Vancouver, British Columbia, Canada, 3 Department of Physical Therapy, University of British Columbia, Vancouver, British Columbia, Canada, 4 Department of Occupational Science and Occupational Therapy, University of British Columbia, Vancouver, British Columbia, Canada, 5 Department of Mechanical Engineering, University of British Columbia, Vancouver, British Columbia, Canada

Abstract

Background: The objective of this analysis was to systematically review the evidence for virtual reality (VR) therapy in an adult post-stroke population in both custom built virtual environments (VE) and commercially available gaming systems (CG).

Methods: MEDLINE, CINAHL, EMBASE, ERIC, PSYCInfo, DARE, PEDro, Cochrane Central Register of Controlled Trials, and Cochrane Database of Systematic Reviews were systematically searched from the earliest available date until April 4, 2013. Controlled trials that compared VR to conventional therapy were included. Population criteria included adults (>18) post-stroke, excluding children, cerebral palsy, and other neurological disorders. Included studies were reported in English. Quality of studies was assessed with the Physiotherapy Evidence Database Scale (PEDro).

Results: Twenty-six studies met the inclusion criteria. For body function outcomes, there was a significant benefit of VR therapy compared to conventional therapy controls, $G = 0.48$, 95% CI = [0.27, 0.70], and no significant difference between VE and CG interventions ($P = 0.38$). For activity outcomes, there was a significant benefit of VR therapy, $G = 0.58$, 95% CI = [0.32, 0.85], and no significant difference between VE and CG interventions ($P = 0.66$). For participation outcomes, the overall effect size was $G = 0.56$, 95% CI = [0.02, 1.10]. All participation outcomes came from VE studies.

Discussion: VR rehabilitation moderately improves outcomes compared to conventional therapy in adults post-stroke. Current CG interventions have been too few and too small to assess potential benefits of CG. Future research in this area should aim to clearly define conventional therapy, report on participation measures, consider motivational components of therapy, and investigate commercially available systems in larger RCTs.

Trial Registration: Prospero CRD42013004338

Editor: Terence J. Quinn, University of Glasgow, United Kingdom

Funding: This research was funded by #11-079 from the Peter Wall Solutions Initiative at the University of British Columbia awarded to H.F.M. Van der Loos. The funders had no role in study design, data collection and analysis, decision to publish, or preparation of the manuscript.

Competing Interests: The authors have declared that no competing interests exist.

* E-mail: kelopelli@gmail.com

Introduction

Stroke is a leading cause of death and disability around the world, and the majority of survivors experience chronic motor deficits associated with reduced quality of life [1]. Neurophysiological data suggest considerable amounts of practice are required to induce neuroplastic change and functional recovery of these motor deficits [2]–[4]. This requisite high repetition is problematic, however, because observational data show that clients generally perform a very limited number of movement repetitions in traditional therapy sessions [5]. Furthermore, many logistical, financial, environmental, and individual barriers limit the efficacy of conventional therapy for adults post-stroke [6],[7]. Conse-

quently, research is often focused on optimizing an individual's potential amount of recovery for a given amount of time in therapy. One proposed method for optimizing the effects of therapy is the use of virtual reality (VR). VR can be defined as a type of user-computer interface that implements real-time simulation of an activity or environment allowing user interaction via multiple sensory modalities [8]. VR therapies are an appealing avenue of research because they can provide patients and therapists with additional feedback during therapy, increase patient motivation, and dynamically adjust the difficulty of therapy [9]–[11].

Increasingly, VR therapies have been compared to "usual care" or "conventional therapy" (CT) as sophisticated technologies have become more readily available and affordable. VR therapy refers to a broad class of interventions, but can generally be defined as technological interventions that alter properties of the physical world. These properties might be perceptual, such as providing clients with additional sensory feedback about their movement in a virtual environment (VE). At times, VE training is integrated with exogenous forms of support such as robotic assistance or resistance [12],[13], but we restricted our review to interventions that did not include robotic assistance. Moreover, the advent of movement-controlled videogames such as the Wii (Nintendo), Move (Sony), and Kinect (Microsoft) has also allowed therapists to integrate commercial gaming (CG) systems into therapy. Although only a small number of randomized controlled CG studies exist [14]–[17], CG research is appealing because these interventions offer some of the benefits of VE interventions [18], but have greater availability and a significantly reduced cost. Thus, a major objective for the current review was to quantitatively explore the effectiveness of VE and CG interventions compared to CT.

Previous reviews comparing VR therapy to CT exist [19]–[21], and while they indicate moderate positive benefits of VR therapy, overall there is considerable variability in the observed effects. Potential sources of variability include the type and parameters of intervention, the type of outcome being measured, and the demographics of clients being studied, such as the time from stroke to intervention onset and the initial severity of the motor deficit. This review adds to the current body of knowledge about VR therapy by: (1) including new data comparing VR therapies to CT control groups; (2) exploring how VR therapies affect different outcomes according to the International Classification of Function, Disability, and Health (ICF); and (3) exploring how different types of VR therapy affect outcomes, or more specifically, how custom-built VE systems compare to interventions using CG technology.

Methods

Prior to data collection, the review was registered with the Prospero registry for systematic reviews (#CRD42013004338; http://www.crd.york.ac.uk/NIHR_PROSPERO/). Objectives were defined according to a PICO model (Population, Intervention, Comparison, Outcome). The population of interest was adults post-stroke. Interventions considered were VR therapies that did not include exogenous stimulation (such as functional electrical stimulation) or robotic assistance. Comparison groups included "usual care", "standard care" or "conventional therapy", and could involve physical therapy (PT) and/or occupational therapy (OT). (See Table 1 for a description of control therapies.) Primary and secondary outcomes from all studies were considered, provided that these outcomes were behavioural assessments in one of the ICF domains (i.e., body structure, body function, activity, participation). Self-report measures such as the Motor Activity Log (e.g., Housman et al. [22]) or the ABILIHAND inventory (e.g., Piron et al. [23]) were excluded. Restricting our analysis to behavioural measures of function or impairment that compared VR and conventional therapy makes these outcomes more comparable for the purpose of meta-analysis. Further stratifying these results by ICF classification increases comparability, however there are still concerns about differences in the types of CT provided in control groups. These concerns are discussed below.

Search Strategy

Relevant literature was first identified through electronic searches. A liaison librarian within the Faculty of Medicine at the University of British Columbia was consulted in selecting appropriate databases and developing the search strategy, including identifying key words and medical subject headings (MeSH terms). On April 4, 2013, electronic searches were conducted from the earliest available date in Medline, CINAHL, EMBASE, ERIC, PSYCInfo, DARE, PEDro, the Cochrane Central Register of Controlled Trials, and the Cochrane Database of Systematic Reviews. Population search terms were restricted to stroke and stroke synonyms, and intervention search terms included "video game", "virtual reality", and "augmented reality". Further relevant articles were identified by manually searching the bibliographies of retrieved papers. See Appendix S1 for the full search strategy.

Study Selection

Following removal of duplicate publications, 4512 records were screened for eligibility (See Figure 1). The following exclusion criteria were used to screen the studies: (a) studies of children (<18 years old), (b) studies where fewer than 70% of subjects were adults post-stroke (e.g., studies involving cerebral palsy, traumatic brain injury, and other neurological disorders were excluded), (c) studies that did not use CT control conditions (e.g., studies comparing robotic assistance in combination with virtual reality to robotic assistance alone were excluded), (d) studies that did not use randomization or quasi-randomization with an appropriate control (e.g., case reports, case series, and uncontrolled trials were excluded), and (e) studies not published or translated into English were not searched. (Note, non-English studies were not excluded, but only studies published in English or translated into English were searched. Thus, relevant non-English studies may exist, but were not included, in our search. Despite this last criterion, the pool of included studies was highly international with studies from Canada, USA, Japan, Taiwan, Sweden, Italy, and Brazil.)

One author (CH) screened articles by title and abstract according to these criteria. Next, four authors used these criteria to screen the remaining articles by full text for inclusion. When there was disagreement, authors discussed the articles in question until consensus was reached. A total of 26 trials remained and were included in the assessment of study quality, but two of these articles were subsequently excluded for a lack of necessary data [25],[26], leaving 24 randomized controlled trials (RCTs) in the quantitative analysis.

Quality Assessment

Three authors (CH, KC, ST) assessed the methodological quality of individual studies using the Physiotherapy Evidence Database Scale (PEDro; www.pedro.org.au), a criterion based measure of quality for randomized controlled trials. PEDro assesses 11 criteria to determine the selection, performance, detection, and attrition biases present within a study. For this review's quality assessment, a sample of 5 studies was extracted and all authors provided ratings. Across the 5 studies and 11 items of the PEDro Scale, reviewers had 93% initial agreement. Differences were discussed until 100% agreement was reached and authors proceeded to independently code the remaining studies.

Quantitative Analysis

Three authors (CH, KC, ST) extracted data relevant to sample size, participant characteristics, intervention protocols, and outcome measures. One author (KL) extracted initial statistical data. All statistical data were then corroborated by an additional author; CH, KC, or ST. All calculations were based on data in the published manuscript except in one case [27], where additional

Table 1. Characteristics of trials comparing virtual reality therapy to conventional therapy in adults post-stroke.

Reference	Intervention	VR Intervention	Ctrl Intervention	VR Type	Extracted Outcomes	Outcome Classification
Broeren, 2008 [32]	VE training + CT vs. CT*	3-D computer games with UL unsupported, with rehabilitation personnel	Creative crafts, social and physical activities at activity centre.	VE	BBT, movement time, hand-path ratios	ACT, BF, BF
Cho, 2013 [36]	VE walking + standard therapy vs. CT + standard therapy	Virtual walking training program with video recording, Co-intervention: Standard therapy: Therapeutic exercise, functional therapy, OT, FES	Treadmill gait training Co-intervention: Standard therapy: Therapeutic exercise, functional therapy, OT, FES	VE	BBS, TUG	ACT, ACT
Cikajlo, 2012 [37]	VE balance training vs. CT	VR supported balance training in standing frame, (2 week in clinic & 1 week in home) with PT supervision.	Balance training without VR (in clinic only).	VE	BBS, TUG, 10mWT	ACT, ACT, ACT
Crosbie, 2012 [38]	VE therapy vs. CT	VR tasks focused on UL reaching and grasping with therapist.	Standard UL therapy, including muscle facilitation, stretching, strengthening and functional tasks with PT.	VE	Mobility Index, ARAT	BF, ACT
da Silva Cameirao, 2011 [39]	VE game + Standard Therapy vs. CT + Standard Therapy	Rehabilitation gaming system targeting UL speed, range of motion, grasp and release. Co-intervention: Standard OT & PT.	One of two treatments: 1) Pure occupational therapy targeting object displacement, grasp, and release; or 2) Wii games. Co-intervention: Standard OT & PT.	VE	Mobility Index, FMA, CAHAI	BF, BF, ACT
Gil-Gómez, 2011 [15]	Wii balance board therapy vs. CT	Easy balance VR system with Wii balance board (eBaViR).	Traditional rehabilitation balance exercises individually or in group)	CG	BBS, BBA	ACT, ACT
In, 2012 [40]	VE + Standard Therapy vs. Sham + Standard Therapy	VR reflection therapy for UL movements (with caregiver).	UL movements using unaffected limb (no VR component) (with caregiver).	VE	FMA, BBT, JTHF	BF, ACT, PART
Jung, 2012 [30]	VE treadmill vs. treadmill	VR (with head mounted device) treadmill training.	Treadmill training.	VE	TUG	ACT
Katz, 2005 [41]	VE street-crossing vs. visual training	Desktop VR street-crossing cognitive training.	Computer-based visual scanning tasks.	VE	FIM, VR-performance, Real street crossing.	ACT, ACT, PART
Kihoon, 2012 [34]	VE + Standard Therapy vs. CT*	Interactive Rehabilitation & Exercise System (IREX) VR targeting UL and visual impairments.	Traditional therapy (unspecified).	VE	WMFT, MVPT	ACT, BF
Kim, 2009 [33]	VE + CT vs. CT*	IREX VR balance therapy + CT.	Standard PT, involving neurofacilitation.	VE	BBS, MMAS, 10mWT	ACT, ACT, ACT
Kim, 2012 [14]	Wii games vs. no gaming	Nintendo Wii for balance and motor control + general exercise (unspecified) and electrical stimulation before each session.	General exercise (unspecified) and electrical stimulation before each session.	CG	FIM, PASS, MASS	ACT, BF, BF
Kiper, 2011 [42]	VE therapy vs. CT	Virtual Reality Rehabilitation System (VRRS) training targeting UL functional tasks (turning, pouring, using a hammer, etc.) with PT.	Traditional neuromotor rehabilitation (postural control, in-hand manipulation, fine motor control and coordination) with PT.	VE	FIM, FMA, MAS	ACT, BF, BF
Kwon, 2012 [35]	VE + CT vs. CT*	IREX VR UL training with OT + CT.	Routine OT & PT (gait & balance training, tabletop activities, UL strengthening and functional tasks.	VE	FMA, MFT, MBI	BF, ACT, ACT
Lam, 2006 [43]	VE skills training vs. CT vs. no treatment	2-D VR program targeting various cognitive functions over 10 sessions.	Psychoeducational training (instruction + video modeling) over 10 sessions.	VE	Behavioural assessment of mass transit skills.	PART

Table 1. Cont.

Reference	Intervention	VR Intervention	Ctrl Intervention	VR Type	Extracted Outcomes	Outcome Classification
Mirelman, 2010 [44]	VE training vs. Non-VE training	Rutgers ankle rehabilitation system (robotic gait training with VR stimulation), involving various ankle movements, with therapist.	Ankle movements without VR under therapist supervision.	VE	Gait speed, ankle movement, ankle power	ACT, BF, BF
Piron, 2007 [45]	VE therapy vs. CT	Reinforced feedback in VR environment for UL training with PT.	Conventional UL therapy (unspecified) with PT.	VE	FMA, FIM	BF, ACT
Piron, 2009 [23]	VE tele-rehab vs. CT	VR with telemedicine (VRRS.net) for upper limb training. Therapist supported through videoconferencing.	Conventional UL therapy progressing in complexity from postural control to postural control with complex motion.	VE	FMA, Ashworth Scale	BF, BF
Piron, 2010 [46]	VE therapy vs. CT	Reinforced feedback in VR environment for UL training with therapist.	Conventional UL therapy progressing in complexity with PT.	VE	FMA, FIM	BF, ACT
Saposnik, 2010 [16]	Wii games + Standard therapy vs. table top games + Standard therapy	VR Wii therapy targeting UL. Co-intervention: Conventional OT & PT 1 hr each per day.	Leisure activities, such as playing cards, Bingo, or Jenga. Co-intervention: Conventional OT & PT 1 hr each per day.	CG	WMFT, BBT, SIS (hand items)	ACT, ACT, BF
Subramanian, 2013 [27]	VE training vs. physical training	VR based UL training (reaching for 6 targets).	Reaching for 6 targets in non-VR environment.	VE	WMFT, RPSS (close, far items)	ACT, BF, BF
Yang, 2008 [31]	VE treadmill vs. treadmill	VR based treadmill training designed to simulate typical community in Taipei (lane walking, street crossing, stepping over obstacles).	Treadmill training while executing different tasks (lifting legs to simulate walking over obstacles, uphill, downhill and fast walking).	VE	Gait speed, walking time in community	BF, ACT
Yavuzer, 2008 [17]	Playstation EyeToy games + Standard therapy vs. sham + Standard therapy	Playstation EyeToy games targeting UL movements. Co-intervention: Conventional OT, PT, and SLP.	Watched Playstation EyeToy games but did not play. Co-intervention: Conventional OT, PT, and SLP.	CG	FIM (self care items), Brunnstrom stages (hand, UE items)	ACT, BF, BF
You, 2005 [47]	VE exercise games vs. CT	IREX VR system targeting range of motion, balance, mobility, stepping and ambulation.	No treatment.	VE	FAC, MMAS (walking items)	ACT, ACT

Abbreviations: ACT, activity; ARAT, Action Research Arm Test; BBA, Brunel Balance Assessment; BBS, Berg Balance Scale; BBT, Box and Block Test; BF, body function; CAHAI, Chedoke Arm and Hand Activity Inventory; CG, commercial gaming; CT, conventional therapy; FES, Functional Electrical Stimulation; FIM, Functional Independence Measure; FMA, Fugl-Meyer Assessment; ICF, International Classification of Function, Disability, and Health; JTHF, Jebsen-Taylor Hand Function Test; MBI, Modified Barthel Index; MFT, Manual Function Test; MMAS, Modified Motor Assessment Scale; MSS, Motor Status Scale; MVPT, Motor-free Visual Perception Test; OT, occupational therapy; PART, participation; PASS, Postural Assessment Scale; PT, physiotherapy; RA, robotic assisted therapy; RPSS, Reaching Performance for Stroke Scale; SIS, Stroke Impact Scale; SLP, speech and language therapy; TUG, Time Up-and-Go test; UL, upper limb; VE, virtual environments; VR, virtual reality; WMFT, Wolf Motor Function Test; 10mWT, 10-metre Walk Test.
* = control group was not matched for time to the experimental group.

data was requested and subsequently provided from the original authors.

Multiple outcome variables from each study were extracted in order to conduct separate analyses for each ICF category (see Table 1). Because the dependent measures fell into three ICF categories (viz. body function, activity, participation), each study had to contribute at least one and no more than three outcome variables. Outcomes were selected based on ICF category, and then precedence was given to primary outcomes. Thus, a study could report a body function outcome, an activity outcome, and a participation outcome. Or, if a study reported activity outcomes and two body function outcomes, the body function outcomes would be averaged together to create a single standardized effect size. This method was selected because it allows multiple outcomes to be selected from each study up to the maximum of one

participation, one activity, and one body function outcome, or a maximum of three outcome measures from a single study (if not all ICF categories were measured).

Means, standard deviations, and sample sizes for the experimental group and the control group were entered into an Excel 2010 (Microsoft) spreadsheet and standardized effect-sizes (Hedge's G) and effect-size variability (V_G) were calculated according to Borenstein, Hedges, Higgins, and Rothstein [28]. Effect-size calculations were arranged such that effects favouring VR therapy always had a positive value and effects favouring CT had a negative value. An effect size of zero indicating no difference between VR and CT. (The full dataset is provided in Appendix S2.) Effect-size measures and demographic information were imported into the statistical analysis software R (cran.r-project.org) and analyzed using the "metafor" package [29]. Custom scripts

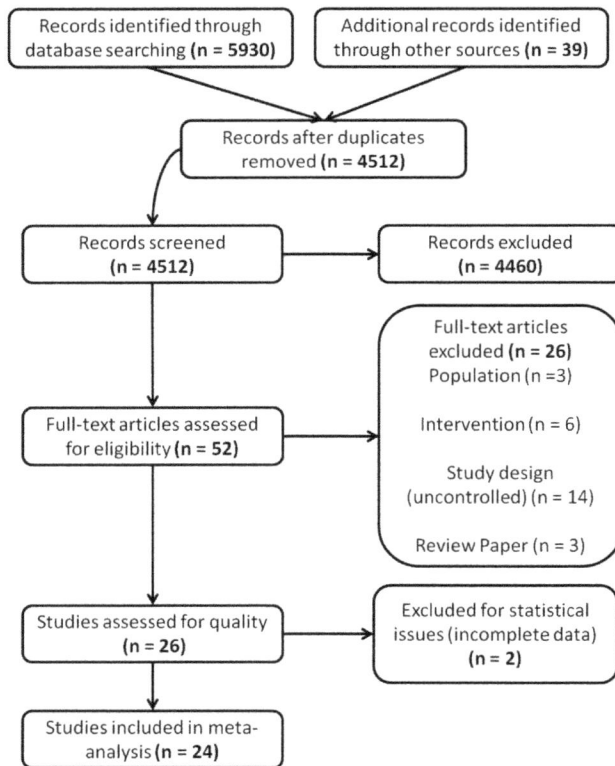

Figure 1. Screening of articles. Four-phase PRISMA flow-diagram for study collection [24], showing the number of studies identified, screened, eligible, and included in the review and analysis.

(Appendix S3) were written to test random-effects models for the overall effect of VR therapy compared to CT and meta-regression models to explore the influence of moderator variables on any VR therapy advantage. In these regressions, we tested the effect VR therapy type (VE versus CG) and the effect of time (in years) from stroke to onset of intervention.

Results

Of the 24 VR studies included in the quantitative analysis, only four studies (16.7%) used CG [14]–[17] and the remaining 20 studies (83.3%) used VE. Often, studies used these VEs in conjunction with another apparatus, such as simulated environments during treadmill walking [30],[31]. In four studies (16.7%) [32]–[35], confounding conditions were present in the experimental methods. In these studies, experimental groups received VE therapy in addition to CT whereas the control group received CT alone, without being matched for time. Consequently, in these four studies, it remains unclear how much of the benefit of therapy can be attributed to the VE versus the additional time in therapy. With respect to the ICF categories that were explored, 32 outcome variables were measures of activity; 24 were measures of body function; and three were measures of participation. See Table 1.

Methodological Quality

PEDro scores for the various studies were moderate, with a mean of 5.42 and SD of 1.60. The number of studies meeting each PEDro criterion is shown in Table 2. Studies generally met criteria for explicitly stating patients' eligibility (88.5%), random allocation

to groups (84.6%), statistical comparisons of treatment and control groups (84.6%), and providing means/SDs for important variables (96.2%). A moderate number of studies met criteria for blinding of assessors (61.5%), achieving follow-up assessments for more than 85% of study participants (76.9%), and having comparable groups determined by baseline measurements (61.5%).

Areas of weakness across studies were concealment of participant allocation (34.6%), blinding of participants (19.2%) and therapists (3.8%) to conditions, and following an intention to treat (ITT) analysis (19.2%). Proper concealment and ITT analysis are particularly important considerations; studies may have actually fulfilled these criteria but lacked explicit description in their Methods sections. Lack of blinding for both participants and therapists was also a limitation of the studies. Although it is not feasible to truly "blind" participants to the fact that they are receiving VR therapy, keeping patients and therapists naive to the experimental hypotheses would be a useful step to add experimental rigour and should be reported if it was achieved. A step further would be to use control conditions that also control for the social context or novelty of the VR therapy. For example, Saposnik and colleagues [16] compared Wii games and CT to a control group who engaged in tabletop games and CT, in an effort to control for the novelty, cognitive demands, and social context of the gaming intervention. Future research should attempt similar controls; the exact nature of these control groups would be dependent on the intervention.

Demographic Characteristics of Included Studies

Sample sizes were quite small in the included studies, ranging from 5 to 40 participants per group (median was 11 participants per group; see Table 3). The intensity (min/day), frequency (days/week) and duration (weeks) of the interventions varied considerably. Interventions across studies ranged from 20-minute sessions [26],[39] to two-five hours of therapy per day (combined VR therapy, occupational and physical therapy) at frequencies of three to five sessions per week [17], and durations from two [16] to 12 weeks [39]. Multiplying intensity × frequency × duration yields total time scheduled for therapy in minutes. For total time, the shortest time scheduled for the VR therapy was 180 min [31] and the longest was 1800 min [45] (the median was 570 min). There was also considerable variability in the average years post-stroke for each study. The shortest average latency between stroke and study onset was 0.04 years [39] and the longest was 6.02 years [31] (the median was 1.05 years). The minimum average age for participants in these studies was 47.45 years and the maximum was 71.37 years (median average age was 61.30 years).

Meta-Analysis: ICF Categories

In order to quantify effects of VR therapy we conducted separate random-effects meta-analyses for each ICF category. Separate analyses were used to ensure that different outcomes from the same study were analyzed independently. When studies had multiple outcomes within the same category (e.g., two activity outcomes) these effect-sizes were averaged together. Thus, each study contributed one data-point (at most) to the body function analysis, the activity analysis, and the participation analysis.

Body Function Outcomes: VE and CG Combined. For body function outcomes combining VE and CG interventions, the overall Hedge's G = 0.48, 95% Confidence Interval = [0.27, 0.70], which was significant, $Z_{obs} = 4.33$, P<0.001. The random-effects model, estimated using restricted maximum likelihood, had a $\tau^2 = 0.05$ (which is the estimate of variance between effects), $I^2 = 24.79\%$ (which is the % of total variability due to heterogeneity), and $H^2 = 1.33$ (which is the proportion of total variability to

Table 2. Studies that meet the criteria of the PEDro scale.

First Author	Year	C1	Selection Bias C2	C3	C4	Performance Bias C5	C6	Detection Bias C7	Attrition Bias C8	C9	C10	C11
Broeren	2008	1	0	0	1	0	0	0	1	0	0	1
Cho	2013	1	1	1	1	0	0	1	1	0	1	1
Cikajlo	2012	1	0	0	0	0	0	1	1	0	1	1
Crosbie	2008	1	1	0	1	0	0	1	1	1	1	0
Crosbie	2012	1	1	1	1	0	0	1	1	1	1	1
da Silva Camiero	2011	1	1	0	0	0	0	1	0	0	1	1
Gil-Gómez	2011	1	1	0	1	0	0	1	1	0	1	1
In	2012	1	1	0	1	0	0	0	0	0	1	1
Jung	2012	1	1	0	0	1	0	1	1	0	1	1
Katz	2005	0	0	0	1	0	0	0	1	0	1	1
Kihoon	2012	1	1	1	1	1	0	0	1	1	0	1
Kim	2011	1	1	0	1	0	0	1	1	0	1	1
Kim	2012	1	1	0	0	0	0	0	0	0	1	1
Kiper	2011	1	1	0	1	0	0	0	1	1	1	1
Kwon	2012	1	1	0	1	1	1	1	1	0	1	1
Lam	2006	1	1	1	1	1	0	0	1	0	0	1
Mirelman	2010	0	1	0	0	1	0	0	1	0	1	1
Piron	2007	0	0	0	0	0	0	0	1	0	0	1
Piron	2009	1	1	1	0	0	0	1	1	0	1	1
Piron	2010	1	1	1	0	0	0	1	1	1	1	1
Saposnik	2010	1	1	0	0	0	0	1	0	0	1	1
Subramanian	2013	1	1	1	1	0	0	1	1	0	1	1
Yang	2008	1	1	1	1	0	0	1	0	0	1	1
Yang	2011	1	1	0	0	0	0	1	0	0	1	1
Yavuzer	2008	1	1	1	1	0	0	1	1	0	1	1
You	2005	1	1	0	1	0	0	0	1	0	1	1

Note. A "1" indicates that a study met that particular criterion, a "0" indicates that a study did not meet that criterion or that not enough information was given to make an assessment. C1 = Eligibility criteria were specified; C2 = Participants were randomly allocated to groups; C3 = Treatment allocation was concealed; C4 = Groups were similar at baseline; C5 = Blinding of participants; C6 = Blinding of therapists administering treatment; C7 = Blinding of assessors for outcome measures; C8 = Measurement of key outcome from >85% of participants; C9 = Intention to treat analysis; C10 = Between-groups statistical comparison is reported for key outcome; C11 = Measures of central tendency and variability are provided. As per PEDro guidelines, the "total" score is based on C2 through C11.

Table 3. Demographic statistics for the included studies.

Reference	VR Type	Time Scheduled for VR Intervention (min)	Experimental Group N	Control Group N	Years Post-Stroke (average)	Average Patient Age (yrs)
Broeren, 2008 [32]	VE	45*3*4 = 540‡	11	11	5.87	NR; range: 44-85
Cho, 2013 [36]	VE	30*3*6 = 540	7	7	0.82	64.85
Cikajlo, 2012 [37]	VE	20*5*3 = 300	6	20	0.36	58.50
Crosbie, 2012 [38]	VE	37.5*3*3 = 337.5	9	9	0.90	60.35
da Silva Cameirao, 2011 [39]	VE	20*3*12 = 720	8	8	0.04	61.37
Gil-Gómez, 2011 [15]	CG	60*20 sessions = 1200	9	8	1.58	47.45
In, 2012 [40]	VE	30*5*4 = 600	11	8	1.11	63.97
Jung, 2012 [30]	VE	30*5*3 = 450	11	10	1.17	62.05
Katz, 2005 [41]	VE	45*3*4 = 540	11	8	0.11	62.85
Kihoon, 2012 [34]	VE	30*3*4 = 360‡	15	14	NR	63.85
Kim, 2009 [33]	VE	30*4*4 = 480‡	12	12	0.07	52.09
Kim, 2012 [14]	CG	30*3*3 = 270	10	10	1.05	48.15
Kiper, 2011 [42]	VE	60*5*4 = 1200	40	40	0.48	64.00
Kwon, 2012 [35]	VE	30*5*4 = 600‡	13	13	0.67	57.54
Lam, 2006 [43]	VE	NR	20	16	4.74	71.37
Mirelman, 2010 [44]	VE	60*3*4 = 720	9	9	>2.00†	62.00
Piron, 2007 [45]	VE	60*5*6 = 1800	25	13	0.22	61.50
Piron, 2009 [23]	VE	60*5*4 = 1200	18	18	1.11	65.20
Piron, 2010 [46]	VE	60*5*4 = 1200	27	20	1.27	60.50
Saposnik, 2010 [16]	CG	60*8 sessions = 480	9	9	0.07	61.30
Subramanian, 2013 [27]	VE	45*3*4 = 540	16	16	3.35	61.00
Yang, 2008 [31]	VE	20*3*3 = 180	9	11	6.01	58.17
Yavuzer, 2008 [17]	CG	30*5*4 = 600	10	10	0.33	61.10
You, 2005 [47]	VE	60*5*4 = 1200	5	5	1.57	57.10

Note. Time scheduled for the VR intervention is given as (min/day) * (days/week) * (weeks) = total time in minutes. NR = 'not reported'.
† = this study did not report an average time post-stroke, so the minimum time was used instead.
‡ = control group was not matched for time to the experimental group.

sampling variability). The test for heterogeneity was not significant, $Q(15) = 21.55$, $P = 0.12$. We tested years post-stroke as a potential moderating factor, but time post-stroke did not significantly affect outcomes ($P = 0.76$). We also tested the type of VR therapy used as a moderating factor (CG interventions were coded as 0 and VE interventions were coded as 1 in the regression), but type of therapy did not significantly affect outcomes ($P = 0.38$). Thus, there was an overall benefit of VR therapy for body function outcomes in adults post-stroke and we found no evidence that this effect was attenuated by the time post-stroke or the type of therapy given. Individual analyses for VE and CG studies are provided below.

Body Function Outcomes: Virtual Environments. For VE studies only (13 studies, 401 total participants, see Figure 2), the overall effect size was $G = 0.43$, 95% CI = [0.22, 0.64], which was significant, $Z_{obs} = 3.97$, $P<0.001$. The random-effects model, estimated using restricted maximum likelihood, had a $\tau^2 = 0.02$, $I^2 = 11.03\%$, and $H^2 = 1.12$. The test for heterogeneity was not significant, $Q(12) = 14.64$, $P = 0.26$.

Body Function Outcomes: Commercial Games. For CG studies only (3 studies, 58 total participants, see Figure 3), the overall effect size was $G = 0.76$, 95% CI = [−0.17, 1.70], which approached significance, $Z_{obs} = 1.60$, $P = 0.10$. The random-effects model, estimated using restricted maximum likelihood,

had a $\tau^2 = 0.45$, $I^2 = 66.30\%$, and $H^2 = 2.97$. The test for heterogeneity approached significance, $Q(2) = 5.85$, $P = 0.05$.

Activity Outcomes: VE and CG Combined. For activity outcomes, the overall effect size was $G = 0.58$, 95% CI = [0.32, 0.85], which was significant, $Z_{obs} = 4.32$, $P<0.001$. The random-effects model had a $\tau^2 = 0.21$, $I^2 = 55.23\%$, and $H^2 = 2.23$. The test for heterogeneity was significant, $Q(21) = 49.18$, $P<0.01$, thus there was significantly more variability in activity outcomes than would be predicted by sampling variability alone. Again, we tested time post-stroke as a moderating factor, but it was not significant ($P = 0.65$). We also tested the type of VR therapy used a moderating factor, but type of therapy did not significantly affect outcomes ($P = 0.66$). Thus, there was an overall benefit of VR therapy for activity outcomes in adults post-stroke and we found no evidence that this effect was attenuated by the time post-stroke or the type of therapy given. Individual analyses for VE and CG studies are provided below.

Activity Outcomes: Virtual Environments. For VE studies only (18 studies, 479 total participants, see Figure 4), the overall effect size was $G = 0.54$, 95% CI = [0.28, 0.81], which was significant, $Z_{obs} = 4.00$, $P<0.001$. The random-effects model, estimated using restricted maximum likelihood, had a $\tau^2 = 0.15$, $I^2 = 49.18\%$, and $H^2 = 1.96$. The test for heterogeneity was significant, $Q(17) = 35.99$, $P<0.01$.

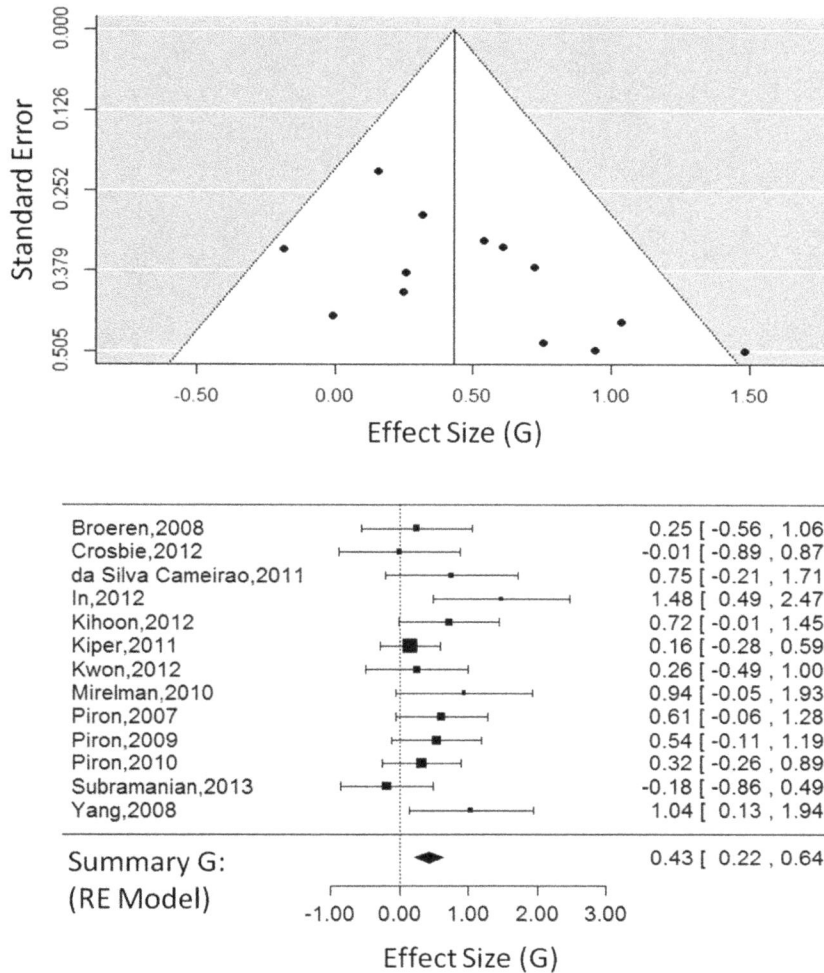

Figure 2. Body function outcomes in VE studies. The funnel plot (top) for body function outcomes showing effect-sizes (G) as a function of precision (standard error) in each virtual environment study. The forest plot (bottom) showing the effect-sizes and 95% confidence intervals for each study and the summary effect-size from the random-effects model. Positive values show a difference in favour of VE therapy. Negative values show a difference in favour of CT. Abbreviations: VE, virtual environments; RE, random effects.

Activity Outcomes: Commercial Gaming. For CG studies only (4 studies, 75 total participants, see Figure 5), the overall effect size was G = 0.76, 95% CI = [−0.25, 1.76], which was not significant, $Z_{obs} = 1.48$, P = 0.14. The random-effects model, estimated using restricted maximum likelihood, had a $\tau^2 = 0.80$, $I^2 = 77.17\%$, and $H^2 = 4.38$. The test for heterogeneity was significant, Q(3) = 12.56, P<0.01.

Participation Outcomes. For participation outcomes (3 studies, 74 total participants, see Figure 6), the overall effect size was G = 0.56, 95% CI = [0.02, 1.10], which was significant, $Z_{obs} = 2.02$, P = 0.04. The random-effects model had a $\tau^2 = 0.06$, $I^2 = 26.75\%$, and $H^2 = 1.37$. The test for heterogeneity was not significant, Q(2) = 2.82, P = 0.24. Also, given the small number of studies in this category, these results should be interpreted with caution. Due to the lack of sufficient data points, we were unable to test the moderating effect of time post-stroke or the effects of different VR interventions (all participation outcomes came from studies using VE interventions). These findings provide preliminary evidence that VR therapy has a positive effect on participation outcomes, but this is an understudied area of research, and more participation outcomes should be included in future studies.

Discussion

This meta-analysis and systematic review is the first to examine the effects of VR across levels of the ICF and to compare effect-sizes as a function of the type of VR therapy implemented. These findings build upon previous reviews that have explored VR therapy compared to CT in general. This review adds to the current body of literature in three key areas: (1) 14 new RCTs have been published since previous reviews and are included in our analysis; (2) this review found positive effects of VR therapy across domains of the ICF; and (3) VR therapies were found to be effective when delivered as VE or CG. In the current analysis, time post-stroke and the type of VR intervention were not found to significantly affect outcomes. However, the small number of CG studies all had poor precision (shown in Figures 3 and 5), so larger trials with carefully designed control groups using CG interventions are needed before conclusions can be drawn about the efficacy of CG interventions.

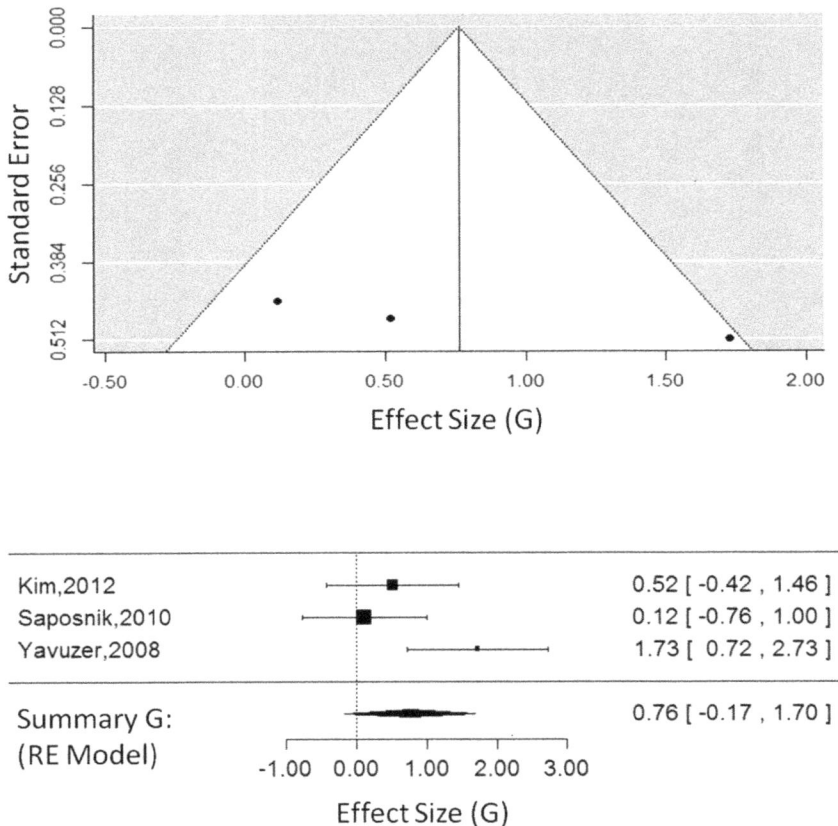

Figure 3. Body function outcomes in CG studies. The funnel plot (top) for body function outcomes showing effect-sizes (G) as a function of precision (standard error) in each commercial gaming study. The forest plot (bottom) showing the effect-sizes and 95% confidence intervals for each study and the summary effect-size from the random-effects model. Positive values show a difference in favour of CG therapy. Negative values show a difference in favour of CT. Abbreviations: CG, commercial gaming; RE, random effects.

Review identifies new trials

The most recent previous reviews summarizing the evidence for VR therapy included searches of the literature up to March and July 2010 [19],[20]. Fourteen trials (58.3%) included in our review were published after 2010 and had not yet been included in a meta-analysis. Furthermore, previous reviews [19] included observational studies, whereas we selected only randomized controlled trials to ensure robustness of the evidence. All previous reviews of this topic have demonstrated a moderate effect in favour of VR therapy over CT [19]–[21] however, the heterogeneity of trial parameters requires that all effect sizes and conclusions be interpreted with caution. Similarly, our review suggests VR therapy has a moderate effect on outcomes for adults after stroke, but many sources of variability exist in the interventions and outcomes of the included trials.

Sources of variability within interventions

There was considerable variability in how VR interventions were delivered with respect to intensity, frequency and duration of the intervention. VR interventions were also inconsistently conducted in conjunction with other PT/OT treatments. As such, we are unable to comment on optimal prescribing dosage for VR therapies.

Studies lacked detail about the content of the CT being compared to VR. Studies were inconsistent in their reporting of the role(s) of therapists, rehabilitation assistants, caregivers, and/or other personnel; future research should ensure sufficient information is given to readers to allow for accurate comparisons. Individual studies did often schedule equal time in therapy for experimental and control groups, but most studies did not ensure true dosage matching of groups (e.g., matching active time in therapy or numbers of repetitions). Subramanian and colleagues [27] explicitly matched arm-reaching repetitions between the experimental and control groups, and they also controlled for the amount of feedback (knowledge of results and performance) provided. Repetitions were controlled in that study, and there was no overall benefit of VR therapy beyond CT. However, VR training did lead to larger improvements in participants with mild impairments compared to CT, and VR training reduced compensatory movements in moderate-to-severely impaired participants compared to CT. Future studies should use similar methods for controlling repetitions when investigating VR therapies to clarify our understanding of the benefits of VR in therapy.

Another source of variability could be the degree to which participants felt motivated and engaged during therapy. It has been suggested that VR therapies are advantageous to CT in part because of the motivating influence of using novel technologies or games [10],[11]. Unfortunately, most of the trials included in this review do not discuss motivation, use motivation as an outcome measure, or control for the motivating or novel components of VR therapy. Some studies did attempt to control for this factor using

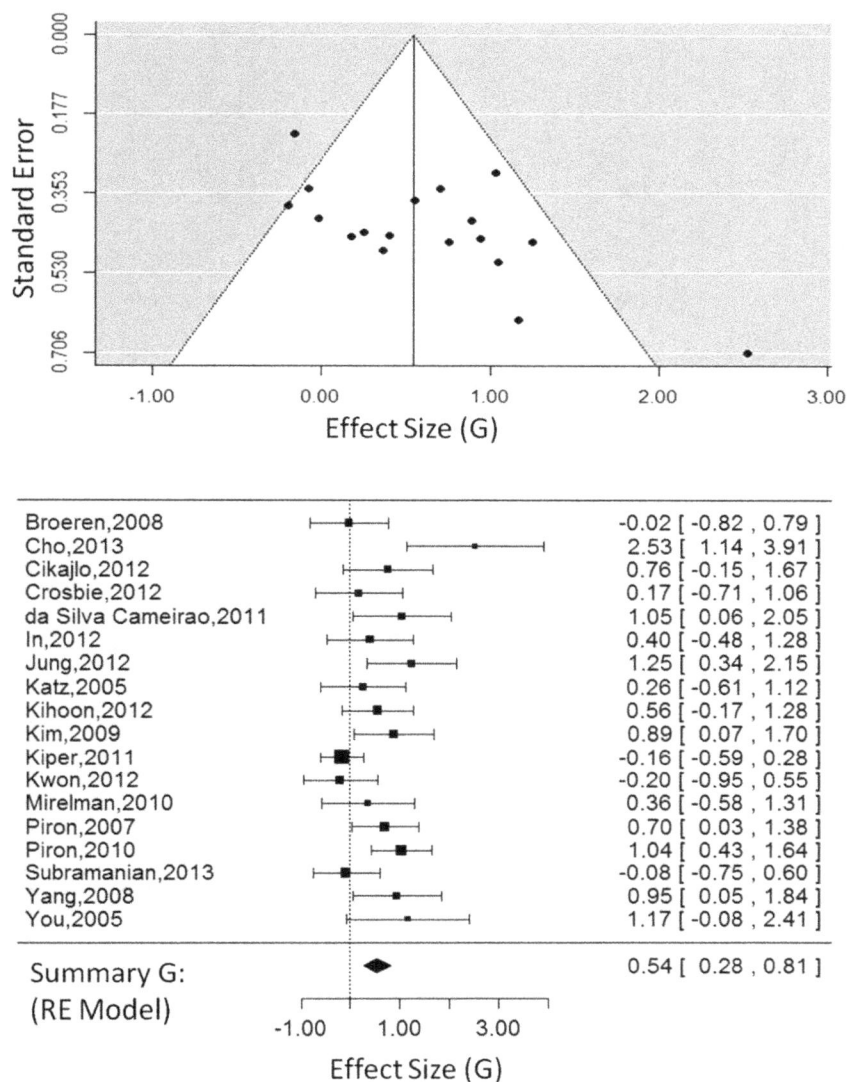

Figure 4. Activity outcomes in VE studies. The funnel plot (top) for activity outcomes showing effect-sizes (G) as a function of precision (standard error) in each virtual environment study. The forest plot (bottom) shows the effect-sizes and 95% confidence intervals for each study and the summary effect-size from the random-effects model. Positive values show a difference in favour of VE therapy. Negative values show a difference in favour of CT. Abbreviations: RE, random effects.

card games [16] or cognitive computer games [33] in their control group. Arguably, interactive video games may still be considered more novel to an older population.

No differences found for VR therapy types

A major objective of our review was to compare the effects of commercial gaming systems (CG) to rehabilitation-specific virtual environments (VE) in a therapy context for adults post-stroke. We found no evidence for differences between VE and CG games in the current analysis, but CG interventions have been too few and too small to draw conclusions. Four trials (16.7%) examined the effects of CG therapy [14]–[17] and 20 trials (83.3%) researched VE therapy compared to CT for adults post-stroke. Our meta-analysis provides strong evidence for the effectiveness of VE interventions and demonstrates promising initial data for the effectiveness of CG interventions. More data needs to be collected to see if gains for CG interventions are reliable and to see if the

moderate effect-sizes observed (from $G = 0.4$–0.7) translate into clinically meaningful results. These results suggest larger RCTs using CG interventions are justified; we recommend RCTs compare CG directly to VE and CT groups.

Movement-controlled games are increasingly investigated as therapeutic tools for individuals with neurological disorders such as cerebral palsy [48] and stroke [49]. An appealing aspect of movement-controlled games is combining aerobic exercise and motor skills practice, which may increase neuroplasticity during motor rehabilitation [50]. As a result, commercial games have been investigated as tools for learning motor skills and for improving cardiovascular fitness. For example, the game Dance Dance Revolution has been shown to increase energy expenditure in adolescents up to 5.4 (1.8 SD) Metabolic Equivalent Tasks (METs) [51]. In healthy adults, Wii Sports tennis requires 2.1 (1.2 SD) METs, baseball 2.8 (0.9 SD) METs, and boxing 4.7 (1.4 SD) METs [48]. However, in adults with cerebral palsy, the same

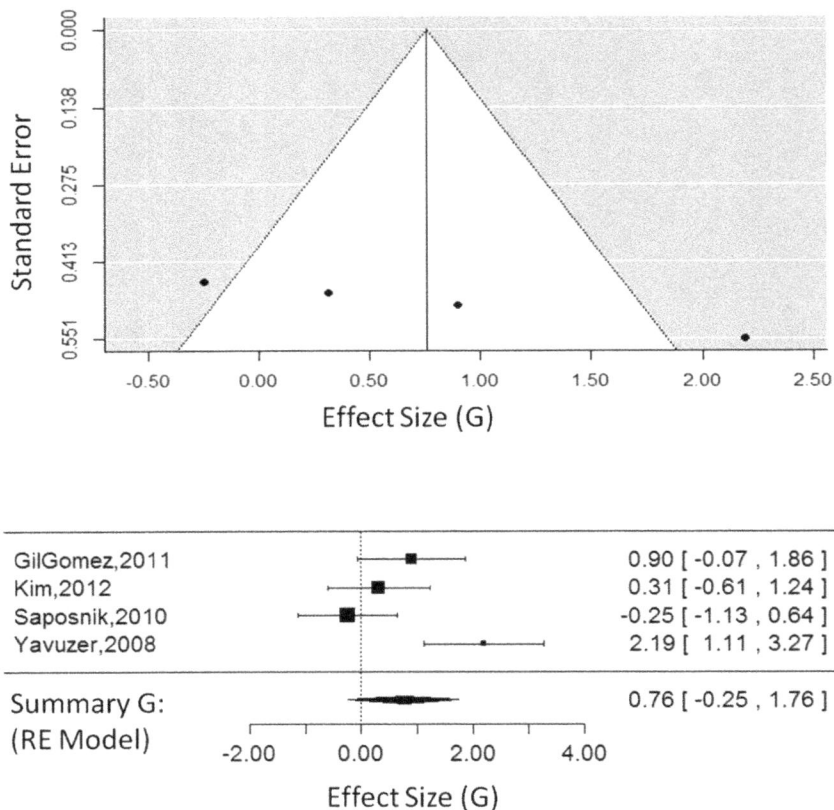

Figure 5. Activity outcomes in CG studies. The funnel plot (top) for activity outcomes showing effect-sizes (G) as a function of precision (standard error) in each commercial gaming study. The forest plot (bottom) shows the effect-sizes and 95% confidence intervals for each study and the summary effect-size from the random-effects model. Positive values show a difference in favour of CG therapy. Negative values show a difference in favour of CT. Abbreviations: CG, commercial gaming; RE, random effects.

games all increase energy expenditure to over 3 METs [48], suggesting they can help these individuals meet recommended guidelines for physical activity. In addition to increasing energy expenditures, commercial movement games have been used therapeutically to improve balance, strength and coordination [49],[52].

Increased availability and lower cost are also potential advantages of using commercial games over virtual reality systems that have been designed specifically for rehabilitation. For example, the Nintendo Wii (Nintendo Co., Kyoto, JP) has been sold to over 100 million customers worldwide [53], and the console retails below US$150. As a comparison, the GestureTek IREX (GestureTek, Toronto, CA) system, used in the study by Kwon et al. in 2012 [35], is only available through specialized rehabilitation equipment distributors and retails at more than US$15,000 [54]. Understanding the benefits of CG and VE systems, relative to their costs, thus has significant implications for therapists and clients facing budget constraints.

Positive effects of VR therapy across ICF categories

The ICF provides a framework and a comprehensive perspective of functioning and disability in research and clinical practice [55]. The overarching goal of rehabilitation for adults post-stroke is to restore the person's ability to participate in normal life roles with as much independence as possible. Impairments at the body structure and function level may influence activity limitations, and activity limitations may influence participation restrictions [56].

However, impairments and activity limitations do not necessarily affect the enjoyment of participation by individuals in various life situations [57],[58]. It is, therefore, important for researchers and clinicians to be clear about which ICF domains an intervention intends to, and actually does, impact.

Our review did not identify any trials that examined outcomes related to body structures, personal factors, or environmental factors and only three trials (12.5%) that examined participation outcomes. There was a moderate but reliable advantage of VR therapy over CT in the categories of body function and activity, but outcomes from other ICF categories should be included in future research.

Limitations

Our review included studies conducted in all stages of stroke recovery, from acute inpatient to chronic outpatient settings (average time post-stroke of the study participants ranged from 0.04 years [39] to 6.02 years [31]). However, our analysis was based on a small number of studies making statistical power a concern for these regression analyses. Furthermore, the small number of studies limits our ability to control for other moderating factors such as the initial severity of stroke and the effect of time post-stroke on conventional therapy outcomes.

This review is limited by some risk of publication bias in the included studies. Visual inspection of the funnel plots in the figures reveals highly positive studies with low precision for both activity and body function outcomes. For activity outcomes, two outlying

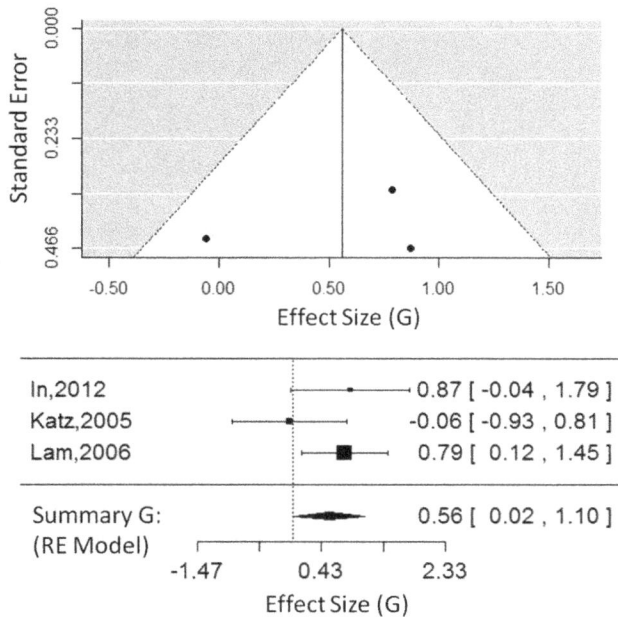

Figure 6. Participation outcomes in VE studies. The funnel plot (top) for participation outcomes showing effect-sizes (G) as a function of precision (standard error) in each study. The forest plot (bottom) shows the effect-sizes and 95% confidence intervals for each study and the summary effect-size from the random-effects model. Positive values show a difference in favour of VE therapy. Negative values show a difference in favour of CT. Abbreviations: VE, virtual environments; RE, random effects.

Conclusions

This review updated the evidence for virtual reality therapy to include the most recent trials, and is the first to investigate the effects of VR therapy across ICF domains and between VR therapy types. Virtual reality therapy demonstrates a significant moderate advantage in body function and activity outcomes when compared to CT. Research on participation outcomes is limited, but initial data show a positive benefit of VR therapy compared to CT. No significant differences were found between the VE and CG therapy types, and there was no evidence that time post-stroke attenuated the benefits of VR therapy, but these findings are limited by a high degree of variability between studies. To date, CG interventions have been too few and too small to draw strong conclusions about their efficacy. Larger RCTs investigating CG interventions would provide better evidence for their use in therapy as a potentially effective and cost-efficient method of increasing motor repetitions in a motivating way. Given the relationship between participation and quality of life, it is also recommended that future trials include participation outcome measures in their investigations.

Author Contributions

Conceived and designed the experiments: KRL. Performed the experiments: KRL CGEH KLC ST. Analyzed the data: KRL CGEH KLC ST. Wrote the paper: KRL CGEH KLC ST HFMVdL.

studies (8.3%) [17],[36] had small numbers of subjects (N = 20 and 14, respectively) but relatively good study quality (7/10 for both studies on PEDro criteria). Similarly for body function outcomes, two studies (8.3%) [17],[40] had small numbers of subjects (N = 20 and 19, respectively) and while Yavuzer et al. [17] had good study quality (7/10), In et al. [40] had poor study quality (4/10).

References

1. Nichols-Larsen DS, Clark PC, Zeringue A, Greenspan A, Blanton S (2005) Factors influencing stroke survivors' quality of life during subacute recovery. Stroke 36(7):1480–4.
2. Nudo RJ, Milliken GW (1996) Reorganization of movement representations in primary motor cortex following focal ischemic infarcts in adult squirrel monkeys. J Neurophysiol 75(5):2144–9.
3. Plautz EJ, Milliken GW, Nudo RJ (2000) Effects of repetitive motor training on movement representations in adult squirrel monkeys: role of use versus learning. Neurobiol Learn Mem Jul;74(1):27–55.
4. Kwakkel G (2006) Impact of intensity of practice after stroke: Issues for consideration. Disabil Rehabil 28(July):823–30.
5. Lang CE, Macdonald JR, Reisman DS, Boyd L, Jacobson Kimberley T, et al. (2009) Observation of amounts of movement practice provided during stroke rehabilitation. Arch Phys Med Rehabil 90(10):1692–8.
6. Langhorne P, Coupar F, Pollock A (2009) Motor recovery after stroke: a systematic review. Lancet Neurol 8(8):741–54.
7. Foley N, Teasell R, Bhogal S, Speechley M (2003) The efficacy of stroke rehabilitation. Top Stroke Rehabil 10(2):1–18.
8. Adamovich SV, Fluet GG, Tunik E, Merians AS (2009) Sensorimotor training in virtual reality: a review. NeuroRehabilitation 25: 29–44.
9. Mirelman A, Bonato P, Deutsch JE (2009) Effects of training with a robot-virtual reality system compared with a robot alone on the gait of individuals after stroke. Stroke 40(1):169–74.
10. Burke JW, McNeill MDJ, Charles DK, Morrow PJ, Crosbie JH, et al. (2009) Optimising engagement strategies for stroke rehabilitation using serious games. Visual Computing 25: 1085–99.
11. Shirzad N, Van der Loos HFM (2012) Error amplification to promote motor learning and motivation in therapy robotics. In: Proceedings of the Annual International Conference of the IEEE Engineering in Medicine and Biology Society: 2012 Aug 28 - Sep 1; San Diego, USA: IEEE Engineering in Medicine and Biology Society.
12. Deutsch JE, Merians AS, Adamovich S, Poizner H, Burdea GC (2004) Development and application of virtual reality technology to improve hand use and gait of individuals post-stroke. Restor Neurol Neurosci 22(3–5):371–386.
13. Patton J, Dawe G, Scharver C, Mussa-Ivaldi F, Kenyon R (2006) Robotics and virtual reality: a perfect marriage for motor control research and rehabilitation. Assist Technol 18: 181–195.
14. Kim EK, Kang JH, Park JS, Jung BH (2012) Clinical feasibility of interactive commercial nintendo gaming for chronic stroke rehabilitation. J Phys Ther Sci 24: 901–3.
15. Gil-Gómez J-A, Lloréns R, Alcañiz M, Colomer C (2011) Effectiveness of a Wii balance board-based system (eBaViR) for balance rehabilitation: a pilot randomized clinical trial in patients with acquired brain injury. J Neuroeng Rehabil 8(1):30.
16. Saposnik G, Teasell R, Mamdani M, Hall J, Mcilroy W, et al. (2010) Effectiveness of virtual reality using Wii gaming technology in stroke rehabilitation. Stroke 1477–84.
17. Yavuzer G, Senel A, Atay MB, Stam HJ (2008) "Playstation eyetoy games" improve upper extremity-related motor functioning in subacute stroke: a randomized controlled clinical trial. Eur J Phys Rehabil Med 44(3):237–44.
18. Lohse KR, Shirzad N, Verster A, Hodges NJ, Van der Loos HFM (2013) Videogames and rehabilitation: Using design principles to enhance patient engagement. J Neurol Phys Ther 37: 166–175.

19. Saposnik G, Levin M (2011) Virtual reality in stroke rehabilitation: a meta-analysis and implications for clinicians. Stroke 42(5):1380–6.

20. Laver K, George S, Thomas S, Deutsch JE, Crotty M (2011) Virtual reality for stroke rehabilitation. Stroke 43(2):e20–e21.

21. Henderson A, Korner-Bitensky N, Levin M, (2007) Virtual reality in stroke rehabilitation: a systematic review of its effectiveness for upper limb motor recovery. Top Stroke Rehabil 14(2):52–61.

22. Housman SJ, Scott KM, Reinkensmeyer DJ (2009) A randomized controlled trial of gravity-supported, computer-enhanced arm exercise for individuals with severe hemiparesis. Neurorehabil Neural Repair 23(5):505–14.

23. Piron L, Turolla A, Agostini M, Zucconi C, Cortese F, et al. (2009) Exercises for paretic upper limb after stroke: a combined virtual-reality and telemedicine approach. J Rehabil Med 41(12):1016–102.

24. Moher D (2009) Preferred reporting items for systematic reviews and meta-analyses: The PRISMA statement. Ann Intern Med 151(4):264.

25. Crosbie JH, Lennon S, Mcgoldrick MC, Mcneill MDJ, Burke JW, et al. (2008) Virtual reality in the rehabilitation of the upper limb after hemiplegic stroke: a randomised pilot study. Clin Rehabil 229–35.

26. Yang S, Hwang W-H, Tsai Y-C, Liu F-K, Hsieh L-F, et al. (2011) Improving balance skills in patients who had stroke through virtual reality treadmill training. Am J Phys Med Rehabil 90(12):969–78.

27. Subramanian SK, Lourenço CB, Chilingaryan G, Sveistrup H, Levin MF (2013) Arm motor recovery using a virtual reality intervention in chronic stroke: randomized control trial. Neurorehabil Neural Repair 27(1):13–23.

28. Borenstein M, Hedges L V., Higgins JPT, Rothstein HR (2011) Introduction to meta-analysis [eBook online]. John Wiley & Sons [cited 2013 Jul 20]. p. 450. Available from: URL: http://books.google.com/books?hl = en&lr = &id = JQg 9jdrq26wC&pgis = 1

29. Viechtbauer W (2010) Conducting meta-analyses in R with the metafor Package. J Stat Softw 36(3):1–48.

30. Jung J (2012) Effects of virtual-reality treadmill training on balance and balance self efficacy in stroke patients with a history of falling. J Phys Ther Sci 24(5):1133–6.

31. Yang Y-R, Tsai M-P, Chuang T-Y, Sung W-H, Wang R-Y (2008) Virtual reality-based training improves community ambulation in individuals with stroke: a randomized controlled trial. Gait Posture 28(2):201–6.

32. Broeren J, Claesson L, Goude D, Rydmark M, Sunnerhagen KS (2008) Virtual rehabilitation in an activity centre for community-dwelling persons with stroke. The possibilities of 3-dimensional computer games. Cerebrovasc Dis 26(3):289–96.

33. Kim JH, Jang SH, Kim CS, Jung JH, You JH (2009) Use of virtual reality to enhance balance and ambulation in chronic stroke: a double-blind, randomized controlled trial. Am J Phys Med Rehabil 88(9):693–701.

34. Kihoon J (2012) Effects of virtual reality-based rehabilitation on upper extremity function and visual perception in stroke patients: A randomized control trial. J Phys Ther Sci 24: 1205–8.

35. Kwon J-S, Park M-J, Yoon I-J, Park S-H (2012) Effects of virtual reality on upper extremity function and activities of daily living performance in acute stroke: a double-blind randomized clinical trial. NeuroRehabil 31(4):379–85.

36. Cho KH, Lee WH (2013) Virtual walking training program using a real-world video recording for patients with chronic stroke: a pilot study. Am J Phys Med Rehabil 92(5):371–84.

37. Cikajlo I, Rudolf M, Goljar N, Burger H, Matjačić Z (2012) Telerehabilitation using virtual reality task can improve balance in patients with stroke. Disabil Rehabil 34(1):13–8.

38. Crosbie JH, Lennon S, McGoldrick MC, McNeill MDJ, McDonough SM (2012) Virtual reality in the rehabilitation of the arm after hemiplegic stroke: a randomized controlled pilot study. Clin Rehabil 26(9):798–806.

39. Da Silva Cameirão M, Bermúdez I, Badia S, Duarte E, Verschure PF (2011) Virtual reality based rehabilitation speeds up functional recovery of the upper extremities after stroke: a randomized controlled pilot study in the acute phase of stroke using the rehabilitation gaming system. Restor Neurol Neurosci 29(5):287–98.

40. In TS, Jung KS, Lee SW, Song CH (2012) Virtual reality reflection therapy improves motor recovery and motor function in the upper extremities of people with chronic stroke. J Phys Ther Sci 24(4):339–43.

41. Katz N, Ring H, Naveh Y, Kizony R, Feintuch U, et al. (2005) Interactive virtual environment training for safe street crossing of right hemisphere stroke patients with unilateral spatial neglect. Disabil Rehabil 27(20):1235–43.

42. Kiper P, Piron L, Turolla A, Sto J, Tonin P (2011) The effectiveness of reinforced feedback in virtual environment in the first 12 months after stroke. Neurol Neurochir Pol 436–44.

43. Lam YS, Man DWK, Tam SF, Weiss PL (2006) Virtual reality training for stroke rehabilitation. NeuroRehabil 21(3):245–53.

44. Mirelman A, Patritti BL, Bonato P, Deutsch JE (2010) Effects of virtual reality training on gait biomechanics of individuals post-stroke. Gait Posture 31(4):433–7.

45. Piron L, Tombolini P, Turolla A, Zucconi C, Agostini M, et al. (2007) Reinforced feedback in virtual environment facilitates the arm motor recovery in patients after a recent stroke. In: Virtual Rehabilitation [serial online]. 2007 Sep 27–29; Venice, Italy. 2007. p 121–3. Available from: URL: http://ieeexplore.ieee.org/lpdocs/epic03/wrapper.htm?arnumber = 4362151

46. Piron L, Turolla A, Agostini M, Tonin P, Dam M (2010) Motor learning principles for rehabilitation: A pilot randomized controlled study in poststroke patients. Neurorehabil Neural Repair 24(6):501–8.

47. You SH, Jang SH, Kim Y-H, Hallett M, Ahn SH, et al. (2005) Virtual reality-induced cortical reorganization and associated locomotor recovery in chronic stroke: an experimenter-blind randomized study. Stroke 36(6):1166–71.

48. Taylor MJD, McCormic D, Shawis T, Impson R, Griffin M (2011) Activity-promoting gaming systems in exercise and rehabilitation. J Rehabil Res Dev 48(10):1171–1186.

49. Deutsch JE, Brettler A, Smith C, Welsh J, John R, et al. (2011) Nintendo Wii Sports and Wii Fit game analysis, validation, and application to stroke rehabilitation. Top Stroke Rehabil 18(6):701–19.

50. Mang CS, Campbell KL, Ross CJD, Boyd LA (2013) Promoting neuroplasticity for motor rehabilitation after stroke: Considering the effects of aerobic exercise and genetic variation on brain-derived neurotrophic factor. Phys Ther [online first] [cited 2013 Sep 14]. Available from: URL: http://ptjournal.apta.org/content/early/2013/07/31/ptj.20130053

51. Bailey BW, McInnis K (2001) Energy cost of exergaming: A comparison of the energy cost of 6 forms of exergaming. Arch Pediatr Adolesc Med 165(7):597–602.

52. Agmon M, Perry CK, Phelan E, Demiris G, Nguyen HQ (2011) A pilot study of Wii Fit exergames to improve balance in older adults. J Geriatr Phys Ther 34: 161–7.

53. Nintendo Co., Ltd. Consolidated sales transition by region. Nintendo Web site: http://www.nintendo.co.jp/ir/library/historical_data/pdf/consolidated_sales_e1306.pdf. Accessed August 21, 2013.

54. Flaghouse.ca. GestureTek IREX systems. Flaghouse.ca Web site: http://www.flaghouse.ca/itemdy00.asp?T1 = 39081. Accessed August 21, 2013.

55. World Health Organization (2002) Towards a common language for functioning, disability and health. World Health Organization Web site: http://www.who.int/classifications/icf/training/icfbeginnersguide.pdf. Accessed September 14, 2013.

56. Sullivan KJ, Cen SY (2011) Model of Disablement and Recovery: Knowledge translation in rehabilitation research and practice. Phys Ther 91: 1892–1904.

57. Harding J, Harding K, Jamieson P, Mullally M, Politi C, et al. (2009) Children with disabilities' perceptions of activity participation and environments: A pilot study. Can J Occup Ther 76(3):133–144.

58. Majnemer A, Shevall M, Law M, Birnbaum R, Chilingaryan G, et al. (2008) Participation and enjoyment of leisure activities in school- aged children with cerebral palsy. Dev Med Child Neurol 50: 751–758.

15

Effect of Transcranial Direct-Current Stimulation Combined with Treadmill Training on Balance and Functional Performance in Children with Cerebral Palsy: A Double-Blind Randomized Controlled Trial

Natália de Almeida Carvalho Duarte[1]*, Luanda André Collange Grecco[2], Manuela Galli[3], Felipe Fregni[4], Cláudia Santos Oliveira[5]

1 Master Program in Rehabilitation Sciences, Movement Analysis Lab, University Nove de Julho, São Paulo, São Paulo, Brazil, 2 Doctoral Program in Rehabilitation Sciences, Movement Analysis Lab, University Nove de Julho, São Paulo, São Paulo, Brazil, 3 Dept. of Electronic Information and Bioengineering, Politecnico di Milano and IRCCS San Raffaele Pisana, Rome, 4 Laboratory of Neuromodulation & Center of Clinical Research Learning, Department of Physical Medicine & Rehabilitation, Spaulding Rehabilitation Hospital and Massachusetts General Hospital, Harvard Medical School, Boston, MA, United States of America, 5 Professor, Master and Doctoral Programs in Rehabilitation Sciences, Movement Analysis Lab, University Nove de Julho, São Paulo, São Paulo, Brazil

Abstract

Background: Cerebral palsy refers to permanent, mutable motor development disorders stemming from a primary brain lesion, causing secondary musculoskeletal problems and limitations in activities of daily living. The aim of the present study was to determine the effects of gait training combined with transcranial direct-current stimulation over the primary motor cortex on balance and functional performance in children with cerebral palsy.

Methods: A double-blind randomized controlled study was carried out with 24 children aged five to 12 years with cerebral palsy randomly allocated to two intervention groups (blocks of six and stratified based on GMFCS level (levels I-II or level III).The experimental group (12 children) was submitted to treadmill training and anodal stimulation of the primary motor cortex. The control group (12 children) was submitted to treadmill training and placebo transcranial direct-current stimulation. Training was performed in five weekly sessions for 2 weeks. Evaluations consisted of stabilometric analysis as well as the administration of the Pediatric Balance Scale and Pediatric Evaluation of Disability Inventory one week before the intervention, one week after the completion of the intervention and one month after the completion of the intervention. All patients and two examiners were blinded to the allocation of the children to the different groups.

Results: The experimental group exhibited better results in comparison to the control group with regard to anteroposterior sway (eyes open and closed; $p<0.05$), mediolateral sway (eyes closed; $p<0.05$) and the Pediatric Balance Scale both one week and one month after the completion of the protocol.

Conclusion: Gait training on a treadmill combined with anodal stimulation of the primary motor cortex led to improvements in static balance and functional performance in children with cerebral palsy.

Trial Registration: Ensaiosclinicos.gov.br/RBR-9B5DH7

Editor: Barry J. Byrne, Earl and Christy Powell University, United States of America

Funding: The authors gratefully acknowledge financial support from the Brazilian fostering agencies Conselho Nacional de Desenvolvimento Científico e Tecnológico (CNPq), Coordenação de Aperfeiçoamento de Pessoal de Nível Superior (CAPES), and Fundação de Amparo á Pesquisa (FAPESP - 2012/24019-0). The funders had no role in study design, data collection and analysis, decision to publish, or preparation of the manuscript.

Competing Interests: The authors have declared that no competing interests exist.

* Email: natycarvalho_fisio@hotmail.com

Introduction

Cerebral palsy (CP) involves a set of neurophysiological impairments caused by a global reduction in subcortical activity that compromises the activity of corticospinal and somatosensory circuits [1], [2], [3], [4], [5], [6]. CP results in diminished activation of the central nervous system during the execution of movements [4]. A reduction in motor cortex excitability in children is associated with poor motor development [7]. Neurophysiological analyses have demonstrated global changes in cortex excitability in children with CP, even when the brain lesion is unilateral [8]. Such children have postural problems due to spasticity, muscle weakness and impaired muscle coordination. These postural problems can also affect motor development, leading to difficulties in performing basic functional actions, such as sitting, standing and walking [9], [10], [11], [12].

Adequate postural control involves a complex network of sensory and motor information. The integration of subcortical systems, such as the vestibular, sensorial and visual systems, is fundamental to the maintenance of balance. Moreover, posture is maintained through the combined efforts of the sensory motor cortex, supplementary motor area and pre-motor cortex [13].

While there is no cure for the brain lesion in CP, the manifestations of this condition can be minimized through neurorehabilitation [14]. Studies involving the administration of functional magnetic resonance on children with CP have demonstrated that rehabilitation resources are capable of promoting the activation of the primary motor cortex (M1) [14]. M1 is an important area of the brain that facilitates cerebral reorganization. Through a better understanding of the relationship between neuropathology and clinical function in CP, interventions can be individualized based on the neurological substrate available for recuperation, thereby maximizing the efficacy of the therapeutic process [15].

Recent studies have reported the benefits of gait training on a treadmill. Grecco et al. describe the positive effects of treadmill training in comparison to over-ground gait training on static and functional balance. The effects were found after 12 sessions of training at the aerobic threshold without body weight support. The benefits included an improvement in functional performance, suggesting that the motor effects can lead to greater independence in children with CP [10],[11].

Marchese et al. [16] suggest that repetitive sensory stimulation may favor the activation of important mechanisms that facilitate the motor learning process. Thus, like treadmill training, motor training may favor proprioceptive feedback, leading to adjustments for adequate postural balance and functional performance.

Transcranial direct-current stimulation (tDCS) is a safe, low-cost resource that can be used during motor therapy sessions and involves the administration of a weak electrical current to the scalp using sponge electrodes moistened with saline solution. The effects of stimulation are achieved by the movement of electrons due to electrical charges. The two poles are the anode (positive) and cathode (negative) electrodes. The electrical current flows from the positive pole to the negative pole, penetrating the skull and reaching the cortex, with different effects on biological tissues. Although most of the current is dissipated among the overlying tissues, a sufficient amount reaches the structures of the cortex and changes of membrane potential of the surrounding cells [17],[18]. tDCS is known to induce lasting changes in cortex excitability in both animals and humans. In rehabilitation processes, the aim of tDCS is to enhance local synaptic efficiency, thereby altering the maladaptive plasticity pattern that emerges following a cortex lesion. Stimulation is used to modulate the cortex activity by opening a pathway to increase and prolong functional gains achieved in physical therapy [19].

The authors believe that the combination of tDCS of the primary motor cortex and treadmill training can potentiate the effects on static balance. The hypothesis is that tDCS leads to the maintenance of the results following the interruption of the gait training protocol by inducing long-lasting changes in cortex excitability, thereby facilitating the learning process.

The aims of the present study were to determine the effects of tDCS applied over the primary motor cortex during ten sessions of treadmill gait training on balance and functional performance in children with PC and investigate whether the effects are maintained one month after the completion of the training sessions.

Materials and Methods

Ethics Statement

The protocol for this trial and supporting CONSORT checklist are available as supporting information; see Checklist S1 and Protocol S1. This study received approval from the Human Research Ethics Committee of the University Nove de Julho (Brazil) under process number 69803/2012 and was carried out in compliance with the ethical standards established by the Declaration of Helsinki. The study is registered with the Brazilian Registry of Clinical Trials under process number RBR-9B5DH7 (URL:http://www.ensaiosclinicos. gov.br/rg/RBR-9b5dh7/). There was a delay in releasing the record number for our study. To avoid delays in the conduct of the project or even loss of the sample, the recruitment of the sample was performed according to the previous schedule of the study. The authors confirm that all ongoing and related trials for this intervention are registered. All parents/guardians agreed to the participation of the children by signing a statement of informed consent.

Design

Full details about the trial protocol have previously been reported [20] and can be found in the supplementary appendix, available at http://www.biomedcentral.com. A phase II, prospective, analytical, double-blind, randomized, placebo-controlled clinical trial was carried out. Figure 1 presents the CONSORT [21] flow chart of the study.

Sample

The study took place at the Movement Analysis Lab, University Nove de Julho, Sao Paulo, Brazil, from November 2012 to September 2013. Twenty-nine children with CP were recruited from specialized outpatient clinics, from the physical therapy clinics of the University Nove de Julho and Center for Pediatric Neurosurgery, São Paulo, Brazil. The following were the inclusion criteria: diagnosis of spastic CP; classification on levels I, II or III of the Gross Motor Function Classification System (GMFCS); independent gait for at least 12 months; age between five and ten years; and degree of comprehension compatible with the execution of the procedures. The following were the exclusion criteria: history of surgery or neurolytic block in the previous 12 months; orthopedic deformities; epilepsy; metal implants in the skull or hearing aids.

All children who met the eligibility criteria (n = 24) were submitted to the initial evaluation and randomly allocated to an experimental group (treadmill training combined with active tDCS) and control group (treadmill training combined with placebo tDCS). Block randomization was used and stratified based on GMFCS level (levels I-II or level III). For each stratum, blocks of six were determined to minimize the risk of imbalance in the size of the separate samples. Numbered opaque envelopes were employed to ensure the concealment of the allocation. Each envelop contained a card stipulating to which group the child was allocated.

Evaluation

All evaluation procedures were carried out by two examiners who were blinded to the allocation of the children to the different groups. All patients were blinded for this study. Evaluations consisted of stabilometric analysis as well as the administration of the Pediatric Balance Scale (PBS) and Pediatric Evaluation of Disability Inventory (PEDI) one week before the intervention (Evaluation 1), one week after the completion of the intervention (Evaluation 2) and one month after the completion of the intervention (Evaluation 3). Each evaluation was held on a single

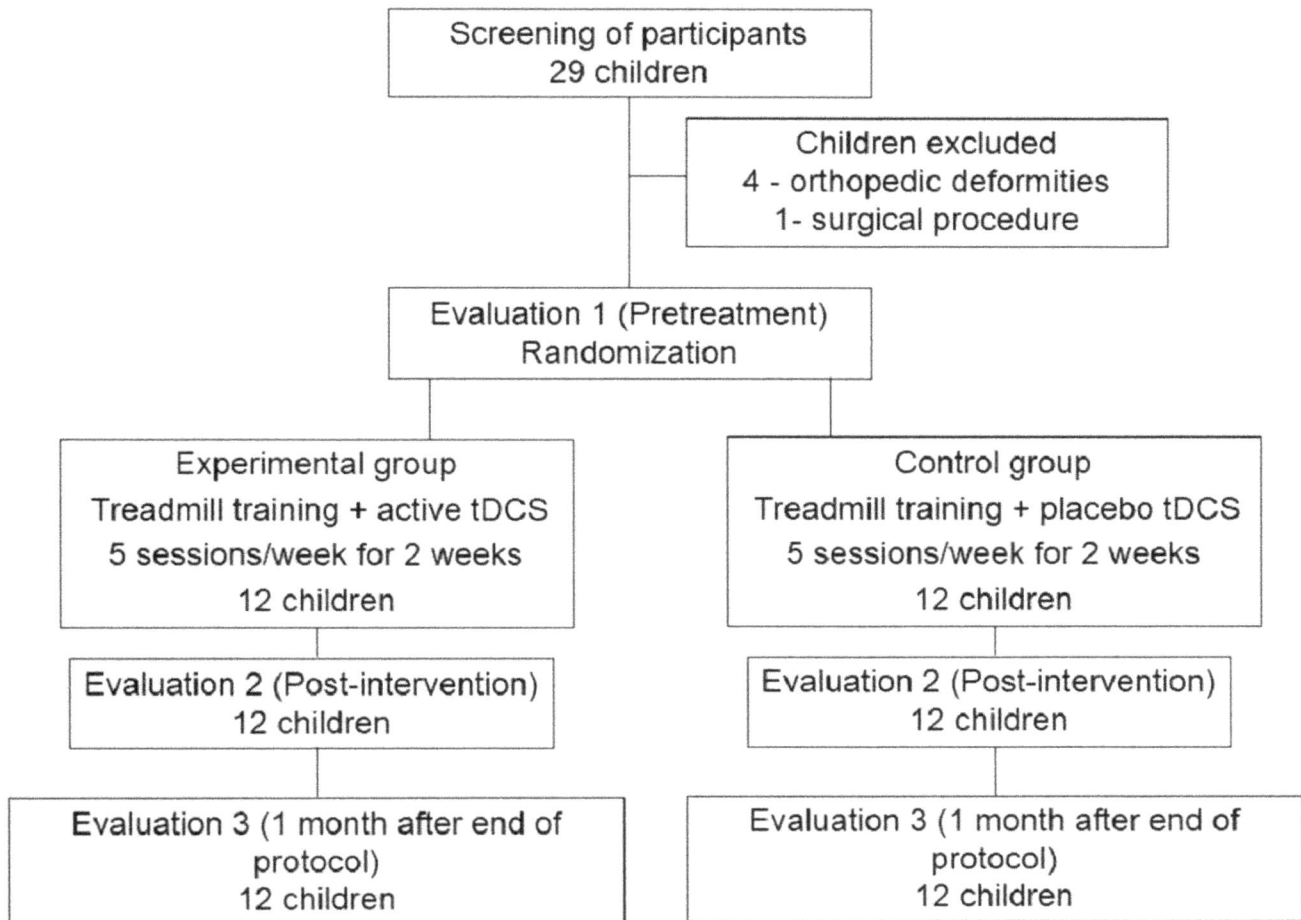

Figure 1. Flowchart of study based on Consolidated Standards of Reporting Trials.

day. The child first rested in a chair for 20 minutes. The stabilometric analysis was then performed, followed by the PBS and then by the PEDI.

Stabilometric analysis was performed for the evaluation of static balance. For such, a force plate (Kistler model 9286BA) was used, which allows the record of oscillations of the center of pressure (COP). The acquisition frequency was 50 Hz, captured by four piezoelectric sensors positioned at the extremities of the force plate, which measured 40×60 cm. The data were recorded and interpreted using the SWAY software program (BTS Engineering), integrated and synchronized to the SMART-D 140 system. The child was instructed to remain in a standing position on the force plate, barefoot, arms alongside the body, with an unrestricted foot base, heels aligned and gazed fixed on a point marked at a distance of one meter at the height of the glabellum (adjusted for each child). Children classified on level III of the GMFCS used their normal gait-assistance device, which was positioned off the force plate. Thirty-second readings were taken under two conditions: eyes open and eyes closed. Displacement of the COP was measured in the anteroposterior (x axis) and mediolateral (Y axis) directions under each visual condition.

The PBS consists of 14 tasks resembling activities of daily living. The items are scored on a five-point scale ranging from 0 (inability to perform the activity without assistance) to 4 (ability to perform the activity independently). The maximum score is 56. Scoring is based on the time in which a position is maintained, the distance to which the upper limb is able to reach out in front of the body and the time required to complete the task [19].

The PEDI allows a quantitative evaluation of functional performance. This questionnaire is administered in interview format to one of the caregivers, who offers information on the child's performance on routine activities and typical tasks of daily living. The test is composed of three parts. The first part addresses abilities in the child's repertoire, which are grouped into three functional domains: self-care (73 items), mobility (59 items) and social function (65 items). Each item on this part receives a score of either 0 (child is unable to perform the activity) or 1 (activity is part of the child's repertoire). The score of each domain is determined by the sum of the items [22], [23].

Intervention

One week after Evaluation 1, the children underwent the 10-session intervention protocol (5 weekly sessions for 2 weeks) involving treadmill training and tDCS (active or placebo). A specific test for children with CP was used to determine the treadmill training speed. This procedure was carried out based on the recommendations of Grecco *et al.* [9]. During the training sessions, the tDCS electrodes were positioned, the equipment was switched on and 20 minutes of gait training was performed simultaneously with anodal stimulation over the primary motor cortex (active or placebo). All children wore their normal braces during training, which were duly placed by the physiotherapist. Heart rate was monitored throughout the entire session to ensure an absence of overload on the cardiovascular system.

Gait training was performed on a treadmill (Inbramed, Millenium ATL, RS, Brazil). Two sessions were performed prior to the beginning of the protocol to familiarize the children with the treadmill. During these trial sessions, the children did not receive tDCS and treadmill speed was gradually increased based on the tolerance of each child. Training velocity was set at 80% of the maximum speed established during the exercise test [9].

Transcranial stimulation was applied with the tDCS Transcranial Stimulation device (Soterix Medical Inc., USA), using two sponge (non-metallic) electrodes (5×5 cm) moistened with saline solution. The anodal electrode was positioned over the primary motor cortex of the non-dominant hemisphere following the 10–20 International Electroencephalogram System [24] and the cathode was positioned in the supra-orbital region on the contralateral side.

To standardize the positioning of the electrodes of the diparetic patients, lower limb dominance was determined through self-reports; the children were asked: "Which leg is easier to move?" [25]. The anodal electrode was positioned over the hemisphere ipsilateral to the dominant lower limb. Thus, the patients were stimulated in the more compromised hemisphere. In cases of hemiparesis, stimulation was standardized over the lesioned hemisphere.

In the experimental group, a 1-mA current was applied over the primary motor cortex for 20 minutes as the children performed the treadmill training. The device has a button that allows the operator to control the intensity of the current. In the first ten seconds, stimulation was gradually increased until reaching 1 mA and gradually diminished in the last ten seconds of the session. In the control group, the electrodes were positioned at the same sites and the device was switched on for 30 seconds, giving the children the initial sensation of the 1 mA current, but no stimulation was administered during the rest of the time. This is a valid control procedure in studies involving tDCS.

The number of sessions attended, maximum speed during treadmill training, duration of treadmill training and distance travelled in each session were recorded on the follow-up chart. Any problems or injuries that occurred during training were also recorded. All participants were instructed to maintain their routine daily activities.

Statistical analysis

The sample size was calculated using the STATA 11 program and based on a study by Grecco *et al.* 2012 [9] [*Effect of treadmill training without partial weight support on functionality in children with cerebral palsy: Randomized controlled clinical trial.*] The PBS was selected as the primary outcome due to its proven validity and reliability in the literature for the evaluation of functional balance in children with CP and was therefore used in the sample size calculation. Based on a mean and standard deviation of 46.7±7.6 in the experimental group and 34.9±6.8 in the control group, 10 children in each group would be necessary for a bi-directional alpha of 0.05 and an 80% power. Twenty percent were added to each group to compensate for possible dropouts. Thus, the final sample was made up of 12 children in each group (total: 24 participants).

The Kolmogorov-Smirnov test was used to determine the adherence of the data to the Gaussian curve. The data proved to be parametric and were expressed as mean and standard deviation values. The effect size was calculated by the difference between

means of the pre-intervention and post-intervention evaluations and was expressed with respective 95% confidence intervals. Repeated-measures ANOVA was used for the intra-group analyses and one-way ANOVA was used for the inter-group analyses. A p-value <0.05 was considered statistically significant. The data were organized and tabulated using the Statistical Package for the Social Sciences v.19.0 (SPSS, Chicago, IL, USA).

Results

Twenty-nine children were screened and 24 were selected for participation in the present study, from November 2012 to September 2013. No losses occurred in either group. Table 1 displays the anthropometric characteristics and functional classification of the participants.

No statistically significant differences between groups were found regarding the anthropometric data, age or data referring to the primary or secondary outcomes at the baseline evaluation (p>0.05). Data as age, body mass, height and body mass index were analyzed by the independent t test. The GMFCS and topography was analyzed by the chi square test.

Table 2 displays the variables analyzed at baseline (Evaluation 1), after training (Evaluation 2) and at the follow up (Evaluation 3).

The PBS was chosen as the primary outcome due to the fact that this scale allows the evaluation of functional balance and has proven validity for use on children with CP. The experimental group exhibited the effect of training with tDCS, as demonstrated by the increase in the final score after training and at the follow up evaluation [F (1.33) = 3.9; p = 0.05] (Figure 2). In contrast, no significant effect on the PBS score was found in the control group after the intervention [F (1.11) = 1.3; p = 0.27].

The stabilometric evaluation revealed positive effects on the reduction in body sway in the anteroposterior direction with eyes open [F (2.33) = 7.1; p = 0.002], anteroposterior direction with eyes closed [F (2.22) = 24.3; p<0.0001], mediolateral direction with eyes open [F (2.33) = 4.0; p = 0.02] and mediolateral direction with eyes closed [F (2.33) = 3.6; p = 0.03] (Figure 3). The experimental group maintained these effects on anteroposterior and mediolateral sway with eyes open and closed after the intervention (p<0.05). In the control group, the effect was maintained at Evaluation 3 only with regard to mediolateral sway with eyes closed [F (1.11) = 18.4; p = 0.001].

Regarding the PEDI, an increase in the final score was found for the mobility [F (2.22) = 19.2; p<0.0001] and self-care [F (2.22) = 9.90; p = 0.0008] subscales. In the intra-group analysis, positive effects were found after treatment regarding self-care in both groups, but these effects were not maintained at Evaluation 3. Moreover, only the experimental group exhibited a positive effect regarding mobility after treatment (Evaluation 2). Figure 4 displays the PEDI results in both groups.

In the intra-group analysis, repeated-measures ANOVA revealed significant differences in both groups following motor training, with a reduction in oscillations of the COP one week after the end of the protocols. However, only the experimental group maintained this reduction one month after the protocol (Evaluation 3). The experimental group also exhibited improvements in regarding the balance scale. No significant intra-group differences were found with regard to self-care and functional mobility following treadmill training with tDCS.

In the inter-group analysis, one-way ANOVA revealed significant differences between groups. The experimental group exhibited significantly lower oscillations of the COP in the anteroposterior (experimental group with eyes open: 18.6±3.9, 14.0±2.7 and 14.2±1.9 mm; experimental group with eyes

Table 1. Anthropometric characteristics and functional classification of children analyzed.

	Experimental group (n = 12)	Control group (n = 12)	
Age (years)*	7.8 (2.0)	8.1 (1.5)	p = 0.74
Body mass (Kg)*	27.9(2.5)	28.3(2.7)	p = 0.58
Height (cm)*	127.7(6.4)	128.2(7.4)	p = 0.73
Body mass index (Kg^2/m)*	17.2(0.8)	17.8(1.5)	p = 0.39
GMFCS (I\II\III)**	(3\6\3)	(2\7\3)	p = 0.17
Topography (hemiparesis\diparesis)**	(3\9)	(2\10)	p = 0.77

Legend: GMFCS: Gross Motor Function Classification System.
*data expressed as mean (standard deviation); ** data representing frequency.

closed: 24.3±5.6, 17.1±4.3 and 17.7±4.6 mm; control group with eyes open: 20.3±4.5, 15.8±3.6 and 18.4±3.7 mm; control group with eyes closed: 24.2±4.8, 22.7±4.1 and 23.2±3.1 mm) and mediolateral (experimental group with eyes open: 20.3±4.5, 14.7±3.6 and 15.3±4.1 mm; experimental group with eyes closed: 25.4±18.9, 18.9±4.3 and 19.7±4.1 mm; control group with eyes open: 20.2±4.3, 18.6±3.2 and 18.8±3.1 mm; control group with eyes closed: 25.1±5.2, 22.9±4.2 and 22.8±3.6 mm) directions. These differences were found both one week and one month after the end of the interventions (Figure 2).

The experimental group also had better scores on the pediatric balance scale (experimental group: 40.5±9.4, 45.3±7.9 and 44.7±6.7; control group: 39.1±9.8, 39.7±8.9 and 39.5±9.3) (Figure 3).

However, no significant differences between groups were found regarding the self-care (experimental group: 46.1±10.8, 48.0±9.5 and 47.3±9.2; control group: 45.0±9.2, 45.5±9.3 and 45.6±8.9) or mobility (experimental group: 38.0±8.5, 41.7±7.4 and 40.9±7.7; control group: 39.3±7.4, 39.5±6.9 and 38.8±7.0) subscales of the PEDI (Figure 4).

Discussion

There has been increasing use of tDCS in the rehabilitation of patients with lasting neurological effects following a brain lesion, especially in cases of stroke. Studies have also demonstrated the benefits of this technique in patients with Parkinson's disease, pain

and depression. The method has proven to be promising and safe on adults [18].

Studies involving children also suggest that the method is safe, but requires lesser intensity of the electrical current. Through computations modeling, Minhas et al. (2012) [26] found that lesser intensity than that conventionally used on adults is capable of cortex stimulation in children. Based on the results achieved with stroke victims and studies that demonstrate an absence of adverse effects in children, the aim of the present investigation was to determine whether anodal stimulation of the primary motor cortex in the dominant hemisphere combined with treadmill training would lead to an increase in or the maintenance of the effect of treadmill training on static and functional balance in children with CP.

Previous studies have demonstrated that treadmill training without body support and at a speed determined by a prior exercise test leads to improvements in both static and functional balance and favors functional performance in children with CP [9]. In the present study, an established treadmill training protocol with effects demonstrated in the literature was used to determine whether tDCS is valid in children with CP classified on levels I, II and III of the GMFCS. The treadmill training had to be adapted to the tDCS procedures reported in the literature. The protocol described by Grecco et al. [9] was used as the basis for the present investigation. However, this protocol involves two weekly sessions of training over a seven-week period (total of 14 sessions). In the present study, five weekly sessions were held over a two-week

Table 2. Comparison of variables between experimental group and control group in three moments: Evaluation 1, Evaluation 2, and Evaluation 3.

	Experimental group			Control group		
	Evaluation 1	Evaluation 2	Evaluation 3	Evaluation 1	Evauation 2	Evaluation 3
PBS*	40.5(9.4)	45.3(7.9)	44.7(7.7)	39.1(9.8)	39.7(8.4)	39.5(9.3)
Oscillation AP EO*	18.6(3.9)	14.0(2.7)	14.2(2.6)	20.3(4.5)	15.8(3.6)	18.4(3.6)
Oscillation AP EC*	24.3(5.6)	17.1(4.3)	17.7(4.6)	24.2(4.8)	22.7(4.1)	23.2(4.1)
Oscillation ML EO*	20.3(4.5)	14.7(3.6)	15.3(4.1)	19.2(4.3)	18.6(3.2)	18.8(3.1)
Oscillation ML EC*	25.4(5.5)	18.9(4.3)	19.7(4.1)	25.1(5.2)	22.9(4.2)	22.8(3.6)
Self-care*	46.1(10.0)	48.0(9.5)	47.8(9.2)	45.0(9.2)	45.5(9.3)	45.6(9.4)
Mobility*	38.0(8.5)	41.7(7.4)	40.9(7.7)	38.3(7.4)	39.5(7.6)	38.8(7.0)

Legend: PBS (Pediatric Balance Scale), AP EO (Anteroposterior Eyes Open); AP EC (Anteroposterior Eyes Closed); ML EO (Mediolateral Eyes Open); ML EC (Mediolateral Eyes Closed).
*Data expressed as mean and standard deviation.

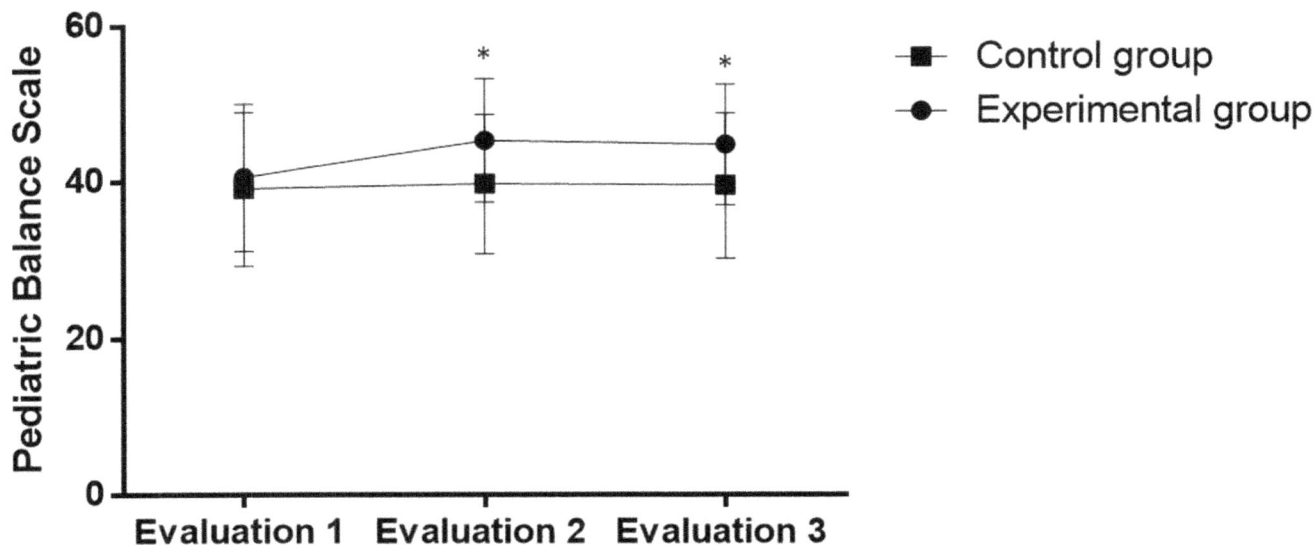

Figure 2. PBS scores in both groups before and after intervention. *statistically significant difference between groups (p<0.05).

period (total of 10 sessions). Thus, it was important to carry out a randomized controlled study involving a control group with placebo tDCS to determine the effects of treadmill training alone.

In a study involving patients with hemiparesis following a stroke, three sessions of anodal stimulation over the damaged motor cortex combined with specific training for the ankle of the paretic limb led to improvements in dorsiflexion and plantar flexion. This

is in agreement with the present findings, as the strategies used by the ankle are fundamental to postural control and balance [27]. Another interesting study carried out by Kashi *et al.* (2013) [28] demonstrated that a single session of anodal stimulation in combination with balance and gait training resulted in improvements in balance, gait velocity and stride length in elderly individuals with leukoaraiosis (cerebral white matter lesion that

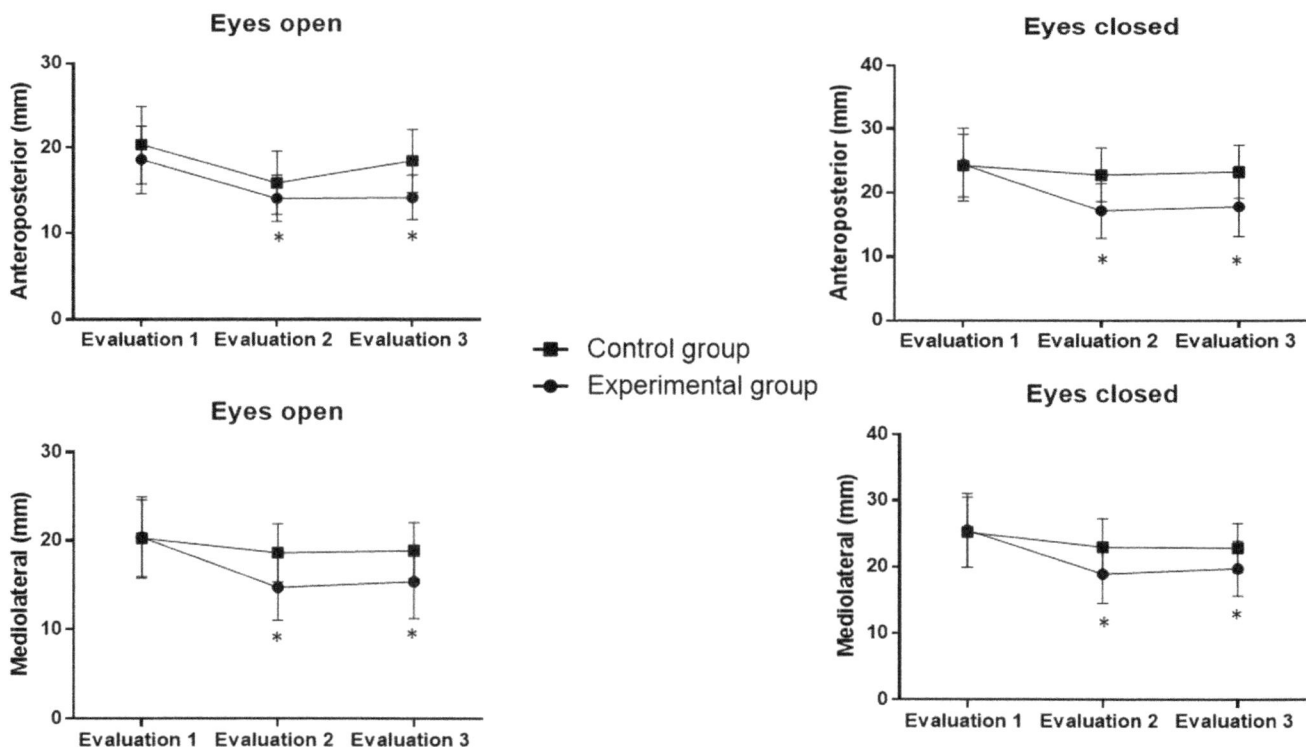

Figure 3. Oscillations of center of pressure. A) anteroposterior sway with eyes open; B) mediolateral sway with eyes open; C) anteroposterior sway with eyes closed; D) mediolateral sway with eyes closed. *Statistically significant difference between groups (p<0.05).

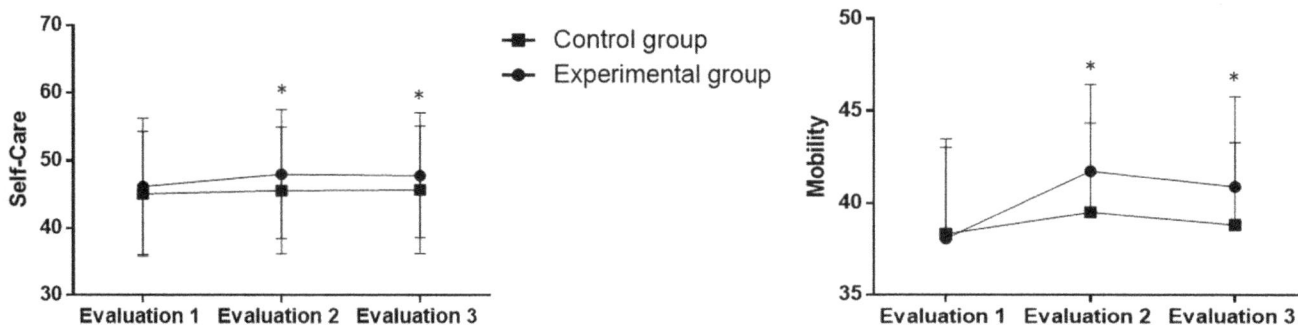

Figure 4. Self-care and mobility scores on PEDI in both groups before and after intervention.

affects gait and balance). In the present study, 10 consecutive sessions of tDCS were performed with the aim of potentiating the neuroplastic changes that occur from the combination of tDCS and motor training to determine whether the effects are persistent modifications of synaptic efficiency similar to long-term potentiation [29].

Kashi et al. (2012) [30] evaluated 30 healthy volunteers who received 15 minutes of anodal stimulation (2 mA; either active or placebo) of the prefrontal cortex while at rest prior to walking on a moving platform. The active group demonstrated improvements in postural control and gait velocity in comparison to the placebo group. These findings demonstrate that anodal tDCS is capable of causing changes in motor cortex excitability, thereby favoring motor control and lower limb movements.

In the present study, both groups demonstrated positive results following the different protocols. However, statistically significant differences between groups were found, with better results in the experimental group regarding anteroposterior sway, mediolateral sway and functional balance (PBS). These findings suggest that anodal stimulation of the primary motor cortex potentiated the results of treadmill training. The randomized, controlled study design allows the determination of the effect size, demonstrating the statistically significant effect of tDCS. One of the most important findings regards the fact that tDCS contributed to the maintenance of the effects of treadmill training. In clinical practice, the effects of physical therapy are often minimized or even completely lost following the interruption of the therapy sessions. In the present study, the gains achieved with the combination of treadmill training and tDCS remained one month after the completion of the protocol, suggesting the potential of tDCS to modify cortex excitability and favor neuroplasticity. The lack of an analysis of cortex excitability constitutes a limitation of this study. Although the aim was to analyze motor results, the measure of excitability could have allowed a more adequate explanation of the findings.

The possible adverse effects of tDCS should be addressed. However, the literature on tDCS in children is scarce and no previous papers involving motor training are found. In the present study, the children and their caregivers were asked about side effects at the end of each session and during the evaluations after the completion of the protocol. Three children in the experimental group experienced redness in the supra-orbital region (site of the cathode). No other adverse effects were reported, such as behavioral changes, headache or discomfort. During the sessions, 18 children (12 in the experimental group and 6 in the control group) reported a tingling sensation at the beginning of stimulation, but this sensation either ceased after a few seconds or was not considered bothersome. No children needed the

intensity to be diminished or the stimulation to be stopped prior to the end of the 20-minute session. No children had difficulty performing treadmill training with tDCS and neither the wires nor the positioning of the electrodes hampered walking.

According to Kashi et al. (2012) [30], anodal tDCS induces changes in the excitability of the motor cortex referring to the lower limbs, with a consequent improvement in gait. Minhas et al. (2012) [26] carried out studies involving the administration of tDCS to children and found that the method is safe, but the current needs to be adjusted from 2 mA, which is used for adults, to 1 mA for children.

As a relatively new technique, few studies have employed tDCS on children with CP. Findings reported in the literature regard the use of transcranial magnetic stimulation as a method for analyzing the evoked potential [31] and cortex map [15]. This method has also been used to reduce spasticity in children with CP [32] in one or both hemispheres [15].

No studies were found addressing the effects of anodal tDCS over M1 on motor function or the combined use of tDCS and physical therapy, such as during gait training. Moreover, a limited number of studies discuss important clinical differences in CP, especially with regard to body sway and functional independence. For the present study, the findings described by Grecco et al. (2013) [20], who used the same treadmill training protocol, were considered clinically relevant.

The authors found no consensus in the literature or studies that specifically address a minimum difference that could be considered clinically important in the population with CP. However, as the present study involved a short intervention (2 weeks), the positive effect regarding the variables analyzed in the experimental group (gait training combined with anodal tDCS) at the follow up evaluation can be considered clinically important. The positive change in the PBS score in the experimental group allows one to infer that the quality of movement was optimized in these children. Indeed, the results demonstrate the effect size on functional balance in the experimental group vs. the control group at Evaluation 2 (5.6) and Evaluation 3 (5.2).

The findings of the present study demonstrate that the combination of treadmill training and anodal stimulation of the primary motor cortex in the dominant hemisphere was capable of potentiating improvements in static and functional balance in the children with cerebral palsy analyzed. Moreover, anodal stimulation favored the maintenance of the gains one month following the completion of the intervention. However, as this was a phase 2 study with a small sample size, further investigations with a larger number of participants and longer follow-up period are needed to confirm the results.

Author Contributions

Conceived and designed the experiments: ND LG MG FF CO. Performed the experiments: ND LG MG FF CO. Analyzed the data: ND LG MG FF CO. Contributed reagents/materials/analysis tools: ND LG MG FF CO. Wrote the paper: ND LG MG FF CO.

References

1. Burton H, Sachin D, Litkowski P, Wingert JR (2009) Functional connectivity for somatosensory and motor cortex in spastic diplegia. Somatosens Mot Res 26: 90–104.
2. Inder TE, Huppi PS, Warfield S, Kikinis R, Zientara GP, et al. (1999) Periventricular white injury in the premature infant is followed by reduced cerebral cortical gray matter volume at term. Ann Neurol 46:755–760.
3. Kurz MJ, Wilson TW (2011) Neuromagnetic activity in the somatosensory cortices if children with cerebral palsy. Neurosci Let 490:1-5.
4. Shin YK, Lee DR, Hwang HJ, You SJ (2012) A novel EEG-based brain mapping to determine cortical activation patterns in normal children and children with cerebral palsy during motor imagery tasks. NeuroRehabil 31: 349–55.
5. Rose S, Guzzetta A, Pannek K, Boyd R (2011) MRI structural connectivity, disruption of primary sensorimotor pathways, and hand function in cerebral palsy. Brain Connect 1: 309–16.
6. Chagas PSC, Mancini MC, Barbosa A, Silva PTG (2004) Análise das intervenções utilizadas para a promoção da marcha em crianças portadoras de paralisia cerebral: uma revisão sistemática da literatura. Rev Bras Fisioter 8: 155–63.
7. Pitcher JB, Schmeider LA, Burns NR, Drysdale JL, Higgins RD, et al. (2012) Reduced corticomotor excitability and motor skills development in children born preterm. J Physiol 590: 5827–44.
8. Nevalainen P, Pihko E, Maenpaa H, Valanne L, Nummenmaa L, et al. (2012) Bilateral alterations in somatosensory cortical processing in hemiplegic cerebral palsy. Dev Med Child Neurol 54:361–7.
9. Grecco LAC, Zanon N, Sampaio LMM, Oliveira CS (2013) A comparison of treadmill training and overground walking in ambulant children with cerebral palsy: randomized controlled clinical Trial. Clin Rehabil 27:674.
10. Rose J, Wolff DR, Jones VK, Bloch DA, Oehlert JW, et al. (2002) Postural balance in children with cerebral palsy. Dev Med Child Neurol 44:58–63.
11. Grecco LA, Tomita SM, Christovão TC, Pasini H, Sampaio LM, et al. (2013) Effect of treadmill gait training on static and functional balance in children with cerebral palsy: a randomized controlled trial. Rev Bras Fisioter 17:17–23.
12. Miranda PC, Lomarev M, Hallett M (2006) Modeling the current distribution during transcranial direct current stimulation. Clin Neurophysiol 117:1623–9.
13. Morris ME, Iansek R, Smithson F, Huxham F (2000) Postural instability in parkinson's disease: a comparison with and without a concurrent task. Gait and Posture 12: 205–216.
14. Dinomais M, Lignon G, Chinier E, Richard I, Ter MInassian A, et al. (2013) Effect of observation of simple hand movement on brain activations in patients with unilateral cerebral palsy: an fMRI study. Res Dev Disabil 34:1928–37.
15. Kesar TM, Sawaki L, Burdette JH, Cabrera MN, Kolaski K, et al. (2012) Motor cortical functional geometry in cerebral palsy and its relationship to disability. Clin Neurophysiol 123:1383–90.
16. Marchese R, Diverio M, Zucchi F, Lentino C, Abbruzzese G (2000) The role of sensory cues in the rehabilitation of parkisonian patients: a comparison of two physical therapy protocols. Movement Disorders 15: 879–883.
17. Wagner T, Fregni F, Fecteau S, Grodzinsky A, Zahn M, et al. (2007) Transcranial direct current stimulation: A computer-based human model study. Neuroimage 35:1113–24.
18. Mendonça ME, Fregni F (2012) Neuromodulação com estimulação cerebral não invasiva: aplicação no acidente vascular encefálico, doença de Parkinson e dor crônica. In:ASSIS, R.D. Manole. Condutas práticas em fisioterapia neurológica. São Paulo, p. 307–39.
19. Ries LGK, Michaelsen Soares PSA, Monteiro VC, Allegretti KMG (2012) Adaptação cultural e análise da confiabilidade da versão brasileira da Escala de Equilíbrio Pediátrica (EEP). Rev Bras Fisioter 16:205–215.
20. Grecco LAC, Duarte NAC, Mendonça ME, Pasini H, Lima VLCC, et al. (2013) Effect of transcranial direct current stimulation combined with gait and mobility training on functionality in children with cerebral palsy: study protocol for a double-blind randomized controlled clinical trial. BMC Pediatrics 13:168.
21. Moher D, Hopewell S, Schulz KF, Montori V, Gøtzsche PC, et al. (2010) CONSORT 2010 Explanation and Elaboration: updated guidelines for reporting parallel group randomised trial. J Clin Epi 63:e1–e37.
22. Feldman AB, Haley SM, Corvell J (1990) Concurrent and construct validity of the Pediatric Evaluation of Disability Inventory. Phys Ther 70:602–10.
23. Haley SM, Coster J, Faas RM (1991) A content validity study of the Pediatric Evaluation of Disability Inventory. Pediatr Phys Ther 3:177–84.
24. Homan RW, Herman J, Purdy P (1987) Cerebral location of international 10–20 system electrode placement. Electroencephalogr Clin Neurophysiol 66:376–82.
25. Sadeghi H, Allard P, Prince H, Labelle H (2000) Symmetry and limb dominance in able-bodied gait: a review. Gait & Posture 12:34–45.
26. Minhas P, Bikson M, Woods AJ, Rosen AR, Kessler SK (2012) Transcranial direct current stimulation in pediatric brain: A computational modeling study. Conf Proc IEEE Eng Med Biol Soc: 859–862
27. Stagg CJ, Bachtiar V, O'Shea J, Allman C, Bosnell RA, et al. (2012) Cortical activation changes underlying stimulation induced behavioral gains in chronic stroke. Brain 135: 276–84.
28. Kashi D, Dominguez RO, Allum JH, Bronstein AM (2013) Improving gait and balance in patients with leukoaraiosis using transcranial direct current stimulation and physical training: An exploratory study. Neurorehabil Neural Repair 27:864–71.
29. Liebetanz D, Nitsche MA, Tergau F, Paulus W (2002) Pharmacological approach to the mechanism of transcranial DC stimulation induced after effects of human motor cortex excitability. Brain 125:2238–47.
30. Kashi D, Quadir S, Patel M, Yousif N, Bronstein AM (2012) Enhanced locomotor adaptation after effect in the "broken escalator" phenomenon using anodal tDCS. J Neurophysiol 107:2493–2505.
31. Garvey MA, Mall V (2008) Transcranial magnetic stimulation in children. Clin. Neurophysiol 119:973–84.
32. Valle AC, Dionisio K, Pitskel NB, Pascual-Leone A, Orsati F, et al. (2007) Low and high frequency repetitive transcranial magnetic stimulation for the treatment of spasticity. Dev Med Child Neurol 49:534–8.

16

Clinical Characteristics and Outcomes of Hospitalized Older Patients with Distinct Risk Profiles for Functional Decline: A Prospective Cohort Study

Bianca M. Buurman[1]*, Jita G. Hoogerduijn[2], Elisabeth A. van Gemert[1], Rob J. de Haan[3], Marieke J. Schuurmans[2,4], Sophia E. de Rooij[1]*

1 Department of Internal Medicine and Geriatrics, Academic Medical Center, Amsterdam, The Netherlands, 2 Research Group Care for the Chronically Ill, Faculty of Health Care, Hogeschool Utrecht, University of Applied Sciences Utrecht, Utrecht, The Netherlands, 3 Clinical Research Unit, Academic Medical Center, Amsterdam, The Netherlands, 4 Department of Nursing Science, University Medical Center, Utrecht, The Netherlands

Abstract

Background: The aim of this research was to study the clinical characteristics and mortality and disability outcomes of patients who present distinct risk profiles for functional decline at admission.

Methods: Multicenter, prospective cohort study conducted between 2006 and 2009 in three hospitals in the Netherlands in consecutive patients of ≥65 years, acutely admitted and hospitalized for at least 48 hours. Nineteen geriatric conditions were assessed at hospital admission, and mortality and functional decline were assessed until twelve months after admission. Patients were divided into risk categories for functional decline (low, intermediate or high risk) according to the Identification of Seniors at Risk-Hospitalized Patients.

Results: A total of 639 patients were included, with a mean age of 78 years. Overall, 27%, 33% and 40% of the patients were at low, intermediate or high risk, respectively, for functional decline. Low-risk patients had fewer geriatric conditions (mean 2.2 [standard deviation [SD] 1.3]) compared with those at intermediate (mean 3.8 [SD 2.1]) or high risk (mean 5.1 [SD 1.8]) ($p < 0.001$). Twelve months after admission, 39% of the low-risk group had an adverse outcome, compared with 50% in the intermediate risk group and 69% in the high risk group ($p < 0.001$).

Conclusion: By using a simple risk assessment instrument at hospital admission, patients at low, intermediate or high risk for functional decline could be identified, with distinct clinical characteristics and outcomes. This approach should be tested in clinical practice and research and might help appropriately tailor patient care.

Editor: Ulrich Thiem, Marienhospital Herne - University of Bochum, Germany

Funding: This study was financed by the Netherlands Organization for Health Research and Development (Zon MW), grant number 13550004. The funders had no role in study design, data collection and analysis, decision to publish, or preparation of the manuscript.

Competing Interests: The authors have declared that no competing interests exist.

* E-mail: B.m.vanes@amc.uva.nl (BB); s.e.derooij@amc.nl (SR)

Introduction

Functional decline, defined as a loss of activities of daily living (ADL), is experienced by 30 to 60% of hospitalized older patients [1,2]. In acutely hospitalized patients, functional decline often precedes hospital admission [3], and hospitalization itself further increases the risk of worsening ADL disabilities [4]. Patients with functional decline are also at risk for other adverse health outcomes, such as institutionalization and death [5].

Preventing functional decline during and after hospitalization is therefore an increasingly important health-care focus in older hospital patients [6,7]. Not all patients are at equal risk of developing functional decline because decline is dependent on (among other factors) patients' premorbid status, including geriatric conditions present at admission [1,8]. The aggregate number of geriatric conditions present at hospital admission determines a patient's individual risk for functional deterioration [1,9].

In studies focusing on assessing the risk of functional decline, the study population is often crudely dichotomized into a low-risk and a high-risk group [5]. Both the International Classification of Functioning (ICF) and expert opinion suggest the need for patient care and research to adopt a more tailored approach, in which different subgroups or categories of older patients are identified.[7–10]. The added value of such an approach is that it might help clinicians define subtle treatment goals at an early stage (for instance, at hospital admission), discuss preferred and expected hospital care outcomes with their patients and it might enhance clinical decision making. Although some studies have attempted to develop an approach using more than two subgroups of patients [11,12], the clinical characteristics and outcomes of these patients groups have not been described and studied thoroughly [13].

The objectives of this multicenter, prospective, observational study were therefore to investigate 1) differences in the clinical characteristics of patients at low, intermediate or high risk for functional decline, 2) the different functional trajectories from baseline to one year after discharge in the risk groups and 3) the association between risk categories and mortality and functional decline at three and twelve months after hospital admission.

Methods

Design and setting

This multicenter prospective cohort study, the DEFENCE study (Develop strategies Enabling Frail Elderly New Complications to Evade) was conducted between April 1, 2006 and April 1, 2008 in three hospitals in The Netherlands: the Academic Medical Center (AMC) in Amsterdam, the University Medical Centre Utrecht (UMCU) in Utrecht and the Spaarne Hospital (SH) in Hoofddorp. The AMC (1,024 beds) and UMCU (1,042 beds) are tertiary university teaching hospitals. The SH (455 beds) is a regional teaching hospital.

In total, five wards in the AMC, three wards in the UMCU and three wards in the SH participated in this study. The staff on the general medical wards consisted of residents, physicians and registered nurses who did not specialize in geriatric medicine or geriatric nursing. A geriatric consultation team consisting of at least one clinical nurse specialist and one geriatrician was available in all hospitals.

The study was approved by the Medical Ethics Committee of the AMC. Local approval was given by the UMCU and SH.

Patients

The study enrolled all consecutive patients aged 65 years and older who were acutely admitted to one of the three participating hospitals' medical wards and hospitalized for at least 48 hours. Patients were excluded if 1) they or their relatives did not give informed consent; 2) they were too ill to participate, as determined by their attending medical doctor; 3) they came from another ward in or outside the hospital; 4) they were transferred to the Intensive Care Unit of the Coronary Care Unit or another ward in or outside the hospital within 48 hours after admission; or 5) they were unable to speak or understand Dutch. Enrollment had to take place within 48 hours after admission, and written informed consent was obtained before inclusion.

Data collection

A research nurse visited the participating wards every weekday seeking eligible patients for the study. After obtaining informed consent from the patient or, in case of cognitive impairment, from the primary caregiver, the patient received a risk assessment, followed by a systematic geriatric assessment on four domains of functioning (somatic, psychological, functional and social) performed by the research nurse. The primary caregiver was also interviewed. The patient assessment had to be completed within 48 hours after admission.

Risk assessment for functional decline

The Identification of Seniors at Risk–Hospitalized Patients (ISAR-HP) was applied to determine which patients were at low, intermediate or high risk for functional decline. The ISAR-HP is based on the original ISAR for the Emergency Department (ED) [14]. The ISAR has been validated to detect a broad range of adverse outcomes after Emergency Department discharge and has been shown to be a clinimetrically sound screening instrument [14–16]. The original ISAR was tested on its predictive accuracy in acutely hospitalized older medical patients, but did not show good discriminative values in this population [17]. Therefore, a new prediction model was developed in an independent population and externally validated to assess the risk of functional

decline three months after hospital admission in older hospitalized patients. The complete procedure is described in another article [18] . Briefly, in the development study (n = 492) potential predictors associated with functional decline were identified using univariate logistic regression. Items of the original ISAR screening instrument [14], of the IADL index of Lawton and Brody [19], of the Short Nutritional Assessment Questionnaire [20] and other predictors known from the literature were analyzed as individual predictors. Next, a multivariate logistic regression was conducted (backward procedure, accepting P-values≤0.05). The four best models were compared and validated in a bootstrap procedure (1000 samples drawn randomly with replacement) using the AUC with 95% CI to determine the discriminative value. The AUC of the best model was 0.71 (95% CI 0.66–0.76) and the Hosmer Lemeshow test showed a p-value of 0.95, indicating a good fitting model. The validation cohort consisted of a retrospective analysis of a cohort of 484 patients acutely admitted to general medicine ward; the AUC of the prediction model in the validation cohort was 0.68 (95% CI 0.63–0.73).

The screening instrument was named ISAR-HP (with permission of the original author) and consists of four variables 1) the need for assistance with instrumental activities of daily living (IADL) two weeks prior to hospital admission, 2) eight years or fewer of formal education, 3) the inability to travel alone two weeks prior to hospital admission and 4) the use of a walking device. The first three items scored one point each, and the last item scored two points. Patients were at risk for functional decline if the ISAR-HP was 2 points or more. Definition of risk categories applied in this article: low risk if patients scored 0 or 1 point on the ISAR-HP, at intermediate risk if they scored 2 or 3 points and at high risk if patients had a score of 4 or 5.

Systematic geriatric assessment

At admission, patients' baseline and clinical characteristics were assessed with a comprehensive geriatric assessment (CGA). Table S1 shows the measurement tools, score ranges and cut-off scores used during this assessment. The CGA started with the eleven-item Minimal Mental State Examination (MMSE) [21] to assess the presence and degree of global cognitive impairment. Patients with a MMSE score ≥21 were interviewed; patients with a MMSE score of 16–20 were also interviewed, but their answers concerning baseline characteristics and ADL performances were cross-checked with their caregiver. In case of a disagreement, the caregiver's answer was included. Data for patients with an MMSE score ≤15 were obtained from their primary caregiver. This latter group was not screened for pain, depression or perceived health status, as the instruments we used have not been validated with cognitively impaired patients.

After administering the comprehensive geriatric assessment, the research nurse reported her findings to the geriatrician. The geriatrician also visited each patient within 48 hours and paid special attention to diagnosing potential psychiatric problems. The patient was screened for delirium using the confusion assessment method (CAM) [22].

After discharge, a geriatrician reviewed the discharge letter to determine the medical diagnoses presented at admission, new diagnoses developed during the patient's hospital stay, comorbidities and medication. Charlson comorbidity index scores were derived from this information [23], indicating the number and severity of comorbidities. Charlson comorbidity index scores range from 0 to 31, with a higher score indicating an increased number of severe comorbidities. International Classification of Diseases-9 diagnostic criteria were used to score these diagnoses.

Follow-up and definition of outcomes

Three and twelve months after admission, a research nurse from each center phoned the patient and/or primary caregiver to assess the patient's current ADL functioning. ADL status was collected from the same person (patient or informal caregiver) from whom the baseline information was obtained. Functional decline was defined as a loss of at least one point on the original Katz ADL index score [24] three or twelve months after admission, compared with the premorbid Katz ADL index score two weeks prior to hospital admission.

The mortality rate at three months and twelve months after admission was based on information from the Municipal Data Registry.

Functional trajectories were defined as the course of functioning from admission up to one year after discharge and were constructed using mortality and functional decline data at each time point. Patients who were still alive at three and twelve months and did not demonstrate decreased ADL functioning remained at their baseline level of function.

Statistical analysis

Baseline characteristics and outcomes were summarized using descriptive statistics. To determine the differences in the prevalence of geriatric conditions and outcomes among patients at low, intermediate and high risk for functional decline, dichotomous variables and categorical data were tested with a chi-squared test, and continuous variables were tested using ANOVA. For some geriatric conditions there were missing values.

To gain more insight in the functional trajectories until one year after admission in relation to the ISAR-HP two strategies were followed. One strategy was to calculate the individual responses to the ISAR-HP questions, and to compute the mean number of baseline and follow up scores on the Katz ADL index and the mean number of ADL functions that were lost between baseline and follow up. To establish functional trajectories including mortality at three and twelve months, the number of patients who had died and who demonstrated functional decline in each risk group was calculated. Patients who improved in activities of daily living were added to the group that remained at baseline functional levels. This was set out in figure 1.

To determine the relationship between risk category and mortality and functional decline at three and twelve months, regression analyses were performed. For mortality, Cox regression analyses were performed. Crude and adjusted (for age, sex and Charlson comorbidity index) models were calculated. For functional decline, logistic regression analyses were conducted

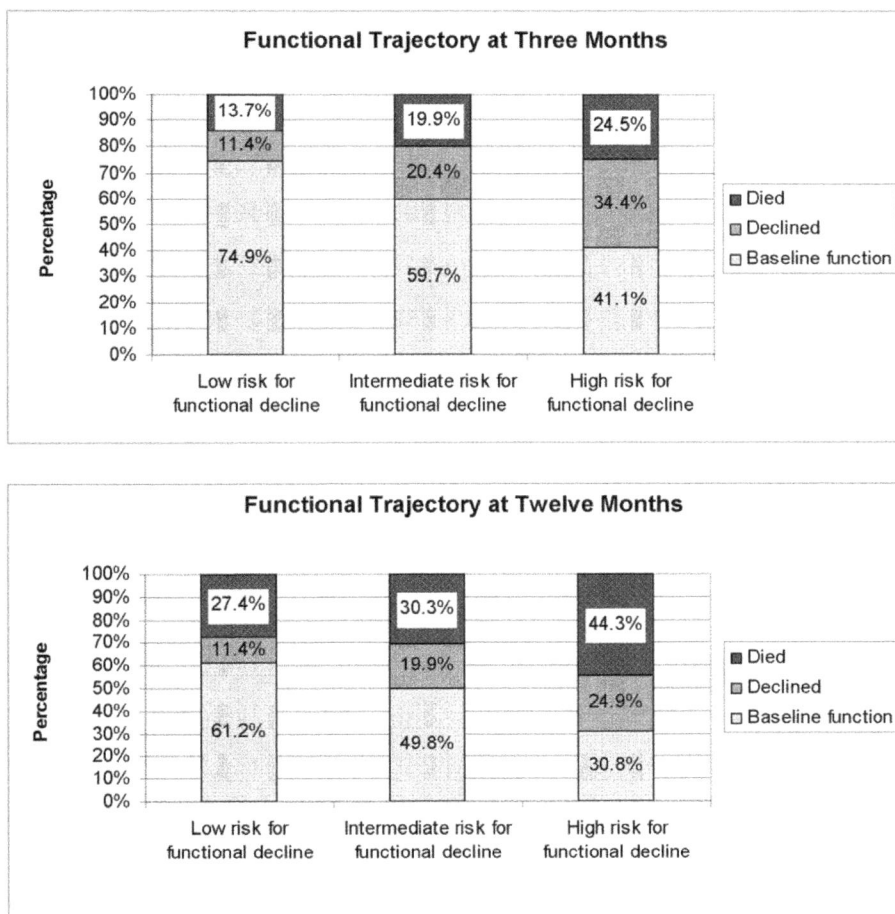

Figure 1. Functional trajectories for patients at low, intermediate or high risk for functional decline three and twelve months after admission. "Baseline function" refers to the level of premorbid functioning on the Katz ADL index score two weeks prior to hospital admission. A decline in function was defined as a loss of at least one point at three or twelve months on the six-item Katz ADL index compared with premorbid functioning.

and crude and adjusted models were computed, adjusting for the same factors. Patients in the low-risk group were used as a reference category.

Results

There were 1,031 consecutive patients eligible for participation in this study, 639 (62%) of whom were included after informed consent. Reasons for exclusion were refusal to participate (n = 222), insufficient Dutch language capabilities (n = 86), transfer from another ward (n = 36), transfer to Intensive Care Unit or Coronary Care Unit within 48 hours (n = 28) and terminal illness (n = 20). Compared with included patients, excluded patients were significantly younger (75 years vs. 78 years, p<0.001) and died more frequently within one year (48% vs. 35%, p<0.001).

Baseline characteristics of the three risk groups

Table 1 presents the baseline characteristics of the complete study population. The mean age was 78 years; 72% lived independently before hospital admission and approximately half the patients lived alone. The most common reason for admission was infection (41%). ISAR-HP scores showed that 27%, 33% and 40% of the patients were at low, intermediate or high risk for functional decline, respectively. There was a significant relationship between higher risk levels and older age, female sex, fewer years of education/lower social status, living alone, and care dependency.

Clinical characteristics

Table 2 shows the clinical characteristics of patients at low, intermediate or high risk for functional decline. Patients at high risk

for functional decline had more geriatric conditions (mean 5.1 [SD 1.8]) than those at low risk (mean 2.2 [SD 1.3]) or intermediate risk (mean 3.8 [SD 2.1]) for decline (p<0.001). In the high-risk group, patients frequently presented geriatric syndromes, such as fall risk, incontinence, premorbid cognitive impairment and delirium. As expected, there was also a substantial caregiver burden in the high-risk group.

We could not demonstrate clear differences between the subgroups with regard to malnutrition, obesity, pain, constipation or depressive symptoms.

Functional trajectories at three and twelve months

The mean number of baseline impairments on the modified Katz ADL index differed significantly between the three risk groups (0.1, 1.2, 2.4, p<0.001, Table 3). In the low risk group only 13% experienced one or more dependencies in ADL, whereas in the high risk group this was 77%, with 11% demonstrating complete dependence. The mean decline experienced until one year after discharge was also significantly different. Outcomes in terms of mortality and functional decline three and twelve months after hospital admission differed significantly between the groups (Figure 1). After three months, 25% of the low-risk group had a poor outcome (mortality or functional decline), compared with 40% and 59% in the intermediate- and high-risk groups, respectively (p<0.001). At twelve months, these rates were 39%, 50% and 69% for the low-, intermediate- and high-risk group, respectively (p<0.001). Only 30% of the patients in the high-risk group remained at their baseline level of functioning at twelve months. Although the high-risk patients had the most premorbid

Table 1. Baseline characteristics of acutely hospitalized older patients in three risk categories for physical functional decline.

	Patients n = 639	Low risk (n = 175)	Intermediate risk (n = 211)	High risk (n = 253)	p-value
Age in years	78.2 (7.8)	73.8 (6.4)	77.4 (7.1)	82.0 (7.5)	<0.001
Male (%)	46.2	60.0	46.9	36.0	<0.001
Education in years	9.9 (3.9)	11.4 (3.8)	10.2 (3.9)	8.6 (3.6)	<0.001
Caucasian (%)	92.8	95.4	91.9	91.7	0.35
Social status (%)					<0.001
Living alone	47.9	37.1	46.7	56.3	
Living arrangement (%)					<0.001
Independent	72.4	93.7	78.6	52.6	
Senior residence	10.3	4.6	9.0	15.4	
Supported living community	10.3	0.6	6.7	20.2	
Nursing home/intermediate care	7.0	1.1	5.8	11.8	
Diagnosis at admission (%)					0.76
Infectious disease	40.9	42.9	45.5	35.9	
Digestive system disease	22.8	23.8	21.8	22.9	
Malignancy	6.2	8.3	4.5	6.1	
Cardiovascular disease	4.3	4.8	2.7	5.3	
Water and electrolyte disturbance	10.5	9.5	8.2	13.0	
Other	15.4	10.7	17.3	16.8	
Charlson comorbidity index*	3.5 (2.3)	3.9 (2.7)	3.8 (2.4)	3.5 (2.2)	0.27
Length of hospital stay in days (median [range])	7 (2–100)	5 (2–100)	7 (2–77)	8 (2–80)	0.01

Mean (SD) are given for continuous variables.
*Range 0–31; a higher score indicates more or more severe comorbidities.

Table 2. Clinical characteristics of acutely hospitalized older patients in the three risk categories for physical functional decline.

	Low risk n = 175% (n/total number of observations)	Intermediate risk n = 211% (n/total number of observations)	High risk n = 253% (n/total number of observations)	p-value
Somatic domain				
Polypharmacy	46.6 (81/174)	64.8 (136/210)	66.3 (167/252)	<0.001
Malnutrition	45.2 (76/168)	50.5 (105/208)	54.6 (136/249)	0.17
Obesity	8.9 (15/168)	13.8 (26/188)	12.7 (27/213)	0.33
Pain*	42.3 (58/137)	44.5 (77/173)	42.8 (74/173)	0.91
Fall risk	4.2 (7/165)	27.9 (57/204)	30.0 (72/240)	<0.001
Presence of a pressure ulcer	0.0 (0/141)	3.6 (7/196)	4.1 (10/245)	0.06
Indwelling urinary catheter	7.6 (13/172)	20.0 (42/210)	37.3 (94/252)	<0.001
Incontinence	14.5 (24/165)	23.8 (49/206)	24.3 (60/247)	0.04
Constipation	20.3 (35/172)	14.9 (31/208)	22.0 (55/250)	0.15
Psychological domain				
Premorbid cognitive impairment	7.4 (9/121)	24.7 (43/174)	42.1 (91/216)	<0.001
Cognitive impairment at time of admission	10.9 (19/175)	34.6 (73/211)	64.8 (164/253)	<0.001
Depressive symptoms*	18.2 (25/137)	20.3 (35/172)	24.7 (42/170)	0.36
Prevalent delirium	2.3 (4/175)	19.2 (40/208)	29.7 (71/239)	<0.001
Functional domain				
Premorbid ADL impairment	13.1 (23/175)	50.2 (106/211)	77.3 (194/251)	<0.001
Vision impairment	9.5 (16/169)	20.7 (41/198)	30.5 (75/246)	<0.001
Hearing impairment	13.0 (21/161)	18.1 (35/193)	23.3 (55/236)	0.04
Low health status score*	31.1 (42/135)	38.0 (65/171)	44.0 (74/168)	0.07
Social domain				
High perceived caregiver burden	26.3 (31/118)	41.7 (70/168)	50.2 (111/221)	<0.001
Total number of geriatric conditions† (mean (SD))	2.2 (1.3)	3.8 (2.1)	5.1 (1.8)	<0.001

*Not assessed in patients with severe cognitive impairment, defined as an MMSE score ≤15 at admission.
†not including pain, depressive symptoms and low health status score, as those were most frequently not measured in high risk patients. Only cognitive impairment at admission was included in the total number of geriatric conditions.
ADL = activities of daily living, IADL = instrumental activities of daily living.

impairments in ADL, they also deteriorated the most at three and twelve months.

Risk profiles in relation to mortality and functional decline

Tables 4 and 5 show that in both the crude and adjusted models, being at high risk for functional decline was significantly associated with mortality and poor functional health at both time points. Among patients at intermediate risk, the only significant association was found for functional decline at three and twelve months. However, when adjusting for age, sex and level of comorbidity, we could not demonstrate an association between moderate risk and functional decline one year after discharge.

Discussion

This multicenter study showed that by applying a simple risk assessment instrument at admission, three subgroups of older patients with distinct clinical characteristics and outcomes could be identified. Twenty-seven percent of the patients were at low risk for functional decline, 33% were at intermediate risk and 40% were at high risk for developing new disabilities. Patients at high risk for further functional decline presented with the highest number of geriatric conditions. High-risk patients were also at the

highest risk for poor outcomes in terms of mortality and deterioration in ADL functioning and their mean overall decline in functioning was significantly greater.

The low-risk group, as expected, presented with the fewest geriatric conditions and ADL impairments at admission but still had an average of two geriatric conditions besides the acute and chronic diseases leading to hospital admission. The number of geriatric conditions and premorbid ADL impairments gradually increased in the intermediate- and high-risk groups. The findings on the differences between the subgroups are consistent with other studies that used a more detailed risk classification for functional decline or frailty [9,13].

The geriatric conditions most often present in the high-risk group (cognitive impairment, delirium, premorbid ADL impairment, urine incontinence and fall risk) reflect the patients' frailty [25,26] and are known risk factors for future functional decline [1,8,26,27] . The high-risk group presented with the most baseline impairments and the greatest deterioration of ADLs both in percentage and the mean number of decline over the follow-up period. Lost functions are difficult to recover, and new disabilities or impairment reported at discharge that are still present at one month of follow-up are especially difficult to rehabilitate [27]. Patients discharged with new or additional disabilities also have the highest probability of dying in the year after admission [27].

Table 3. Response to the ISAR-HP questions, baseline impairments and functional outcomes at three and twelve months in the three risk groups for functional decline.

	Low risk (n = 175)	Intermediate risk (n = 211)	High risk (n = 253)
Response to ISAR-HP questions			
1. Needed more help in IADL (% yes)	16.6	32.5	47.6
2. Eight years or fewer of formal education (% yes)	20.8	37.8	58.7
3. Needed help with travelling (% yes)	5.7	48.6	91.3
4. Use of a walking device (% yes)	0.0	56.4	100.0
Baseline functional characteristics			
Katz ADL index* (mean/SD)	0.14 (0.39)	1.16 (1.64)	2.36 (2.10)
No of baseline impairments on Katz ADL index (%)			
0	86.9	49.8	22.7
1	12.6	23.7	24.7
2	0.0	10.0	11.2
3	0.6	5.2	8.8
4	0.0	3.8	10.8
5	0.0	3.8	12.0
6	0.0	3.8	10.0
Functional outcome at three months			
Katz ADL index* (mean/SD)	0.36 (0.76)	1.32 (1.87)	3.05 (2.10)
Functional decline† (mean/SD)	0.20 (0.77)	0.34 (1.47)	0.83 (1.83)
Functional outcome at twelve months			
Katz ADL index* (mean/SD)	0.41 (0.73)	1.40 (1.94)	2.77 (2.13)
Functional decline† (mean/SD)	0.24 (0.70)	0.51 (1.85)	0.68 (1.88)

ISAR-HP = identification of seniors at risk-hospitalized patients, IADL = instrumental activities of daily living, ADL = activities of daily living, SD = standard deviation.
*Katz ADL index; range of scores between 0–6, with a higher score indicating more dependence.
†Functional decline was measured with the Katz ADL index and the outcome at three or twelve months was compared to premorbid functioning two weeks prior to hospital admission. These data were only available for those patients still alive at follow up.

The severity of the acute illness leading to admission is an important risk factor for mortality [28,29]. This risk factor might explain the still relatively high mortality rates of 27% and 30% in the low- and intermediate-risk groups, respectively, up to one year after admission.

Compared with the low-risk group, the intermediate group showed an increased risk for functional decline at three months, but this increased risk disappeared at one year. A clear association between the high-risk group and mortality and functional decline was demonstrated at both time points. Only one-third of this group maintained baseline function one year after admission. This finding could indicate that the intermediate group has more potential for further rehabilitation after admission compared with the high-risk group, which might be too frail. Research has demonstrated that once patients begin to decline, they are more prone to further decline, even if they have regained their initial level of functioning [30,31]. More interestingly, one large study on functional decline at the end of life clearly demonstrated that functional trajectories for patients with both organ failure and frailty in the last year of life demonstrated an almost continuous decline in ADL functioning, starting with already many baseline impairments, whereas in patients with end-stage cancer, this decline only starts in the last two or three months of life and these patients predominantly have a good level of ADL functioning [32]. In our study this might also be visible; in the low risk group, many patients died, but did not have much premorbid dependencies. These patients were more fre-

Table 4. Cox regression models for three- and twelve-month mortality in relation to risk categories.

Risk category	Three-month mortality Unadjusted HR (95% CI)	Three-month mortality Adjusted* HR (95% CI)	Twelve-month mortality Unadjusted HR (95% CI)	Twelve-month mortality Adjusted* HR (95% CI)
Low risk	Ref	Ref	Ref	Ref
Intermediate risk	1.49 (0.90–2.45)	1.43 (0.85–2.42)	1.15 (0.79–1.67)	1.10 (0.75–1.62)
High risk	1.82 (1.13–2.91)	1.71 (1.01–2.90)	1.81 (1.29–2.54)	1.62 (1.11–2.35)

HR = hazard ratio; CI = confidence interval.
*Adjusted for age, sex and Charlson comorbidity index.

Table 5. Logistic regression models for functional decline at three and twelve months in relation to risk categories.

Risk category	Functional decline at three months Unadjusted OR (95% CI)	Functional decline at three months Adjusted* OR (95% CI)	Functional decline at twelve months Unadjusted OR (95% CI)	Functional decline at twelve months Adjusted* OR (95% CI)
Low risk	Ref	Ref	Ref	Ref
Intermediate risk	2.19 (1.21–3.95)	2.07 (1.11–3.89)	2.07 (1.13–3.80)	1.60 (0.81–3.14)
High risk	5.31 (3.04–9.27)	4.48 (2.41–8.35)	4.29 (2.38–7.75)	3.22 (1.63–6.36)

OR = odds ratio; CI = confidence interval.
*Adjusted for age, sex and Charlson comorbidity index.

quently cancer patients, whereas in the high risk group, many baseline impairments were present, and these patients demonstrated most decline in the year after hospital admission.

An important question is whether risk status can identify the patients most likely to benefit from multidisciplinary intervention by a geriatric consultation team. Results of a meta analysis of inpatient geriatric rehabilitation argued that subgroup evidence in favor of providing geriatric rehabilitation during and after hospital admission is warranted [33] and that more tailored approaches to patient selection still need to be tested. A recent randomized clinical trial (RCT) focusing on disease management in older heart failure patients divided participants into three risk groups and found that there was a difference in intervention benefits, in terms of both outcomes and costs, in favor of the intermediate-risk group [34]. The authors argued that the low-risk group was too healthy and that the high-risk group too ill to profit from the intervention.

Further research should focus on testing this risk-based approach in acutely hospitalized older patients. This research could be implemented in two ways. The first is an impact study, testing the clinical usefulness of the approach by determining whether the risk assessment outcomes influence decision making and goal setting in both physicians and patients [35]. The second study that could be performed is an RCT using the three risk groups as a basis for goal setting and intervention. The ICF rehabilitation model could inform goals for the low-, intermediate- and high-risk groups [10]. The ICF rehabilitation model identifies several different health strategies, which can be used to determine rehabilitation outcomes. The three health strategies that might be relevant in relation to this study are the preventive health strategy, in which the main purpose is to prevent health conditions and remain functioning. The second strategy is aimed at rehabilitation in which the primary goal should be to restore functioning and the third strategy is supportive care direct towards maintaining quality of life and preservation of autonomy. These strategies might be relevant for the low, intermediate and high risk group, respectively.

Some limitations need to be addressed. First, in our study, we made a predefined selection with one risk assessment instrument, the ISAR-HP. Our main purpose was to demonstrate that a risk assessment instrument can be helpful to detect low-, intermediate- and high-risk patients. Although our study is a multicenter study, using the ISAR-HP for this purpose in other settings might produce different arising from differences in the case mix of patients, leading to a different distribution of the outcome and predictive factors [35]. We clearly demonstrated that this risk-based approach revealed differences in baseline (clinical) charac-

teristics and health outcomes, further enhancing the validity of this screening instrument.

Second, functional decline was operationalized as a one-point decline at follow-up functioning compared with premorbid functioning. For further analyses, we dichotomized the outcome as present or absent. Although this approach is used in most studies of functional decline in hospitalized older patients [2], it leads to a loss of information about the ADL functioning level after hospitalization.

Third, the inclusion percentage was 62%. This expected but still low inclusion rate is a common problem in studies of acutely hospitalized older patients, and most trials conducted in this population demonstrated equal or lower participation rates [36–38]. We did conduct a small non-respondent analysis in which we demonstrated that the patients that were excluded were often younger and died more frequently after discharge. Presumably, these patients more frequently had end stage diseases or were very frail older patients. It would have strengthened the validity of study results, if we would have collected more baseline information on these patients.

Conclusion

In conclusion, by using an easily applied risk assessment instrument at hospital admission, three patients groups (low, intermediate and high risk for functional decline) with distinct clinical characteristics could be distinguished. This approach might contribute to better defining of treatment goals at hospital admission, earlier initiation of appropriate (preventive) interventions and better communication with patients and caregivers about the preferred outcomes of admission. The application of this approach and the effectiveness of risk-based clinical interventions should further be tested in clinical practice and randomized clinical trials.

Author Contributions

Conceived and designed the experiments: MS SR. Performed the experiments: BB JH EG SR. Analyzed the data: BB RH SR. Wrote the paper: BB. Critical revision of manuscript: JH EG RH MS SR. Study supervision: RH SR.

References

1. Buurman BM, van Munster BC, Korevaar JC, de Haan RJ, de Rooij SE (2011) Variability in measuring (instrumental) activities of daily living functioning and functional decline in hospitalized older medical patients: a systematic review. J Clin Epidemiol 64: 619–627.

2. McCusker J, Kakuma R, Abrahamowicz M (2002) Predictors of functional decline in hospitalized elderly patients: a systematic review. J Gerontol A Biol Sci Med Sci 57: M569–M577.
3. Covinsky KE, Palmer RM, Counsell SR, Pine ZM, Walter LC, et al. (2000) Functional status before hospitalization in acutely ill older adults: validity and clinical importance of retrospective reports. J Am Geriatr Soc 48: 164–169.
4. Sager MA, Franke T, Inouye SK, Landefeld CS, Morgan TM, et al. (1996) Functional outcomes of acute medical illness and hospitalization in older persons. Arch Intern Med 156: 645–652.
5. De Saint-Hubert M, Schoevaerdts D, Cornette P, D'Hoore W, Boland B, et al. (2010) Predicting functional adverse outcomes in hospitalized older patients: a systematic review of screening tools. J Nutr Health Aging 14: 394–399.
6. Boltz M, Capezuti E, Shabbat N, Hall K (2010) Going home better not worse: older adults' views on physical function during hospitalization. Int J Nurs Pract 16: 381–388.
7. Ferrucci L, Guralnik JM, Studenski S, Fried LP, Cutler GB, et al. (2004) Designing randomized, controlled trials aimed at preventing or delaying functional decline and disability in frail, older persons: a consensus report. J Am Geriatr Soc 52: 625–634.
8. Fried LP, Ferrucci L, Darer J, Williamson JD, Anderson G (2004) Untangling the concepts of disability, frailty, and comorbidity: implications for improved targeting and care. J Gerontol A Biol Sci Med Sci 59: 255–263.
9. Health Council of the Netherlands (2009) Prevention in the elderly; focus on functioning in daily life.
10. Stucki G, Cieza A, Melvin J (2007) The International Classification of Functioning, Disability and Health (ICF): a unifying model for the conceptual description of the rehabilitation strategy. J Rehabil Med 39: 279–285. 10.2340/16501977-0041 [doi].
11. Jones DM, Song X, Rockwood K (2004) Operationalizing a frailty index from a standardized comprehensive geriatric assessment. J Am Geriatr Soc 52: 1929–1933.
12. Sager MA, Rudberg MA, Jalaluddin M, Franke T, Inouye SK, et al. (1996) Hospital admission risk profile (HARP): identifying older patients at risk for functional decline following acute medical illness and hospitalization. J Am Geriatr Soc 44: 251–257.
13. Ellis G, Langhorne P (2004) Comprehensive geriatric assessment for older hospital patients. Br Med Bull 71: 45–59.
14. McCusker J, Bellavance F, Cardin S, Trepanier S (1998) Screening for geriatric problems in the emergency department: reliability and validity. Identification of Seniors at Risk (ISAR) Steering Committee. Acad Emerg Med 5: 883–893.
15. Dendukuri N, McCusker J, Belzile E (2004) The identification of seniors at risk screening tool: further evidence of concurrent and predictive validity. J Am Geriatr Soc 52: 290–296.
16. McCusker J, Bellavance F, Cardin S, Trepanier S, Verdon J, et al. (1999) Detection of older people at increased risk of adverse health outcomes after an emergency visit: the ISAR screening tool. J Am Geriatr Soc 47: 1229–1237.
17. Hoogerduijn JG, Schuurmans MJ, Korevaar JC, Buurman BM, de Rooij SE (2010) Identification of older hospitalised patients at risk for functional decline, a study to compare the predictive values of three screening instruments. J Clin Nurs 19: 1219–1225.
18. Hoogerduijn JG, Buurman BM, Korevaar JC, Grobbee DE, de Rooij SE, et al. (2011) The prediction of functional decline in older hospitalized patients. Age Ageing; [in press].
19. Lawton MP, Brody EM (1969) Assessment of older people: self-maintaining and instrumental activities of daily living. Gerontologist 9: 179–186.
20. Kruizenga HM, Seidell JC, de Vet HC, Wierdsma NJ, van Bokhorst-de van der Schueren MA (2005) Development and validation of a hospital screening tool for malnutrition: the short nutritional assessment questionnaire (SNAQ). Clin Nutr 24: 75–82.
21. Folstein MF, Folstein SE, McHugh PR (1975) "Mini-mental state". A practical method for grading the cognitive state of patients for the clinician. J Psychiatr Res 12: 189–198.
22. Inouye SK, van Dyck CH, Alessi CA, Balkin S, Siegal AP, et al. (1990) Clarifying confusion: the confusion assessment method. A new method for detection of delirium. Ann Intern Med 113: 941–948.
23. Charlson ME, Pompei P, Ales KL, MacKenzie CR (1987) A new method of classifying prognostic comorbidity in longitudinal studies: development and validation. J Chronic Dis 40: 373–383.
24. Katz S, Ford AB, Moskowitz RW, Jackson BA, Jaffe MW (1963) Studies of illness in the aged. The index of ADL: A standardized measure of biological and psychosocial function. JAMA 185: 914–919.
25. Fried LP, Tangen CM, Walston J, Newman AB, Hirsch C, et al. (2001) Frailty in older adults: evidence for a phenotype. J Gerontol A Biol Sci Med Sci 56: M146–M156.
26. Inouye SK, Studenski S, Tinetti ME, Kuchel GA (2007) Geriatric syndromes: clinical, research, and policy implications of a core geriatric concept. J Am Geriatr Soc 55: 780–791.
27. Boyd CM, Landefeld CS, Counsell SR, Palmer RM, Fortinsky RH, et al. (2008) Recovery of activities of daily living in older adults after hospitalization for acute medical illness. J Am Geriatr Soc 56: 2171–2179.
28. Buurman BM, van Munster BC, Korevaar JC, Abu-Hanna A, Levi M, et al. (2008) Prognostication in Acutely Admitted Older Patients by Nurses and Physicians. J Gen Intern Med 23: 1883–1889.
29. Walter LC, Brand RJ, Counsell SR, Palmer RM, Landefeld CS, et al. (2001) Development and validation of a prognostic index for 1-year mortality in older adults after hospitalization. JAMA 285: 2987–2994.
30. Hardy SE, Gill TM (2004) Recovery from disability among community-dwelling older persons. JAMA 291: 1596–1602.
31. Hardy SE, Gill TM (2005) Factors associated with recovery of independence among newly disabled older persons. Arch Intern Med 165: 106–112.
32. Lunney JR, Lynn J, Foley DJ, Lipson S, Guralnik JM (2003) Patterns of functional decline at the end of life. JAMA 289: 2387–2392.
33. Bachmann S, Finger C, Huss A, Egger M, Stuck AE, et al. (2010) Inpatient rehabilitation specifically designed for geriatric patients: systematic review and meta-analysis of randomised controlled trials. BMJ 340: c1718.
34. Pulignano G, Del SD, Di LA, Tarantini L, Cioffi G, et al. (2010) Usefulness of frailty profile for targeting older heart failure patients in disease management programs: a cost-effectiveness, pilot study. J Cardiovasc Med (Hagerstown) 11: 739–747.
35. Moons KG, Altman DG, Vergouwe Y, Royston P (2009) Prognosis and prognostic research: application and impact of prognostic models in clinical practice. BMJ 338: b606.
36. Counsell SR, Holder CM, Liebenauer LL, Palmer RM, Fortinsky RH, et al. (2000) Effects of a multicomponent intervention on functional outcomes and process of care in hospitalized older patients: a randomized controlled trial of Acute Care for Elders (ACE) in a community hospital. J Am Geriatr Soc 48: 1572–1581.
37. Kircher TT, Wormstall H, Muller PH, Schwarzler F, Buchkremer G, et al. (2007) A randomised trial of a geriatric evaluation and management consultation services in frail hospitalised patients. Age Ageing 36: 36–42.
38. Naylor MD, Brooten D, Campbell R, Jacobsen BS, Mezey MD, et al. (1999) Comprehensive discharge planning and home follow-up of hospitalized elders: a randomized clinical trial. JAMA 281: 613–620.

17

Can Falls Risk Prediction Tools Correctly Identify Fall-Prone Elderly Rehabilitation Inpatients? A Systematic Review and Meta-Analysis

Bruno Roza da Costa[1], Anne Wilhelmina Saskia Rutjes[1], Angelico Mendy[2], Rosalie Freund-Heritage[3], Edgar Ramos Vieira[3,4]*

1 Division of Clinical Epidemiology and Biostatistics, Institute of Social and Preventive Medicine, University of Bern, Bern, Switzerland, 2 Department of Epidemiology and Biostatistics, Robert Stempel School of Public Health, Florida International University, Miami, Florida, United States of America, 3 Glenrose Rehabilitation Hospital, Edmonton, Alberta, Canada, 4 Department of Physical Therapy, Florida International University, Miami, Florida, United States of America

Abstract

Background: Falls of elderly people may cause permanent disability or death. Particularly susceptible are elderly patients in rehabilitation hospitals. We systematically reviewed the literature to identify falls prediction tools available for assessing elderly inpatients in rehabilitation hospitals.

Methods and Findings: We searched six electronic databases using comprehensive search strategies developed for each database. Estimates of sensitivity and specificity were plotted in ROC space graphs and pooled across studies. Our search identified three studies which assessed the prediction properties of falls prediction tools in a total of 754 elderly inpatients in rehabilitation hospitals. Only the STRATIFY tool was assessed in all three studies; the other identified tools (PJC-FRAT and DOWNTON) were assessed by a single study. For a STRATIFY cut-score of two, pooled sensitivity was 73% (95%CI 63 to 81%) and pooled specificity was 42% (95%CI 34 to 51%). An indirect comparison of the tools across studies indicated that the DOWNTON tool has the highest sensitivity (92%), while the PJC-FRAT offers the best balance between sensitivity and specificity (73% and 75%, respectively). All studies presented major methodological limitations.

Conclusions: We did not identify any tool which had an optimal balance between sensitivity and specificity, or which were clearly better than a simple clinical judgment of risk of falling. The limited number of identified studies with major methodological limitations impairs sound conclusions on the usefulness of falls risk prediction tools in geriatric rehabilitation hospitals.

Editor: Hamid Reza Baradaran, Tehran University of Medical Sciences, Islamic Republic of Iran

Funding: This work was supported by the Alberta Health Services. Funding for publishing this paper was provided by the College of Nursing and Health Sciences, Florida International University, Miami. The funders had no role in study design, data collection and analysis, decision to publish, or preparation of the manuscript.

Competing Interests: The authors have declared that no competing interests exist.

* E-mail: evieira@fiu.edu

Introduction

Patient falls is a predominant patient safety issue in hospitals accounting for up to 32.3% of all reported patient safety incidents [1]. Fall-related complications lead to a prolonged rehabilitation period and increased health care costs [2,3]. It is estimated that just in the United Kingdom, patient falls in acute care hospitals cost approximately 92 million pounds per year [4]. The actual costs of inpatient falls may be even higher as falls are frequently underreported [1]. Other than the cost of falls to hospitals, patients incur additional costs as 35% of the patients who fall suffer physical harm or even death [1]. Falls may also cause fear of falling, which may lead to immobility and its complications such as muscle weakness, contracture, postural hypotension, and thrombogenic events [5,6].

Falls are the first leading cause of unintentional injury-related death among the elderly (i.e. people 65 years and older) [7]. Falls cause more than 95% of all hip fractures in the elderly; 20% of the

elderly people who suffer hip fractures die within a year [8]. The prevalence rate of falls in acute hospitals is around two to six percent, [9] in general rehabilitation settings is 12.5%, [3,10] and in geriatric rehabilitation hospitals is 24 to 30% [11,12]. The higher prevalence of falls in geriatric rehabilitation hospitals may be explained by the fact that elderly patients are generally frailer, are more exposed to risk factors for falling than younger patients, and are encouraged in rehabilitation settings to be physically active, independent, and involved in rehabilitation activities [3,13]. These circumstances challenge their physical abilities, and places them in situations where they are more likely to fall [3]. Thus, elderly patients in rehabilitation hospitals are particularly at risk for falls.

Although there is a clear need to implement strategies to prevent elderly inpatient falls in rehabilitation hospitals, it is unclear which strategies are the most effective for fall prevention in this population [14]. A common strategy is the use of falls risk prediction tools [4]. Identifying fall-prone patients on admission may help prevent falls by guiding implementation of targeted fall prevention strategies. However, the accuracy of the available prediction tools in actually identifying fall-prone patients is debated [15,16]. Using inaccurate falls prediction tools may create a false sense of safety on both patients and staff, leaving patients at risk exposed to the potential adverse effects of falling and consequent injuries [15]. It is not clear at the moment if there is an efficient tool to assess the risk of falls among rehabilitation hospital elderly inpatients. Therefore, the objective of this study was to systematically review the literature to identify the falls prediction tools available for assessing elderly inpatients in rehabilitation hospitals, and to assess the prediction usefulness of these tools.

Methods

Literature Search

To identify eligible studies we undertook a systematic search of 6 databases (MEDLINE, CINAHL, SCOPUS, Web of Science, Rehab data, and CIRRIE Database of International Rehabilitation Research). The search strategy used a combination of terms for rehabilitation hospital inpatient, falls, risk assessment, prediction, and older age. The terms included text words, keywords and subject headings specific to each database (Appendix S1). Similar strategies were used to identify previously published systematic reviews in three databases (Cochrane Database of Systematic Reviews, OTseeker, and PEDro). To try and minimize the chance of publication bias, we conducted a thorough search of unpublished studies. We searched ProQuest Dissertations for unpublished studies and searched conference proceedings on OCLC ProceedingsFirst. We also screened reference lists of included papers and contacted authors and experts in the field. All searches were conducted from databases inception to July 2011. Our systematic review has no published protocol available.

Study Selection and Outcomes of Interest

To be included in our review, studies must have conducted a prospective investigation of the predictive properties of prediction tools for falls of elderly (i.e. ≥65 years of age) inpatients in rehabilitation hospitals. Only studies published in the English language were considered for inclusion. In addition, studies should have either reported our primary outcome of interest with respective confidence intervals (i.e. sensitivity and specificity of prediction tools of falls among elderly rehabilitation inpatients) or have reported enough data so that we could construct 2×2 tables and directly calculate these estimates. Positive and predictive values were secondary outcomes of interest, and were also extracted whenever available. Two reviewers (BRDC, ERV) independently screened the titles and abstracts of all identified citations and subsequently assessed full text versions of potentially eligible studies for inclusion. Disagreements regarding study eligibility were resolved through discussion.

Data Collection

Two reviewers (BRDC, ERV) trained in health research methodology extracted data independently and in duplicate using a standardized form. Data regarding participants' characteristics, prediction tools used, main findings, and methodological quality were extracted and tabulated. Disagreements regarding extracted data were resolved through discussion.

Methodological Quality Assessment

We assessed the following study characteristics deemed important for the development of risk prediction tools: [17,18] (1) Fall or faller clearly defined: Was a clear definition of the outcome "fall" or "faller" explained and standardized among staff? (e.g. an incident in which a patient suddenly and involuntarily came to rest upon the ground or surface lower than their original station) [19]; (2) Blinded adjudication of event: Were staff responsible for counting falls/identify fallers blinded to the estimates produced by the prediction tool?; (3) Confounding assessed: Were other relevant patient characteristics taken into account when interpreting results? (i.e. difference between groups regarding relevant risk factors not covered by the predicting tool); (4) Cut-score predefined: If a single cut-score was used to report estimates, was it based on previous evidence and defined *a priori*?; (5) Prediction tool compared to clinical judgment: Was the prediction tool compared to staff's intuitive estimates (best guess)?

Statistical Analysis

Description of the characteristics of the included studies were tabulated and presented in terms of absolute and relative frequencies, sensitivities and specificities, negative- and positive predictive values and corresponding 95% confidence intervals. We illustrated the data by plotting sensitivities and specificities in ROC space graphs, which allows the visual inspection of between-study heterogeneity. For meta-analytical purposes, we pre-specified to summarize the data applying the cut-scores that were either considered standard or were reported to optimally balance sensitivity against specificity. Only the STRATIFY tool had enough data to be meta-analyzed in the present investigation. It ranges from zero to five and the cut-score of ≥2 was considered for meta-analysis [20]. We meta-analyzed sensitivities and specificities using the 'metandi' module in STATA (version 11.2) [21]. To perform a meta-analysis of sensitivities and specificities with three studies, we used a univariate version of 'metandi', which was kindly provided to us by the University of Bristol.

Results

We identified 1257 references in our literature search and considered 786 to be potentially eligible (Figure 1). After full text screening, three studies met our inclusion criteria.

Description of the Included Studies

Overall, three studies including 754 elderly inpatients in rehabilitation wards/hospitals were identified by our search strategy (Table 1). The median year of publication was 2006 (range, 2003 to 2008). The average age of the patients ranged from 79 to 81 years, the percentage of female subjects ranged from 62 to 69%, and the proportion of fallers ranged from 26 to 51%. Cooker & Oliver did not report the number of fallers in their study. All included studies used a prospective cohort design. Two studies reported diagnosis of study participants which consisted mostly of orthopedic and neurological conditions [20,22]. Fall rates per 1000 patient-days were 13.4 in the study of Cooker & Oliver and 14.7 in the study of Haines et al [20,22]. Vassallo et al. did not report length of follow-up [23].

Quality Assessment

The methodological limitations of the studies are presented on Table 2. In two out of three studies adjudicators were unblinded or it was unclear whether adjudicators were blinded to the baseline score of the predicting tools which was established at study entry. One out of three studies did not report whether a "fall" definition

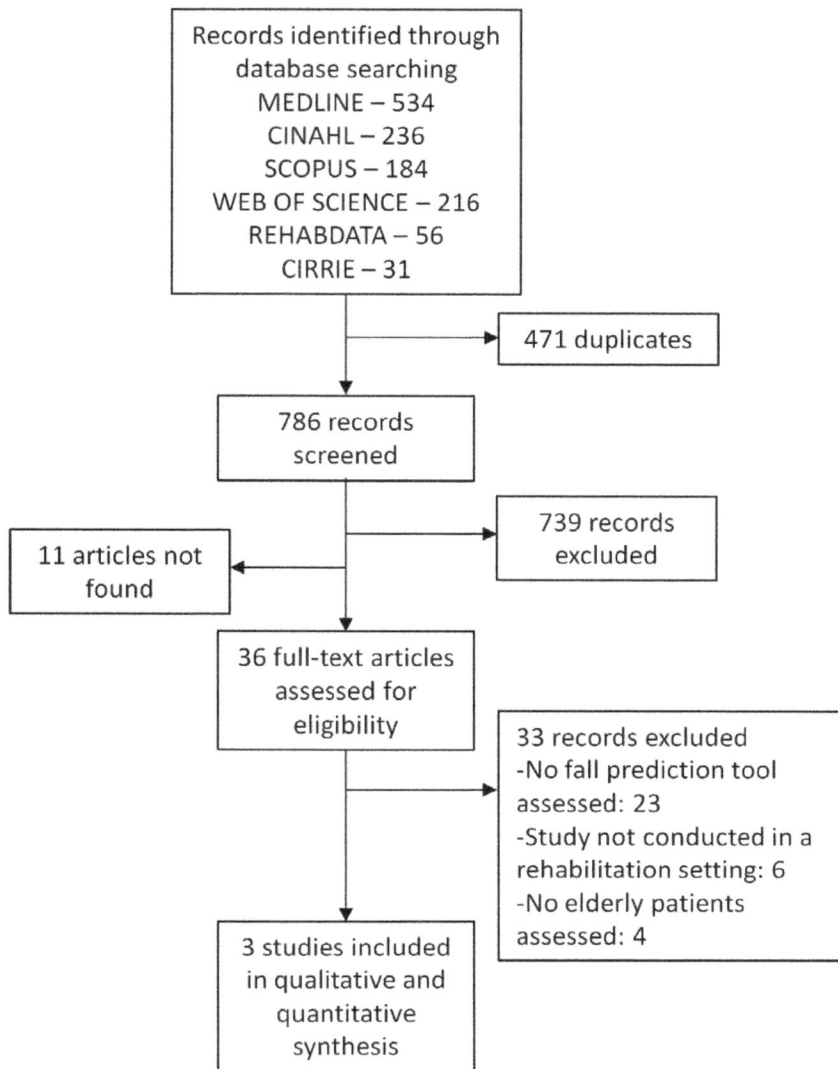

Figure 1. Flow-diagram depicting the selection process of studies investigating risk assessment tools for elderly inpatient falls in rehabilitation hospitals.

was pre-established. Two out of three studies did not compare the performance of the prediction tool to staff's intuitive estimates (best guess).

Fall Prediction Tools

All three studies investigated the predictive properties of the STRATIFY tool. Two of the studies also used other fall prediction tools: Haines et al. also used the PJC-FRAT, and Vassallo et al. also used the DOWNTON Fall Risk Index and "clinical judgment" [22,23].

Estimates

Table 1 displays results extracted from the three studies. In general, Haines et al. reported higher sensitivity but lower specificity of the STRATIFY tool compared to the PJC-FRAT [22]. Vassallo et al. examined the STRATIFY tool, the DOWNTON Fall Risk Index, and clinical judgment and reported that the DOWNTON Fall Risk Index showed the highest sensitivity and clinical judgment the highest specificity [23]. Cooker & Oliver

examined exclusively the STRATIFY tool, and reported similar estimates of sensitivity and specificity reported by Haines et al., but somewhat different estimates than those reported by Vassallo et al [20].

Cooker & Oliver and Haines et al. reported estimates of sensitivity and specificity for different cut-scores of the STRATIFY tool, whereas Vassalo et al. reported these estimates only for a cut-score of two or more points (figure 2). Figure 2(A) displays sensitivity and specificity for different cut-scores of the STRATIFY tool. The closer estimates are to the top left corner, the better are their sensitivity-specificity. All three studies reported sensitivity and specificity for the STRATIFY cut-score ≥ 2 which allowed pooling of these estimates. Pooled sensitivity across the three studies was 73% (95%CI 63 to 81%) and pooled specificity was 42% (95%CI 34 to 51%). Visual inspection of figure 2(A) indicates moderate between-study heterogeneity in estimates. Figure 2(B) displays estimates of sensitivity and specificity for each prediction tool according to cut-scores defined by developers of these tools as their optimal cut-score. It can be seen from this graph that the

Table 1. Overview of included studies showing studies characteristics and summary of findings.

Ref.	Sampling	n*	Mean Age	%♀	Fall data source	#falls	Fallers (%)	Reported findings
Cooker 2003	Patients admitted to a Geriatric Assessment and Rehabilitation Unit. Mean length of patient stay was 50 days.	432	81	69	Patient incident report	13.4 falls/1000 patient days	–	**STRATIFY (cut-off score ≥1)** sensitivity: 95% (95%CI 90–99) specificity: 17% (95%CI 13–21) positive predictive value: 28% (95%CI 24–33) negative predictive value: 90% (95%CI 83–98) **STRATIFY (cut-off score ≥2)** sensitivity: 66% (95%CI 57–75) specificity: 47% (95%CI 41–52) positive predictive value: 30% (95%CI 24–36) negative predictive value: 80% (95%CI 74–85) **STRATIFY (cut-off score ≥3)** sensitivity: 36% (95%CI 27–45) specificity: 85% (95%CI 81–89) positive predictive value: 45% (95%CI 35–55) negative predictive value: 79% (95%CI 75–84) **STRATIFY (cut-off score ≥4)** sensitivity: 11% (95%CI 5–17) specificity: 96% (95%CI 94–98) positive predictive value: 50% (95%CI 30–70) negative predictive value: 76% (95%CI 72–80) **STRATIFY (cut-off score =5)** sensitivity: 9% (95%CI −0.9–3) specificity: 100% (95%CI 99–100) positive predictive value: 50% (95%CI −19–119) negative predictive value: 74% (95%CI 70–79)
Haines 2006	Patients consecutively admitted at a hospital. metropolitan rehabilitation and aged care Rate of falls per 1000 patient-days was reported but exact length of follow-up is unclear.	122	79	69	Patient incident report	14.7 falls/1000 patient days	26	**STRATIFY (cut-off score ≥1)** sensitivity: 96% (95%CI 86–100) specificity: 20% (95%CI 12–29) **STRATIFY (cut-off score ≥2)** sensitivity: 77% (95%CI 59–92) specificity: 51% (95%CI 41–61) **STRATIFY (cut-off score ≥3)**

Table 1. Cont.

Ref.	Sampling	n*	Mean Age	%♀	Fall data source	#falls	Fallers (%)	Reported findings
Vassallo 2008	Consecutive patients from rehabilitation ward of a rehabilitation hospital admitting elderly patients. Length of follow-up unclear.	200	81	62	Falls diary compiled by nurses		51 (length of follow-up unclear)	sensitivity: 42% (95%CI 24–63)
								specificity: 78% (95%CI 70–86)
								STRATIFY (cut-off score ≥4)
								sensitivity: 4% (95%CI 0–14)
								specificity: 93% (95%CI 88–98)
								PJC-FRAT (Falls risk alert card)
								sensitivity: 73% (95%CI 55–90)
								specificity: 75% (95%CI 66–83)
								PJC-FRAT (Exercise program)
								sensitivity: 12% (95%CI 3–27)
								specificity: 84% (95%CI 77–91)
								PJC-FRAT (Education program)
								sensitivity: 27% (95%CI 12–46)
								specificity: 68% (95%CI 58–77)
								PJC-FRAT (Hip protectors)
								sensitivity: 31% (95%CI 14–48)
								specificity: 90% (95%CI 83–95)
								STRATIFY (cut-off score ≥2)
								sensitivity: 82% (95%CI 69–90)
								specificity: 34% (95%CI 27–42)
								positive predictive value: 30% (95%CI 23–38)
								negative predictive value: 85% (95%CI 73–91)
								DOWNTON (score ≥3)
								sensitivity: 92% (95%CI 82–97)
								specificity: 36% (95%CI 28–43)
								positive predictive value: 33% (95%CI 25–41)
								negative predictive value: 93% (95%CI 83–97)
								Clinical judgment (observation of wandering behavior)
								sensitivity: 43% (95%CI 30–56)
								specificity: 91% (95%CI 84–94)
								positive predictive value: 61% (95%CI 44–75)
								negative predictive value: 82% (95%CI 75–87)

*Number of patients;
♀Number of females.

Table 2. Assessment of potential threats to internal/external validity of included studies.

Study	Fall or faller clearly defined	Blinded adjudication of event	Confounding assessed	Cut-score pre-defined	Prediction tool compared to clinical judgment*
Coker 2003					
STRATIFY	+	?	−	NA	−
Haines 2006					
STRATIFY	+	+	+	NA	−
PJC-FRAT	+	−	+	NA	−
Vassallo 2008					
STRATIFY	?	?	−	+	+
DOWNTON	?	?	−	+	+
Clinical Judgement	?	?	−	+	NA

+: the criterion was satisfied; −: the criterion was not satisfied; ?: it was unclear whether the criterion was satisfied; NA: Not applicable; *comparison of sensitivity.

DOWNTON tool has the highest sensitivity (92%), while the PJC-FRAT offers a good balance between sensitivity and specificity (73% and 75%, respectively).

Discussion

The present systematic review identified three studies that investigated the prediction properties of different prediction tools for falls of elderly inpatients in rehabilitation hospitals: the STRATIFY, the DOWNTON, and the PJC-FRAT. The combined estimates for the three studies at the optimal cut-score of the STRATIFY tool (score ≥2) indicated that this tool has less than optimal sensitivity and specificity when applied to a population of elderly rehabilitation inpatients. The paucity in data did not allow meta-analysis of either the PJC-FRAT or DOWNTON tool. The STRATIFY gives a score which can range from zero to five, and its authors reported that a cut-score of ≥2 offers the best combination of sensitivity and specificity [20]. The PJC-FRAT is composed of four elements (falls risk alert card, additional exercise program, education program, hip protectors); the element "falls risk alert card", which yields a simple dichotomous score "high risk of fall" or "low risk of fall", was reported by its authors to have the best combination sensitivity-specificity [22]. The DOWNTON score can range from zero to

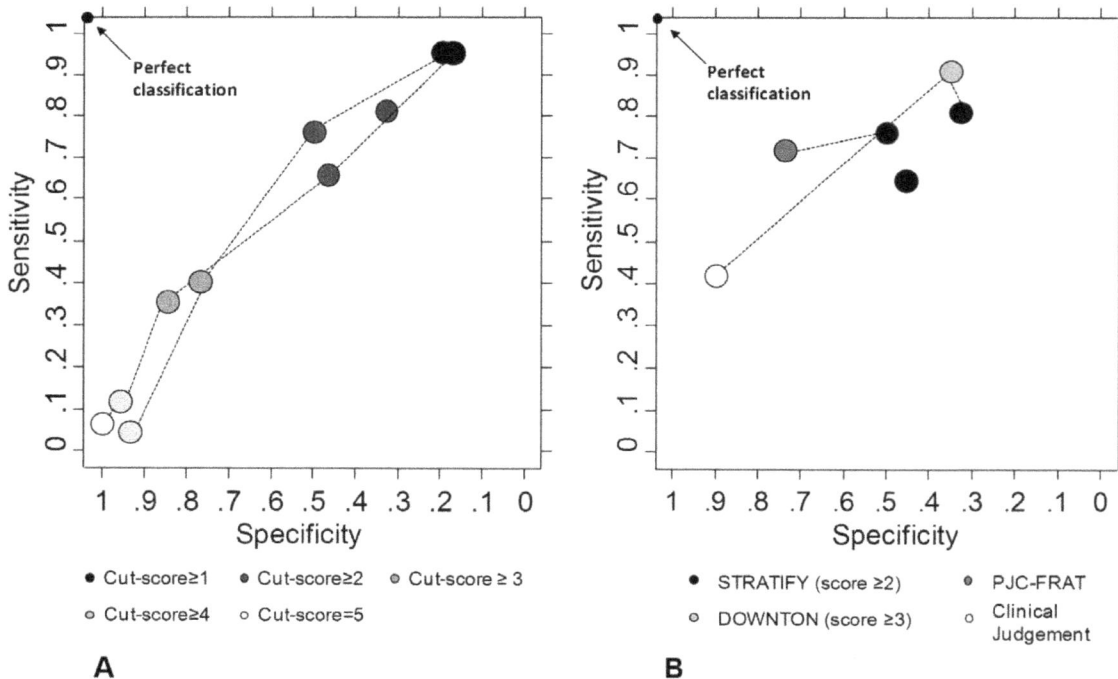

Figure 2. ROC space showing sensitivity and specificity of the STRATIFY tool per study for different cut-scores (A), and for fall prediction based on clinical judgment and on the optimal cut-off score of STRATIFY, DOWNTON and PJC-FRAT (B). Estimates originated from the same studies are connected with dashed lines. Estimates closer to the top left corner have better sensitivity-specificity.

eleven, and a cut-score of ≥ 3 has been determined to result in the best balance between sensitivity and specificity [23].

Two of the included studies reported sensitivity and specificity for multiple cut-scores of the STRATIFY [20,22]. It can be seen from figure 2(A) that also in an elderly rehabilitation setting a cut-score ≥ 2 results in the best combination of sensitivity and specificity for this particular tool. Two studies reported sensitivity and specificity for more than one prediction tool, allowing the direct comparison of their performance to identify patients with high risk of falling. This comparative design is optimal to draw conclusions regarding which tool performs best for the identification of patients at high risk of falling. Haines et al. compared the prediction performance of the STRATIFY (cut-score ≥ 2) and of the PJC-FRAT (falls risk alert card) in the same patients, and reported similar values of sensitivity and specificity for both tools (figure 2(B)) [22]. Vassalo et al. also used a comparative design to assess the prediction properties of the STRATIFY (cut-score ≥ 2) and of the DOWNTON (cut-score ≥ 3) and reported that these tools had similar values of specificity but that the DOWNTON had a better sensitivity (figure 2(B)) [23]. As shown in figure 2(B), the indirect comparison of sensitivity and specificity between the falls prediction tools across all studies indicate that no single tool clearly stands out from the others as the optimal prediction tool. When identifying patients at high risk of falling, the trade-off between sensitivity and specificity is optimal when the tool correctly discriminates patients at high risk of falling from those at low risk. If we assume that sensitivity should be at least 80% to be clinically relevant when predicting fall risk, we observe that the corresponding specificity is very low, leading to many falsely labeled persons at high risk of falling which unnecessarily burdens patients and staff. It is important to stress that comparison across studies of estimates shown in figure 2(B) is indirect in nature and therefore may be misleading and must be interpreted with caution.

We observed some variation between estimates of the same tool and cut-score across studies which must also be considered when interpreting our findings. Previous reviews have linked such variation to methodological and clinical heterogeneity. A systematic review of fall prediction tools identified 35 studies conducted in acute care settings [24]. The authors reported great variation between the studies and concluded that different settings, populations, and study designs (retrospective or prospective) were responsible for the reported variation. Oliver et al. (2008) conducted a systematic review to identify all studies that had prospectively investigated the predictive property of the STRAT-IFY tool [17]. They identified 8 studies that reported considerably different results regarding the predictive properties of the tool. The authors also associated such variation to different settings and populations between studies. Our results show that results can vary between studies even in a similar population, setting and design. In fact, creators of the STRATIFY tool themselves have contested the usefulness of such tools claiming that it may be much better to address reversible risk factors to try and avoid patients from falling, which is supported by others [17] [23]. Oliver advocates the identification and modification of risk factors as the optimal strategy to prevent falls as opposed to "risk prediction, which may be inaccurate and does not of itself do anything to stop patients falling" [15]. Nonetheless, other creators of well known fall-risk prediction tools defend their use [16].

This is the first review to search for studies investigating the predictive properties of different fall prediction tools in an elderly population in a rehabilitation hospital setting. Our findings reveal the scarcity of effective falls risk prediction tools for this specific population which may be particularly at risk. We found only one tool (PJC-FRAT) that was developed and tested in an elderly population of a rehabilitation hospital [22]. Moreover, implementation of such tools in the clinical setting is time and money consuming and to be worth the process, they must be at least significantly better than clinicians' clinical judgment (best guess). Vassalo et al. reported that the STRATIFY and DOWNTON had better sensitivity (82% and 92%, respectively) than clinical judgment (43%), and that both had worse specificity (34% and 36%, respectively) than clinical judgment (91%), which makes the usefulness of the these two falls prediction tools questionable [23].

Strengths of our review include an extensive search of six general and field-specific databases with a sensitive search strategy and thorough assessment of methodological quality of included studies. The major limitation of our study concern the low number of studies included. Although not a limitation which concerns the design of our review, the limited number of identified studies impairs sound conclusions to be made at this point concerning usefulness of falls risk prediction tools in geriatric rehabilitation hospitals. Moreover, we only included studies published in the English language, which have been reported to have different results than studies published in other languages [25]. However, the evidence for this potential bias is based only on studies of therapeutic interventions. Because there is currently no study which investigated whether this bias exists in systematic reviews of screening intervention studies, we do not know whether this language restriction may be indeed a potential threat to the validity of our findings [26].

Future studies with the purpose of developing new falls prediction tools should follow the rigorous steps required for such a purpose, taking into consideration the methodological issues discussed in the present review, and including suggestions for interventions rather than simply classifying the level of falls risk. In addition, future studies using prediction tools in falls prevention programs should investigate whether prediction tools are better than either simply addressing reversible risk factors or clinical judgment.

Acknowledgments

We thank Penny Whitting for providing us with a univariate version of the STATA command 'metandi'. We also thank Yemisi Takwoingi for the helpful discussions concerning meta-analysis of estimates of sensitivity and specificity.

Author Contributions

Conceived and designed the experiments: BRdC AWSR RFH ERV. Performed the experiments: BRdC AWSR AM ERV. Analyzed the data: BRdC AWSR. Wrote the paper: BRdC AWSR AM RFH ERV.

References

1. Healey F, Scobie S, Oliver D, Pryce A, Thomson R, et al. (2008) Falls in English and Welsh hospitals: a national observational study based on retrospective analysis of 12 months of patient safety incident reports. Qual Saf Health Care 17: 424–430.

2. Bates DW, Pruess K, Souney P, Platt R (1995) Serious falls in hospitalized patients: correlates and resource utilization. Am J Med 99: 137–143.

3. Saverino A, Benevolo E, Ottonello M, Zsirai E, Sessarego P (2006) Falls in a rehabilitation setting: functional independence and fall risk. Eura Medicophys 42: 179–184.

4. National Patient Safety Agency (2007) Slips, trips and falls in hospital. Available: http://www.npsa.nhs.uk/nrls/alerts-and-directives/directives-guidance/slips-trips-falls/. Accessed 2011 Nov 5.

5. Rousseau P (1993) Immobility in the aged. Arch Fam Med 2: 169–177; discussion 178.

6. Vellas BJ, Wayne SJ, Romero LJ, Baumgartner RN, Garry PJ (1997) Fear of falling and restriction of mobility in elderly fallers. Age Ageing 26: 189–193.

7. Centers for Disease Control and Prevention (2007) Preventing falls among older adults. Available: http://www.cdc.gov/ncipc/duip/preventadultfalls.htm. Accessed 2011 Mar 21.

8. PHAC - Public Health Agency of Canada. Division of Aging and Seniors. (2005) Report on Seniors' falls in Canada. Available: http://www.phac-aspc.gc.ca/seniors-aines/alt-formats/pdf/publications/pro/injury-blessure/seniors_falls/seniors-falls_e.pdf. Accessed 2011 Nov 5.

9. Evans D, Hodgkinson B, Lambert L, Wood J, Kowanko I (1998) Falls in acute hospitals: a systematic review. The Joanna Briggs Institute for Evidence Based Nursing and Midwifery.

10. Vlahov D, Myers AH, al-Ibrahim MS (1990) Epidemiology of falls among patients in a rehabilitation hospital. Arch Phys Med Rehabil 71: 8–12.

11. Uden G (1985) Inpatient accidents in hospitals. J Am Geriatr Soc 33: 833–841.

12. Vassallo M, Sharma JC, Briggs RS, Allen SC (2003) Characteristics of early fallers on elderly patient rehabilitation wards. Age Ageing 32: 338–342.

13. Vieira ER, Freund-Heritage R, da Costa BR (2011) Risk factors for geriatric patient falls in rehabilitation hospital settings: a systematic review. Clin Rehabil 25: 788–799.

14. Gillespie LD, Gillespie WJ, Robertson MC, Lamb SE, Cumming RG, et al. (2003) Interventions for preventing falls in elderly people. Cochrane Database Syst Rev: CD000340.

15. Oliver D (2006) Assessing the risk of falls in hospitals: time for a rethink? Can J Nurs Res 38: 89–94; discussion 95–86.

16. Morse JM (2006) The safety of safety research: the case of patient fall research. Can J Nurs Res 38: 73–88.

17. Oliver D, Papaioannou A, Giangregorio L, Thabane L, Reizgys K, et al. (2008) A systematic review and meta-analysis of studies using the STRATIFY tool for prediction of falls in hospital patients: how well does it work? Age Ageing 37: 621–627.

18. Hayden JA, Cote P, Bombardier C (2006) Evaluation of the quality of prognosis studies in systematic reviews. Ann Intern Med 144: 427–437.

19. Oliver D, Britton M, Seed P, Martin FC, Hopper AH (1997) Development and evaluation of evidence based risk assessment tool (STRATIFY) to predict which elderly inpatients will fall: case-control and cohort studies. BMJ 315: 1049–1053.

20. Coker E, Oliver D (2003) Evaluation of the STRATIFY falls prediction tool on a geriatric unit. Outcomes Manag 7: 8–14; quiz 15–16.

21. Harbord RM, Whiting P (2009) Metandi: Meta–analysis of diagnostic accuracy using hierarchical logistic regression. Stata Journal 9: 211–229.

22. Haines TP, Bennell KL, Osborne RH, Hill KD (2006) A new instrument for targeting falls prevention interventions was accurate and clinically applicable in a hospital setting. J Clin Epidemiol 59: 168–175.

23. Vassallo M, Poynter L, Sharma JC, Kwan J, Allen SC (2008) Fall risk-assessment tools compared with clinical judgment: an evaluation in a rehabilitation ward. Age Ageing 37: 277–281.

24. Haines TP, Hill K, Walsh W, Osborne R (2007) Design-related bias in hospital fall risk screening tool predictive accuracy evaluations: systematic review and meta-analysis. J Gerontol A Biol Sci Med Sci 62: 664–672.

25. Higgins JP, (editors) GS (2009) Meta-analyses with continuous outcomes. In: Collaboration TC, editor. Cochrane Handbook for Systematic Reviews of Interventions.

26. Macaskill P, Gatsonis C, Deeks J, Harbord R, Takwoingi Y (2010) Cochrane Handbook for Systematic Reviews of Diagnostic Test Accuracy. Chapter 10 Analysing and Presenting Results. In: Deeks JJ, Bossuyt PM, Gatsonis C, editors: The Cochrane Collaboration.

18

Behavioural Distinction between Strategic Control and Spatial Realignment during Visuomotor Adaptation in a Viewing Window Task

Jane M. Lawrence-Dewar*, Lee A. Baugh, Jonathan J. Marotta

Perception and Action Laboratory, Department of Psychology, University of Manitoba, Winnipeg, Manitoba, Canada

Abstract

We must frequently adapt our movements in order to successfully perform motor tasks. These visuomotor adaptations can occur with or without our awareness and so, have generally been described by two mechanisms: strategic control and spatial realignment. Strategic control is a conscious modification used when discordance between an intended and actual movement is observed. Spatial realignment is an unconscious recalibration in response to subtle differences between an intended and efferent movement. Traditional methods of investigating visuomotor adaptation often involve simplistic, repetitive motor goals and so may be vulnerable to subject boredom or expectation. Our laboratory has recently developed a novel, engaging computer-based task, the *Viewing Window*, to investigate visuomotor adaptation to large, apparent distortions. Here, we contrast behavioural measures of visuomotor adaptation during the *Viewing Window* task when either gradual progressive rotations or large, sudden rotations are introduced in order to demonstrate that this paradigm can be utilized to investigate both strategic control and spatial realignment. The gradual rotation group demonstrated significantly faster mean velocities and spent significantly less time off the object compared to the sudden rotation group. These differences demonstrate adaptation to the distortion using spatial realignment. Scan paths revealed greater after-effects in the gradual rotation group reflected by greater time spent scanning areas off of the object. These results demonstrate the ability to investigate both strategic control and spatial realignment. Thus, the *Viewing Window* provides a powerful engaging tool for investigating the neural basis of visuomotor adaptation and impairment following injury and disease.

Editor: Joy J. Geng, University of California, Davis, United States of America

Funding: This work was supported by a Natural Sciences and Engineering Research Council of Canada (NSERC) grant to JJM and Riverview Health Centre Research Grant to JMLD and JJM. JMLD is supported by a Manitoba Health Research Council (MHRC) postdoctoral research fellowship. LAB was a recipient of a MHRC graduate studentship. The funders had no role in study design, data collection and analysis, decision to publish, or preparation of the manuscript.

Competing Interests: The authors have declared that no competing interests exist.

* E-mail: dewarja@tbh.net

Introduction

We must frequently adapt our movements to successfully complete everyday tasks. These adaptations are sometimes conscious modifications in our motor plan in reaction to large distortions in order to achieve a desired output. At other times, the altered movements may be so subtle that we may not be aware they are occurring. Two mechanisms of visuomotor adaptation have generally been agreed upon: strategic control and spatial realignment. These mechanisms have also recently been described as 'fast' and 'slow' processes of motor adaptation [1]. Strategic control, or the fast component, involves a recalibration or the selection and learning of specific movements in order to successfully complete the desired action [2]. Whereas spatial realignment, or the slow component, is an automatic spatial remapping due to a detected discrepancy between an intended movement and the resulting sensory feedback [3,4,5]. During tasks of subtle distortions, it is believed that proprioceptive sensory feedback updates an internal model [6]. As an example of these two strategies, a car may develop a subtle and progressive problem with the steering column. A person who drives the car everyday may not notice this issue because as the distortion progresses over time, they automatically adapt their movements to match – this is

spatial realignment. In contrast, a person who seldom uses that car may notice the distortion right away and adjust the direction of the steering wheel in order to compensate for this change – this is strategic control.

Visuomotor adaption has classically been studied through prism experiments [7]. In these studies, subjects view objects through prism lenses, which alter the perception of an object's location. Healthy individuals can adapt their motor movements to accommodate the dissociation between their visual perception and the object's actual location. More recently, computer based tasks have supplemented these experiments and allowed more flexibility in their design as well as the acquisition of more precise and detailed behavioural information. In general, these tasks have tended to use target-based pointing [8] movements.

By introducing rotational distortions either incrementally, or suddenly, behaviour during spatial realignment and strategic control has been investigated during prism studies [9] and computer based point-to point or target tasks [8,10,11]. Kagerer et al [8] used a digitized point-to-point task on a touch sensitive tablet to show that participants exposed to a gradual, incremental rotation of $10°$, up to a maximum of $90°$, demonstrated faster movements with less spatial error and showed larger after effects than those who experienced a $90°$ rotation throughout the experiment. In their task, participants moved a marker to one of four targets while having no vision of their moving arm or hand. Klassen et al. [10] used an out-and back target task to one of eight targets where in a gradual condition increments of $0.125°$ were introduced to a maximum of $30°$ in a gradual distortion group. Even though these tasks have revealed important information regarding visuomotor adaptation behaviour and its neural basis, they are simplistic as they require one trajectory of movement therefore limiting the internal model a participant is capable of building during adaptation. In order to investigate visuomotor adaptation in a more natural, enriched setting, our lab has developed a computer-based task, the *Viewing Window* [12,13,14]. The paradigm is a visuomotor experiment hidden within a perceptual task. Subjects view a blurred or masked image of an object on a computer screen with the instruction to identify the object as quickly and accurately as possible. To accomplish this, they must move a small, circular region, the *Viewing Window*, around the screen using a touch sensitive screen, trackball or joystick. The task has previously been used during reading and text comprehension tasks [15,16], as well as scene exploration [17], to investigate visual attention and perception. More recently, our lab has used to this task to investigate visuomotor adaptation by manipulating the relationship between the actions of the participant and the resulting movement of the window [14]. By restricting the region of an object that can be viewed clearly, the visuomotor scanning pattern can be analyzed. The benefits of the *Viewing Window* over traditional prism experiments is that this task requires minimal experimenter instruction, distortions can be presented in finer and progressive increments, it can be performed on a compact tablet PC therefore it is highly portable, and precise timing and spatial information regarding viewing window movement and object identification can be recorded.

Our previous studies with the *Viewing Window* task have utilized large distortions in the form of flips in *Viewing Window* movement in the horizontal and vertical direction and so it would be anticipated that strategic control would be the predominant mechanism of visuomotor adaptation [12,13,14]. The use of this task has revealed novel recruitment of the claustrum, not found in previous studies of visuomotor adaptation [12]. The purpose of the present study is to demonstrate that the *viewing window* paradigm can be used to investigate both strategic control and spatial realignment.

We hypothesize that distinct behaviours between participants using strategic control and those who adapt using spatial realignment can be measured using the *Viewing Window* paradigm. In line with our previous Viewing Window studies, we anticipate participants in the sudden rotation group will demonstrate difficulty in controlling the window when the distortion is initially introduced, which will be reflected by more complicated paths of movement, slower velocities of movement, and more time spent off the object during the first half (early phase) of the trials. As the experiment progresses, we hypothesize the participants will adapt and their performance evaluated by these measures will improve during the second half of the distortion trials (late phase) and will continue to do so once the distortion is removed. In contrast, we hypothesize that participants in the gradual rotation group will not notice the introduced distortion and so changes in behaviour in the form of movement velocities, the time taken to identify the viewed object (scan time), and the time that the *Viewing Window* spent on areas that did not contain object image (time off object), will be minimal during the early and late phase distortion trials and the paths of window movement will be more simple with fewer changes in direction compared to the sudden rotation group. However, once the distortion is removed in the post-distortion

phase, we hypothesize that participants in the gradual rotation group will show greater after-effects in the form of decreased performance of these measures. The ability to distinguish and measure behavioural differences between groups will demonstrate that the Viewing Window task can be used to evaluate performance of both strategic control and spatial realignment.

The ability to use the *Viewing Window* to measure behaviour during strategic control and spatial realignment would provide a novel, powerful tool for examining visuomotor adaptation. This would expand the repertoire of experimental designs available for investigating visuomotor adaptation in healthy individuals and in decline due to natural aging, and neural injury and degenerative disease.

Methods

Subjects

Written informed consent was obtained from all subjects prior to the study. Fifty-eight right-handed, first year psychology students with normal or corrected-to-normal vision (15 male) were recruited from the University of Manitoba psychology participant pool. Subjects received course credit for participating in the study. This research was approved by the Human Research Ethics Board at the University of Manitoba.

Prior to start of the experiment, subjects were familiarized with the response equipment, a track ball, used in the study. Participants were presented with a medium difficulty maze (set 5) acquired from www.printablemazes.net and asked to guide a computer cursor through the maze to get acquainted with the sensitivity of the trackball. Participants were aware that no data were being collected during this time and that it was self-paced.

The Viewing Window Task

The *Viewing Window* task [14], is an in-house software program written in Matlab® (2007b, MathWorks, Natick, MA), run on a Dell tablet computer and presented to the participant on a 19″ LCD monitor. During the present study our methods were modified slightly from our previously published studies [12,13,14]. During pilot testing, the sudden rotation distortions were not apparent to all subjects when a blurred image was presented. Therefore, clear images of the objects were overlaid with a black mask. As a result, subjects could not obtain any additional cues as to where useful information may be, resulting in a much more difficult task. The number of trials therefore had to be reduced to maintain an acceptable duration of experiment and prevent subject fatigue. In the present study, 40 trials were presented which all subjects completed in less than one hour. During each trial a masked picture of an everyday object would appear at 1280×1024 resolution. All participants viewed the same 40 images however, to control for order effects, 2 counterbalanced lists were used so that half the participants in each experimental group would view the list in one order, and the other half would view the list in the reverse order. No images were viewed more than once by each participant. Even though there was some variation in the size of the image of the object, all images were larger than the size of the Viewing Window so that no object could be seen in its entirety without moving the Window. The goal of the task was to identify the object as quickly and accurately as possible. To do this, subjects used a trackball to control the *Viewing Window*, a small circular region through which part of the object could be seen completely clearly (Figure 1). During the first 9 and last 4 trials the movement of the viewing window was controlled normally by the trackball (Figure 2). During the 27 trials in between, a distortion was introduced between the movement of the trackball and the resulting movement of the *Viewing Window*. Subjects were divided into two groups according to the way in which this distortion was presented. To evoke strategic control, distortions had to be presented large enough to be noticeable, and in enough variety to avoid becoming predictable. In a previous pilot study we had utilized two large distortions in the counter-clockwise direction, pseudo-randomized with no distortion. However, to an adapted subject, a change from a counter-clockwise distorted trial to one with no distortion is similar to adapting to a change in the clockwise rotation. More problematic was that with only three conditions it was difficult to pseudo-randomize the change in control from one trial to another. In the present study, we aimed to pseudo-randomize the change experienced by the subject and so used two large distortions, but in either direction (four in total). Therefore, the group in which we aimed to evoke strategic control in, received large noticeable distortions of 0°, 34°, or 68° in either direction, so that the change in rotation from the previous trial was pseudo-randomized. In the second group, distortions incrementally increased in each trial by 2.5° in the counter-clockwise direction. In this distortion group, changes were cumulative in one direction as we wanted to end the distortion period at a large rotation, so that return to normal control in the post-distorted trial would be evident.

Subjects received verbal instruction to try to identify the images as quickly and accurately as possible by using the trackball to move the window around the computer screen. Once subjects knew the identity of the object, they were to press the space bar on a keyboard and enter the name in a text box that appeared on the computer screen. The task would then move onto the next trial with a new masked image. The task therefore proceeded at the subject's own pace. Feedback regarding accuracy was not provided to the participant.

To account for order effects, two lists of objects were used that were counterbalanced. Therefore, in each rotation group, ten subjects received one list of items and the other ten received the same list but the order of items in the experimental (distortion) period was reversed.

Data Analysis

All participants knew that the task was self-paced and so while they received the instruction to identify the object "as quickly and accurately as possible", time was not a limiting factor. It is possible that participants, motivated by the goal to identify the object, guessed at the object identity. To account for this, an accuracy threshold of 60% was applied to consider data from participants who were fully engaged in the task and the highest performing. This type of threshold was selected because it was the most objective. The use of a threshold more specific to the motor component of the task rather than the perceptual component may be more desirable in examining adaptation behaviour such as movement velocity, or the time off the object. However, establishing the level of this threshold is subjective. This is an interesting topic for further examination. As a result of the accuracy threshold, 18 subjects were excluded and so a total of 58 participants had to be recruited to obtain group sizes of 20 subjects for each experimental group. The resulting data analyzed was from 40 participants (14 male, mean age 19.5±1.9 years, range 18–26 years). An additional analysis of all 58 participants is presented in Supplementary Information S1.

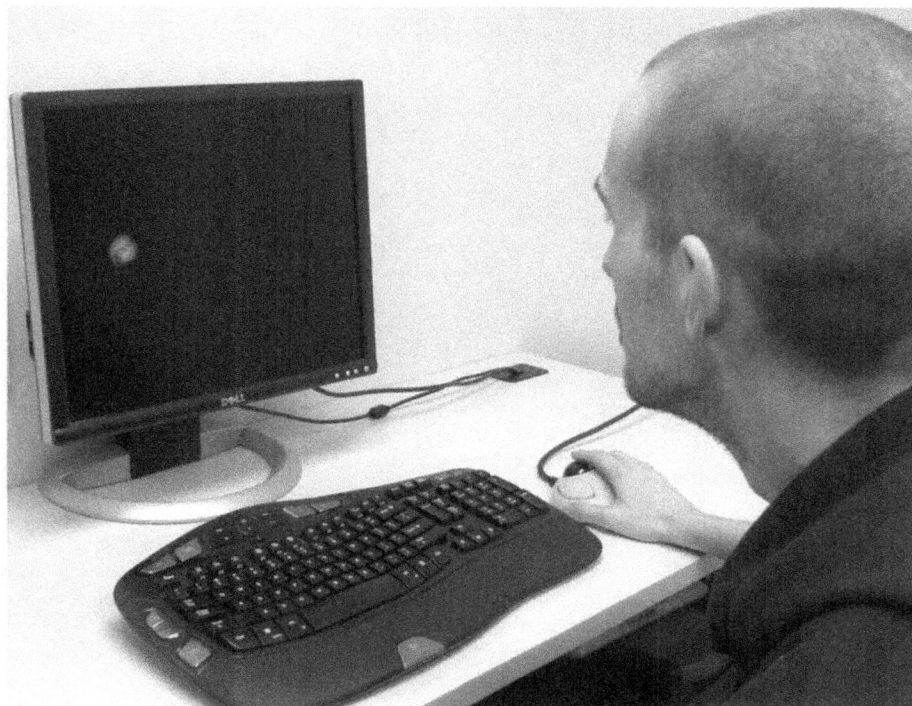

Figure 1. Experimental setup of the *Viewing Window* task. Subjects sat at a desktop workstation and viewed masked images on a 19″ monitor. In order to identify the images, subjects used a trackball to control the movement of the Viewing Window that would allow part of the image to be seen clearly. Subjects were instructed to, upon identification of the image, press the space bar on the keyboard and enter the name of the object in a text box that would appear on the computer screen. The photographed subject has given written informed consent, as outlined in the PLoS consent form, to publication of their photograph.

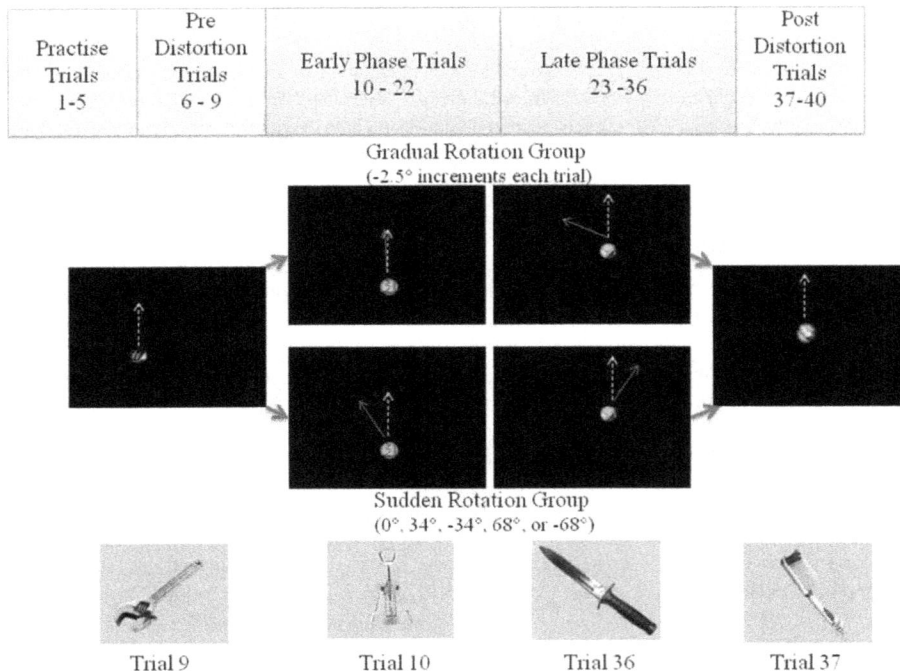

Figure 2. Experimental design of the *Viewing Window* **task.** The first five trials were used as practise and therefore excluded from all analysis. No distortion was present in movement of the *Viewing Window* during trials 6–9. During trials 10–36, in two separate groups, participants either received a gradual progressive distortion of 2.5° in the counter-clockwise direction on each trial, or a large sudden distortion in either direction. For analysis, these trials were divided in half in two phases (early and late). On trial 37 the distortion was removed and control of the *Viewing* Window returned to normal for the remainder of the study to examine after-effects.

The first five trials were removed as practice trials. The remaining data sets were exported to SPSS 13.0. Data was filtered to exclude trials in which the object was incorrectly identified and to consider only data acquired after movement of the window was first initiated for each trial. Measures of movement behaviour examined included the velocity of the Viewing Window, time the image was viewed (scan time), and the percentage of the time the Viewing Window spent on the object. For each subject, trials were identified as outliers by calculating the Z scores for each of the examined behavioural measures and excluding data beyond 2.5 standard deviations from all subsequent analyses. To examine differences between groups during the distortion trials, the movement velocities, scan times and percentage of time spent off the object were analyzed with ANOVA with Bonferroni correction (alpha 0.05). To examine changes in behaviour over the course of the experiment the trials were then divided into the pre-distortion phase (trials 6–9), early distortion phase (trials 10–22), late distortion phase (trials 23–36), and post distortion phase (trials 37–40). To examine phase interactions within groups, a repeated-measures ANOVA was conducted. For each subject, data were normalized by subtracting the mean of the appropriate behavioural measure obtained during the pre-distortion period. For example, to normalize the measurement of mean scan time during the early distortion period for subject X, the mean scan time found during the pre-distortion phase (trials 6–9) was subtracted from the mean scan time found during the early distortion phase (trials 10–22). This process was repeated for each phase, for each behavioural measure, and for each subject. The normalized data were then analyzed with a repeated measures ANOVA with Bonferroni correction using a factor structure for each behavioural measure of a 2 [Group:Gradual vs Sudden distortion] × 3 [Phase:

Early, Late, Post distortion]. The scan paths of *Viewing Window* movement were visually inspected.

Results

Group comparisons revealed several anticipated behavioural differences (Figure 3). Subjects in the gradual rotation group demonstrated significantly faster mean velocities of movement compared to the sudden rotation group ($F(1,38) = 5.406$, $p<0.05$ Figure 3A). No significant difference in scan times were identified ($F(1,38) = 1.185$, $p>0.05$, Figure 3B). The gradual rotation group spent significantly less time scanning areas off the object ($F(1, 38) = 4.620$, $p<0.05$, Figure 3C). The faster velocities and ability to keep the window on the object, suggest that the gradual rotation group experienced less difficulty in controlling the movement of the window and adapted easily to the distortions. The slower movement velocities and greater time off the object observed in the sudden rotation group suggest that participants did experience some difficulty in controlling the *Viewing Window* movement.

When data were divided into pre, early, late, and post distortion periods, several behavioural differences between groups were visible. Figure 4 depicts sample scan paths from one representative subject in the gradual rotation group and another representative subject from the sudden rotation group. The gradual rotation subject demonstrates fairly simple scan paths during the distortion trials indicating good control over window movement. However, once the distortion is removed, the same participant shows after-effects in the form of difficulty in keeping the *Viewing Window* on the object. In contrast to this behaviour, the participant in the distortion group shows a complicated scan path and therefore more difficulty when the distortion is first introduced. By the last distortion trial, the same participant has adapted and shows

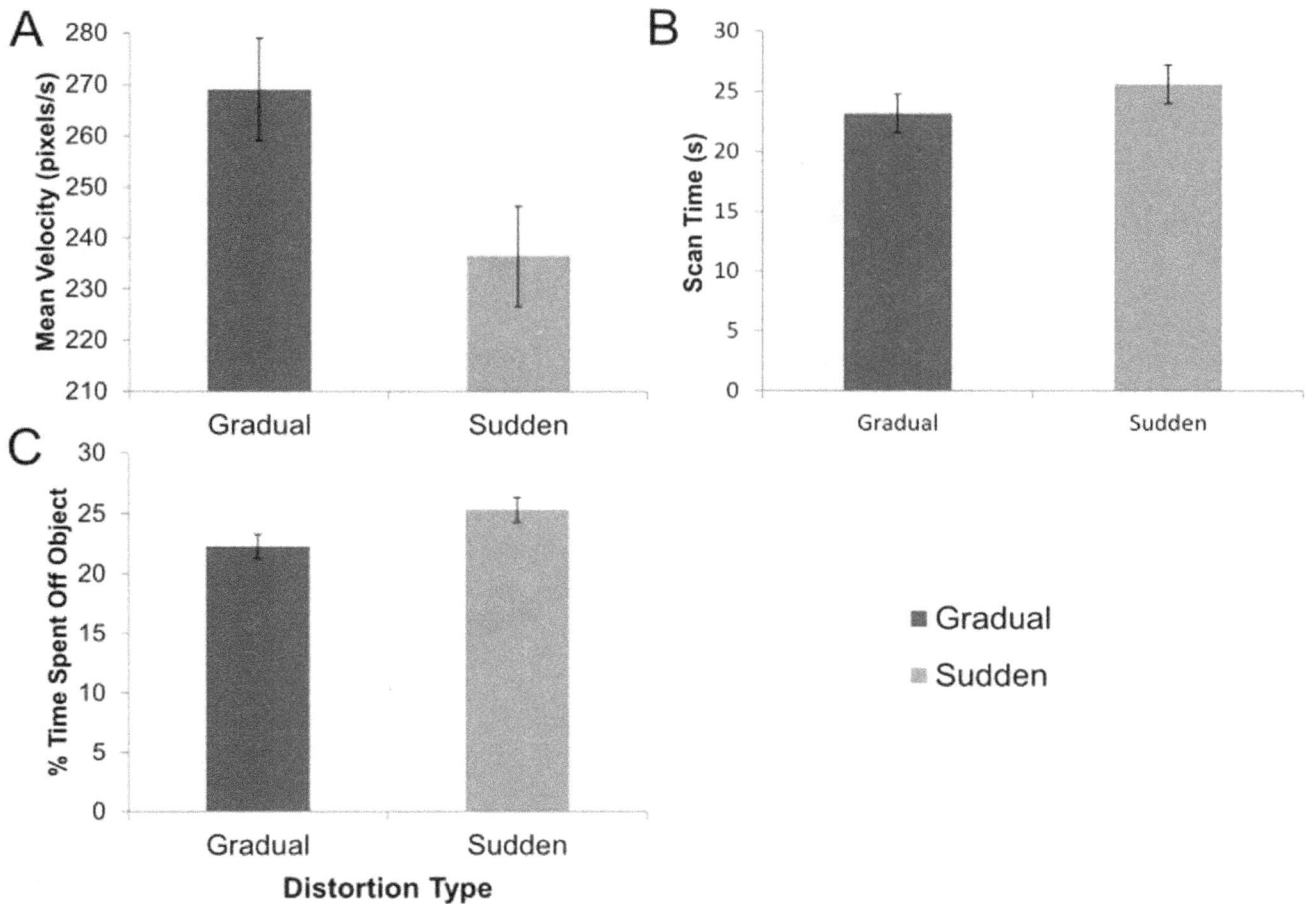

Figure 3. Comparisons of behavioural measures between groups during distorted trials. A) Subjects in the gradual rotation group demonstrated significantly faster ($F(1,38) = 5.406$, $p<0.05$) mean velocities than those in the sudden rotation group. B) Subjects in the sudden rotation group spent a slightly longer (but not significant) time scanning the images prior to indicating their identification. C) Subjects in the sudden rotation group spent significantly more time ($F(1,38) = 4.620$), $p<0.05$) with the *Viewing Window* off of the object than those in the gradual rotation group.

a simpler scan path with fewer changes in direction. When the distortion is removed, the sudden rotation subject shows a much smaller after-effect compared to that observed in the gradual rotation subject.

Quantitatively, these observations can also be made with the examined behavioural measures. Both groups demonstrated reductions in movement velocity that were significant by phase (Figure 5A, $F(2,76) = 14.890$, $p<0.01$). Overall, there was not a significant interaction between phase with distortion type for mean movement velocity ($F(2,76) = 1.486$, $p>0.05$). Relative to the pre distortion period, a slight (but not significant, $p = 0.078$) increase in scan time was observed in the sudden rotation group in the early phase (Figure 5B). Both groups demonstrated significant reductions in scan times in the post distortion phase ($p<0.05$), however, this reduction was slightly larger in the sudden rotation group. Overall, there was a significant effect of phase ($F(2,76) = 43.396 = p<0.01$) but not a significant interaction between phase with distortion type for mean scan time ($F(2,76) = 2.463$, $p>0.05$). A significant interaction between phase and distortion type was found for the amount of time that the *Viewing Window* spent off the object ($F(2,76) = 10.320$, $p<0.001$, Figure 5C). Relative to the early phase, subjects in the sudden rotation group demonstrated greater difficulty in controlling *Viewing Window*

movement compared to those in the gradual rotation group as evidenced by a greater percentage of time spent off the object (Figure 5C). Both groups demonstrated significant differences compared to their baseline values ($p<0.05$). During the post distortion phase, subjects in the sudden rotation group spent significantly less time off the object ($p<0.05$).

Discussion

We hypothesized that the *Viewing* Window task could be used to investigate two mechanisms of adaptation. To do this, we identified measurable differences in behaviour in two experimental groups eliciting strategic control and spatial realignment. When comparing behavioural measures during all distortion trials of the two groups, we found significant differences in the movement velocities, and time that the *Viewing Window* spent on areas in which there was no object. This demonstrates the ability to distinguish quantitative differences in behaviour between the use of strategic control and spatial realignment within a novel, engaging computer-based task for studying visuomotor adaptation. *No significant difference was observed between scan times however, this aspect of behaviour is also influenced by the perceptual component of the task. While the existence of between group differences during distortion trials is interesting,*

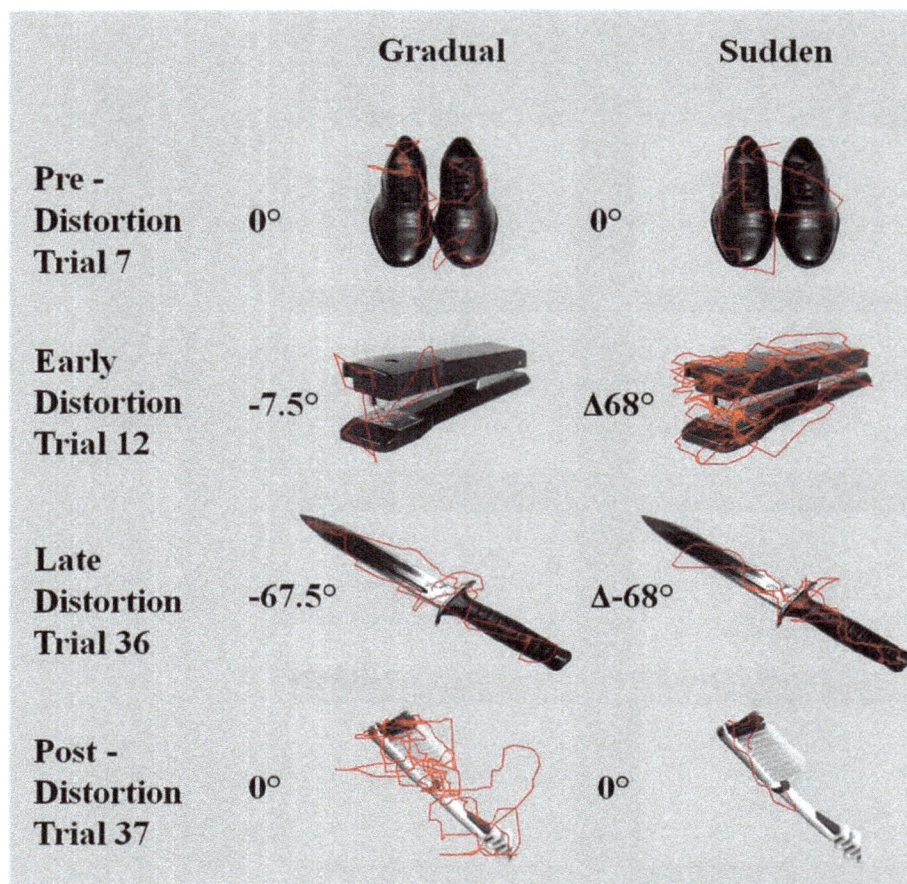

Figure 4. Sample scan paths from representative participants. A) gradual rotation group and B) sudden rotation group. The line represents the pathway of the viewing window from image onset until participant signal of image identification.

of more relevance is how behaviour changes over the course of study, therefore, an examination of behaviour by phase was also conducted.

When the trials were divided into four phases: pre, early, late, post distortion phases; no significant interaction between distortion type and phase of the experiment were found for movement velocities and scan times. However, a significant effect of phase was found. We anticipate that scan time is not only influenced by the ability to move the *Viewing* Window to the desired areas of the computer screen but also by the participant's familiarity with the type of object. The item list contained a variety of everyday objects that most people would encounter including, fruits, vegetables, tools, office supplies, and musical instruments. However, how quickly these are identified can be expected to be influenced by how often a participant encounters these particular items. For example, a person who does not often interact with tools may have more difficulty identifying the image of the vice grips. The ability to recognize the objects may also be influenced by the perspective of the images. The items were displayed with variable orientation which could affect the difficulty of the task. Even though this strengthens the task in terms of increasing the variability of the location of valuable information on the computer screen, the changing perspective could also affective the ability to identify the objects. This is not something that was controlled, however, it was one reason for using counterbalanced lists in the two groups so that any effects would not drive the results of any particular phase of the study. In addition, it is possible that participants may have

improved their scan times over the course of the experiment as they because more familiar with the task. We excluded the first items to account for practice trials. It is possible that subjects are more likely to hesitate in signalling their response at the start of the experiment while the task is still novel and answer more quickly later in the study when they become more confident. These influences contributed to the observation of decreased mean scan time between the late and post distortion phases (Figure 5B) despite the mean velocities also decreasing (Figure 5 A). The decreased velocity indicates increased difficulty in controlling the window movement, however, participants were still able to quickly identify the masked objects. In the analysis of time spent off the object, a significant difference between groups was found indicating larger after effects in the gradual rotation group.

The present study demonstrates that the *Viewing Window* is capable of distinguishing performance of both strategic control and spatial realignment and therefore is a powerful tool for measuring visuomotor adaptation behaviour. Even though subjects in the gradual rotation group did not report observing a change during the distortion trials, the large after-effects observed in their scan behaviour indicate adaptation took place. This is consistent with previous studies investigating gradual rotations [8].

In addition to behavioural differences, the neural basis of strategic control and spatial realignment are believed to differ. Strategic control primarily recruits posterior parietal cortex

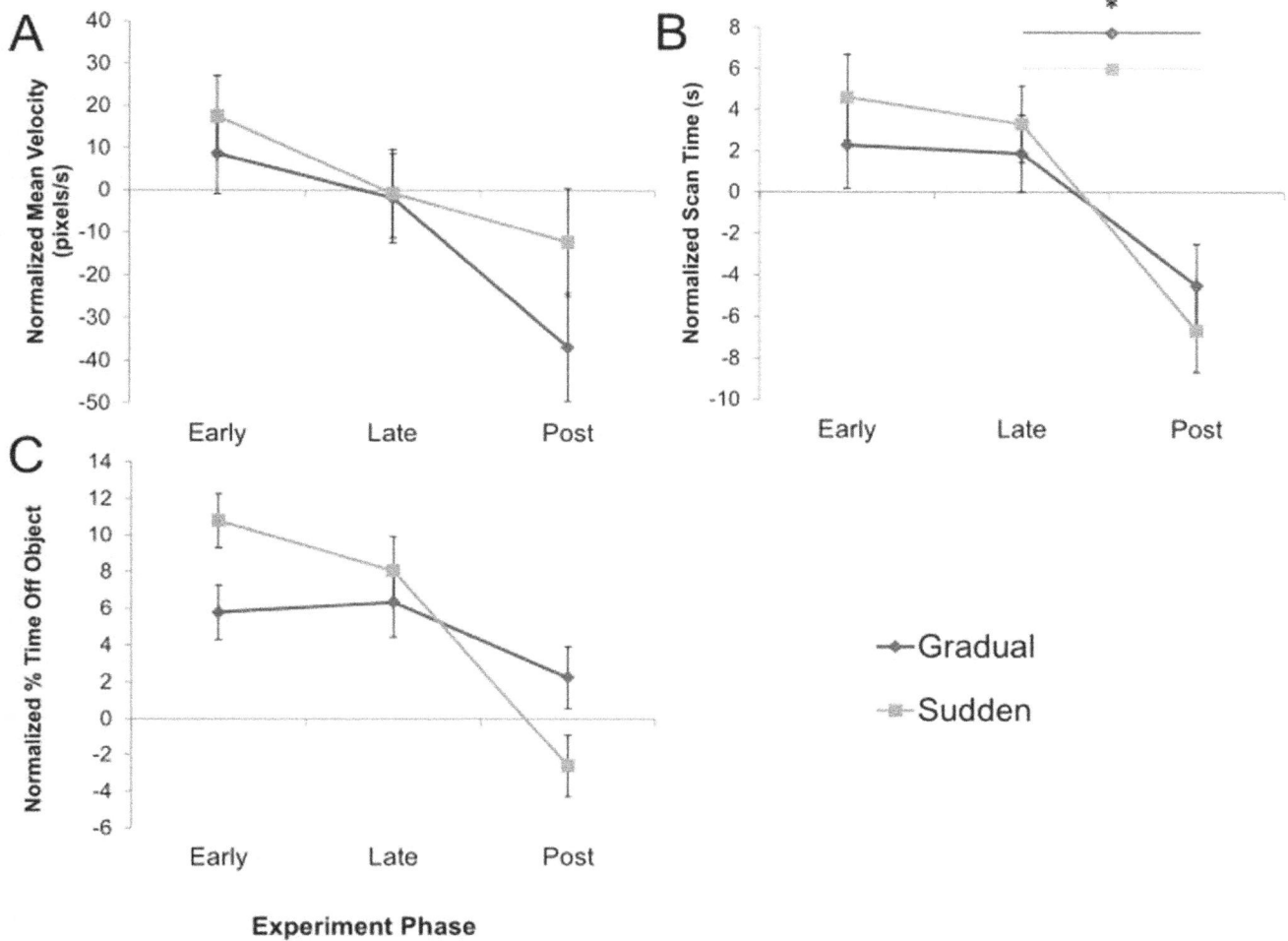

Figure 5. Normalized mean behavioural measures by phase. Behavioural measures of the early, late, and post distortion values are presented relative to the baseline (measures during the pre distortion phase) of each group. A) Velocity of Viewing Window movement. B) Scan Time required to identify object *Both distortion groups demonstrated a significant reduction in scan time in the post distortion phase (p<0.05). C) Percentage of Time off Object. A significant interaction was found between phase and distortion type was found in the percentage of time spent off the object (p<0.001).

[18,19], whereas, spatial realignment is believed to rely on the cerebellum [4,20,21,22]. However, to date there have only been a handful of neuroimaging studies investigating the neural correlates of visual motor adaptation [18,23,24,25,26]. We have recently employed the *Viewing* Window task with large distortions in the form of flips in direction to investigate the neural basis of strategic control using functional magnetic resonance imaging (fMRI) and found in addition to traditional areas associated with visuomotor adaptation, novel recruitment of the claustrum. This task presents several advantages over other tasks previously used as it is computer-based therefore easier to manipulate a range of distortions over a short period of time. This would be difficult to do using prism glasses in an environment such as that during a functional magnetic resonance imaging (fMRI) study. In the future, we will utilize this paradigm to investigate the neural correlates that underlie both mechanisms of visuomotor adaptation.

Incremental rotations have previously been used to investigate visuomotor adaptation without the awareness of the participant [10,11,25]. However, there are some differences between our

experimental design and those used in the past. Kagerer et al. [8] used a rotated mouse task with 10° increments during their gradual rotation condition to a maximum rotation of 90°. In their study, they suggest that using a gradual feedback distortion allows for a more complete adaptation compared to a sudden onset of the distortion [8]. During our 27 trials of distortion we kept increments as small and uniform as possible in order to ensure that distortions would not be apparent to the subject. Therefore, we selected an incremental change of 2.5° to a maximum rotation of 67.5°. The present study task differs from both Kagerer et al [8] and Klassen et al [10] in that subject naturally explored the computer screen without restrictions on directions. Kagerer et al [8] used a target task where subjects used a pen to start a center point and were instructed to draw a line in one of four directions. Similarly, Klassen et al [10] used a point-to-point task in eight directions. The use of the *Viewing Window* task has several advantages over previous prism studies and anti-pointing tasks. First, the adaptation task is hidden within a perceptual task. Subjects do not know that the motor relationship is altered ahead of time. Second, the *Viewing Window* investigates visuomotor adaptation in a more natural visual scanning environment in which the directions of motion are not restricted. In point-to-point tasks, subjects make directed movements in a restricted number of directions. One may anticipate that the increased freedom in direction used in the present study allows for more detailed remapping and would contribute to more complete adaptation.

The results of the present study broaden the research applications of the *Viewing Window* as a tool for investigating disturbances in spatial realignment more specifically. This is not only useful in the context of changes due to natural aging but also in the study of impairment following injury and neurodegenerative disease. The use of a visuomotor rotation task has previously been used in patients with cerebellar degeneration [27]. Computer-based point-to-point tasks have previously been used for investigating adaptation behaviour in children with Developmental Coordination Disorder (DCD) [28]. Historically, rehabilitation methods using prism lenses have shown to be beneficial for patients with unilateral neglect (see [29] for review). The development of novel, valid techniques that are simple to administer may advance rehabilitative medicine for these conditions. A restricted focus task such as the Viewing Window may also show to be beneficial in the assessment and rehabilitation of patients with unilateral neglect or hemianopia. The application of

the *Viewing Window* within patient work may help further elucidate the roles of specific cerebellar structures in visuomotor adaptation in a more natural setting. We are currently exploring the use of the *Viewing Window* as part of a dual-task paradigm in a combined cognitive/motor rehabilitation therapy program. In summary, we demonstrate that distinct behaviours used during strategic control and spatial realignment can be measured using the *Viewing* Window. This provides a powerful, engaging tool for investigating the neural basis of visuomotor adaptation and impairment following injury and disease.

Supporting Information

Supporting Information S1   Supplementary methods and results. We examined behaviour of all of the 58 recruited participants in a separate analysis. The analysis methods and results are described.

Author Contributions

Conceived and designed the experiments: JMLD LAB JJM. Performed the experiments: JMLD. Analyzed the data: JMLD. Contributed reagents/materials/analysis tools: JMLD LAB. Wrote the paper: JMLD LAB JJM.

References

1. Keisler A, Shadmehr R (2010) A shared resource between declarative memory and motor memory. The Journal of neuroscience 30: 14817–14823.
2. Redding GM, Rossetti Y, Wallace B (2005) Applications of prism adaptation: a tutorial in theory and method. Neuroscience and biobehavioral reviews 29: 431–444.
3. Redding GM, Wallace B (1996) Adaptive spatial alignment and strategic perceptual-motor control. Journal of experimental psychologyHuman perception and performance 22: 379–394.
4. Weiner MJ, Hallett M, Funkenstein HH (1983) Adaptation to lateral displacement of vision in patients with lesions of the central nervous system. Neurology 33: 766–772.
5. Redding GM, Wallace B (2006) Generalization of prism adaptation. Journal of experimental psychologyHuman perception and performance 32: 1006–1022.
6. Roby-Brami A, Burnod Y (1995) Learning a new visuomotor transformation: error correction and generalization. Brain researchCognitive brain research 2: 229–242.
7. Rock IG, Goldberg J, Mack A (1966) Immediate correction and adaptation based on viewing a prismatically displaced scene. Perception and Psychophysics 1: 351–354.
8. Kagerer FA, Contreras-Vidal JL, Stelmach GE (1997) Adaptation to gradual as compared with sudden visuo-motor distortions. Experimental brain research-Experimentelle HirnforschungExperimentation cerebrale 115: 557–561.
9. Michel C, Pisella L, Prablanc C, Rode G, Rossetti Y (2007) Enhancing visuomotor adaptation by reducing error signals: single-step (aware) versus multiple-step (unaware) exposure to wedge prisms. J Cogn Neurosci 19: 341–350.
10. Klassen J, Tong C, Flanagan JR (2005) Learning and recall of incremental kinematic and dynamic sensorimotor transformations. Experimental brain researchExperimentelle HirnforschungExperimentation cerebrale 164: 250–259.
11. Buch ER, Young S, Contreras-Vidal JL (2003) Visuomotor adaptation in normal aging. Learning & memory (Cold Spring Harbor, NY) 10: 55–63.
12. Baugh LA, Lawrence JM, Marotta JJ (2011) Novel claustrum activation observed during a visuomotor adaptation task using a viewing window paradigm. Behavioural brain research.
13. Baugh LA, Marotta JJ (2009) When what's left is right: visuomotor transformations in an aged population. PloS one 4: e5484.
14. Baugh LA, Marotta JJ (2007) A new window into the interactions between perception and action. Journal of neuroscience methods 160: 128–134.
15. Just MA, Carpenter PA, Woolley JD (1982) Paradigms and processes in reading comprehension. Journal of experimental psychologyGeneral 111: 228–238.
16. Osaka N, Oda N (1994) Moving window generator for reading experiments. Behav Res Meth Ins C 26: 49–53.
17. van Diepen PM, Wampers M (1998) Scene exploration with Fourier-filtered peripheral information. Perception 27: 1141–1151.
18. Clower DM, Hoffman JM, Votaw JR, Faber TL, Woods RP, et al. (1996) Role of posterior parietal cortex in the recalibration of visually guided reaching. Nature 383: 618–621.
19. Rossetti Y, Rode G, Pisella L, Farne A, Li L, et al. (1998) Prism adaptation to a rightward optical deviation rehabilitates left hemispatial neglect. Nature 395: 166–169.
20. Marr D (1969) A theory of cerebellar cortex. The Journal of physiology 202: 437–470.
21. Baizer JS, Kralj-Hans I, Glickstein M (1999) Cerebellar lesions and prism adaptation in macaque monkeys. Journal of neurophysiology 81: 1960–1965.
22. Ito M (1993) Synaptic plasticity in the cerebellar cortex and its role in motor learning. The Canadian journal of neurological sciencesLe journal canadien des sciences neurologiques 20 Suppl 3: S70–74.
23. Danckert J, Ferber S, Goodale MA (2008) Direct effects of prismatic lenses on visuomotor control: an event-related functional MRI study. The European journal of neuroscience 28: 1696–1704.
24. Luaute J, Schwartz S, Rossetti Y, Spiridon M, Rode G, et al. (2009) Dynamic changes in brain activity during prism adaptation. The Journal of neuroscience : the official journal of the Society for Neuroscience 29: 169–178.
25. Diedrichsen J, Hashambhoy Y, Rane T, Shadmehr R (2005) Neural correlates of reach errors. The Journal of neuroscience : the official journal of the Society for Neuroscience 25: 9919–9931.
26. Chapman HL, Eramudugolla R, Gavrilescu M, Strudwick MW, Loftus A, et al. (2010) Neural mechanisms underlying spatial realignment during adaptation to optical wedge prisms. Neuropsychologia 48: 2595–2601.
27. Rabe K, Livne O, Gizewski ER, Aurich V, Beck A, et al. (2009) Adaptation to visuomotor rotation and force field perturbation is correlated to different brain areas in patients with cerebellar degeneration. Journal of neurophysiology 101: 1961–1971.
28. Kagerer FA, Contreras-Vidal JL, Bo J, Clark JE (2006) Abrupt, but not gradual visuomotor distortion facilitates adaptation in children with developmental coordination disorder. Human movement science 25: 622–633.
29. Newport R, Schenk T (2012) Prisms and neglect: what have we learned? Neuropsychologia 50: 1080–1091.

19

Socioeconomic Status, Functional Recovery, and Long-Term Mortality among Patients Surviving Acute Myocardial Infarction

David A. Alter[1,2,4,5,7]*, Barry Franklin[6], Dennis T. Ko[1,3,7], Peter C. Austin[1,7], Douglas S. Lee[1,7], Paul I. Oh[2], Therese A. Stukel[1,7], Jack V. Tu[1,3,7]

1 The Institute for Clinical Evaluative Sciences, Toronto, Ontario, Canada, 2 The Cardiac Rehabilitation and Secondary Prevention Program, Toronto Rehabilitation Institute, Toronto, Ontario, Canada, 3 The Schulich Heart Centre and the Clinical Epidemiology Unit of Sunnybrook Health Science Centre, Toronto, Ontario, Canada, 4 The Li Ka Shing Knowledge Institute of St. Michaels' Hospital, Toronto, Ontario, Canada, 5 Department of Medicine, University of Toronto, Toronto, Ontario, Canada, 6 Cardiac Rehabilitation and Exercise Laboratories, William Beaumont Hospital, Royal Oak, Michigan, United States of America, 7 Department of Health Policy, Management and Evaluation, University of Toronto, Toronto, Ontario, Canada

Abstract

Objectives: To examine the relationship between socio-economic status (SES), functional recovery and long-term mortality following acute myocardial infarction (AMI).

Background: The extent to which SES mortality disparities are explained by differences in functional recovery following AMI is unclear.

Methods: We prospectively examined 1368 patients who survived at least one-year following an index AMI between 1999 and 2003 in Ontario, Canada. Each patient was linked to administrative data and followed over 9.6 years to track mortality. All patients underwent medical chart abstraction and telephone interviews following AMI to identify individual-level SES, clinical factors, processes of care (i.e., use of, and adherence, to evidence-based medications, physician visits, invasive cardiac procedures, referrals to cardiac rehabilitation), as well as changes in psychosocial stressors, quality of life, and self-reported functional capacity.

Results: As compared with their lower SES counterparts, higher SES patients experienced greater functional recovery (1.80 ml/kg/min average increase in peak V02, P<0.001) after adjusting for all baseline clinical factors. Post-AMI functional recovery was the strongest modifiable predictor of long-term mortality (Adjusted HR for each ml/kg/min increase in functional capacity: 0.91; 95% CI: 0.87–0.94, P<0.001) irrespective of SES (P = 0.51 for interaction between SES, functional recovery, and mortality). SES-mortality associations were attenuated by 27% after adjustments for functional recovery, rendering the residual SES-mortality association no longer statistically significant (Adjusted HR: 0.84; 95% CI:0.70–1.00, P = 0.05). The effects of functional recovery on SES-mortality associations were not explained by access inequities to physician specialists or cardiac rehabilitation.

Conclusions: Functional recovery may play an important role in explaining SES-mortality gradients following AMI.

Editor: Benjamin Van Tassell, Virginia Commonwealth University, United States of America

Funding: This study was supported by a grant from the Canadian Institute for Health Research (MOP#119956). The Institute for Clinical Evaluative Sciences is supported in part by a grant from the Ontario Ministry of Health. The funders had no role in study design, data collection and analysis, decision to publish, or preparation of the manuscript.

Competing Interests: Dr. Alter received an honorarium from Forest Laboratories Canada for attending one advisory board meeting, and an honorarium from Boehringer-Ingelheim Canada for speaking at one CME event.

* E-mail: david.alter@ices.on.ca

Introduction

Socioeconomic status (SES) has been shown to be an important determinant of survival after acute myocardial infarction (AMI) in countries with and without universal health care. [1] The reasons for socioeconomic-mortality disparities after AMI remain unclear. [2–12] Available evidence has demonstrated that SES-outcome disparities have been partially attributable to differences in baseline cardiovascular risk-factor profiles that existed prior to AMI [2,13].

Socioeconomic differences in functional capacity have been shown to partially account for SES-mortality associations in populations with suspected coronary artery disease. [14] Moreover, available evidence from our group and others have demonstrated that access to secondary prevention services such as cardiac rehabilitation and specialty physician services after AMI are poorer among socioeconomically disadvantaged than among their socially-advantaged counterparts. [15–17] Accordingly, one may reasonably hypothesize that socioeconomic disparities in functional capacity recovery may exist after AMI, and that such disparities may help explain why lower SES patients experience higher long-term mortality after AMI [18,19].

Accordingly, the objective of our study was to examine the relationship between SES, self-reported functional recovery, and long-term survival following AMI. We hypothesized that differences in access to secondary prevention service delivery may help explain SES-differences in self-reported functional recovery, and accordingly, may partially account for long-term SES-mortality associations through changes in functional capacity among AMI survivors [20].

Methods

Health System Context

Canada's universal health insurance system provides comprehensive coverage for most medical and hospital services without user fees at point of service. Under such provisions, patients are entitled to equitable access to medical care based on medical need, regardless of age, SES, or financial circumstances. [21] Medication costs are covered by provinces for individuals 65 years of age and older and those whose annual incomes fall at or below the poverty line. However, access to multidisciplinary secondary prevention services and related interventions are severely constrained, and have not significantly changed throughout the decade. At the time of the study, cardiac rehabilitation programs served as the only available multidisciplinary secondary prevention service program in Ontario. While some cardiac rehabilitation programs required that patients pay modest administrative fees (e.g., $25 per month) for participation, the vast majority of cardiac rehabilitation programs were funded by the Ontario government, with capacity for approximately 16,000 patients per year at the time of the study period, representing fewer than 30% of the eligible post-hospitalized cardiac population [22,23].

Data Sources

The Socio-Economic Status and Acute Myocardial Infarction Study (SESAMI) study is a prospective, observational investigation of patients hospitalized for AMI between December 1, 1999 and February 28, 2003 in 53 large volume acute hospitals throughout Ontario, Canada. [15] Details about SESAMI have been previously published. [2,15,24] Briefly, the study consisted of baseline surveys, in-hospital chart abstraction, and telephone follow-up at 30-days and one-year post AMI. Mortality over the 9.6 year follow-up was assessed using vital statistics data (the Registered Persons Data Base), as has been used previously and whose accuracy has been verified [2,13,15,25].

Study Sample

Details of SESAMI recruitment and eligibility have been previously described. [15] All patients were English-speaking and were enrolled if 2 of 3 AMI criteria were met: presence of symptoms, abnormal electrocardiographic findings (ST elevation or depression), or elevated serum levels of cardiac enzymes (CK-MB and/or Tropinin I levels). Patients were excluded if they were <19 or >101 years of age, lacked a valid health card number issued by the province of Ontario, or were transferred to the recruiting hospital. In total, 2829 consecutive participants were enrolled and underwent detailed clinical information abstracted from medical charts pertaining to the index hospitalization. Given severe access constraints and significant waiting-time delays for

multidisciplinary secondary prevention programs, this sub-study required that all SESAMI patients survive for at least one year following AMI to ensure each patient had equal opportunity for referral and participation into the program. All patients had to be available and agree to participate in follow-up interviews at one-year to evaluate self-reported functional capacity, medication compliance, psychosocial status, and quality of life (see below). Among the 1859 (65.7%) remaining patients who were alive and eligible for the one-year follow-up telephone interview, 1463 (78.7%) patients participated; 95 patients were excluded because of missing data, leaving 1368 patients available for final analyses. Despite attrition due to death and follow-up, previous work has determined that the distribution and prevalence of ethno-demographic and comorbid characteristics across income and education categories were similar between the current study sample and the original SESAMI cohort from which it was derived. [26] The Sunnybrook Health Sciences Centre Research Ethics Board approved the study protocol and methodology and all subjects gave informed consent to participate.

Socioeconomic Status

Previous studies have demonstrated the importance of self-reported income as an independent determinant of mortality after AMI. Accordingly, annual self-reported income served as our primary socioeconomic indicator for this study. Self-reported household annual income (from all sources) in Canadian (C) dollars was ascertained using a 7-level categorical scale ranging from <C$15 000 to >C$80 000; income categories were then re-aggregated into three age-specific categories (i.e., <$30 000; $30000-$59999; $60000+ for patients younger than 65 years; <$20000; $20000-39 999; $40000+ for patients 65 years and older), as has been done previously. [2] These cut-points corresponded to the low, medium, and high-income taxation thresholds for Canadian citizens in the labour force, as previously described. [15] A repeat analysis in which income aggregation ignored age-specific income rankings did not alter our results.

Our study also collected information on education. Self-reported educational status incorporated a 5-level categorical variable ranging from incomplete high school to university degree. All our analyses examining income-mortality associations adjusted for patient-level education. However, as a sensitivity analysis, we re-analyzed our data using education (as opposed to income) as our primary SES indicator. While the magnitude of association between unadjusted education and mortality was smaller than that for income, the relationships between education, functional recovery, and post-AMI survival were similar as for income.

Other Baseline Characteristics

Information on ethnicity was obtained via self-report from one or more categories of 13 ethno-racial subgroups. [27] For the purposes of this study, ethno-racial data were re-aggregated a priori into five variables: White, Black, South Asian, First Nations, and Other (Other here includes East Asian/Chinese respondents), as in our previous studies. [26,28] Several clinical and comorbid factors were identified and incorporated into the data base. We examined other clinical markers of disease severity (e.g., acute pulmonary edema, resting blood pressure, sinus tachycardia), cardiovascular risk factors (diabetes, hypertension, hyperlipidemia, and current or former smoking use), comorbidity (total number as well as type), [13,29] during the index AMI hospitalization. In addition to these factors, we calculated the Global Registry of Acute Coronary Events (GRACE) prognostic index on each patient. The GRACE prognostic index was used to calculate a 6-month predicted post-AMI mortality risk-score based on age, development (or history) of

Table 1. Baseline characteristics of study participants according to income tertile.

	Income			
	Low(N = 331)	Intermediate (N = 472)	High(N = 565)	P value
ETHNO-GEO-DEMOGRAPHIC				
Age in years, mean (STD)	65.1 (12.4)	63.9 (12.4)	60.5 (12.1)	<0.001
Sex, female (%)	157 (47.4)	127 (26.9)	112 (19.8)	<0.001
Caucasian (%)	252 (76.1)	405 (85.8)	517 (91.5)	<0.001
Rural residence (%)	28 (8.5)	28 (5.9)	18 (3.2)	<0.001
PSYCHOSOCIAL				
Lives alone (%)	100 (30.5)	86 (18.3)	46 (8.2)	<0.001
Chronic stress, mean (STD)	2.8 (2.7)	2.4 (2.1)	2.2 (2.0)	0.05
Education (%)				
Incomplete high-school	171 (52.5)	162 (34.5)	96 (17.0)	<0.001
Complete high-school	76 (23.3)	158 (33.6)	181 (32.1)	
University or college degree	79 (24.2)	150 (31.9)	287 (50.9)	
CLINICAL CHARACTERISTICS				
Predicted 6 month mortality rate, mean (STD)	3.45 (4.3)	3.13 (3.96)	2.51 (3.8)	0.01
Heart rate on admission, mean (STD)	82.2 (23.0)	80.6 (23.2)	79.2 (22.3)	0.04
Systolic blood pressure on admission, mean (STD)	150.7 (30.9)	148.2 (31.9)	147.2 (30.2)	0.01
Diastolic blood pressure on admission, mean (STD)	83.3 (18.5)	83.4 (19.1)	84.8 (19.1)	0.77
Respiratory rate on admission, mean (STD)	20.3 (4.8)	19.7 (4.3)	19.3 (4.4)	0.01
Acute pulmonary edema on admission (%)	9 (2.7)	12 (2.5)	10 (1.8)	0.32
ST elevation myocardial infarction (%)	128 (39.0)	193 (40.9)	252 (44.8)	0.08
Total number of comorbid conditions, mean (STD)	2.23 (0.93)	2.1 (0.99)	1.95 (1.03)	0.03
Previous AMI (%)	93 (28.1)	121 (25.6)	113 (20.0)	0.004
Previous angina (%)	167 (20.2)	223 (47.3)	241 (42.7)	0.02
Previous Heart failure (%)	67 (20.2)	67 (14.2)	61 (10.8)	<0.001
Diabetes (%)	100 (30.2)	107 (22.7)	96 (17.0)	<0.001
Hypertension (%)	177 (53.5)	213 (45.1)	248 (43.9)	0.009
Hyperlipidemia (%)	124 (37.5)	193 (40.9)	246 (43.6)	0.07
Smoking (%)	132 (39.9)	183 (38.8)	209 (37.0)	0.37
Asthma (%)	31 (9.4)	27 (5.7)	22 (3.9)	0.001
COPD (%)	67 (20.2)	44 (9.3)	40 (7.1)	<0.001
Cancer (%)	2 (0.6)	7 (1.5)	11 (1.95)	0.11
Dementia (%)	6 (1.8)	3 (0.6)	1 (0.18)	0.007
Dialysis (%)	1 (0.3)	2 (0.42)	1 (0.18)	0.67
Peripheral artery disease (%)	21 (6.3)	31 (6.6)	31 (5.5)	0.55
Stroke or TIA (%)	10 (3.0)	20 (4.2)	22 (3.9)	0.58
Previous depression (%)	26 (7.0)	16 (3.4)	19 (3.4)	0.004
PROCESSES OF CARE DURING HOSPITALIZATION				
Length of stay during index hospitalization, mean (STD)	8.9 (5.6)	8.9 (6.5)	8.5 (5.3)	0.67
Aspirin on discharge (%)	233 (70.4)	352 (74.6)	426 (75.4)	0.12
Nitrates on discharge (%)	126 (38.1)	139 (29.5)	169 (29.9)	0.02
Beta blockers on discharge (%)	218 (65.9)	337 (71.4)	414 (73.3)	0.02
Statins on discharge (%)	181 (54.7)	258 (54.7)	316 (55.9)	0.69

heart failure, peripheral vascular disease, systolic blood pressure, Killip class, baseline serum creatinine concentration, elevated initial cardiac markers, cardiac arrest on admission, and ST segment deviation. The GRACE index has been previously validated in SESAMI patients. [28] Substituting the GRACE index with their original comprised clinical variables did not meaningfully alter the results.

Table 2. Functional recovery, depression, psychosocial stress, emotional and physical well-being according to income tertile during the year following AMI hospitalization.

	Low income (N = 331)	Intermediate income (N = 472)	High income (N = 565)	P value
Functional recovery (Duke Activity Status Index)				
Baseline V02 peak in ml/kg/min, mean score (STD)	15.4 (4.2)	17.4 (4.8)	18.6 (5.1)	<0.001
Change in VO2 peak in ml/kg/min between 30-days and 1-year after AMI, mean score (STD)	2.1 (5.1)	3.2 (5.8)	4.5 (5.7)	<0.001
Depression (Carroll-Depression Inventory)				
Baseline Chronic Depression Inventory, mean score (STD)	0.19 (0.4)	0.12 (0.33)	0.08 (0.27)	0.01
One-year changes in Chronic Depression Inventory following hospitalization, mean score (STD)	−0.76 (0.44)	−0.08 (0.34)	−0.02(0.28)	0.03
Chronic stress				
Baseline chronic stress, mean score (STD)	2.8 (2.7)	2.4 (2.1)	2.2 (2.0)	<0.001
One-year change in chronic stress following hospitalization, mean score (STD)	−0.14 (2.3)	−0.025 (2.1)	0.08 (1.0)	0.12
Emotional well-being (SF-12)				
Baseline SF-12 emotional, mean (STD)	17.1 (3.9)	18.1 (3.6)	18.5 (3.4)	0.03
One-year change in SF-12 emotional following hospitalization, mean score (STD)	0.61 (3.9)	0.99 (3.4)	1.2 (3.4)	0.01
Physical well-being (SF-12)				
Baseline SF-12 physical, mean score (STD)	12.9 (3.3)	13.8 (3.2)	14.4 (3.1)	<0.001
Changes in SF-12 physical, following hospitalization, mean score (STD)	0.98 (3.5)	1.5 (3.3)	2.0 (3.2)	<0.002

Multidisciplinary Secondary Prevention Service Delivery

Referrals to cardiac rehabilitation within the first year following hospital discharge were identified using self-report. All revascularization procedures (angioplasty or coronary bypass surgery), as well as physician visits (stratified according to physician specialty of general practitioner, internal medicine, and cardiology) were also assessed within the first year following the index AMI hospitalization. [30] We examined the prescribing of cardiovascular medications (aspirin, beta-blockers, statins, ACE inhibitors, and nitrates) at hospital discharge. We also assessed the utilization of, and adherence to, cardiovascular medications throughout the year

following hospitalization on the assumption that self-management behaviours reflect the quality and effectiveness of secondary prevention service delivery. The utilization of, and adherence to, pharmacological therapies over the first year were ascertained through serial telephone interviews in which patients were asked to collect and read the names of all medications currently taken. There was moderate to good agreement between self-reported medication use and drug-claims for SESAMI patients aged 65 years and older for which drug claims data were available (Kappas ranging from 0.43 to 0.60 for beta-blockers and statins, respectively).

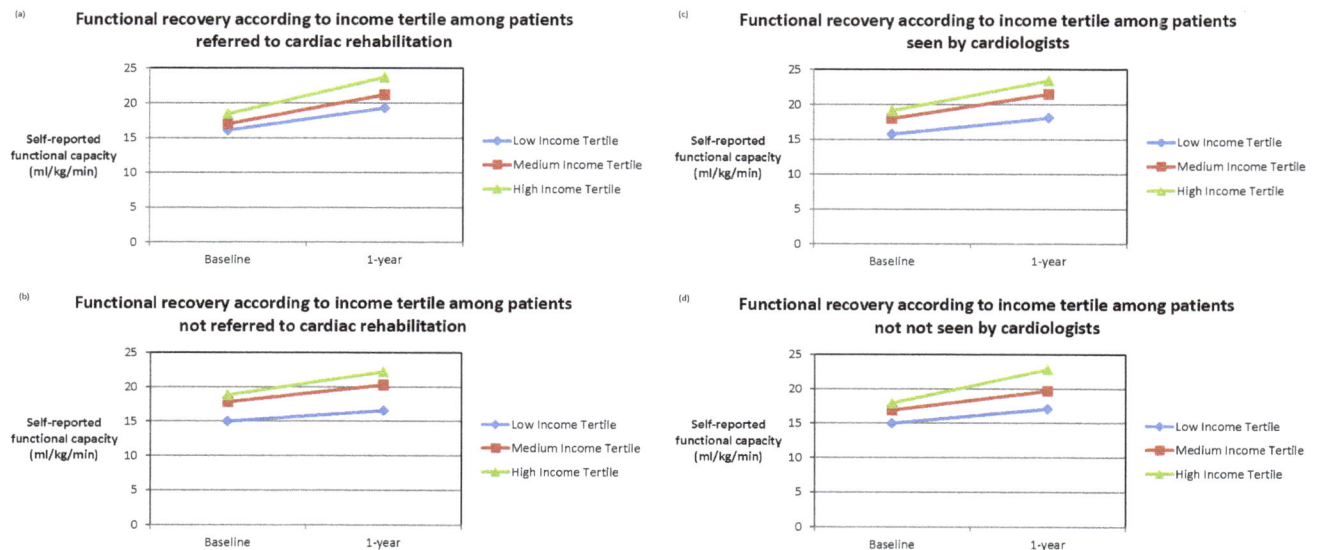

Figure 1. Function recovery according to income tertile among patients referred to cardiac rehabilitation (Figure 1a), not referred to cardiac rehabilitation (Figure 1b), seen by a cardiologist in follow-up (Figure 1), not seen by a cardiologist in follow-up (Figure 1d).

Table 3. Health service delivery according to income tertile during the year following AMI hospitalization.

	Low income (N = 331)	Intermediate income (N = 472)	High income (N = 565)	P value
Cardiac rehabilitation				
Cardiac rehabilitation participation by 30-days post-hospitalization (%)	93 (29.3)	151 (32.4)	242 (43.7)	<0.001
Cardiac rehabilitation participation by 1-year post-hospitalization (%)	120 (37.3)	213 (45.7)	333 (59.6)	<0.001
Cardiology visits				
Cardiology visit within 30-days of hospitalization (%)	163 (50.3)	243 (51.8)	312 (55.5)	0.11
Cardiology visit within 1 year of hospitalization (%)	261 (78.9)	381 (81.4)	510 (90.3)	<0.001
Internal Medicine visits				
Internal medicine visit within 30-days of hospitalization (%)	24 (7.7)	39 (8.7)	59 (9.0)	0.55
Internal medicine visit within 1 year of hospitalization (%)	47 (17.2)	94 (19.5)	94 (16.1)	0.66
General Practice visits				
GP visit within 30-days of hospitalization (%)	267 (81.4)	397 (84.1)	466 (82.5)	0.80
GP visit within 1 year of hospitalization (%)	323 (97.6)	456 (96.6)	551 (97.5)	0.92
Cardiac interventions				
Percutaneous Coronary Intervention within 30 days of hospitalization (%)	81 (25.6)	116 (25.0)	196 (34.8)	0.001
Percutaneous Coronary Intervention within 1 year of hospitalization (%)	99 (29.9)	151 (32.0)	223 (39.5)	0.002
Coronary artery bypass surgery within 30 days of hospitalization (%)	43 (13.4)	65 (13.9)	78 (13.9)	0.85
Coronary artery bypass surgery within 1 year of hospitalization (%)	59 (17.8)	88 (18.6)	113 (20)	0.41
Beta Blockers				
No B-blockers taken at 30-days or at 1 year (%)	44 (13.3)	40 (8.5)	29 (5.1)	<0.001
B-blockers taken at 30-days but not at 1 year (%)	29 (8.8)	45 (9.5)	48 (8.5)	
B-blockers taken at 1 year but not at 30-days (%)	26 (7.9)	35 (7.4)	34 (6.0)	
B-blockers taken at 30-days and 1 year (%)	232 (70.1)	352 (74.6)	454 (80.4)	
ACE Inhibitors				
No ACE inhibitors taken at 30-days or at 1 year (%)	73 (22.1)	76 (16.1)	92 (16.3)	0.01
ACE inhibitors taken at 30-days but not at 1 year (%)	30 (9.1)	46 (9.8)	41 (7.3)	
ACE inhibitors taken at 1 year but not at 30-days (%)	43 (13.0)	93 (19.7)	79 (14.0)	
ACE inhibitors taken at 30-days and 1 year (%)	185 (55.9)	257 (54.5)	353 (62.5)	
Statins				
No statins taken at 30-days or at 1 year (%)	67 (20.2)	94 (19.9)	96 (17.0)	0.008
Statins taken at 30-days but not at 1 year (%)	37 (11.2)	43 (9.1)	42 (7.4)	
Statins taken at 1 year but not at 30-days (%)	52 (15.7)	75 (15.9)	71 (12.6)	
Statins taken at 30-days and 1 year (%)	173 (52.9)	260 (55.1)	356 (63.1)	
Aspirin				
No Aspirin taken at 30-days or at 1 year (%)	29 (8.8)	26 (5.5)	27 (4.8)	0.01
Aspirin taken at 30-days but not at 1 year (%)	22 (6.7)	37 (7.8)	35 (6.2)	
Aspirin taken at 1 year but not at 30-days (%)	35 (10.6)	46 (9.8)	46 (8.1)	
Aspirin taken at 30-days and 1 year (%)	245 (74.0)	363 (76.9)	457 (80.9)	
Nitrates				
No Nitrate taken at 30-days or at 1 year (%)	160 (58.3)	247 (52.3)	332 (58.8)	<0.001
Nitrates taken at 30-days but not at 1 year (%)	67 (20.2)	114 (24.2)	128 (22	
Nitrates taken at 1 year but not at 30-days (%)	35 (10.6)	40 (8.5)	52 (9.2)	
Nitrates taken at 30-days and 1 year (%)	69 (20.9)	71 (15.0)	53 (9.4)	

Functional Recovery

Functional recovery was assessed using the Duke Activity Status Index (DASI), as measured at baseline (i.e., 30 days post-AMI) and at follow-up (i.e., 1-year post AMI), and expressed as peak oxygen consumption (peak VO_2). [31] The DASI questionnaire and its derived functional capacity, expressed as ml/kg/min, have been validated against objectively measured peak VO_2 from cardiopulmonary exercise testing, [32,33] and therefore, served as our primary indicator for functional recovery. (See Appendix S1).

As other surrogates of functional recovery, we examined changes in psychosocial stress, including depression, social support, chronic stress, as well as other measures of self-rated

Table 4. The relationship between income and long-term survival after sequential adjustments for factors associated with one-year recovery[i].

Model	Income	Hazard Ratio +/−95% Confidence Interval)	95% Confidence Interval
Unadjusted model[ii]			
	Low income	2.19 (1.69–2.83)	<0.001
	Medium income	1.59 (1.24–2.04)	<0.001
	High income	1.00 (Reference)	Reference
	Overall wealth-mortality-gradient[iii]	0.62 (0.54–0.71)	<0.001
Adjusted for all baseline and follow-up factors with the exception of functional recovery[iv]			
	Low income	1.46 (1.06–2.03)	0.02
	Medium income	1.45 (1.07–1.96	0.02
	High income	1.00 (Reference)	Reference
	Overall wealth-mortality-gradient[‡]	0.78 (0.65–0.93)	0.005
Adjusted for all baseline and follow-up factors as well as functional recovery[v]			
	Low income	1.40 (1.00–1.95)	0.05
	Medium income	1.33 (0.99–1.81)	0.06
	High income	1.00 (Reference)	Reference
	Overall wealth-mortality-gradient[‡]	0.84 (0.70–1.00)	0.05

[i]Functional recovery was defined using self-reported DASI score. Statistical survival models incorporated Cox Proportional hazards and adjusted for clinical and process factors using backward stepwise regression.
[ii]The unadjusted mortality model examines the crude relationship between income and long-term mortality with no adjustment for any concomitant factors.
[iii]Overall wealth-mortality gradient examines income in tertiles but with one degree of freedom.
[iv]The partially adjusted mortality model examines the relationship between income and long-term mortality after adjustments for age, sex, education, ethnicity, rurality, predicted 6 month mortality from the time of hospitalization, hypertension, diabetes, hyperlipidemia, comorbidities, smoking history, social isolation, history of depression, depression at 30-days, depression change between 30-days and 1-year, quality of life (SF-12) at 30-days and changes between 30-days and 1-year, chronic stress at 30-days and changes between 30-days and 1-year, Percutaneous Coronary Intervention within 1 year of hospitalization, Coronary artery bypass surgery within 1 year of hospitalization, physician visits (cardiologist, internal medicine and general practitioner), cardiac rehabilitation referral. as well as pharmacotherapies (beta-blockers, statins, ACE inhibitors, aspirin, nitrates) at hospital discharge, 30-days, and 1 year post-MI.
[v]All factors included in the partially adjusted mortality model+functional capacity at 30-days and changes in functional capacity between 30-days and 1-year.

physical and mental health status at 30-days and one-year after AMI. Chronic stress incorporated the National Population Health Survey questions related to stressful life events. [34] Self-rated physical and mental health status was assessed using the short-form 12 questionnaire while depression was assessed using the Brief Carroll Depression Rating Scale [35–37].

Outcome

Long-term mortality (as of December 31, 2010, representing a mean follow-up of 9.6 years) served as the primary outcome for our study, which corresponded to 11,765 patient life-years of follow-up. No patients were lost to follow-up.

Statistical Analysis

Income was analyzed as a continuous variable, to examine the main-effect of income across the 3 income tertiles using one degree of freedom, and categorically to allow for the comparison between tertiles, where overall income associations where statistically significant. The Mantel-Haenszel test for trend was used for categorical data and ANOVA (or nonparametric tests where relevant) were used for continuous data to detect differences in baseline characteristics between income categories. Multiple Least Squares Regression analyses (using backward stepwise regression) were used to examine the relationship between SES and self-reported functional recovery, after adjusting for all baseline

characteristics (including age, sex, baseline functional capacity, cardiac risk, comorbidity, chronic stress, depression, and medication use) as well as for referrals and use of cardiac specialty services (including cardiac rehabilitation referral, cardiology visits, cardiac procedures, and evidence-based medications).

Cox proportional hazards models were used to examine which factors throughout the first year of AMI recovery were most strongly associated with long-term survival irrespective of patient SES, cardiac specialty use, or cardiac rehabilitation referrals. The mortality hazard associated with each dataset variable including SES, ethnicity, rurality, age, sex, cardiac risk factors, prior medical history, total numbers and types of medical comorbidities, predicted 6 month mortality (using the GRACE predictive risk index), medications at hospital discharge, as well as primary care and specialty care physician visits, coronary interventions, medication adherence, changes in quality of life, depression, chronic stress, and changes in functional capacity during the year of AMI follow-up were assessed using backwards stepwise regression.

To examine the extent to which baseline and follow-up factors modulated or altered the relationship between SES and mortality, sequential risk adjustment was undertaken for each baseline and follow-up factor using backward stepwise regression techniques, while forcing income into each mortality model. To quantify the relative contribution of functional recovery to the observed association between income and mortality, we used the formulae:

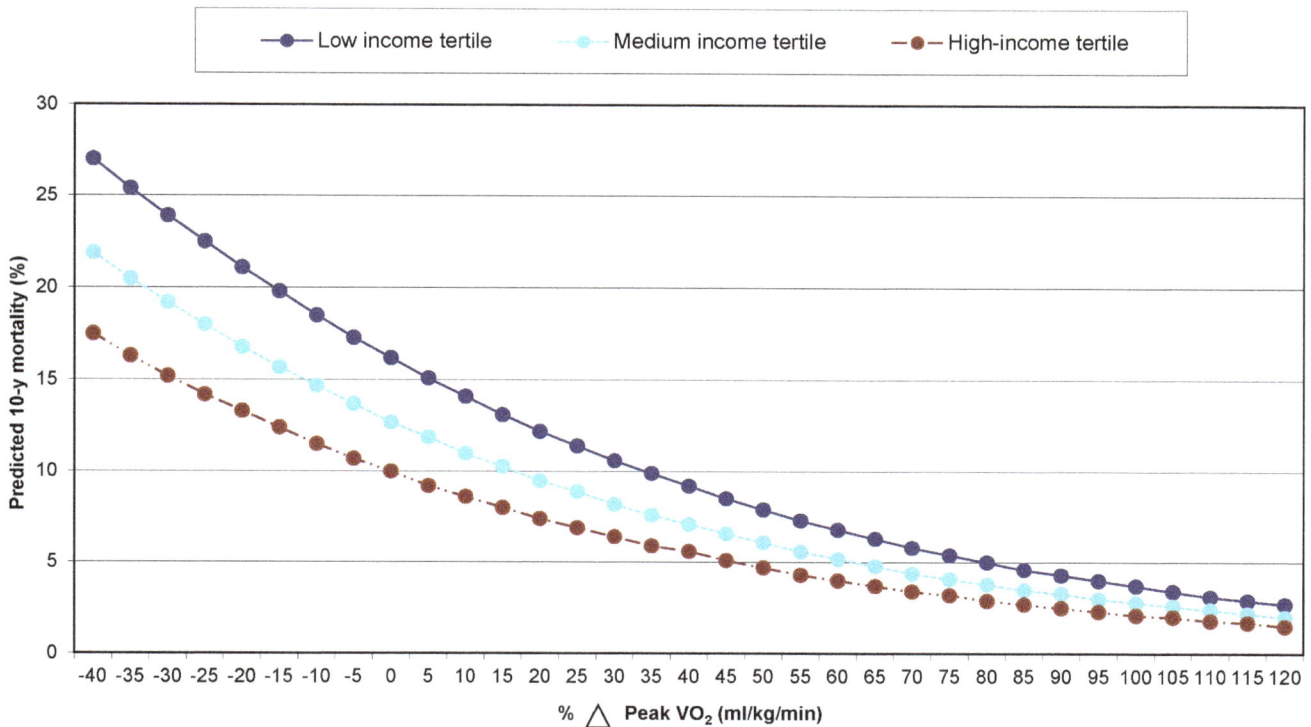

Figure 2. Relationship between functional recovery (i.e., % 1-year changes in self-reported peak VO₂) and expected 10-year mortality according to income after risk-adjustment for all remaining factors.

$$HR_{income} - HR_{income + functionalrecovery} / (HR_{income} - 1) \quad (38)$$

The relative contribution of functional recovery on income-mortality associations were examined incrementally over and beyond other baseline and recovery factors (i.e,. all models adjusted for self-reported functional capacity, self-reported physical health, emotional health, chronic stress, depression at baseline, as well as one-year changes in chronic stress and depression. However, given the high correlation between the DASI and SF-12 self-rated physical health measures (r = 0.73, P<0.001), a risk-adjustment model did not include change scores for both the DASI and the SF-12 self-rated physical health score within the same statistical model. Statistical models in which functional recovery were derived from changes in DASI yielded similar results as those in which functional recovery were derived using the SF-12 self-rated physical health composite score. Formal diagnostic testing revealed no evidence of multi-collinearity in any of our statistical models. A sensitivity analysis using non-parsimonious modeling did not meaningfully alter our results. We tested for violations of the proportionality assumption in all proportional hazard model specifications. All analyses were performed using SAS statistical software, version 9.1 (SAS Institute, Cary, NC).

Results

Baseline Characteristics

Socioeconomically disadvantaged patients were significantly older, more likely to be women, have fewer social supports, greater comorbidities, and higher predictive 6-month mortality rates than their more affluent counterparts. Income disadvantaged patients

were also significantly less likely to receive beta blockers and more likely to receive nitrates at hospital discharge (**Table 1**).

SES and Functional Recovery

Socially disadvantaged patients had poorer baseline self-reported functional capacity and achieved less improvement in one-year post-AMI functional recovery than did their higher SES counterparts. Patients of higher incomes also experienced better recovery from chronic stress, depression, self-rated physical and mental health than did patients who had lower annual earnings (P<0.001 for all), although the magnitude of changes for all of these other variables were less marked than the DASI-derived self-reported functional capacity. (**Table 2**).

Functional recovery improved among all patients regardless of SES or referral to cardiac rehabilitation, but did so more markedly among patients in higher SES tertiles (i.e. highest SES tertile patients on average, experienced a 1.80 ml/kg/min increase in peak VO2 as compared with lowest SES tertile patients, P<0.001) (**Figure 1**), and did so even after adjustment for all baseline factors irrespective of whether functional recovery was assessed as a continuous or a categorical variable. For example, patients in lowest as compared with highest income tertile patients were 44% less likely to experience functional recovery gains exceeding levels corresponding to the sample median, even after adjusting for all remaining factors (Adjusted OR: 0.56; 95% CI:0.38–0.84, P = 0.005).

SES and Secondary Prevention Services

Patients within highest income tertiles were 60% more likely to be referred to cardiac rehabilitation than those in lowest income tertiles. Income disadvantaged patients were significantly less likely to be followed up by a cardiologist, to receive cardiac rehabilitation, and to be taking evidence-based pharmacotherapies (B-blockers, aspirin, statins, and ACE inhibitors) during the year following AMI than were their higher SES counterparts. (**Table 3**).

Secondary Prevention Services and Functional Recovery

Neither cardiac rehabilitation referrals nor specialty care visits were significantly associated with functional recovery after adjusting for all baseline factors. Among all secondary prevention factors examined, only 30-day post-AMI coronary revascularization (PCI or CABG) significantly predicted functional recovery after AMI (P<0.001).

SES, Functional Recovery and Long-term Mortality

After adjusting for baseline and follow-up factors, functional recovery was the strongest modifiable predictor of long-term mortality based on the rank-order magnitude of the Chi-Square, and remained so irrespective of SES strata, cardiac rehabilitation referral or physician specialty service use (interaction terms between SES strata or cardiac rehabilitation referral or physician specialty service utilization, functional recovery, and mortality were all P>0.5). Each 1 ml/kg/min increase in estimated peak VO_2 was associated with a 9% reduction in long-term mortality (Adjusted HR: 0.91; 95% CI: 0.88–0.94, P<0.001).

There was a strong association between income and long-term mortality (Unadjusted HR for income with one-degree of freedom: 0.62; 95% CI: 0.54–0.71, P<0.001) was attenuated by 42% after adjustment for all post-AMI baseline and follow-up variables, excluding functional recovery (Adjusted HR: 0.78; 95% CI:0.65–0.93; P = 0.005). Adding functional recovery further reduced the magnitude of this association explaining an additional 27% of income's association with mortality, rendering the relationship between income and mortality no longer statistically significant (Adjusted HR: 0.84; 95% CI:0.70–1.00, P = 0.05) (**Table 4**). In contrast, sequential risk-adjustments for access to cardiac rehabilitation and specialty service had no significant impact on SES-mortality associations.

After adjusting for all factors, lowest income-tertile patients whose functional recovery exceeded that of the sample median had similar predicted long-term mortality as high-income tertile patients whose functional recovery improvements were less than the 20th percentile. (**Figure 2**).

Discussion

Our study demonstrated that higher SES patients experienced significantly greater post-AMI functional recovery than did their socioeconomically disadvantaged counterparts. Functional recovery was the strongest modifiable predictor of long-term mortality irrespective of SES, and explained nearly 30% of the association between SES and long-term mortality after AMI, as demonstrated through sequential risk-adjustment. The effects of functional recovery on SES-mortality associations were not explained by access inequities to physician specialists or cardiac rehabilitation.

Our results are consistent with other studies which have demonstrated that patients of lower SES have poorer functional capacity. [39–41] For example, Shishehbor and colleagues in which differences in functional capacity explained as much as 47% of the SES-mortality associations among patients with suspected coronary artery disease. [14] Moreover, the 9% reduction in long-term mortality associated with each increased calculated MET, as derived using a self-reported functional capacity survey is comparable to studies that examined the relationship between

METs and survival as measured objectively from exercise testing [42].

Our study builds upon previous studies by examining the relationship between SES and functional recovery during the transitional year of AMI convalescence, where the baseline risk of death and the needs for specialized cardiovascular services are highest. Our study also examined functional recovery within a context of other psychosocial, clinical, process of care and self-rated physical and mental health measures. The consistency by which SES correlated with functional recovery and the magnitude by which self-reported functional recovery explained SES-mortality associations underscores the importance of physical activity and exercise as social determinants of cardiovascular health.

We had hypothesized that SES access inequities to specialized cardiovascular services, such as cardiac rehabilitation and physician specialists, might have explained why socially-disadvantaged patients experience fewer gains in functional recovery after AMI as compared with their socially-advantaged counterparts. However, such was not the case. While patients in lowest income tertiles were 60% less likely to be referred to cardiac rehabilitation following AMI, cardiac rehabilitation was not independently associated with functional recovery after adjusting for patient factors. Indeed, functional recovery remained systematically lower among socially-disadvantaged irrespective of access to cardiac rehabilitation and/or cardiac specialists, which may partially explain why access to specialized cardiac services did not explain post-AMI SES-mortality associations.

Socioeconomically disadvantaged patients may experience poorer post-AMI functional recovery for several reasons. First, available evidence has shown that lower socioeconomic patients are generally less behaviourally engaged in healthy lifestyle choices, [43] in part, due to poorer awareness and insights into their health and disease. [44] Second, some have argued that socioeconomically-disadvantaged patients may have fewer social supports and networks. [45] Such networks may serve to act on the community culture of healthy life-style living, [7] resulting in such patients participating less frequently in physical activity and exercise as compared with their more affluent counterparts. [45] Third, socioeconomically-disadvantaged patients may be functionally limited by other co-existing medical illnesses and/or disabilities, which impede the ability of a patient to exercise. [46] Finally, lower SES patients may be challenged by employment constraints or finances to gain access to community resources and/or exercise accessories [47].

Our results support the need for innovative solutions to improve exercise and physical activity patterns among socio-economically disadvantaged patients. However, such innovative solutions may not necessarily simply reside with the broader implementation of established health services, such as cardiac rehabilitation programs and access to physician specialists. Instead, such strategies may necessitate other health and social policies, which may necessitate more integrative solutions into the workplace, tax-incentives, community-networks, and investments into the built-environment.

Our study has several important limitations which warrant discussion. First, functional recovery data were obtained using self-reported Questionnaires. While the functional capacity derived from DASI has been validated, [32,33] and while our study's use of the DASI questionnaire yielded similar results as did the self-rated physical health score as derived from the SF-12, it is possible that our findings may have differed had we estimated or directly measured peak VO_2 during progressive exercise testing. Second, ours was an observational study and some clinical details, such as left ventricular function were unavailable. Moreover, all of our survey data was confined to the first year of AMI recovery. We acknowledge that residual unmeasured confounding, particularly throughout the multiple years of follow-up, might have partially explained our results. That being said, our study did adjust for over 40 clinical, psychosocial, and process of care. Furthermore, we believe that the magnitude of associations between factors collected during the year following the index AMI and survival throughout the many years that follow would have if anything attenuated over time. Therefore, we believe that the associations between SES, functional recovery, and long-term mortality are conservative. Moreover, available evidence has demonstrated that the transitional period following AMI is important given the prevalence of cardiovascular specialty care-gaps, fragmentation and discontinuity in health care delivery as patients navigate from hospitals to community-based ambulatory care settings. [15,48–51] Finally, our study was conducted among a sample of AMI patients who survived and participated in one year interviews. While the distribution of sociodemographic factors among our AMI sub-sample was similar to the original SESAMI cohort, [26] the extent to which our results are applicable to all AMI populations remains unclear. That said, the original SESAMI cohort did enrol 70% of consecutive AMI patients from 95% of the large volume hospitals throughout Ontario - - a province which comprises 40% of the Canadian population. [26] These limitations must be counter-balanced against the strengths of this study, which include the comprehensiveness of our clinical, psychosocial, behavioural, and health service utilization data, as well as the duration and completeness of follow-up.

In conclusion, our study demonstrated the importance of functional recovery on explaining long-term SES-mortality associations. Post-AMI functional recovery may therefore represent an important intermediary causal pathway determinant of SES-outcome gradients after AMI. Given that the relationships between SES, functional recovery, and outcomes occurred independently of, and irrespective to, exposure to specialty cardiac services, innovative solutions must look beyond improvements in access to cardiac rehabilitation to improve SES-outcomes gradients after AMI. Such solutions may require novel policies that better integrate physical activity and exercise-based interventions into communities to better target and improve functional recovery and outcomes among socioeconomically-disadvantaged populations.

Supporting Information

Appendix S1 The Duke Activity Status Index is a self-administered questionnaire that measures a patient's functional capacity. It can be used to estimate the patient's peak oxygen uptake.

Acknowledgments

Drs. Alter and Tu are Career Investigators with the Heart and Stroke Foundation of Ontario. Dr. Tu is Canada Research Chair. Dr. Ko is a New Investigator with the Canadian Institute for Health Research.

Author Contributions

Conceived and designed the experiments: DA. Performed the experiments: DA. Analyzed the data: DA. Contributed reagents/materials/analysis tools: DA. Wrote the paper: DA. Contributed to critical revision of the manuscript for important intellectual content: DA BF DK PA DL PO TS JT.

References

1. Mackenbach JP, Stirbu I, Roskam AJ, Schaap MM, Menvielle G et al (2008) Socioeconomic inequalities in health in 22 European countries. N Engl J Med 358: 2468–2481.
2. Alter DA, Chong A, Austin PC, Mustard C, Iron K et al (2006) Socioeconomic status and mortality after acute myocardial infarction. Ann Intern Med 144: 82–93.
3. Bloch KV, Klein CH, de Souza e Silva NA, Nogueira AR, Salis LH (2003) Socioeconomic aspects of spousal concordance for hypertension, obesity, and smoking in a community of Rio de Janeiro, Brazil. Arq Bras Cardiol 80: 179–8.
4. Danenberg HD, Marincheva G, Varshitzki B, Nassar H, Lotan C (2009) Stent thrombosis: a poor man's disease? Isr Med Assoc J 11: 529–532.
5. Ganova-Iolovska M, Kalinov K, Geraedts M (2009) Quality of care of patients with acute myocardial infarction in Bulgaria: a cross-sectional study. BMC Health Serv Res 9: 15.
6. Gerber Y, Benyamini Y, Goldbourt U, Drory Y (2009) Prognostic importance and long-term determinants of self-rated health after initial acute myocardial infarction. Med Care 47: 342–349.
7. Gerber Y, Benyamini Y, Goldbourt U, Drory Y (2010) Neighborhood socioeconomic context and long-term survival after myocardial infarction. Circulation 121: 375–383.
8. Lynch JW, Kaplan GA, Cohen RD, Tuomilehto J, Salonen JT (1996) Do cardiovascular risk factors explain the relation between socioeconomic status, risk of all-cause mortality, cardiovascular mortality, and acute myocardial infarction? Am J Epidemiol 144: 934–942.
9. Menec VH, Roos NP, Black C, Bogdanovic B (2001) Characteristics of patients with a regular source of care. Can J Public Health 92: 299–303.
10. Pitsavos C, Kavouras SA, Panagiotakos DB, Arapi S, Anastasiou CA et al (2008) Physical activity status and acute coronary syndromes survival The GREECS (Greek Study of Acute Coronary Syndromes) study. J Am Coll Cardiol 51: 2034–2039.
11. Rosvall M, Chaix B, Lynch J, Lindstrom M, Merlo J (2008) The association between socioeconomic position, use of revascularization procedures and five-year survival after recovery from acute myocardial infarction. BMC Public Health 8: 44.
12. Sihm I, Dehlholm G, Hansen ES, Gerdes LU, Faergeman O (1991) The psychosocial work environment of younger men surviving acute myocardial infarction. Eur Heart J 12: 203–209.
13. Alter DA, Stukel T, Chong A, Henry D (2011) Lesson from Canada's Universal Care: socially disadvantaged patients use more health services, still have poorer health. Health Aff (Millwood) 30: 274–283.
14. Shishehbor MH, Litaker D, Pothier CE, Lauer MS (2006) Association of socioeconomic status with functional capacity, heart rate recovery, and all-cause mortality. JAMA 295: 784–792.
15. Alter DA, Iron K, Austin PC, Naylor CD (2004) Socioeconomic status, service patterns, and perceptions of care among survivors of acute myocardial infarction in Canada. JAMA 291: 1100–1107.
16. Clark RA, Coffee N, Turner D, Eckert KA, van GD et al (2012) Application of geographic modeling techniques to quantify spatial access to health services before and after an acute cardiac event: the Cardiac Accessibility and Remoteness Index for Australia (ARIA) project. Circulation 125: 2006–2014.
17. Raine R, Hutchings A, Black N (2003) Is publicly funded health care really distributed according to need? The example of cardiac rehabilitation in the UK. Health Policy 63: 63–72.
18. Clark AM, Hartling L, Vandermeer B, McAlister FA (2005) Meta-analysis: secondary prevention programs for patients with coronary artery disease. Ann Intern Med 143: 659–672.
19. Taylor RS, Brown A, Ebrahim S, Jolliffe J, Noorani H et al (2004) Exercise-based rehabilitation for patients with coronary heart disease: systematic review and meta-analysis of randomized controlled trials. Am J Med 116: 682–692.
20. Morey MC, Pieper CF, Crowley GM, Sullivan RJ, Puglisi CM (2002) Exercise adherence and 10-year mortality in chronically ill older adults. J Am Geriatr Soc 50: 1929–1933.
21. [Anonymous] (1984) Canada Health Act. C-6.
22. Candido E, Richards JA, Oh P, Suskin N, Arthur HM et al (2011) The relationship between need and capacity for multidisciplinary cardiovascular risk-reduction programs in Ontario. Can J Cardiol 27: 200–207.
23. Suaya JA, Shepard DS, Normand SL, Ades PA, Prottas J et al (2007) Use of cardiac rehabilitation by Medicare beneficiaries after myocardial infarction or coronary bypass surgery. Circulation 116: 1653–1662.
24. Candido E, Kurdyak P, Alter DA (2011) Item nonresponse to psychosocial questionnaires was associated with higher mortality after acute myocardial infarction. J Clin Epidemiol 64: 213–222.
25. Alter DA, Naylor CD, Austin P, Tu JV (1999) Effects of socioeconomic status on access to invasive cardiac procedures and on mortality after acute myocardial infarction. N Engl J Med 341: 1359–1367.
26. Alter DA, Iron K, Austin PC, Naylor CD (2004) Influence of education and income on atherogenic risk factor profiles among patients hospitalized with acute myocardial infarction. Can J Cardiol 20: 1219–1228.
27. Statistics Canada (1999) 1996 National Population Health Survey Documentation. Ottawa:

28. Alter DA, Venkatesh V, Chong A (2006) Evaluating the performance of the Global Registry of Acute Coronary Events risk-adjustment index across socioeconomic strata among patients discharged from the hospital after acute myocardial infarction. Am Heart J 151: 323–331.
29. Ko DT, Mamdani M, Alter DA (2004) Lipid-lowering therapy with statins in high-risk elderly patients: the treatment-risk paradox. JAMA 291: 1864–1870.
30. Buurman BM, Parlevliet JL, van Deelen BA, de Haan RJ, de Rooij SE (2010) A randomised clinical trial on a comprehensive geriatric assessment and intensive home follow-up after hospital discharge: the Transitional Care Bridge. BMC Health Serv Res 10: 296.
31. Hlatky MA, Boineau RE, Higginbotham MB, Lee KL, Mark DB et al (1989) A brief self-administered questionnaire to determine functional capacity (the Duke Activity Status Index). Am J Cardiol 64: 651–654.
32. Bairey Merz CN, Olson M, McGorray S, Pakstis DL, Zell K et al (2000) Physical activity and functional capacity measurement in women: a report from the NHLBI-sponsored WISE study. J Womens Health Gend Based Med 9: 769–777.
33. Carter R, Holiday DB, Grothues C, Nwasuruba C, Stocks J et al(2002) Criterion validity of the Duke Activity Status Index for assessing functional capacity in patients with chronic obstructive pulmonary disease. J Cardiopulm Rehabil 22: 298–308.
34. Allison KR, Adlaf EM, Ialomiteanu A, Rehm J (1999) Predictors of health risk behaviours among young adults: analysis of the National Population Health Survey. Can J Public Health 90: 85–89.
35. Koenig HG, George LK, Larson DB, McCullough ME, Branch PS et al (1999) Depressive symptoms and nine-year survival of 1,001 male veterans hospitalized with medical illness. Am J Geriatr Psychiatry 7: 124–131.
36. Melville MR, Lari MA, Brown N, Young T, Gray D (2003) Quality of life assessment using the short form 12 questionnaire is as reliable and sensitive as the short form 36 in distinguishing symptom severity in myocardial infarction survivors. Heart 89: 1445–1446.
37. Kurdyak PA, Gnam WH, Goering P, Chong A, Alter DA (2008) The relationship between depressive symptoms, health service consumption, and prognosis after acute myocardial infarction: a prospective cohort study. BMC Health Serv Res 8: 200.
38. Birkmeyer JD, Stukel TA, Siewers AE, Goodney PP, Wennberg DE et al (2003) Surgeon volume and operative mortality in the United States. N Engl J Med 349: 2117–2127.
39. Cohen B, Vittinghoff E, Whooley M (2008) Association of socioeconomic status and exercise capacity in adults with coronary heart disease (from the Heart and Soul Study). Am J Cardiol 101: 462–466.
40. Shishehbor MH, Gordon-Larsen P, Kiefe CI, Litaker D (2008) Association of neighborhood socioeconomic status with physical fitness in healthy young adults: the Coronary Artery Risk Development in Young Adults (CARDIA) study. Am Heart J 155: 699–705.
41. Sulander T, Heinonen H, Pajunen T, Karisto A, Pohjolainen P et al (2012) Longitudinal changes in functional capacity: effects of socio-economic position among ageing adults. Int J Equity Health 11: 78.
42. Kokkinos P, Myers J, Faselis C, Panagiotakos DB, Doumas M et al (2010) Exercise capacity and mortality in older men: a 20-year follow-up study. Circulation 122: 790–797.
43. Hillier FC, Batterham AM, Nixon CA, Crayton AM, Pedley CL et al (2012) A community-based health promotion intervention using brief negotiation techniques and a pledge on dietary intake, physical activity levels and weight outcomes: lessons learnt from an exploratory trial. Public Health Nutr 15: 1446–1455.
44. Harkins C, Shaw R, Gillies M, Sloan H, Macintyre K et al (2010) Overcoming barriers to engaging socio-economically disadvantaged populations in CHD primary prevention: a qualitative study. BMC Public Health 10: 391.
45. Hunt J, Marshall AL, Jenkins D (2008) Exploring the meaning of, the barriers to and potential strategies for promoting physical activity among urban Indigenous Australians. Health Promot J Austr 19: 102–108.
46. Sainio P, Martelin T, Koskinen S, Heliovaara M (2007) Educational differences in mobility: the contribution of physical workload, obesity, smoking and chronic conditions. J Epidemiol Community Health 61: 401–408.
47. Brownson RC, Boehmer TK, Luke DA (2005) Declining rates of physical activity in the United States: what are the contributors? Annu Rev Public Health 26: 421–443.
48. Ayanian JZ, Landrum MB, Guadagnoli E, Gaccione P (2002) Specialty of ambulatory care physicians and mortality among elderly patients after myocardial infarction. N Engl J Med 347: 1678–1686.
49. Ghosh R, Pepe P (2009) The critical care cascade: a systems approach. Curr Opin Crit Care 15: 279–283.
50. Lee DS, Stukel TA, Austin PC, Alter DA, Schull MJ et al (2010) Improved outcomes with early collaborative care of ambulatory heart failure patients discharged from the emergency department. Circulation 122: 1806–1814.
51. Oberg EB, Fitzpatrick AL, Lafferty WE, LoGerfo JP (2009) Secondary prevention of myocardial infarction with nonpharmacologic strategies in a Medicaid cohort. Prev Chronic Dis 6: A52.

20

Step-to-Step Variability in Treadmill Walking: Influence of Rhythmic Auditory Cueing

Philippe Terrier[1,2]*

1 IRR, Institut de Recherche en Réadaptation, Sion, Switzerland, **2** Clinique romande de réadaptation SuvaCare, Sion, Switzerland

Abstract

While walking, human beings continuously adjust step length (SpL), step time (SpT), step speed (SpS = SpL/SpT) and step width (SpW) by integrating both feedforward and feedback mechanisms. These motor control processes result in correlations of gait parameters between consecutive strides (statistical persistence). Constraining gait with a speed cue (treadmill) and/or a rhythmic auditory cue (metronome), modifies the statistical persistence to anti-persistence. The objective was to analyze whether the combined effect of treadmill and rhythmic auditory cueing (RAC) modified not only statistical persistence, but also fluctuation magnitude (standard deviation, SD), and stationarity of SpL, SpT, SpS and SpW. Twenty healthy subjects performed 6×5 min. walking tests at various imposed speeds on a treadmill instrumented with foot-pressure sensors. Freely-chosen walking cadences were assessed during the first three trials, and then imposed accordingly in the last trials with a metronome. Fluctuation magnitude (SD) of SpT, SpL, SpS and SpW was assessed, as well as NonStationarity Index (NSI), which estimates the dispersion of local means in the times series (SD of 20 local means over 10 steps). No effect of RAC on fluctuation magnitude (SD) was observed. SpW was not modified by RAC, what is likely the evidence that lateral foot placement is separately regulated. Stationarity (NSI) was modified by RAC in the same manner as persistent pattern: Treadmill induced low NSI in the time series of SpS, and high NSI in SpT and SpL. On the contrary, SpT, SpL and SpS exhibited low NSI under RAC condition. We used relatively short sample of consecutive strides (100) as compared to the usual number of strides required to analyze fluctuation dynamics (200 to 1000 strides). Therefore, the responsiveness of stationarity measure (NSI) to cued walking opens the perspective to perform short walking tests that would be adapted to patients with a reduced gait perimeter.

Editor: Adrian L.R. Thomas, University of Oxford, United Kingdom

Funding: The study was supported by the Swiss accident insurance company SUVA, which is an independent, non-profit company under public law. The IRR (Institute for Research in Rehabilitation) is supported by the State of Valais and the City of Sion. The funders had no role in study design, data collection and analysis, decision to publish, or preparation of the manuscript.

Competing Interests: The author has declared that no competing interests exist.

* E-mail: philippe.terrier@crr-suva.ch

Introduction

For walking, human beings produce a series of alternating, rhythmical movements of the trunk and limbs, which result in the forward progression of the body. By alternating the stance and oscillation phases of lower limbs, the body moves over a given distance (step length, SpL) in a given duration (step time, SpT) twice during a full gait cycle (or stride = two steps). The resulting speed is the ratio between step length and time (step speed: SpS = SpL/SpT). Theoretically, an infinite combination of SpL and SpT, and hence highly variable gait patterns, could result in a steady speed. On the contrary, it is observed that motor control provides highly consistent gait pattern from one stride to the next, with small residual step-to-step fluctuations [1,2,3]. At a given speed, it has been shown that preferred (spontaneously chosen) SpL and SpT coincide with minimal energy expenditure [4,5]. In an experiment that induced visual perturbations, increased step-to-step variability of SpL has been associated with higher energy cost [6]: the causes are likely twofold: a) an increased number of steps with energetically sub-optimal combination of SpL and SpT; b) increased cost induced by active feedback adjustments to restore optimal gait parameters, that require higher muscular activity [5,6,7]. Therefore, it is very likely that –by integrating both

feedforward (from internal models) and feedback (from sensory inputs) mechanisms – continuous adjustments of basic gait parameter (SpL and SpT) are performed by motor control in order to produce low step-to-step fluctuations and hence an optimal level of energy expenditure.

Apart energy aspects, motor control must also adjust gait to deal with the inherent instability of bipedial locomotion. It has been shown that lateral stabilization plays a central role in this context [8]: lateral foot placement seems actively controlled step-by-step in order to counteract constitutive instability in the frontal plane. Consequently, Step Width (SpW, i.e. the maximal lateral distance between feet during one step) has been extensively studied as a proxy for global dynamic stability and fall risk [9,10,11,12].

The quantification of step-to-step fluctuations has been realized with classical statistical methods that assess the dispersion of data around central trend, such as Standard Deviation (SD) [10], Root Mean Square (RMS) [6], or Coefficient of Variation (CV, defined as SD/mean) [3]. However, these methods assume that gait parameters are purely random processes with no correlation between successive strides, what is unlikely to be the case, because feedback loops are involved in the regulation mechanisms. As a result, alternative methods have been proposed to quantify the temporal dependences in the time series of gait parameters. For instance, the short-term stationarity of the mean throughout a long recording of gait parameters can by assessed (NonStationarityIndex, NSI [13,14]). Detrended Fluctuation Analysis (DFA) is also used to describe the statistical persistence that exists across consecutive strides [15,16]. "Persistence" means that deviations are statistically more likely to be followed by subsequent deviations in the same direction (i.e. persist across subsequent data points). Conversely, "Anti-persistence" means that deviations in one direction are statistically more likely to be followed by subsequent deviations in the opposite direction.

To better understand how humans regulate their steps in order to comply with energy and stability requirements, a possibility is to submit individuals to external constraints and to examine the resulting change in step-to-step fluctuation pattern. Here we wish to introduce two type of constraints, namely temporal constraints, induced by Rhythmic Auditory Cueing (RAC), and speed constraints, induced by motorized treadmill. The synchronization of body movements to external rhythm (auditory-motor coordination) is a remarkable ability of the human brain [17,18]. Step time modulations driven by RAC have been studied in the context of different clinical disorders, such as head injuries, Parkinson's disease or stroke [19]. It can induce a substantial beneficial effect on gait performance [19,20]. Motorized treadmills are widely used in biomechanical studies of human locomotion. They allow the performance of a large number of successive strides under controlled environment, with a selectable steady-state locomotion speed. In the rehabilitation field, treadmill walking is used in locomotor therapy, for instance with partial body weight support in spinal cord injury or stroke rehabilitation [2].

We [3,21], and others [22] observed that RAC deeply modifies statistical persistence of stride time, while fluctuation magnitude (CV) remained unchanged. We concluded that, when the walking pace is controlled by an auditory signal, the feedback loop between the planned movement (at supraspinal level) and the sensory inputs induces a continual shifting of stride time around the mean (anti-persistence), but with no effect on the fluctuation dynamics of the other parameters (stride length and stride speed) [1]. The same anti-persistent pattern has been described by Dingwell and Cusumano for stride speed during treadmill walking [23]. The authors proposed that humans use sub-optimal control to correct stride-to-stride deviations: in order to follow the speed imposed by the treadmill, individuals consistently slightly over-correct small deviations in walking speed at each stride [23]. They also proposed a general model of gait regulation based on redundancy theory (Goal Equivalent Manifold, GEM) and Minimum Intervention Principle (MIP).

Recently, we analyzed the combination of both RAC and treadmill walking [21]. Under this dual constraints condition, we observed that stride time, stride length and stride speed exhibited an anti-persistent pattern. Anti-persistent dynamics may be related to a tighter control: deviations are followed by a rapid over-correction that produces oscillations around target values. Under single constraint condition, while stride speed is tightly regulated in order to follow the treadmill speed, redundancy between ST and SL would likely allow persistent pattern to occur. Conversely, under dual constraint conditions, the absence of redundancy among SL, ST and SS would explain the generalized anti-persistent pattern [21].

In the present study, we further documented step-to-step variability in healthy individuals walking on a treadmill, with and without RAC. In the previous study [21], we assessed statistical persistence and variability (CV) in consecutive strides over 5 min. walking. Here, we re-analyzed the same raw data to study variability in 200 consecutive steps. The methodological goal

was to explore whether fluctuation dynamics could be analyzed with shorter walking test in the perspective to analyze gait impaired patients in future studies. In addition to basic spatio-temporal parameters (SpT, SpL, SpS), we also compute step width (SpW). The hypothesis was that SpW and SpW variability would be not modified by RAC, because variability in the frontal plane is related to dynamic stability and regulated separately. Standard deviation (SD) among steps was used as variability index. In addition, an index of the sationarity of local means (NonStationarity Index) was also computed. We hypothesized that anti-persistence induced by RAC should be associated with more stationary gait parameters (less variation of local means among consecutive steps). Finally, we assess the strength of the association among variability indexes, including scaling exponents from previous study [21]. Because GEM model assumed that SpT and SpL are cross-regulated, we assumed that variability indexes, as well as statistical persistence, would be correlated.

Methods

Participants

In the present article, we re-analyzed data obtained in a previous study [21]. Please refer to this article to obtain supplementary information about the experimental procedure and data analysis. Twenty healthy subjects (10 females, 10 males) participated in the study. The participants' characteristics were (mean (SD): age 36 yr (11), body mass 71 kg (15), and height 171 cm (9). All participants gave written informed consent to take part in the study. The experimental procedure was approved by the local ethics committee (Commission Cantonale Valaisanne d'Ethique Médicale, Sion, Switzerland), in accordance with the ethical standards in the Declaration of Helsinki.

Experimental procedure

Treadmill speeds imposed to the subjects were: Preferred Walking Speed (PWS), $0.7 \times$ PWS (low speed) and $1.3 \times$ PWS (high speed). The sequence of the trials was randomly designed. Each walking trials lasted 5 m30: 30 s of habituation to the speed, and 5 min of measurement. Then, the trials with "metronome" condition were performed at the same speeds as the first 3 trials. The imposed cadences were the preferred cadences, which were measured during the first trials without metronome.

Instrument

The instrumented treadmill was a FDM-TDL (Scheinworks/Zebris, Schein, Germany). The sensor surface contained 7168 (128×56) pressure sensors on a 108.4×47.4 cm grid (1.4 sensors per cm2). Pressure data were sampled at 100 Hz. The raw data consisted for each trial in 30'000 frames of 56×128 points: they were exported for subsequent analysis with Matlab (Mathworks, USA).

Data analysis

The first 90 sec of each test was not analyzed in order to avoid starting effect. A constant number of 200 steps (100 gait cycles) was kept for the subsequent analysis. The time series of Step Time (SpT), Step length (SpL) and Step Speed, (SpS = SpL/SpT) were obtained by specifically detecting the heel strikes in the frames, and hence calculating time and distance between consecutive steps. From the raw data corresponding to the selected 200 steps, continuous (100 Hz) trajectory of the center of pressure was computed as the weighted average of pressure data, with the standard method for determining barycentre (Sum of mass*position)/(Sum of mass). By using a peak detection algorithm, Step

Widths (SpW) were assessed as the maximal left/right distance (medio-lateral signal) reached at each step by the pressure centre.

Central tendencies and fluctuation magnitudes among individuals (N = 20) and conditions (N = 3×2) were assessed by computing Means and Standard Deviations of the time series (M and SD, N = 200). We were also interested to characterize the local, time dependent, fluctuations in the series, irrespectively of the global fluctuation magnitude. Therefore, we computed NonStationarity Index (NSI), which estimates the dispersion of normalized local means [13]: each series is first standardized (by subtracting mean and dividing by SD); then the standardized series is divided in 20 segments of 10 steps; the local average of each segment is computed; the NSI is the SD of these 20 means. NSI provides an estimation of the consistency of the local average values, high NSI indicating more inconsistent local averages [13]. In order to characterize the potential persistent/anti-persistent pattern (auto-correlation) present in the series, we used scaling exponents (α) computed by Detrended Fluctuation Analysis [1,2,21]. Alpha-values obtained in our previous study [21] were used. An overall view of the variables included in the statistical analyses is shown in table 1.

Statistical analysis

For each speed (low, PWS, high) and condition (without and with RAC), descriptive statistics consisted in notched boxplots (median and quartiles of the sample, fig. 1, 2, 3, 4). In addition, means and SD (N = 20 participants) are presented. The effect of RAC was assessed by using standardized Hedge's g: this standardized Effect Size (ES = delta(mean)/SD) is a modified version of the Cohen's d for inferential measure [24,25]. The precision of the effect sizes was estimated with 95% Confidence Intervals (CI). CI were ±1.96 times the asymptotic estimates of the standard error of g. Graphical representation of ES and corresponding CI are given for each variable (see table 1) and speed condition, except for scaling exponents, which were already shown in our previous study [21]. Arbitrary thresholds for small (0.2), medium (0.5) and large (0.8)

effects are also shown to ease the interpretation. It is worth noting that no effects of RAC were expected for average SpT, SpL and SpS, because, by design, the participants performed the two conditions at identical speed (imposed by the treadmill) and cadence (imposed by the metronome), what induced an identical SpL. As a result, descriptive statistics are given only for the "treadmill only" condition (fig. 1).

The strength of the association among variability indexes (SD, NSI, α), taking into account a potential speed effect, was estimated by computing partial Pearson's correlation coefficients (pr). The partial correlation between two variables x and y, controlling for a third one (z), is numerically equivalent to the correlation between the residuals from the regression of x and z and the residuals from the regression of y and z [24]. Thus, pr removes the variance explained by the third variables (z) from the variables of interest (x and y) and then quantifies the remaining correlation [24]. Practically, M-SpS was systematically controlled as the third variable (z) in pr computation: the result can be interpreted as correlation between variables holding speed constant. We also assessed the 95% CI based on an asymptotic normal distribution of $0.5 * \log((1+pr)/(1-pr))$, with an approximate variance equal to $1/(N-4)$, N = 60. Given the eleven variability variables (table 1), 55 pairwise combinations were possible $(11!/(2! \times (11-2)!) = 55)$. We computed pr separately for both conditions (treadmill only and RAC). We arbitrarily chose to present only correlation with $|pr| > 0.3$, a threshold which corresponds to an association of moderate strength, according to Cohen [25] (fig. 5).

Results

In order to ease the understanding of figures, the reader will find in table 1 a summary of the measured variables and their abbreviations.

Figure 1 presents the basic gait parameters measured in the 20 participants. By experimental design, the values are the same for both conditions (treadmill only, and treadmill + RAC). As

Table 1. Summary of the gait parameters.

Abbreviation	Definition	Formulae	Comments
M-SpT	Average values of the times series of the gait parameters, i.e. Step Time (SpT), Step Length (SpL), Step Speed (SpS = SpL/SpT) and Step Width (SpW)	<SpT>, N = 200	See fig. 1 and 2.
M-SpL		<SpL>, N = 200	
M-SpS		<SpS>, N = 200	
M-SpW		<SpW>, N = 200	
SD-SpT	Fluctuation magnitude (SD) of the times series of the gait parameters	SD(SpT), N = 200	See fig. 3
SD-SpL		SD(SpL), N = 200	
SD-SpS		SD(SpS), N = 200	
SD-SpW		SD(SpW), N = 200	
NSI-SpT	NonStationarity Index (NSI). Fluctuation of local standardized averages	SD(<SpT>loc), N = 20	See fig. 4
NSI-SpL		SD(<SpL>loc), N = 20	
NSI-SpS		SD(<SpS>loc), N = 20	
NSI-SpW		SD(<SpW>loc), N = 20	
α-ST	DFA results: Scaling exponent in times series of Stride Time (ST), Stride Length (SL) and Stride Speed (SS = SL/ST)	$F(n) = \sqrt{\frac{1}{N}\sum_{k=1}^{N}[y(k)-y_n(k)]^2}$ $F(n) \sim n^{\alpha}$	Results from [21] Used in correlation analyses (fig. 5)
α-SL			
α-SS			

The table summarizes the gait parameters analyzed in the study.

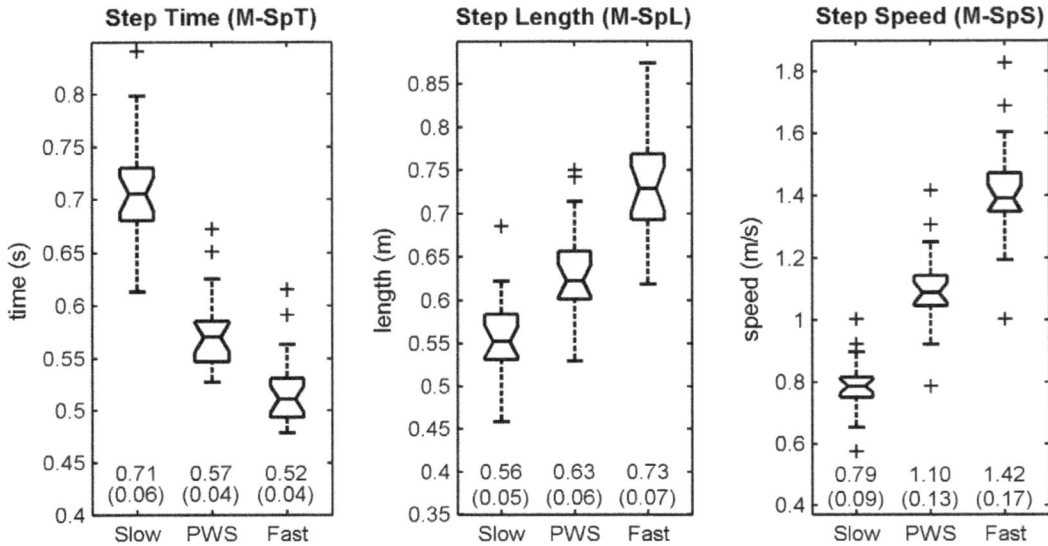

Figure 1. Basic gait parameters. Twenty healthy subjects walked 3×5 min. on a motorized treadmill. 100 strides (200 steps) were analyzed. Step Ttime (M-SpT i.e mean duration of the 200 steps), Step Length (M-SpL, i.e. mean length of the 200 steps) and Step Speed (M-SpS, i.e. mean speed of the 200 steps) are shown. The selected speeds were Preferred Walking Speed (PWS), 0.7x PWS (Slow) and 1.3x PWS (Fast). The range of individual results (N = 20) is presented with notched boxplots. Printed values are mean(SD).

expected, the increase in SpS induced a concomitant increase in SpL and decrease in SpT, because SpS = SpL/SpT. The inter-individual variability, expressed as CV (N = 20), was M-SpT: slow 8%, PWS 7%, fast 8%; M-SpL: slow 9%, PWS 10%, fast 10%; M-SpS: slow 11%, PWS 12%, fast 12%.

Step width was not constrained between conditions by the experimental protocol, and hence could be influenced by RAC.

Figure 2 shows the extent of the results among participants, as well as the Effect Size (ES) of RAC. A substantial inter-individual variability was observed, ranging from 21% (fast speed) to 27% (slow speed). No RAC effect was found, with small and not significant ES.

Figure 3 shows the results for variability among gait parameters. Comparing the notched box, speed seemed to have a high impact

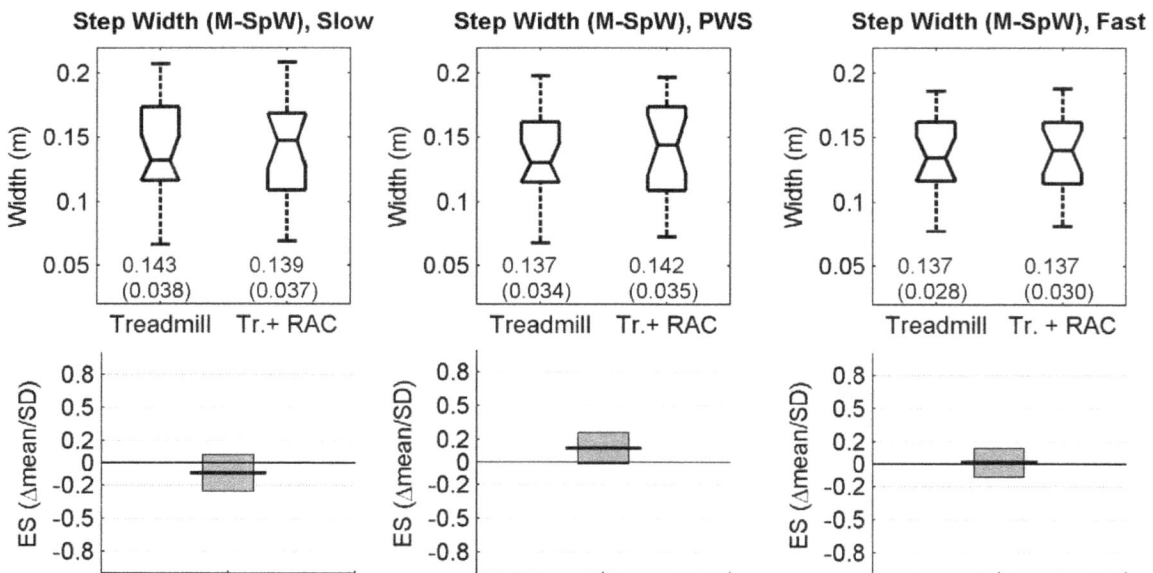

Figure 2. Step Width. Twenty healthy subjects walked 6×5 min. on a motorized treadmill without (Treadmill) and with Rhythmic Auditory Cueing (Tr. + RAC) at their preferred cadence for the given speed. 100 strides (200 steps) were analyzed. Step Width (M-SpW) is the mean of widths between consecutive steps (N = 200). Selected speeds were Preferred Walking Speed (middle, PWS), 0.7x PWS (left, Slow) and 1.3x PWS (right, Fast). The range of individual results (N = 20) is presented with notched boxplots. Printed values are mean(SD). Bottom panels show the Effect Size (ES, Hedge's g, variant of Cohen's d) of the auditory cueing, i.e. the mean difference normalized by SD. Boxes are the 95% confidence intervals for the effect size estimations.

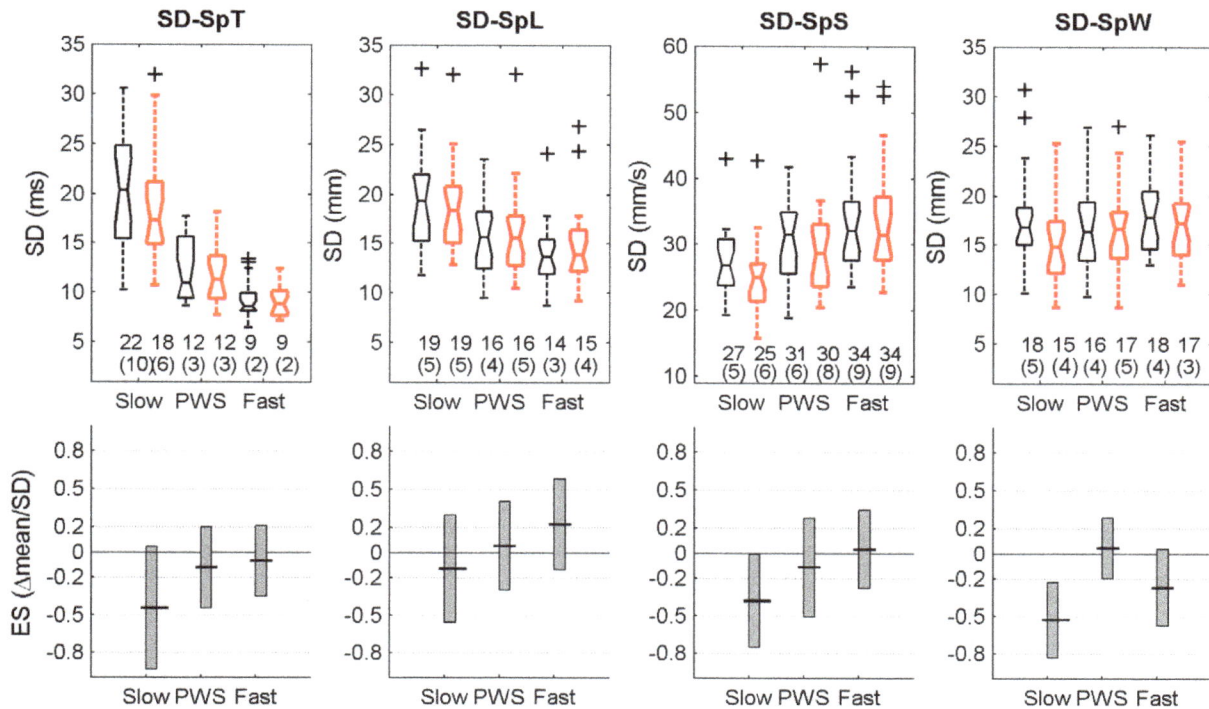

Figure 3. Step-to-step variability. Twenty healthy subjects walked 6×5 min. on a motorized treadmill without (left, black) and with Rhythmic Auditory Cueing (RAC, (metronome), right, red) at their preferred cadence for the given speed. 100 strides (200 steps) were analyzed. Variability indexes are Standard Deviations (SD, N = 200) of step time (SD-SpT), step length (SD-SpL), step speed (SD-SpS), and step width (SD-SpW). Selected speeds were Preferred Walking Speed (middle, PWS), 0.7x PWS (left, Slow) and 1.3x PWS (right, Fast). The range of individual results (N = 20) is presented with notched boxplots. Printed values are means (SD). Bottom panels show the effect size (Hedge's g, variant of Cohen's d) of the auditory cueing, i.e. the mean difference normalized by SD. Vertical boxes are the 95% confidence intervals for the effect size estimations.

on SD-SpT, but a moderate (SD-SpL, SD-SpS) or low (SD-SpW) effect on the other parameters. A high inter-individual variability is observed, which ranged from 19% (normal, slow, SD-SpS) to 45% (normal, Slow, SD-SpT). With one exception (SD-SpW, slow ES = −0.53), RAC did not produce a significant effect on gait variability. However, medium effect size are observed at slow speed for SD-SpT (ES = −0.45) and SD-SpS (ES = −0.38).

Results for NonStationarity Index (NSI) are presented in figure 4. Local fluctuations of speed (NSI-SpS) seemed not influenced by RAC, with low NSI (0.05) at every imposed speed and ES close to zero. In the same manner, no RAC effect was observed for step width (NSI-SpW), but higher values (0.13–0.16) and speed dependence are noted. Conversely, a very strong effect of RAC on step length (NSI–SpL) and step time (NSI–SpT) is evident (ES >>0.8). Under dual constraints conditions (treadmill + RAC), NSI remained rather low (0.07–0.08) for both SpL and SpT under every speed conditions. In contrast, higher NSI values (0.10–0.15) and speed dependence are evident in the treadmill only condition.

The figure 5 synthesizes the results of partial correlations (normalized for speed) among analyzed variables. Among 55 possible combinations, 11 and 16 partial correlation coefficients (pr) were higher than 0.3 in respectively treadmill only and treadmill + RAC conditions. A strong association was observed between scaling exponents of stride length and stride time under both conditions (α-ST vs. α-SL: pr = 0.88 and pr = 0.77). Other outstanding relationship concerns step length and speed variability (SD-SpL vs. SD-SpS: pr = 0.68 and pr = 0.79). It is also worth noting that local stationarity (NSI) seems moderately correlated

with scaling exponents (α), with pr ranging from 0.33 to 0.66 among the different comparisons. Conversely, step width variability exhibited only few relevant (moderate) associations with other variables: treadmill only: SD-SpW vs. α-SL, pr = −0.4; treadmill+RAC: SD-SpS vs. SD-SpW, pr = 0.35; SD-SpL vs. NSI-SpW, pr = 0.32.

Discussion

The present study is the follow-up of a previous study concerning persistent and anti-persistent pattern in gait fluctuations [21]. In this previous study, we observed that treadmill induced anti-persistent dynamics (α<0.5) in the time series of stride speed, but preserved the persistence (α>0.5) of stride time and length. On the contrary, all the three parameters were anti-persistent under dual-constraints (treadmill+RAC) condition. We suggested, according to the results and the previous literature, [1,23,26,27], that two modalities of gait control co-exist: 1) a more automated/unconscious mode, which produces persistent, fractal-like pattern across numerous successive strides, what is likely related to the redundancy among the gait parameters to achieve steady gate; 2) a more voluntary/conscious mode relying upon fast over-correction of deviations in the controlled variable, which produces anti-persistent pattern among successive strides. In addition, the combination of two constraints (time and speed) induces anti-persistence in the three gait variables, what is likely the result of the cross-regulation of stride length and stride time and the absence of redundancy among the gait parameters to achieve the dual goal function.

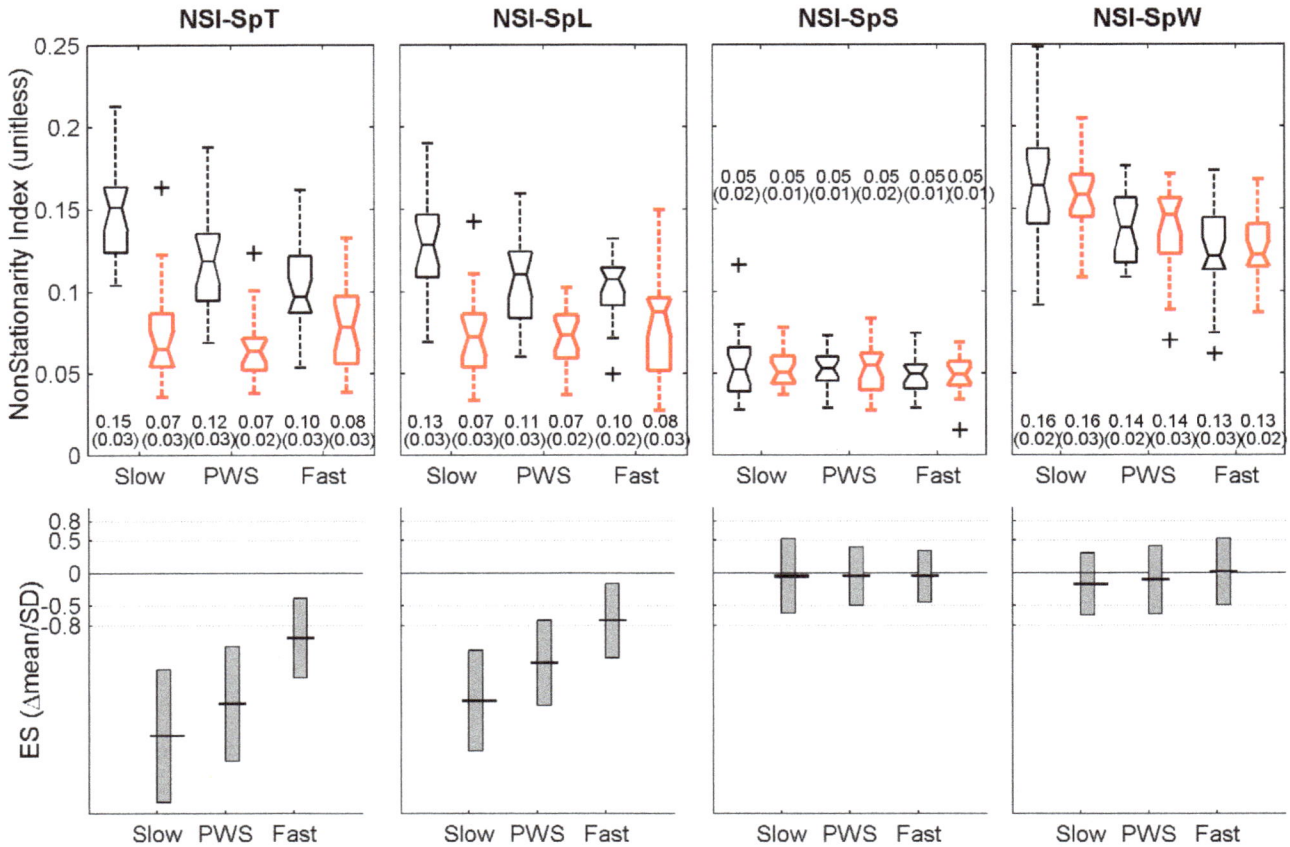

Figure 4. NonStationarity Index. Twenty healthy subjects walked 6×5 min. on a motorized treadmill without (left, blackl) and with Rhythmic Auditory Cueing (RAC, (metronome), right, red) at their preferred cadence for the given speed. 100 strides (200 steps) were analyzed. NonStationarity Index (NSI) is the variability (SD, N = 20) of the local means computed over 10 consecutive steps. Variables are step time (NSI-SpT), step length (NSI-SpL), step speed (NSI-SpS), and step width (NSI-SpW). Selected speeds were Preferred Walking Speed (middle, PWS), 0.7x PWS (left, Slow) and 1.3x PWS (right, Fast). The range of individual results (N = 20) is presented with notched boxplots. Printed values are mean(SD). Bottom panels show the effect size (Hedge's g, variant of Cohen's d) of the auditory cueing, i.e. the mean difference normalized by SD. Vertical boxes are the 95% confidence intervals for the effect size estimations.

Based on the same raw data, the present study explore in more details different variability indexes and their inter-relationships. To summarize the results, we observed that variability of the local means of gait parameters, expressed as Non-Stationarity index (NSI), was responsive to RAC in a similar was as scaling exponent described in our previous study [21]. Furthermore, we found that step width was not modified by RAC. In addition, RAC did not significantly change the variability (expressed as SD) of gait parameter, except for Step width variability at low speed. Concerning correlation results, we found a strong association between scaling exponents of stride length and stride width, as well moderate correlations between NSI and scaling exponents.

Methodological considerations

The main methodological difference between this study and our previous study was that, here, we analyzed step-to-step variability, as compared to stride-to-stride fluctuations in the previous study. Furthermore, we used a constant number of 200 steps for the computation of variability index, as compared to the use of the full 5 min. time series in the previous study (360 to 626 steps). Auto correlation properties of time series, such as statistical persistence or long-range correlations as evidenced by DFA, are typically analyzed over several hundred consecutive points. Some studies

used up to 1000 consecutive strides [1,16]. Five minutes seems already a very short duration to capture reliably the scaling properties of the signal. On the other hand, research in the potential use of RAC in the rehabilitation of neurological disorders [19] requires experimental procedures that are adapted for patients with poor gait capacities and reduced gait perimeter. Therefore, the choice of smaller samples to analyze variability properties of the gait was made in the perspective to design future experiments with short walking tests (1–2 min) in gait disabled patients: because we observed that both NSI and scaling exponent respond similarly to RAC (see below for further explanation), it is likely that NSI would be useful in this perspective.

As we already mentioned in our previous study [21], the experimental design was not aimed at thorough analysis of speed effects. The design was build in order to ensure that the potential auditory cueing effect was not limited to PWS, but was also acting at slow and high speed. It has been observed that scaling exponents exhibited quadratic dependence (U-shaped form) as a function of speed [28]. Step time variability decrease exponentially or quadratically with speed [29,30,31]. It has also been suggested that slow speed alters gait pattern as compared to PWS (higher walk ratio [3]). Such non linear dependences and threshold effects cannot be satisfactorily analyzed with only 3 different speeds. As a

Treadmill only

Treadmill + RAC

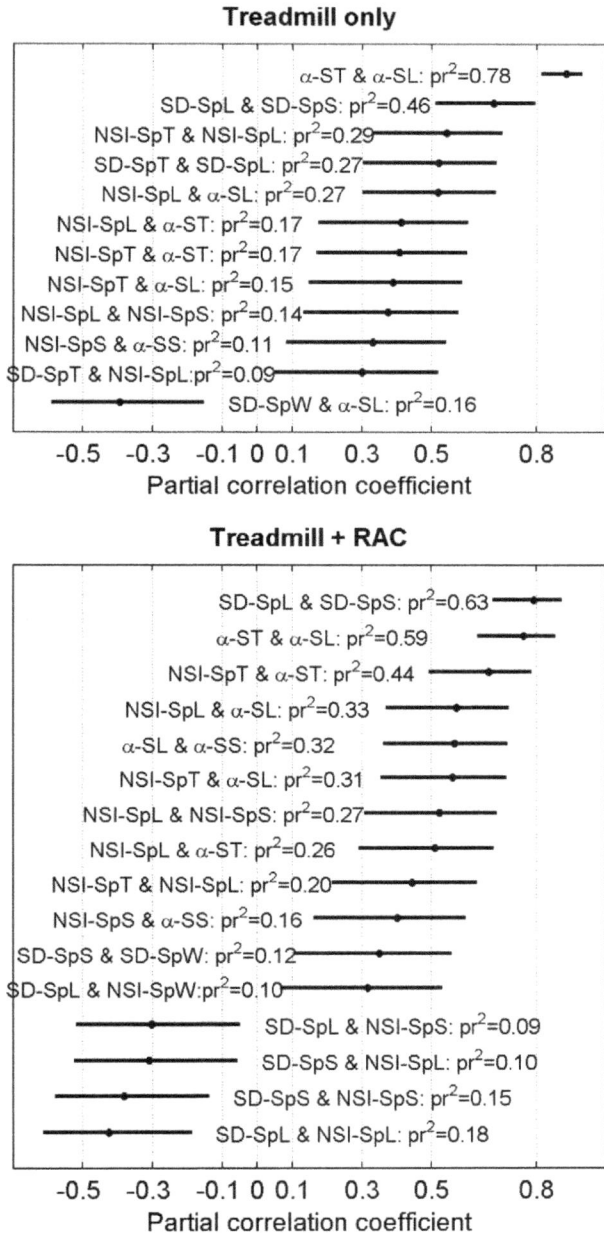

Figure 5. Partial correlations among gait variability indexes, controlled for walking speed. Partial correlation coefficients (pr) were computed among the 55 pairwise combinations of variability indexes (SD, NSI, α, see table 1). Pr's were assessed separately for treadmill only (top, N = 60), and treadmill + Rythmic Auditory Cueing (RAC, bottom, N = 60) conditions. Only pr absolute values greater than 0.3 are shown. Results are classified in decreasing order from top to bottom. Pr's were calculated by systematically taking speed (i.e. M-SpS) as the controlled variable. Horizontal continuous lines indicate 95% Confidence Intervals (CI) of the pr estimations. The definition of the abbreviations is presented in table 1. Pr^2 are numeric values of the Coefficient of Determination, i.e. the percentage of variance explained by the linear regression model.

result, we did not perform specific analysis of speed effects. In short, our results (fig. 3) confirm that low speed induces higher step time variability [3,28,29,30,32]. Moreover, speed seemed to have

no significant effect on step width (fig. 2) and step width variability (fig. 3), what is in line with previous studies [30].

Non Stationarity Index

A process is stationary when its statistical properties are time invariant. Stationarity of gait parameters, and especially stride time, has been extensively studied with various methodologies [13,33,34,35]. It has been reported that the major source of non-stationarities in time series of stride time could be attributed to a change in the mean over time [34]. Consequently, we focused on mean fluctuations by using the NonStationarity Index (NSI). NSI is a simple measure of the consistency of the local average values, independent of the fluctuation magnitude of the original time series. Higher NSI values indicate more inconsistent local averages [13]. We observed (fig. 4) that NSI was highly responsive to RAC, in a similar way as scaling exponents [21]. It is very likely that the switch to a more conscious/voluntary mode of gait control not only produced anti-persistent dynamics [21,23] but also less variable local means. This result is in accordance with the GEM (Goal Equivalent Manifold) model developed by Dingwell and Cusumano [23] based on redundancy theory. Motor redundancy refers to the fact that the motor control has numerous alternatives to perform a given task. It is thought that motor control allows high variability (more freedom) to parameters, which do no affect the desired value of the variable. On the contrary, it restricts the variability of parameters that are essentials for achieving the task [36,37]. Accordingly, in order to maintain the constant speed imposed by the treadmill, a walking individual could choose an infinite combination of stride time and stride length. As a result, statistical persistence and less locally stable means (high NSI) are observed in step time and length fluctuations, because there is a redundancy among these parameters in achieving a given speed. Conversely, statistical anti-persistence and more locally stable means (low NSI) are observe in speed fluctuations. When treadmill and auditory cueing are combined, a degree of freedom is lost: the redundancy between length and time regulation disappears and the three parameters (time, length, speed) exhibit statistical anti-persistence [21] and more locally consistent means (low NSI).

Step width

Regarding step width, modeling approach demonstrated that active lateral stabilization is needed to ensure stable walking, whereas gait is passively stable in the sagittal plane [8]. It has been suggested that lateral stabilization require high-level integration of sensory information, whereas passive stability in antero-posterior direction require far less sensing and control [8,9]. Our results seem to indicate that RAC had no effect on average step width (M-SpW, fig. 2). While participants controlled their steps to be in time with the metronome, they did not significantly modify the lateral placement of the feet as compared to the "treadmill only" situation. Similarly, RAC did not change local mean variability of step width (identical NSI, fig. 4, right); however, higher values than for the other parameters (SpT, SpL, SpS) were observed. The only significant change (ES = −0.53) concerned step width variability under low speed condition (SD-SpW, fig. 3 right), that could be induced by the particularity of slow walking [3,21]. It is likely that active balance control in the frontal plane –which results in optimized lateral foot placement– is independently regulated from the control in the sagittal plane (step length): in order to follow speed (treadmill) and time (metronome) constraints, individuals seem able to perform complex gait regulation in the antero-posterior direction, implying visual, auditory and proprioceptive integrative processes, with no concomitant change in lateral control.

Step-to-step variability

It is very likely that motor control maintains a low magnitude of step-to-step variability in order to ensure minimal energy expenditure and optimal stability [6,7,8]. In overground, free walking, low variability (>3% CV) has been observed in SpT, SpL, SpS, even in long duration walking (30 min) [1]. In this previous study, no difference between free walking and metronome walking was observed regarding variability. Conversely, in our recent study [21], we showed that RAC markedly reduced stride to stride variability of stride time at low speed, with lower effect at higher speeds. We attributed this "low speed" effect to the high variability induced by slow walking [29]: it is likely that slow walking induces a specific spatial and temporal adaptation (higher walk ratio [3]) that was "un-natural" for many subjects, what induced a larger variability. The reference offered by RAC allowed individuals to reduce this variability. The present results did not confirm the RAC effect on gait variability. A general trend to lower variability with RAC was observed, but the large incertitude on ES values produced inconclusive results (fig. 3). The difference between the present analysis and the previous one is that step-to-step variability was analyzed rather stride-to-stride. Moreover, shorter samples (200 steps) were used. Although further studies are needed on this topic, it is evident that the fluctuation magnitude (CV or SD) are by far less responsive to RAC than scaling exponents or NSI. In response to the need of tighter gait control, it is likely that motor control seek to maintain low average fluctuation magnitude while step-to-step fluctuation dynamics is altered (as evidenced by scaling exponents or NSI).

Correlations

In view of the numerous combinations (55) among the analyzed parameters (risks of type I statistical errors), and of the potential non-linear speed effects, caution is required in the interpretation of the partial correlations results (fig. 5). Therefore we limit the discussion to strong associations that seems physiologically grounded and that are coherent with our preliminary assumptions (GEM model).

In the frame of the GEM model [23], phase-randomized surrogate data analysis [21,23] suggests that both stride length and stride time are simultaneously controlled (cross-regulated) stride after stride to ensure stride speed that match treadmill speed. Here, we showed a strong association between scaling exponents of stride time and stride length (α-ST vs. α-SL: pr = 0.88 and pr = 0.77): individuals exhibiting a high α-ST have a high probability to exhibit also a high α-SL value. In other words, deviations are allowed to persist (or to "anti-persist" under dual constraint conditions) in a similar way for both stride time and stride length. Therefore, this confirms that persistence characteristics are likely the result of the simultaneous, coordinated spatial and temporal regulation of the gait at each stride.

Corroborating the hypothesis that associates redundancy, statistical persistence and stationarity (see above), significant positive correlations between NSI and scaling exponents under both conditions were observed (NSI-SpT vs. α-ST: $r^2 = 0.17$, $r^2 = 0.44$. NSI-SpL vs. α-SL: $r^2 = 0.27$, $r^2 = 0.33$): when motor control allows deviations to persist (high α), local means exhibit higher variability (high NSI); accordingly, a more anti-persistent pattern (low α) is associated with more consistent local means (low NSI).

Step width variability (SD-SpW) and stationarity (NSI-SpW) exhibited only one moderate association under treadmill only condition (SD-SpW vs α-SL, pr = −0.40), and two moderate positive under treadmill + RAC conditions (SD-SpS vs. SD-SpW, pr = 0.35; SD-SpL vs. NSI-SpW, pr = 0.32). These inconsistent relationships tend to confirm that a lateral foot placement and antero-posterior gait modulations (i.e. SpL and SpT) are separately regulated.

Conclusion

Externally cued walking is extensively studied because it exhibits positive effects on various gait characteristics of neurologically impaired patients, such as patients with Parkinson's disease [19], hemiparesis [38], or stroke [39]. RAC might be efficient because they would stimulate intact auditory-motor system, which would substitute to impaired gait control [40]. Furthermore, it has been shown that treadmill training also produced improvement in motor performance and ambulation in patients with Parkinson's disease [41]. It has been suggested that the treadmill (i.e. speed cueing) may be acting as an external cue to enhance gait rhythmicity and reduce gait variability [42]. As evidenced by our results, it is likely that the same type of mechanism is acting in healthy individuals: by activating alternative sensory-motor processes as compared to free (overground) walking, treadmill and RAC induced specific changes in step-to-step fluctuations. As far as we know, the simultaneous measurement of SpT, SpL and SpS and their fluctuation dynamics have never been performed in neurologically impaired patients. Future studies comparing the adaptation to external cues in patients with different pathologies would likely help to improve the use of cued walking in gait rehabilitation. The responsiveness of stationarity measure (NSI) to cued walking opens the perspective to perform shorter walking tests (1–2 min.) that would be adapted to patients with a reduced gait perimeter.

Acknowledgments

The author thanks Mr. Philippe Kaesermann for the loan of the instrumented treadmill.

Author Contributions

Conceived and designed the experiments: PT. Performed the experiments: PT. Analyzed the data: PT. Contributed reagents/materials/analysis tools: PT. Wrote the paper: PT.

References

1. Terrier P, Turner V, Schutz Y (2005) GPS analysis of human locomotion: further evidence for long-range correlations in stride-to-stride fluctuations of gait parameters. Human movement science 24: 97–115.
2. Terrier P, Deriaz O (2011) Kinematic variability, fractal dynamics and local dynamic stability of treadmill walking. Journal of Neuroengineering & Rehabilitation 8: 12.
3. Terrier P, Schutz Y (2003) Variability of gait patterns during unconstrained walking assessed by satellite positioning (GPS). Eur J Appl Physiol 90: 554–561.
4. Zarrugh MY, Todd FN, Ralston HJ (1974) Optimization of energy expenditure during level walking. Eur J Appl Physiol Occup Physiol 33: 293–306.
5. Donelan JM, Kram R, Kuo AD (2001) Mechanical and metabolic determinants of the preferred step width in human walking. Proc Biol Sci 268: 1985–1992.
6. O'Connor SM, Xu HZ, Kuo AD (2012) Energetic cost of walking with increased step variability. Gait Posture 36: 102–107.
7. Donelan JM, Shipman DW, Kram R, Kuo AD (2004) Mechanical and metabolic requirements for active lateral stabilization in human walking. J Biomech 37: 827–835.
8. Bauby CE, Kuo AD (2000) Active control of lateral balance in human walking. J Biomech 33: 1433–1440.
9. Dean JC, Alexander NB, Kuo AD (2007) The effect of lateral stabilization on walking in young and old adults. IEEE Trans Biomed Eng 54: 1919–1926.
10. Owings TM, Grabiner MD (2004) Step width variability, but not step length variability or step time variability, discriminates gait of healthy young and older adults during treadmill locomotion. J Biomech 37: 935–938.

11. Brach JS, Berlin JE, VanSwearingen JM, Newman AB, Studenski SA (2005) Too much or too little step width variability is associated with a fall history in older persons who walk at or near normal gait speed. J Neuroeng Rehabil 2: 21.
12. Nordin E, Moe-Nilssen R, Ramnemark A, Lundin-Olsson L (2010) Changes in step-width during dual-task walking predicts falls. Gait Posture 32: 92–97.
13. Hausdorff JM, Lertratanakul A, Cudkowicz ME, Peterson AL, Kaliton D, et al. (2000) Dynamic markers of altered gait rhythm in amyotrophic lateral sclerosis. J Appl Physiol 88: 2045–2053.
14. Malatesta D, Simar D, Dauvilliers Y, Candau R, Borrani F, et al. (2003) Energy cost of walking and gait instability in healthy 65- and 80-yr-olds. J Appl Physiol 95: 2248–2256.
15. Hausdorff JM, Peng CK, Ladin Z, Wei JY, Goldberger AL (1995) Is walking a random walk? Evidence for long-range correlations in stride interval of human gait. Journal of Applied Physiology 78: 349–358.
16. Hausdorff JM, Purdon PL, Peng CK, Ladin Z, Wei JY, et al. (1996) Fractal dynamics of human gait: stability of long-range correlations in stride interval fluctuations. Journal of Applied Physiology 80: 1448–1457.
17. Repp BH (2005) Sensorimotor synchronization: a review of the tapping literature. Psychon Bull Rev 12: 969–992.
18. Zatorre RJ, Chen JL, Penhune VB (2007) When the brain plays music: auditory-motor interactions in music perception and production. Nat Rev Neurosci 8: 547–558.
19. Lim I, van Wegen E, de Goede C, Deutekom M, Nieuwboer A, et al. (2005) Effects of external rhythmical cueing on gait in patients with Parkinson's disease: a systematic review. Clin Rehabil 19: 695–713.
20. Nieuwboer A, Kwakkel G, Rochester L, Jones D, van Wegen E, et al. (2007) Cueing training in the home improves gait-related mobility in Parkinson's disease: the RESCUE trial. J Neurol Neurosurg Psychiatry 78: 134–140.
21. Terrier P, Dériaz O (2012) Persistent and anti-persistent pattern in stride-to-stride variability of treadmill walking: influence of rhythmic auditory cueing. Human Movement Science. In press.
22. Delignieres D, Torre K (2009) Fractal dynamics of human gait: a reassessment of the 1996 data of Hausdorff et al. J Appl Physiol 106: 1272–1279.
23. Dingwell JB, John J, Cusumano JP (2010) Do humans optimally exploit redundancy to control step variability in walking? PLoS Comput Biol 6: e1000856.
24. Nakagawa S, Cuthill IC (2007) Effect size, confidence interval and statistical significance: a practical guide for biologists. Biol Rev Camb Philos Soc 82: 591–605.
25. Cohen J (1992) A power primer. Psychol Bull 112: 155–159.
26. Dingwell JB, Cusumano JP (2010) Re-interpreting detrended fluctuation analyses of stride-to-stride variability in human walking. Gait Posture 32: 348–353.
27. Zijlstra A, Rutgers AW, Hof AL, Van Weerden TW (1995) Voluntary and involuntary adaptation of walking to temporal and spatial constraints. Gait Posture 3: 13–18.
28. Jordan K, Challis JH, Newell KM (2007) Walking speed influences on gait cycle variability. Gait Posture 26: 128–134.
29. Bollens B, Crevecoeur F, Detrembleur C, Guillery E, Lejeune T (2012) Effects of age and walking speed on long-range autocorrelations and fluctuation magnitude of stride duration. Neuroscience 210: 234–242.
30. Agiovlasitis S, McCubbin JA, Yun J, Mpitsos G, Pavol MJ (2009) Effects of Down syndrome on three-dimensional motion during walking at different speeds. Gait Posture 30: 345–350.
31. Beauchet O, Annweiler C, Lecordroch Y, Allali G, Dubost V, et al. (2009) Walking speed-related changes in stride time variability: effects of decreased speed. J Neuroeng Rehabil 6: 32.
32. Kang HG, Dingwell JB (2008) Separating the effects of age and walking speed on gait variability. Gait & Posture 27: 572–577.
33. Sejdic E, Jeffery R, Vanden Kroonenberg A, Chau T (2011) An investigation of stride interval stationarity while listening to music or viewing television. Hum Mov Sci 31: 695–706.
34. Fairley JA, Sejdic E, Chau T (2010) An investigation of stride interval stationarity in a paediatric population. Hum Mov Sci 29: 125–136.
35. Dingwell JB, Cusumano JP (2000) Nonlinear time series analysis of normal and pathological human walking. Chaos 10: 848–863.
36. Latash ML, Scholz JP, Schoner G (2002) Motor control strategies revealed in the structure of motor variability. Exercise & Sport Sciences Reviews 30: 26–31.
37. Todorov E (2004) Optimality principles in sensorimotor control. Nature Neuroscience 7: 907–915.
38. Pelton TA, Johannsen L, Huiya C, Wing AM (2010) Hemiparetic stepping to the beat: asymmetric response to metronome phase shift during treadmill gait. Neurorehabil Neural Repair 24: 428–434.
39. Roerdink M, Lamoth CJ, van Kordelaar J, Elich P, Konijnenbelt M, et al. (2009) Rhythm perturbations in acoustically paced treadmill walking after stroke. Neurorehabil Neural Repair 23: 668–678.
40. McIntosh GC, Brown SH, Rice RR, Thaut MH (1997) Rhythmic auditory-motor facilitation of gait patterns in patients with Parkinson's disease. J Neurol Neurosurg Psychiatry 62: 22–26.
41. Miyai I, Fujimoto Y, Ueda Y, Yamamoto H, Nozaki S, et al. (2000) Treadmill training with body weight support: its effect on Parkinson's disease. Arch Phys Med Rehabil 81: 849–852.
42. Frenkel-Toledo S, Giladi N, Peretz C, Herman T, Gruendlinger L, et al. (2005) Treadmill walking as an external pacemaker to improve gait rhythm and stability in Parkinson's disease. Mov Disord 20: 1109–1114.

21

Persistent Fluctuations in Stride Intervals under Fractal Auditory Stimulation

Vivien Marmelat[1,2], Kjerstin Torre[1], Peter J. Beek[2,3], Andreas Daffertshofer[2]*

1 Movement to Health Laboratory, Montpellier-1 University, EuroMov, Montpellier, France, **2** MOVE Research Institute Amsterdam, Faculty of Human Movement Sciences, VU University Amsterdam, Amsterdam, Netherlands, **3** School for Sport and Education, Brunel University, Uxbridge, Middlesex, United Kingdom

Abstract

Stride sequences of healthy gait are characterized by persistent long-range correlations, which become anti-persistent in the presence of an isochronous metronome. The latter phenomenon is of particular interest because auditory cueing is generally considered to reduce stride variability and may hence be beneficial for stabilizing gait. Complex systems tend to match their correlation structure when synchronizing. In gait training, can one capitalize on this tendency by using a fractal metronome rather than an isochronous one? We examined whether auditory cues with fractal variations in inter-beat intervals yield similar fractal inter-stride interval variability as isochronous auditory cueing in two complementary experiments. In Experiment 1, participants walked on a treadmill while being paced by either an isochronous or a fractal metronome with different variation strengths between beats in order to test whether participants managed to synchronize with a fractal metronome and to determine the necessary amount of variability for participants to switch from anti-persistent to persistent inter-stride intervals. Participants did synchronize with the metronome despite its fractal randomness. The corresponding coefficient of variation of inter-beat intervals was fixed in Experiment 2, in which participants walked on a treadmill while being paced by non-isochronous metronomes with different scaling exponents. As expected, inter-stride intervals showed persistent correlations similar to self-paced walking only when cueing contained persistent correlations. Our results open up a new window to optimize rhythmic auditory cueing for gait stabilization by integrating fractal fluctuations in the inter-beat intervals.

Editor: Alfonso Fasano, University of Toronto, Italy

Funding: This work was supported by SKILLS, an Integrated Project (FP6-IST Contract #035005) of the Commission of the European Community. Andreas Daffertshofer received financial support from the Netherlands Organisation for Scientific Research (NWO grant #400-08-127). The funders had no role in study design, data collection and analysis, decision to publish, or preparation of the manuscript.

Competing Interests: The authors have declared that no competing interests exist.

* E-mail: a.daffertshofer@vu.nl

Introduction

The assessment of mean and standard deviation alone often does not suffice to discriminate between optimal and constrained behavior or between healthy and pathological performances [1–3]. The temporal structure of fluctuations, here synonym for the serial-lag correlation of consecutive events, may contain valuable information about the functional organization of the system generating these events [4–6]. The presence of long-range correlations or *1/f noise*, be it in cortical activity, EMG activity, or macroscopic gait dynamics, is considered a generic marker for systems that can adequately adapt to perturbations in their environment [5,7–9]. Many clinical studies revealed dependencies of the correlation structure of gait to different pathologies like amyotrophic lateral sclerosis [1], Huntington's disease [1–2], and Parkinson's disease [1,9].

External cueing may alter the temporal correlation structure of gait. Isochronous auditory cues are particularly known for changing the typical fractal dynamics of healthy gait [10–11]. Persistent (positive) long-range correlations in stride intervals of self-paced gait may switch to anti-persistent (negative) correlations if an isochronous metronome is present [12]. This qualitative change of gait dynamics may be indicative of 'local' (i.e. short-term) coupling processes, allowing for cycle-by-cycle entrainment

of the movements with the metronome. Isochronous pacing thus constrains the locomotor system to (a narrow band around) the isolated metronome frequency, which is contrary to self-paced walking where the locomotion covers a broad range of frequencies with a power-law distribution [9,12–13]. In spite of this constraining feature, the beneficial capacity of isochronous auditory cueing for gait rehabilitation in the presence of neurodegenerative diseases has been demonstrated in several studies. For instance, stride length, cadence, and speed all increase [14], whereas inter-stride variability and occurrence of freezing decrease (see, e.g., [2], and for a systematic review [15]). Could this beneficial capacity be amplified if cueing contains variability similar to that of healthy gait? And does the presence of fractality in the cueing streams prepare walkers to cope with potential future irregularities in the natural environment?

Introducing variability and fractality in cueing streams is not new. Kaipust and co-workers [16] submitted that isochronous cueing might not be optimal for gait rehabilitation. They showed that participants were sensitive to the correlation structure of cueing fluctuations. However, their participants were not instructed to synchronize their gait to the metronome. It might be that subjects just ignored the metronome and fell back to their own, fractal gait structure, which would question the effect of fractal cueing. Hove and co-workers [17] showed that the correlation structure of stride times in patients suffering Parkinson's disease changed towards that of healthy gait when using an interactive rhythmic auditory stimulation, i.e. when stimulus timing changed in response to the participant's instant tempo. However, why this adjustment occurred remains unclear. Was it because the patients synchronized to the stimulus or vice versa?

We investigated the effect of fractal cueing when subjects were explicitly asked to synchronize with the metronome. We hypothesized that, unlike isochronous pacing, persistent long-range correlated auditory cueing preserves the fractal dynamics of stride intervals in healthy subjects. To test this hypothesis, we conducted two complementary experiments in which we measured inter-stride intervals (ISIs). In Experiment 1 participants walked when paced by either isochronous or fractal cues with different inter-beat interval (IBIs) coefficients of variation to determine the 'optimal' amount of variation in the cueing. In Experiment 2 participants walked when paced by either isochronous or non-isochronous cues with different scaling exponents characterizing the IBIs's correlation structure. We expected that subjects would synchronize with any metronome but we expected stride intervals to present persistent, long-range correlations only when cues resemble the fractal fluctuations present in voluntary, self-paced walking.

Assessing the Correlation Structure

Central to our data analysis are estimates of the scaling behavior of serial-lag correlations that we briefly summarize before outlining our experimental approach. We employed the detrended fluctuations analysis (DFA) [18], which was deemed suitable here in view of its applicability to relatively short time series [19]. DFA assesses the relationship between the magnitude of fluctuations of the variable and the duration over which these fluctuations are observed. If the correlation structure is scale free (fractal), then this relationship should obey the form

$$F(n) \propto n^{\alpha} \qquad (1)$$

where F denotes the fluctuation strength and n is a time interval that provides a measure of the aforementioned duration. The scaling exponent α is of essential interest: a fully random series (white noise) corresponds to $\alpha = 0.5$; time series containing anti-persistent correlations have $\alpha < 0.5$, and persistent correlations imply $\alpha > 0.5$. The exponent α should be bounded to the interval [0,1] because otherwise the time series under study is non-stationary rendering subsequent, conventional statistics invalid. We also note that α is closely related to the Hurst exponent that is often used to characterize fractal stochastic processes – α equals the Hurst exponent if the to-be-analyzed time series has been generated by stationary series, i.e. fractal Gaussian noise.

Detrended Fluctuation Analysis

To obtain the scaling exponent α one first integrates the mean-centered time series under study, which reads for the discrete time series Y:

$$Y(k) = \sum_{i=1}^{k} [y(i) - \bar{y}] \qquad (2)$$

where N corresponds to the number of samples in the series. Then, the integrated time series is divided into non-overlapping intervals of n data points (here $10 < n < N/2$). Within every interval the time series $[Y(k),...,Y(k+n)]$ is fitted by a line $Y_{trend}(k,n)$, which can be interpreted as a linear, local trend. That trend is subsequently

removed yielding per interval of length n, the mean characteristic magnitude of fluctuation $F(n)$ as

$$F(n) = \sqrt{\frac{1}{N} \sum_{k=1}^{N} (Y(k) - Y_{trend}(k,n))^2} \qquad (3)$$

As $\log(n^{\alpha}) = \alpha \cdot \log(n)$, the scaling exponent α can be estimated by a slope of the diffusion plot, i.e. the log-log plot of F as a function of n (Figure 1, left panel) – we note that when determining α on that logarithmic scale, n should be sampled exponentially in order to avoid a bias in the fit towards larger n-values (Figure 1, right panel).

Short-term and Long-term Correlations

We expected what may be referred to as 'complexity matching': when two complex systems interact, they are likely to entrain [20–22]. That is, we expected a strong correlation between fractal exponents of ISIs and IBIs. Because complexity matching is more likely to be manifest on long-term scales [23], we also examined the short- and long-term regions of the diffusion plots, in addition to the overall scaling exponent α (Figure 1, right panel). While the precise separation of short- and long-term regions might be somewhat arbitrary, one may state as a rule of thumb that short-term fluctuations account for local (brief) adaptations, whereas long-term fluctuations reveal more global (durable) changes, possibly in coordination. To guarantee proper sample sizes for reliable exponent estimates, we defined $\alpha_{short-term}$ as the slope of the first half of the diffusion plot and $\alpha_{long-term}$ as the slope of the second half. More precisely, $\alpha_{short-term}$ and $\alpha_{long-term}$ included $F(n)$-values over the intervals $n = 10 \ldots 31$ and $n = 50 \ldots 128$, respectively, for time series with 256 data-points. Note that $\alpha_{short-term}$ does not refer to short-term gait events, e.g., one or two strides, but to the length of the time series under study.

Experiment 1 – Determining the Optimal Coefficient of Variation

We used an isochronous and a set of fractal auditory pacing signals that differed in fluctuation strength (the coefficients of variation of the inter-beat interval were 0.5%, 1%, 1.5%, and 2%, respectively) to determine the conditions in which subjects gait was influenced by the presence of fractal cues, here synonym of cues with persistent, long-range correlations.

Methods

Participants. After giving written informed consent, twelve healthy volunteers (seven female, age = 28±6 years) participated in the experiment.

Ethics. The ethics committee of the Faculty of Human Movement Sciences, VU University Amsterdam, approved the experiment prior to its conductance.

Apparatus and equipment. Participants walked on a treadmill in which a single large force platform was embedded (ForceLink, Culemborg, The Netherlands), allowing for online detection of foot contact [24]. Computer-generated rhythmic auditory stimuli (pitch 600 Hz) were administered through earphones (right ear), to pace the right heel strikes. IBIs were generated containing fractal Gaussian noise with corresponding scaling exponent (Hurst exponent H). Short audio samples of metronomes are available in Audio S1, and the Table S2 provides mean and standard deviations of IBIs series.

Tasks and procedure. We first determined the individual preferred walking speeds. The treadmill speed was increased every

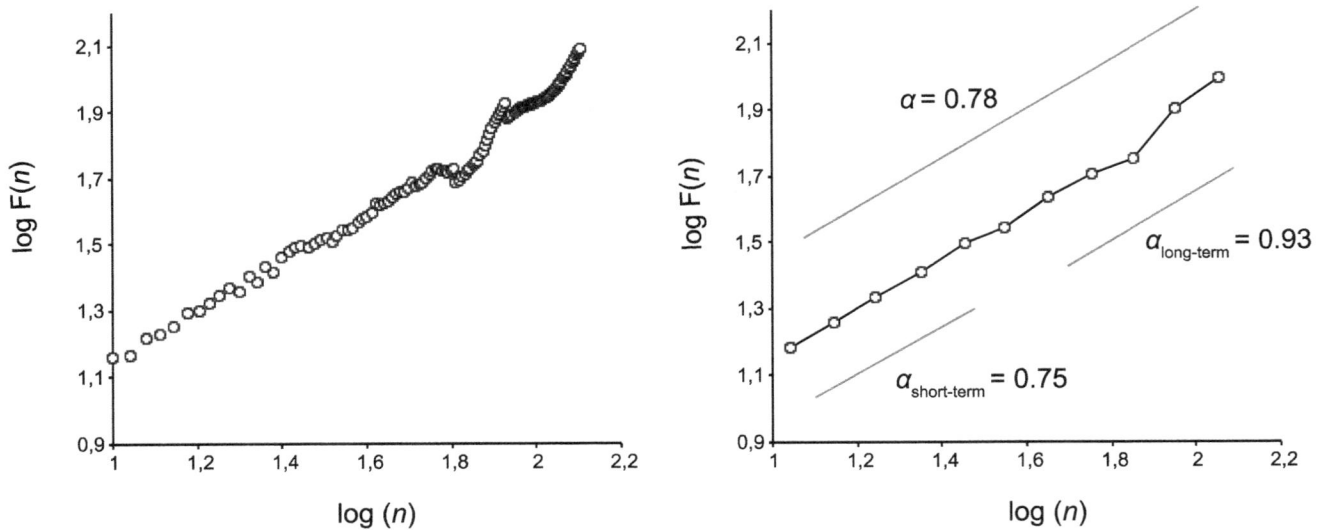

Figure 1. *Left panel:* **Representative example of the average diffusion plots in bilogarithmic coordinates, obtained by performing DFA on inter-stride interval series (condition *CV* 1%).** The average plots are computed by point-by-point averaging over the twelve participants performing under the same experimental condition. *Right panel:* Corresponding plot obtained with the 11-point averaging method. Solid line corresponds to the slope for the 11 points (α), the dashed lines correspond to the slope of the short-term ($\alpha_{\text{short-term}}$) and long-term ($\alpha_{\text{long-term}}$) regions of the diffusion plot.

10 s in steps of 0.1 km/h. When participants indicated that they reached their most comfortable speed (defined as "a speed at which you may continue walking for an hour"), the treadmill's speed was further increased until participants indicated that the speed was too high. Then the speed was decreased until participants again indicated they reached their most comfortable speed again. The individual preferred walking speed was defined as the mean between the two speeds indicated by the participant, and used for all subsequent experimental conditions.

The experiment involved six walking conditions: self-paced walking (SP): participants walked at their previously determined preferred speed, without auditory stimuli (but wearing the earphones in order to create standardized conditions); isochronous metronome pacing with equidistant IBIs; and four fractal metronome pacing conditions with the scaling exponent of IBI series set at $H = 0.9$ (corresponding to very persistent fluctuations), and the coefficients of variation chosen as of $CV\,0.5\%$, $CV\,1\%$, CV 1.5%, and $CV\,2\%$. That range was chosen because the coefficient of variation of natural gait has been found to be lower than 3% [13,25–26]. Each participant received individual metronome sequences. All sequences were generated using a fractional Gaussian noise generator with $H = 0.9$, meaning that the α-value of that sequence converges towards 0.9 for large samples sizes. The short sequences that we employed in the experiment had thus α-values distributed around the mean $H = 0.9$. Not using a single metronome sequence allowed for correlating IBIs and ISIs fractal exponents. For all pacing conditions the mean IBI delivered by the metronome was equal to the mean ISIs of each participant in the SP condition. Metronomes and recordings started at the same time, a few seconds after the treadmill was switched on and participants were walking. Each condition lasted six minutes yielding a sufficiently large number of strides (at least 256) to apply DFA after removing the first ten stride intervals to avoid transients [19].

Participants were explicitly instructed to synchronize the right heel strikes with the beats of the metronome and to maintain this synchronization as accurately as possible while keeping a natural and relaxed gait in case the metronome would present some variations. SP was the first condition for all participants; the order of the five pacing conditions was randomized. The same sampling frequency (300 Hz) was fixed for the generation of IBIs and force platform recording.

Data processing.   Three main variables were analyzed: IBIs; ISIs, defined as the time intervals between two successive right heel strikes; and asynchronies to the metronome (ASYNs). These asynchronies were defined as the time intervals between right heel strikes and corresponding metronome beat onsets, so that negative asynchronies indicate anticipated heel strikes. The final 256 points of IBIs and ISIs were submitted to the subsequent DFA (time series available in Data S1). That is, next to the means and standard deviations of the collected time series our primary outcome measures were the α, $\alpha_{\text{short-term}}$, and $\alpha_{\text{long-term}}$ exponents, as explained above.

Statistics.   To examine the ISIs correlation structure as a function of metronome conditions, we applied a 1×6 repeated measures ANOVA to α exponents. Tukey's HSD was used for post-hoc analysis, and results were considered statistically different for $p < 0.05$. To further assess the nature of adaptive processes occurring in fractal-pacing conditions, we tested for an individual matching of ISIs correlations to IBIs correlations using a linear correlation analysis between $\alpha_{\text{short-term}}$, and $\alpha_{\text{long-term}}$ exponents of IBIs and ISIs.

Results

ANOVA revealed no significant differences in mean ISIs ($F(5, 66) = 1.99$, $p = 0.09$), implying that the walking speed was largely constant across conditions. Also mean ASYNs did not differ significantly over conditions ($F(4, 55) = 0.88$, $p = 0.48$). Mean values ranged from about -50 ms to about -40 ms (Table S1), that is, participants slightly anticipated the metronome as has often been observed in sensorimotor synchronization [27]. This suggests that in all conditions participants were able to adapt to the cueing.

Mean α exponents obtained in IBIs and ISIs series are summarized in Table 1. For the ISIs series the ANOVA revealed a significant effect of pacing conditions on the global α-exponents ($F(5, 66) = 36.34$; $p<0.001$, Figure 2, left panel). Tukey's HSD analysis indicated that α differed between SP and ISO conditions ($p<0.001$) with persistent long-range correlations for SP but anti-persistent correlations for ISO (mean $\alpha = 0.75\pm0.12$ and $\alpha = 0.23\pm0.13$, respectively). ISO was also significantly different from all of the fractal-pacing conditions (CV 0.5% to CV 2% all $p<0.001$). The mean α exponent in the CV 0.5% condition (mean $\alpha = 0.59\pm0.17$) was close to white noise, and significantly smaller than those of all other fractal-pacing conditions (CV 1%, $p = 0.004$; CV 1.5%, $p<0.001$; and CV 2%, $p<0.001$).

In-depth analysis revealed however, that the mean α exponent obtained for CV 0.5% did not correspond to any of the individual series' exponents. In fact the group showed a bimodal distribution: Eight participants switched from anti-persistent to persistent long-range correlations at CV 0.5%, whereas the remaining four participants switched at CV 1%. To address this bimodality we performed an additional 2(sub-groups)×6(pacing) ANOVA with repeated measures and found a significant effect of interaction between sub-groups and pacing conditions ($F(5, 55) = 2.56$; $p = 0.038$, see Figure 2, right panel). Tukey's HSD analysis showed that in CV 0.5% the first sub-group produced long-range correlations in CV 0.5% (mean $\alpha = 0.69\pm0.11$), which were qualitatively different from ISO ($p<0.001$) but not from other pacing conditions. The second sub-group produced anti-persistent ISIs (mean $\alpha = 0.40\pm0.02$) that were qualitatively similar to correlations obtained in ISO pacing ($p = 0.426$). Post-hoc analysis confirmed that the two sub-groups differed only in CV 0.5% condition ($p = 0.031$).

The results of the linear correlation analysis on $\alpha_{short-term}$ and $\alpha_{long-term}$ exponents of IBIs and ISIs series are depicted in Figure 3. We found no significant correlation between $\alpha_{short-term}$ exponents for all fractal-pacing conditions (Figure 3, upper panel), while α_{long-}

α_{term} exponents were positively correlated for all fractal-pacing conditions (r_{10} ranging from 0.76 to 0.98, Figure 3, lower panel). This suggests that the observed complexity matching cannot be the consequence of the aggregation of short-term corrections.

Experiment 2–Varying the Metronome Correlation

Our next step in investigating our participants' ability to synchronize to fractal versus isochronous cueing was to compare different IBIs correlation structures for a fixed coefficient of variation. We expected that the fractal structure of ISIs would only be preserved for fractal-pacing conditions that agree with the correlation structure of self-paced walking. We therefore used metronomes with different IBI structures: anti-persistent, uncorrelated, and persistent.

Methods

Participants. Twelve volunteers (five female, age 28 ± 6 years) participated in the experiment after providing informed written consent. As in Experiment 1, all participants were healthy and none had any neuromuscular disorder or recent injury at the time of study. One participant of Experiment 2 also took part in Experiment 1.

Ethics. The ethics committee of the Faculty of Human Movement Sciences, VU University Amsterdam, The Netherlands, approved the experiment prior to its conductance.

Apparatus and equipment. The equipment was the same as in Experiment 1.

Tasks and procedure. The protocol was identical to Experiment 1 except for the use of different fractal cueing sequences. The conditions were: SP (see Experiment 1); ISO (see Experiment 1); and four non-isochronous cueing sequences with distinct scaling exponents, H 0.2, H 0.5, H 0.6, and H 0.9. In the latter four conditions, the IBIs coefficient of variation was fixed to 1%. Isochronous and non-isochronous conditions were sought to present the least differences. We thus chose the lowest CV in which

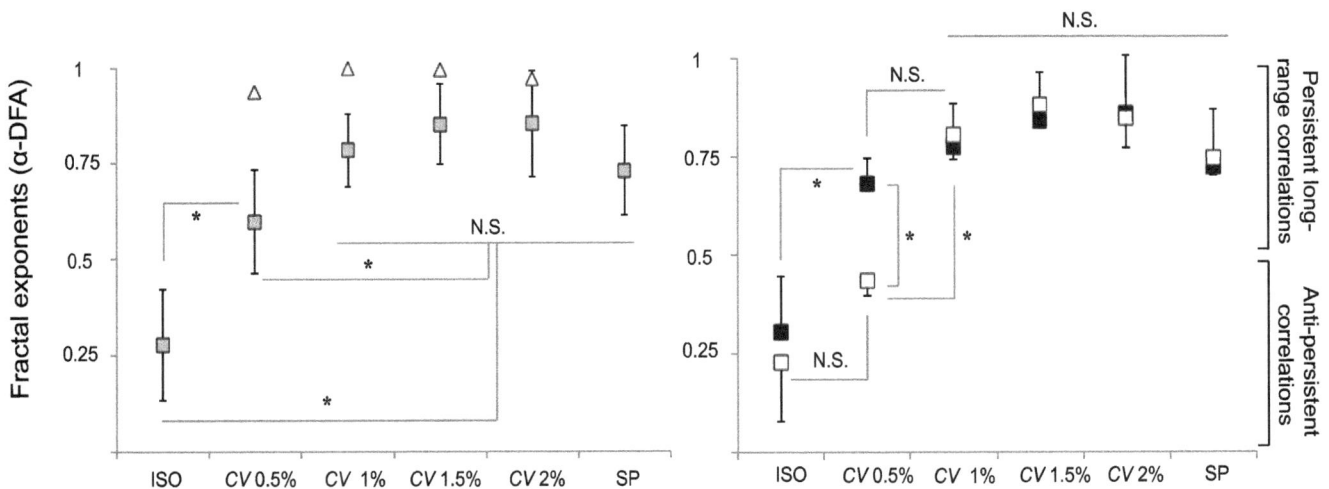

Figure 2. Mean α exponent (DFA) of inter-beat intervals (white triangles) and inter-stride intervals (squares) in Experiment 1. (*: $p<$ 0.05; N.S.: non-significant differences; error bars: standard deviation). *Left panel*: The evolution of α for all participants taken together ($n = 12$) could be interpreted as a progressive increase with increasing CV. *Right panel*: Qualitatively different changes in α exhibited by two subgroups: group 1 (black squares, $n = 8$) shows an abrupt switch from anti-persistent to persistent long-range correlations at $CV = 0.5$%, while group 2 (white squares, $n = 4$) switches at $CV = 1$%.

Table 1. Mean fractal exponents (α_{DFA}) and standard deviation (italics) of inter-beat intervals and inter-stride intervals estimated from all conditions in Experiment 1.

Experiment 1	ISO	CV 0.5%	CV 1%	CV 1.5%	CV 2%	SP
Inter-beat intervals (IBI)	–	0.94	1.00	0.99	0.97	–
	–	*0.11*	*0.10*	*0.11*	*0.10*	–
Inter-stride intervals (ISI)	0.28[a]	0.60[a]	0.78	0.85	0.85	0.73
	0.14	*0.13*	*0.10*	*0.10*	*0.14*	*0.12*

[a]$p < 0.05$ when compared to SP condition.

we observed persistent fluctuations in ISIs for all participants in Experiment 1.

Data processing. Signal processing and estimates of IBIs, ISIs, and ASYNs agreed entirely with Experiment 1.

Statistics. We applied a 1×6 repeated measures ANOVA to all outcome measures. As in Experiment 1, Tukey's HSD was used for post-hoc analysis. Results were considered statistically different for $p < 0.05$. We also used a linear correlation analysis between α, $\alpha_{short-term}$, and $\alpha_{long-term}$ exponents of IBIs and ISIs.

Results

Mean α exponents obtained in IBIs and ISIs series are given in Table 2. For ISIs series, ANOVA revealed a significant effect of pacing conditions on α exponents ($F(5, 66) = 33.33$; $p < 0.001$). Tukey's HSD analysis showed that α differed between SP and ISO conditions ($p < 0.001$) with persistent long-range correlations for SP (mean $\alpha = 0.79 \pm 0.09$) and anti-persistent correlations for ISO (mean $\alpha = 0.25 \pm 0.15$). SP differed from the three non-fractal non-isochronous conditions (H 0.2, H 0.5, and H 0.6 all $p < 0.001$). The α exponents in the H 0.9 condition differed from all other pacing conditions (ISO, $p < 0.001$; H 0.2, $p < 0.001$; H 0.5, $p = 0.004$; H 0.6, $p = 0.004$), but not from the SP condition (H 0.9, $p = 0.099$).

The results of linear correlation analysis on $\alpha_{short-term}$ and $\alpha_{long-term}$ exponents of IBIs and ISIs series in the four non-isochronous conditions are shown in Figure 4. The correlation between $\alpha_{short-term}$ exponents (Figure 4, upper panel) was significant only for H 0.5 ($r_{10} = 0.61$). The correlation between $\alpha_{long-term}$ exponents (Figure 4, lower panel) was significant only for H 0.6 ($r_{10} = 0.66$) and H 0.9 ($r_{10} = 0.90$). This result suggests a sensitivity of ISIs for the long-range structure of fluctuations of IBIs only when persistent fluctuations were present.

Experiments 1 & 2– Revisited

In order to assess possible contributions of short-term behavioral correction to the matching of IBIs and ISIs long-term correlation properties, we further determined the cross-correlation between IBIs and ISIs series. Since the conventional cross-correlation is highly sensitive to the presence of persistent trends in the time series, which would lead to a systematic overestimation of the local co-variations between IBIs and ISIs [20], we used a windowed cross-correlation analysis (WCC): the cross-correlation between the first windows of 15 samples of IBIs and ISIs series was determined after locally detrending each series. These windows were shifted sample-by-sample yielding a series of N–15 cross-correlation coefficients at lag 0 (with N = length of the time series).

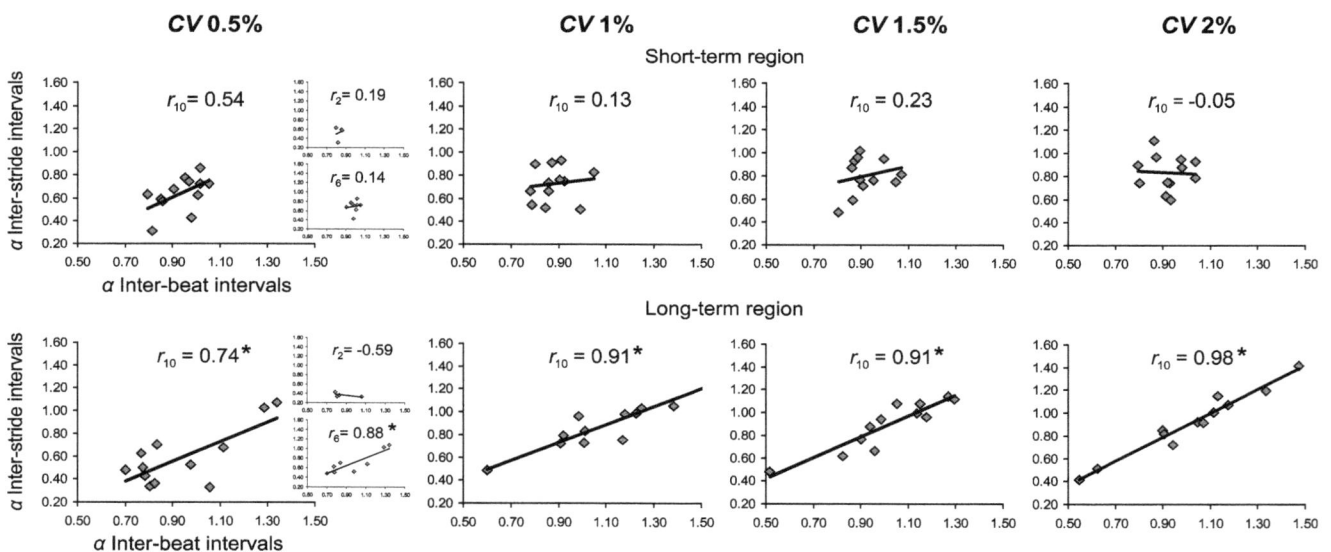

Figure 3. Correlation between α exponents (DFA) of inter-beat intervals and inter-stride intervals obtained in the four conditions with fractal metronome in Experiment 1. *Upper panel:* short-term region of diffusion plots. *Lower panel:* long-term region of diffusion plots. Significance threshold (*) for correlation coefficients is set at $p < 0.05$ ($r_{10} = 0.58$). For the $CV = 0.5\%$ condition, subpanels separately show the correlations for the two subgroups of participants ($n = 4$, upper subpanel, and $n = 8$, lower subpanel).

Table 2. Mean fractal exponents (α_{DFA}) and standard deviation (italics) of inter-beat intervals and inter-stride intervals estimated from all conditions in Experiment 2.

Experiment 2	ISO	H 0.2	H 0.5	H 0.6	H 0.9	SP
Inter-beat intervals (IBI)	–	0.23	0.52	0.57	0.91	–
	–	*0.04*	*0.03*	*0.08*	*0.15*	–
Inter-stride intervals (ISI)	0.25[a]	0.26[a]	0.44[a]	0.44[a]	0.64	0.79
	0.15	*0.11*	*0.13*	*0.09*	*0.17*	*0.09*

[a]$p < 0.05$ when compared to SP condition.

The same procedure was repeated by considering different lags between IBIs and ISIs series, from lag -10 to lag 10 samples. We note that a significant cross-correlation coefficient at lag 0 would evidence that current ISI and IBI have similar lengths. The threshold of significance for 15-point windowed cross-correlation was given as $r_{13} = 0.51$ ($p < 0.05$).

WCC revealed no significant correlation between IBIs and ISIs series in Experiment 1 (Figure 5). Overall, correlations increased with increasing variability (CV) in fractal IBIs with a maximum at lag two. In Experiment 2, WCC also showed no significant correlation between IBIs and ISIs series, and the maximum correlation was again found at lag two.

Discussion

The findings of both experiments support our central hypothesis that when paced by a fractal metronome the correlation structure of stride intervals presents persistent fluctuations, contrary to isochronous cueing when the correlation structure of stride intervals presents anti-persistent fluctuations. We found a negative mean asynchrony in all cueing conditions, suggesting that participants were able to synchronize to the metronome irrespective of its correlation structure: even anti-persistent cueing could be followed. $\alpha_{\text{long-term}}$ exponents of ISIs and IBIs agreed only

when IBIs presented fractal fluctuations implying that the persistent fluctuations in stride intervals were mainly influenced by the long-term correlations in the cueing.

In line with earlier reports [11–13] stride intervals exhibited persistent long-range correlations during self-paced walking and were anti-persistent during isochronous paced walking. The presence of long-range correlations is often considered a hallmark of healthy and adaptive complex systems [5,28]. When the system is altered (by pathology or external constraints imposed on the subjects), deviations from this optimal behavioral dynamics may occur [8,29]. In this respect, anti-persistence in stride intervals during isochronous pacing reveals a more rigid behavior: the gait dynamics is reduced to the regular tempo (single scale) of the metronome. For rehabilitation this may imply that patients only 'learn' to walk to the isolated cueing beat without the capacity to flexibly adapt to potential perturbations [16].

Stride intervals also presented anti-persistence when the IBIs presented anti-persistent or random fluctuations. Unlike isochronous, anti-persistent or random pacing, the use of a fractal metronome enables the locomotor system to maintain the fractal dynamics of gait, similar to self-paced gait dynamics (see Figure 2). The results of Experiment 2 suggest that this is due to the persistent, long-range correlations of inter-beat variations and not to the fact that the presented metronomes were merely variable

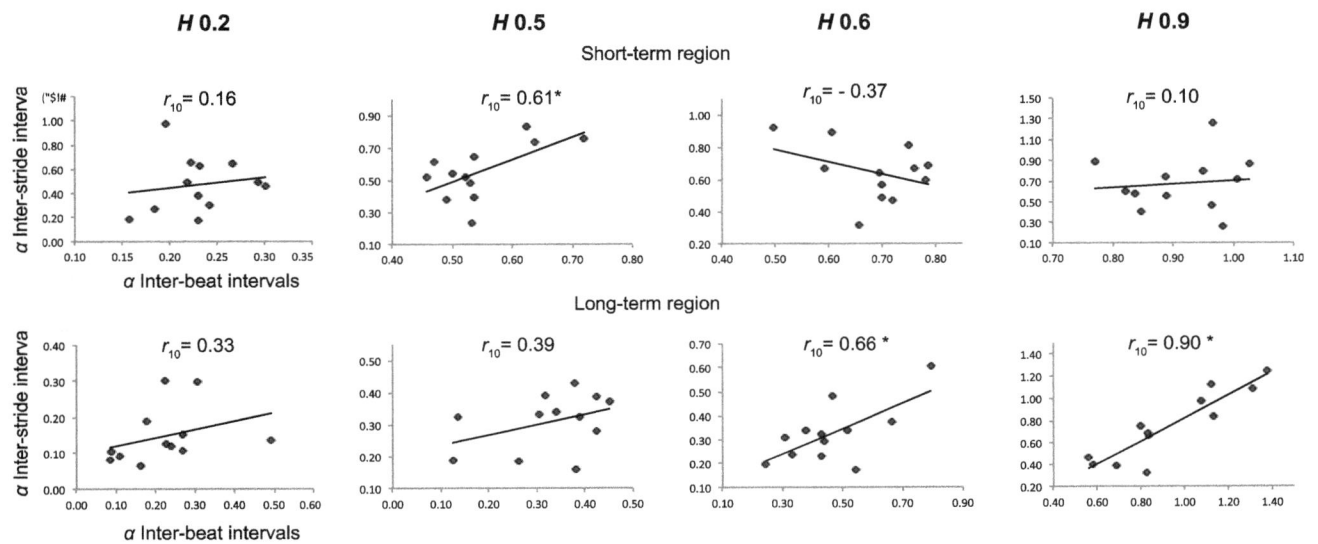

Figure 4. Correlation between α exponents (DFA) of inter-beat intervals and inter-stride intervals obtained in the four conditions with non-isochronous metronome in Experiment 2. *Upper panel*: short-term region of diffusion plots. *Lower panel*: long-term region of diffusion plots. Significance threshold (*) for correlation coefficients is set at $p < 0.05$ ($r_{10} = 0.58$).

Windowed (15 points) cross-correlation

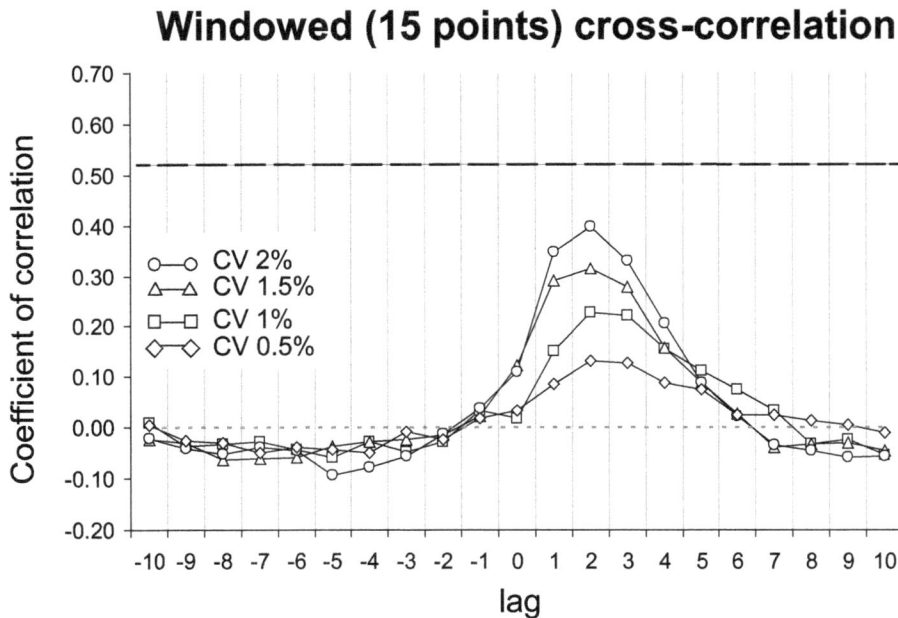

Figure 5. Mean coefficients of windowed (15-point window) cross-correlation functions (from lag −10 to lag 10) between inter-beat intervals series and inter-stride intervals series, for the four fractal-metronome pacing conditions in Experiment 1. The black dashed line shows the significance threshold ($r_{13} = 0.5139$, $p < .05$).

(Figure 4). This agrees with recent findings that ISIs in elderly that listened to a chaotic metronome contained persistent correlations similar to those with no metronome [16]. According to Experiment 1, the fractal exponents of stride intervals between isochronous pacing and increasingly variable, fractal-pacing conditions were either anti-persistent or persistent, revealing that stride dynamics differed completely between isochronous and fractal pacing. Inter-individual differences in the CV 0.5% condition might be explained by differences in the perception of inter-beat variations of the metronome [29,30].

The results in the fractal-pacing conditions (i.e., all conditions in Experiment 1, and H 0.9 in Experiment 2) revealed that, in general, the average fractal exponents of stride intervals tended toward the exponents of the inter-beat intervals presented. In both experiments this largely agreed with the exponents observed in self-paced stride intervals (Figures 2 & 4). In H 0.9 condition the mean fractal exponent decreased compared to self-paced condition. This might be due to individuals that produced anti-persistent fluctuations: a candidate, albeit speculative, explanation is that $CV = 1\%$ did not suffice for these participants (as $CV = 0.5\%$ was not enough for some others in Experiment 1). Hence, at first glance, participants could just have walked at their preferred speed without any effective synchronization to the auditory stimuli rendering this finding not necessarily indicative of adaptive behavior (like in [16]). In fact, synchronization with a fractal metronome (i.e. a largely unpredictable signal) appears quite counterintuitive. However, mean asynchronies obtained in the four fractal-pacing conditions in Experiment 1 and the four non-isochronous pacing conditions in Experiment 2 were similar to asynchronies obtained for isochronous pacing ($\approx$ −40 ms, which is in line with earlier reports, e.g., [11,27]), thus indicating effective synchronization with slight anticipation. Importantly, the CV of IBIs were below the mean asynchronies: the mean deviations were about 6, 12, 18 and 23 ms for CV 0.5, CV 1, CV 1.5 and CV 2, respectively. Consequently the negative mean asynchrony may

have occurred by chance because participants simply adjusted the mean stride intervals to the mean beat intervals. If it was the case, however, we should not have observed any difference in the structure of stride intervals between isochronous and fractal pacing. Our results clearly demonstrate that the presence of fractal fluctuations in the metronome influenced the statistical signature of stride intervals.

Recent findings [31] underscored that the locomotor system cannot be 'healthy' by producing persistent fluctuations when self-paced and – by the same token – 'unhealthy' by producing anti-persistent fluctuations with isochronous cueing. Dingwell and co-workers [31] suggested that the diminution of the fractal structure in cueing conditions in elderly and in pathology might reflect an increase in stride-to-stride gait control ('cautious gait'). Our results do not support this idea. We argue that participants controlled their strides at least as much (and maybe even more) with isochronous conditions as in non-isochronous conditions. In particular in Experiment 1, the metronomes with coefficient of variations of 2% were more variable so that we expected participants to be more careful to not miss any beats (as they were instructed to do so). Participants succeeded and asynchronies were about −50 ms, similar to those in isochronous conditions. However, ISIs were persistent ($\alpha = 0.85$, see Table 1) and similar to the self-paced conditions. That is, our results are not in favor of the hypothesis that fractal exponents decrease with increased control. We are aware that the results presented here are not sufficient to discard this interesting hypothesis and further studies should examine it in more detail. Simulations of stride intervals in non-isochronous conditions may indeed help to unravel the control mechanisms that are at work here. These numerical assessments are beyond the scope of the present paper but will be reported elsewhere.

Our results further provide evidence for a ubiquitous, strong correlation between the individual ISIs exponents and those of the corresponding IBIs series over the long-term region of the DFA plot (Figures 3 & 4). We consider this matching of fractal exponents a hallmark of strong anticipation. Strong anticipation is described as a global synchronization on a broad range of time scales instead of local step-to-step corrections to achieve synchronization [20–22]. We verified that the matching of the temporal correlation structures occurred mainly on the long-term part of the DFA plot: for the four fractal-pacing conditions of Experiment 1, our results showed very high correlations between DFA exponents of individual ISIs and IBIs series computed over the long-term region, but no significant correlation between exponents computed over the short-term region. Importantly, this correlation between DFA exponents on the long-term region occurred in Experiment 2 only when the IBIs series contained fractal long-range correlations (H 0.6 and H 0.9), but not in the case of anti-persistent correlations (H 0.2) or random fluctuations (H 0.5).

To our knowledge, the distinction between short-term and long-term regions of the diffusion plot represents an original methodological approach, which allows one to identify the relative contributions of local short-term and global long-term fluctuations to sensorimotor synchronization. To complement this analysis, we used windowed cross-correlation analysis, which specifically assesses the local co-variations of inter-stride and -beat intervals. This analysis showed no significant cross-correlation at any lag (from lag −10 to +10), nor in any of the four fractal-pacing conditions in Experiments 1 and 2. Synchronization with a variable stimulus has been described as "a mix of reaction, proaction, and synchrony" ([22], p. 5274). Recall that the maximum (lag two) coefficient increased as the variance in the inter-beat intervals increased, suggesting that too much variability might involve more and more reactive processes. Taken together, we may suggest that persistence of the long-range correlated gait dynamics in fractal-pacing conditions mainly results from the matching of the long-range correlation structure of stride intervals performed onto the IBIs series presented.

Our interpretation strongly capitalizes on the estimated scaling exponents α, which brings us to the study's major weakness: the brevity of pacing sequences profoundly limits the reliability of α estimates. DFA and related methods like the rescaled-range analysis, power spectral density estimates, wavelet-based scaling estimates, etc. all require a large number of samples, in particular if the expected (or generated) scaling exponents are larger than 0.5. The persistent long-range correlations do not only camouflage possible non-stationarities in the data but also cause a significant spread of α estimates. For instance, in the case of $H=0.9$, numerical simulations of fractal Gaussian noise with $N=256$ samples may yield standard deviations that can readily exceed $\Delta\alpha=0.15$. Although DFA appears to be the most reliable approach to assess the presence of long-range correlations [19,32] we realize that our results should be interpreted with great caution although this lack of reliability is not necessarily reflected in the group statistics. We note that these considerations do not only apply to the estimates of α but also to those of $\alpha_{\text{short-term}}$ and $\alpha_{\text{long-term}}$. That is, future studies should aim for significantly longer pacing sequences, i.e. much longer walking protocols (preferably $N \geq 600$ strides, see [33]). Given the plenitude of conditions in our experimental design, however, such extended protocols were not deemed feasible for answering our research questions.

Another limitation that should be mentioned is that the participants in the present study walked on a treadmill, which is known to be different from over-ground walking, putatively due to differences in the perceptual information generated. In particular, compared to over-ground walking, treadmill walking appears to be characterized by a less correlated pattern in the stride intervals and greater gait stability [25]. This could imply that the results of the present study would have been even more pronounced over ground; however, this remains speculation as long as a direct empirical comparison remains absent. Hence, also in this regard, the present results must be qualified.

In conclusion, the presence of long-range correlations in auditory cues enabled participants to maintain their 'normal', fractal gait pattern. This complexity matching of inter-stride intervals structures seemed to rely on strong anticipation processes with the attunement of ISIs and IBIs fractal exponents on the long-term region of DFA diffusion plots (supported by the absence of local cross-correlations). Our results may form a first step towards a better understanding of the effect of (correlations in) auditory cueing on gait. The present findings may open new opportunities for optimizing cueing protocols in gait rehabilitation. In particular, further investigations should verify a potential "carry-over" effect of a fractal metronome to stride-time dynamics.

Supporting Information

Table S1 Means and standard deviations of the series of asynchronies (standard deviations in italics) from all conditions in Experiment 1 (upper panel) and Experiment 2 (lower panel).

Table S2 Means and standard deviations of the series of inter-beat intervals (standard deviations in italics) from all conditions in Experiment 1 (upper panel) and Experiment 2 (lower panel).

Audio S1 Audio examples of pacing signals (only 15 seconds). File names corresponds to the conditions (for example : Exp1_CV1 correspond to a fractal metronome used in Experiment 1, in condition $CV=1\%$).

Data S1 Time series from Experiment 1 and Experiment 2 (.xls files). Each sheet correspond to a particular condition for a particular variable (for example : in the file « data_expe1_multipleCV », the sheet ISI CV 1% corresponds to stride-time series of participants in the condition CV = 1% in Experiment 1). Each column corresponds to an individual participant.

Acknowledgments

The authors thank Melvyn Roerdink for technical assistance and comments and Didier Delignières for valuable discussions.

Author Contributions

Conceived and designed the experiments: VM PB AD. Performed the experiments: VM. Analyzed the data: VM KT AD. Contributed reagents/materials/analysis tools: VM AD. Wrote the paper: VM KT PB AD.

References

1. Hausdorff JM, Lertratanakul A, Cudkowicz ME, Peterson AL, Kaliton D, et al. (2000) Dynamic markers of altered gait rhythm in amyotrophic lateral sclerosis. J Appl Physiol 88: 2045–2053.

2. Hausdorff JM, Mitchell SL, Firtion R, Peng CK, Cudkowicz ME, et al. (1997) Altered fractal dynamics of gait: Reduced stride-interval correlations with aging and Huntington's disease. J Appl Physiol 82: 262–269.

3. Vaillancourt DE, Newell KM (2002) Changing complexity in human behavior and physiology through aging and disease. Neurobiol Aging 23: 1–11.
4. Madison G (2001) Variability in isochronous tapping: Higher order dependencies as a function of intertap interval. J Exp Psychol Human 27: 411–422.
5. Van Orden GC, Holden JG, Turvey MT (2003) Self-organization of cognitive performance. J Exp Psychol Gen 132: 331–350.
6. Werner G (2010) Fractals in the nervous system: conceptual implications for theoretical neuroscience. Front Physio 1: 15. doi: 10.3389/fphys.2010.00015.
7. Barnes A, Bullmore ET, Suckling J (2009) Endogenous human brain dynamics recover slowly following cognitive effort. PLoS ONE 4(8): e6626. doi:10.1371/journal.pone.0006626.
8. Goldberger AL (2006) Complex systems. Proc Am Thorac Soc 3: 467–472.
9. Hausdorff JM (2007) Gait dynamics, fractals and falls: Finding meaning in the stride-to-stride fluctuations of human walking. Hum Mov Sci 26: 555–589.
10. Hausdorff JM, Purdon PL, Peng CK, Ladin Z, Wei JY, et al. (1996) Fractal dynamics of human gait: stability of long-range correlations in stride interval fluctuation. J Appl Physiol 80: 1448–1457.
11. Terrier P, Dériaz O (2012) Persistent and anti-persistent pattern in stride-to-stride variability of treadmill walking: influence of rhythmic auditory cueing. Hum Mov Sci 31(6): 1585–97.
12. Delignières D, Torre K (2009) Fractal dynamics of human gait: a reassessment of the 1996 data of Hausdorff et al. J Appl Physiol 106: 1272–1279.
13. Hausdorff JM, Peng CK, Ladin Z, Wei JY, Goldberger AR (1995) Is walking a random walk? Evidence for long-range correlations in stride interval of human gait. J Appl Physiol 78: 349–358.
14. McIntosh GC, Brown SH, Rice RR, Thaut MH (1997) Rhythmic auditory-motor facilitation of gait patterns in patients with Parkinson's disease. J Neurol Neurosur Ps 62: 22–26.
15. Lim I, van Wegen E, de Goede C, Deutekom M, Nieubower A, et al. (2005) Effects of external rhythmical cueing on gait in patients with Parkinson's disease: a systematic review. Clin Rehabil 19 (7): 695–713.
16. Kaipust JP, McGrath D, Mukherjee M, Stergiou N (2012) Gait variability is altered in older adults when listening to auditory stimuli with differing temporal structures. Ann Biomed Eng 41(8): 1595–1603.
17. Hove MJ, Suzuki K, Uchitomi H, Orimo S, Miyake Y (2012) Interactive rhythmic auditory stimulation reinstates natural 1/f timing in gait of Parkinson's patients. PLoS one 7(3): e32600.
18. Peng CK, Mietus J, Hausdorff JM, Havlin S, Stanley HE, et al. (1993) Long-range anti-correlations and non-Gaussian behavior of the heart-beat. Phys Rev Lett 70: 1343–1346.
19. Delignières D, Ramdani S, Lemoine L, Torre K, Fortes M, et al. (2006) Fractal analysis for short time series: a reassessement of classical methods. J Math Psychol 50: 525–544.
20. Marmelat V, Delignières D (2012) Strong anticipation: complexity matching in interpersonal coordination. Exp Brain Res 222: 137–148.
21. Stephen DG, Dixon J (2011) Strong anticipation: multifractal cascade dynamics modulate scaling in synchronization behaviors. Chaos Solitons Fract 44: 160–168.
22. Stephen DG, Stepp N, Dixon J, Turvey MT (2008) Strong anticipation: sensitivity to long-range correlations in synchronization behavior. Physica A 387: 5271–5278.
23. Delignières D, Marmelat V (2013) Strong anticipation and long-range cross-correlation: Application of Detrended Cross-Correlation Analysis to human behavioral data. Physica A 394: 47–60.
24. Roerdink M, Coolen H, Clairbois HE, Lamoth CJC, Beek PJ (2008) Online gait event detection using a large force platform embedded in a treadmill. J Biomech 41: 2628–32.
25. Terrier P, Dériaz O (2011) Kinematic variability, fractal dynamics and local dynamic stability of treadmill walking. J Neuroeng Rehab 8: 12, doi:10.1186/1743-0003-8-12.
26. Terrier P, Turner V, Schutz Y (2005) GPS analysis of human locomotion: Further evidence for long-range correlations in stride-to-stride fluctuations of gait parameters. Hum Mov Sci 24(1): 97–115.
27. Repp BH (2005) Sensorimotor synchronization: a review of the tapping literature. Psychon Bull Rev 12: 969–992.
28. Lipsitz LA, Goldberger AL (1992) Loss of 'Complexity' and ageing. J Am Med Assoc 267: 1806–1809.
29. Goldberger AL, Amaral LAN, Hausdorff JM, Ivanov PC, Peng CK, et al. (2002) Fractal dynamics in physiology: alterations with disease and aging. Proc Natl Acad Sci USA 99: 2466–2472.
30. Ehrlé N, Samson S (2005) Auditory discrimination of anisochrony: Influence of the tempo and musical backgrounds of listeners. Brain Cognition 58: 133–147.
31. Dingwell JB, Cusumano JP (2010) Re-interpreting detrended fluctuation analyses of stride-to-stride variability in human walking. Gait Posture 32: 348–353.
32. Weron R (2002) Estimating long-range dependence: finite sample properties and confidence intervals. Physica A 312: 285–299.
33. Damouras S, Chang MD, Seijdic E, Chau T (2010) An empirical examination of detrended fluctuation analysis for gait data. Gait Posture 31: 336–340.

22

The Effect of Additional Training on Motor Outcomes at Discharge from Recovery Phase Rehabilitation Wards: A Survey from Multi-Center Stroke Data Bank in Japan

Nariaki Shiraishi[1,2]*, Yusuke Suzuki[3], Daisuke Matsumoto[4], Seungwon Jeong[5], Motoya Sugiyama[6], Katsunori Kondo[7], Masafumi Kuzuya[1]

1 Department of Geriatrics, Medicine in Growth and Aging, Program in Health and Community Medicine, Nagoya University Graduate School of Medicine, Nagoya, Japan, 2 Department of Rehabilitation, Faculty of Health Science, Nihon Fukushi University, Nagoya, Japan, 3 Department of Comprehensive Community Care Systems, Nagoya University Graduate School of Medicine, Nagoya, Japan, 4 Department of Physical Therapy, Faculty of Health Science, Kio University, Koryo, Japan, 5 Department of Social Science Center for Gerontology and Social Science, Chubu Rosai Hospital, Nagoya, Japan, 6 Department of Rehabilitation, Chubu Rosai Hospital, Nagoya, Japan, 7 Center for Well-being and Society, Nihon Fukushi University, Nagoya, Japan

Abstract

Objectives: The purpose of the present study was to examine the potential benefits of additional training in patients admitted to recovery phase rehabilitation ward using the data bank of post-stroke patient registry.

Subjects and Methods: Subjects were 2507 inpatients admitted to recovery phase rehabilitation wards between November 2004 and November 2010. Participants were retrospectively divided into four groups based upon chart review; patients who received no additional rehabilitation, patients who were added with self-initiated off hours training, patients who were added with off hours training by ward staff, patients who received both self-initiated training and training by ward staff. Parameters for assessing outcomes included length of stay, motor/cognitive subscales of functional independent measures (FIM) and motor benefit of FIM calculated by subtracting the score at admission from that at discharge.

Results: Participants were stratified into three groups depending on the motor FIM at admission (≤ 28, 29~56, $57 \leq$) for comparison. Regarding outcome variables, significant inter-group differences were observed in all items examined within the subgroup who scored 28 or less and between 29 and 56. Meanwhile no such trends were observed in the group who scored 57 or more compared with those who scored less. In a decision tree created based upon Exhaustive Chi-squared Automatic Interaction Detection method, variables chosen were the motor FIM at admission (the first node) additional training (the second node), the cognitive FIM at admission (the third node).

Conclusions: Overall the results suggest that additional training can compensate for the shortage of regular rehabilitation implemented in recovery phase rehabilitation ward, thus may contribute to improved outcomes assessed by motor FIM at discharge.

Editor: Andreas Meisel, Charité Universitaetsmedizin Berlin, Germany

Funding: This study was supported by the Grant-in-Aid for Scientific Research (C) by The Ministry of Education, Culture, Sports, Science and Technology of the Japanese government, issued for the research project entitled "The effect of additional training after stroke: a data base study." The funders had no role in study design, data collection and analysis, decision to publish or preparation of the manuscript.

Competing Interests: The authors have declared that no competing interests exist.

* E-mail: n-shira@n-fukushi.ac.jp

Introduction

Stroke is one of primary debilitating events that affect health status and functional capacity, and is reportedly ranked second or third cause of mortality or condition leading to functional impairments in most developed countries [1]. Japan is no exception that stroke is the first cause of conditions requiring care and is ranked the first in medical expenditure nationwide among the older population [2]. Recent advancement has made various therapeutic options including thrombolytic therapy, intravascular therapy or cerebral protective therapy available for stroke patients, however that does not undermine the significance of rehabilitation for functional recovery. It has been confirmed from previous randomized control trials (RCT) or systematic reviews that providing care in stroke units by multidisciplinary team comprising doctors, nurses, physiotherapist (PT), occupational therapist (OT) and speech therapist (ST) leads to improved clinical outcomes, such as long-term prognosis, activities of daily living at discharge, length of hospital stay [3,4]. To date, there had been a dearth of multi-center data base for rehabilitation medicine in Japan, which impeded implementation of studies supported by strong evidences. In order to establish rigorous evidences for the quality improvement and to provide rationales for the revision of reimbursement system in stroke rehabilitation, we have been establishing a data bank (DB) of post-stroke patients receiving rehabilitation since 2005, which was supported by a Grant-in-Aid issued from the

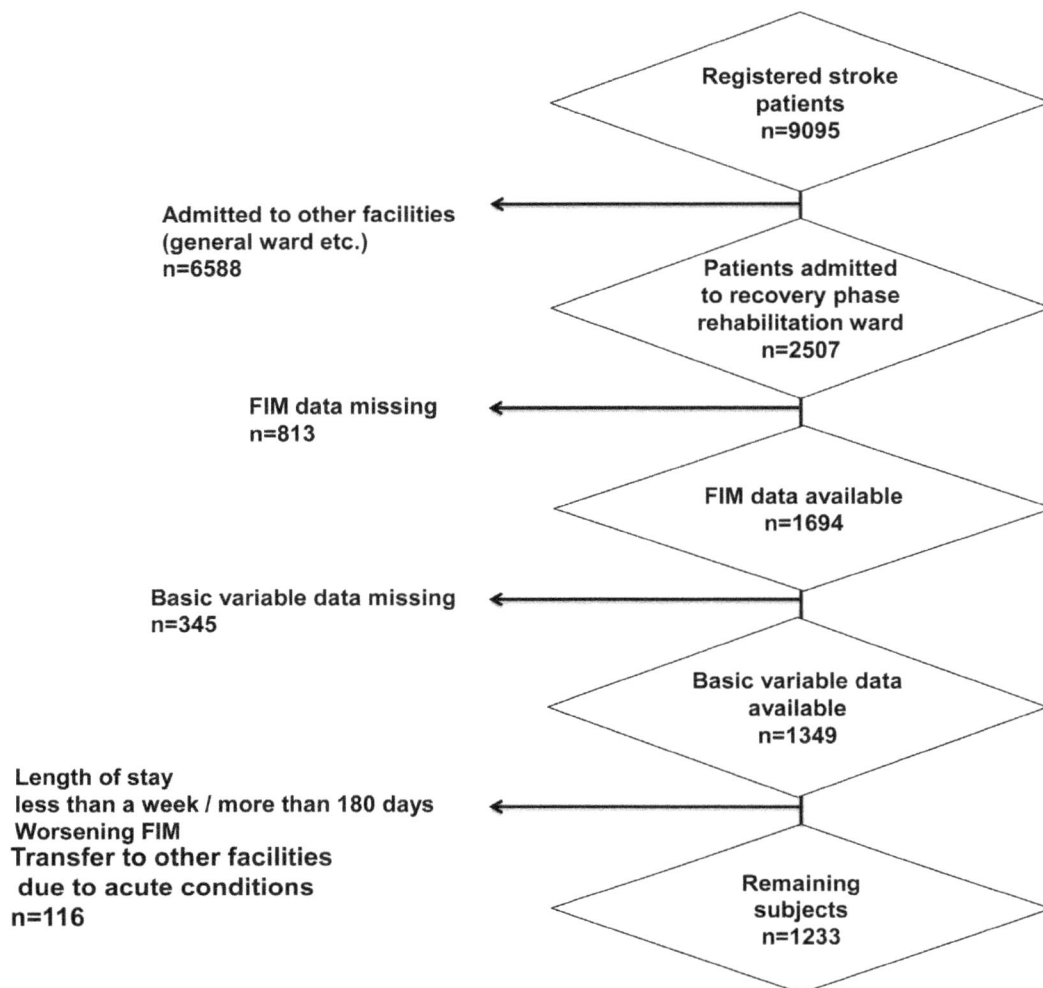

Figure 1. Flow chart showing selection procedure of participants.

Ministry of Health, Labor and Welfare for the research project entitled "The development of data bank for stroke rehabilitation". By November 2011, we collected over 9000 cases from 30 institutions nationwide. In Japan recovery phase rehabilitation ward for patients took effect from the year 2000 and the 2006 revision for reimbursement enabled post stroke patients to receive a maximum of three hours rehabilitation per day by PT, OT and ST. This unique type of ward restricts intake of patient only to medical conditions such as stroke, spinal injuries, head trauma, hip fractures or disuse syndrome. In addition, there are specific regulations regarding the admission criteria, including term of admission. For example, stroke patients have to be admitted within two months after the onset of stroke with maximum length of stay limited until 150 days after the onset. Regarding the time of rehabilitation per day, only those who can tolerate three hours rehabilitation per day are eligible for the entry to rehabilitation programs according to the US Agency for Health Care Policy and Research [5], which is in contrast with the policy applied in Japan. On the other hand, there is a study implemented in a stroke unit that indicated the significance of "off hours" training enhanced by multidisciplinary team for improved activities of daily living (ADL) [1], which suggests a potential benefit of such off hours intervention particularly under the situation where there is a

limitation in authorized volume of training. The "OFF hours" training comprises self-initiated training and training by ward staff. However, little attention to date has been paid to off hours intervention and its effect on functional prognosis [6,7]. As suggested in a recent meta-analysis, the importance of off hours training is a subject to be investigated through further research [8]. Although previous studies regarding off hours training focused on self-initiated training mainly led by patients themselves, there is also a necessity to evaluate additional training provided by ward staff. No studies so far had examined the effect of off hours training (self-initiated training, training by ward staff or both) in recovery phase rehabilitation wards uniquely introduced in Japan.

There is a difficulty in carrying out RCT in rehabilitation medicine. Therefore as an alternative method of investigation, well-designed comparative research with larger samples is considered significant [9]. However, there has been a concern about external validity in previous reports with such method since many of them either came from single institution or had not examined reproducibility in other samples of patients [9,10]. Thus in the present study, in order to endorse external validity, we obtained observational data from multiple sources and randomly assigned the individual data into two groups and examined

Table 1. Characteristics of participants stratified by motor subscales of FIM at admission.

Motor subscales of FIM at admission ≤28 (n=427)

		①No additional training (n=62)	②Self-initiated traning (n=7)	③Training by ward staff (n=203)	④Dual training (n=155)	p value†	multiple comparison‡
Sex	Male	33(14.2%)	2(0.9%)	113(48.7%)	84(36.2%)	0.59	
	Female	29(14.9%)	5(2.6%)	90(46.2%)	71(36.4%)		
Type fo stroke	CI	38(14.7%)	3(1.2%)	132(51.2%)	85(32.9%)	0.02	
	CH	17(13.0)	2(1.5%)	50(38.2%)	62(47.3%)		
	SAH etc.	7(18.4%)	2(5.3%)	21(55.3%)	8(21.1%)		
Informal care resources	NIC	17(18.5%)	2(2.2%)	42(45.7%)	31(33.7%)	0.27	
	OIC	20(13.7%)	4(2.7%)	64(43.8%)	58(39.7%)		
	MTIC	19(10.6%)	1(0.6%)	94(52.5%)	65(36.3%)		
Age		74.5±9.9	73.0±8.0	75.3±9.2	69.4±11.8	<0.001	④<①③
Days after onset at admission		41.1±25.0	48.6±47.3	39.9±21.2	30.9±16.4	<0.001	④<①③

Motor subscales of FIM at admission 29~56 (n=418)

		①No additional training (n=63)	②Self-initiated traning (n=16)	③Training by ward staff (n=71)	④Dual training (n=268)	p value†	multiple comparison‡
Sex	Male	50(18.9%)	13(4.9%)	43(16.2%)	159(60.0%)	0.01	
	Female	13(8.5%)	3(2.0%)	28(18.3%)	109(71.2%)		
Type of stroke	CI	27(10.2%)	11(4.1%)	58(21.8%)	170(63.9%)	<0.001	
	CH	31(13.9%)	2(0.9%)	11(8.9%)	79(64.2%)		
	SAH etc.	5(17.2%)	3(10.3%)	2(6.9%)	19(65.5%)		
Informal care resources	NIC	19(17.3%)	6(5.5%)	23(20.9%)	62(57.3%)	0.46	
	OIC	17(12.4%)	4(2.9%)	23(16.8%)	93(67.9%)		
	MTIC	26(15.7%)	6(3.6%)	23(13.9%)	111(66.9%)		
Age		71.8±9.5	68.1±9.7	75.1±10.7	66.6±12.8	<0.001	④<①③
Days after onset at admission		41.9±21.4	34.9±19.4	36.4±18.4	32.0±14.6	<0.001	④<①③

Motor subscales of FIM at admission 57≤ (n=388)

		①No additional training (n=45)	②Self-initiated traning (n=41)	③Training by ward staff (n=22)	④Dual training (n=280)	p value†	multiple comparison‡
Sex	Male	23(9.3%)	31(12.6%)	13(5.3%)	180(72.9%)	0.12	
	Female	22(15.6%)	10(7.1%)	9(6.4%)	100(70.9%)		
Type of stroke	CI	28(11.2%)	16(6.4%)	16(6.4%)	190(76.0%)	0.003	

Table 1. Cont.

Motor subscales of FIM at admission ≦28 (n = 427)		①No additional training (n = 62)	②Self-initiated traning (n = 7)	③Training by ward staff (n = 203)	④Dual training (n = 155)	p value†	multiple comparison‡
	CH	9(9.8%)	17(18.5%)	2(2.2%)	64(69.6%)		
	SAH etc.	8(17.4%)	8(17.4%)	4(8.7%)	26(56.5%)		
Informal care	NIC	12(12.0%)	13(13.0%)	0(0.0%)	75(75.0%)	0.07	
resources	OIC	15(11.7%)	13(10.2%)	9(7.0%)	91(71.1%)		
	MTIC	16(10.6%)	13(8.6%)	12(7.9%)	110(72.8%)		
Age		72.0±11.1	61.7±15.5	70.9±18.2	64.2±13.7	<0.001	②④<①
Days after onset at admission		35.4±16.8	34.6±14.4	41.6±26.8	30.4±21.9	0.05	

note:SAH = Subarachnoidal hemorrhage; CI = Cerebral infarction; CH = Cerebral hemorrhage; NIC = No informal caregivers; OIC = One informal caregiver; MTIC = More than two informal caregivers.

† p value for one way analysis of variance.

‡multiple comparison: digits refer to group numbers (Tukey multiple comparison procedure).

whether the equation model formulated in one group can also predict the outcomes in the other with statistical significance.

The purpose of the present study was to examine potential benefit of off-hours rehabilitation involving self-initiated training by patients themselves, and training by ward staff in patients admitted to recovery phase rehabilitation wards using the DB of post-stroke patients registered during the term of observation.

Subjects and Methods

The present study was a secondary analysis of the DB of post-stroke patients registered between November 2004 and November 2010. Subjects were 2507 inpatients admitted to recovery phase rehabilitation wards out of 9095 patients registered in post-stroke DB. The DB was managed by the Japan Association of Rehabilitation Database (JARD) and the data was provided after the research protocol was approved by the institutional review board. Thus the data is not publicly available but only those who obtained the approval were authorized access to the DB. Of the subjects, those whose essential data (age, sex, FIM, record of self-initiated off hours training) were either absent or missing in more than 40% of inpatients, length of stay being either less than 7 days or more than 180 days, venue of rehabilitation changed due to acute medical conditions, FIM scores at discharge deteriorated were excluded, eventually 1233 inpatients were subjected to analyses (Fig. 1). Variables included age, sex and type of stroke as basic information. The followings were also included; number of days after admission, number of informal caregivers (none, single person, more than 2 people), total volume of PT and OT counted by Formal Therapy Unit (FTU) and FTU per day were also calculated (1FTU is equivalent to 20 minute Formal Therapy). Parameters for assessing outcomes included length of stay, motor FIM/cognitive FIM and motor benefit of FIM calculated by subtracting the score at admission from that at discharge. Participants were retrospectively divided into four groups based upon chart records; patients who received no additional rehabilitation (no additional training), patients who were added with self-initiated off hours training (self-initiated training), patients who were added with off hours training by ward staff (training by ward staff), patients who received both self-initiated off hours training and training by ward staff (dual additional training) and their outcomes assessed by parameters aforementioned were compared.

Statistical Analysis

Age, length of stay, number of days after the onset of stroke until discharge, FTU, FTU/day, motor FIM, cognitive FIM and motor benefit of FIM of the four intervention groups were compared using analysis of variance followed by Tukey's post-hoc test.It is known that improvement of ADLs during admission can be higher in patients whose physical independence at admission is intermediate compared with patients who have either low or high physical independence, thus exhibits reverse U-shaped trend [11]. Therefore, subjects were divided equally into three subgroups based on the motor FIM at admission for group comparison. Categorical data (sex, types of stroke and presence of informal caregivers) of the four groups were compared using chi-square test. In order to clarify contributing factors to motor FIM at discharge after possible confounding factors (presence of informal caregivers, motor FIM at admission and cognitive FIM at admission) having been adjusted, a decision tree analysis was carried out, making measured variables at admission that indicated significant intergroup differences by univariate analysis explanatory variables. In the present study Exhaustive Chi-Squared Automatic Interaction Detection (ECHAID) was adopted for the analysis. ECHAID is a

Table 2. Outcome parameters of participants at discharge stratified by motor subscales of FIM at admission.

Motor subscales of FIM at admission ≦28 (n=427)	①No additional training	②Self-initiated training	③Training by ward staff	④Dual training	p value†	multiple comparison‡
	(n=62)	(n=7)	(n=203)	(n=155)		
Length of stay	111.3±46.2	105.0±61.4	95.7±43.9	124.9±31.2	<0.001	①④>③
FTU*	358.8±184.0	308.7±252.9	275.3±179.2	474.4±221.4	<0.001	④>①>③
FTU/day*	3.2±1.0	3.2±1.8	2.8±1.2	3.8±1.4	<0.001	④>①③
Motor FIM at admission	17.9±5.0	16.9±3.9	16.3±4.2	20.2±4.9	<0.001	④>①③
Cognitive FIM at admission	11.4±6.4	15.0±8.6	11.9±6.4	17.9±8.3	<0.001	④>①③
Motor FIM at discharge	31.7±16.3	50.6±22.3	33.0±18.4	52.1±21.4	<0.001	④>①③
Cognitive FIM at discharge	15.0±7.7	21.7±8.5	15.9±6.4	24.6±8.3	<0.001	④>①③
Motor benefit of FIM	13.8±12.8	33.7±22.3	16.7±17.0	31.9±19.7	<0.001	④>①③, ②>①

Motor subscales of FIM at admission 29~56 (n=418)	①No additional training	②Self-initiated training	③Training by ward staff	④Dual training	p value†	multiple comparison‡
	(n=63)	(n=16)	(n=71)	(n=268)		
Length of stay	111.2±47.8	100.4±33.1	88.4±38.1	104.1±37.6	0.01	①④>③
FTU*	398.5±222.4	379.4±171.2	248.3±144.3	405.1±242.7	<0.01	①④>③
FTU/day*	3.5±1.0	3.8±0.8	2.8±1.5	3.7±1.5	<0.01	①②④>③
Motor FIM at admission	42.3±8.6	49.5±6.9	39.9±7.5	43.5±8.0	<0.01	②>①③④, ④>③
Cognitive FIM at admission	22.1±7.3	24.5±7.5	19.6±5.9	24.7±7.1	<0.01	④>①③, ②>③
Motor FIM at discharge	61.3±15.7	75.2±7.0	61.0±11.3	72.7±11.5	<0.01	②④>①③
Cognitive FIM at discharge	24.7±7.1	30.0±5.8	22.4±5.8	29.3±5.7	<0.01	②④>①③
Motor benefit of FIM	19.0±11.6	25.7±8.1	21.1±11.6	29.1±11.3	<0.01	④>①③

Motor subscales of FIM at admission 57≦ (n=388)	①No additional training	②Self-initiated training	③Training by ward staff	④Dual training	p value†	multiple comparison‡
	(n=45)	(n=41)	(n=22)	(n=280)		
Length of stay	89.3±46.9	69.4±42.4	75.5±33.2	74.6±39.2	0.10	
FTU*	320.7±210.5	251.0±176.3	175.6±78.7	296.0±207.6	0.02	①④>③
FTU/day*	3.5±1.1	3.6±1.0	2.4±0.7	3.9±1.6	<0.01	①②④>③
Motor FIM at admission	71.4±10.3	76.7±9.8	67.3±9.7	70.8±9.2	<0.01	②>③④
Cognitive FIM at admission	27.4±6.3	29.0±5.7	19.8±6.3	29.2±5.9	<0.01	①②④>③

Table 2. Cont.

Motor subscales of FIM at admission ≦28 (n=427)	①No additional training	②Self-initiated traning	③Training by ward staff	④Dual training	p value[†]	multiple comparison[‡]
	(n=62)	(n=7)	(n=203)	(n=155)		
Motor FIM at discharge	82±7	86.0±6	81.2±7.9	82.2±6.8	0.07	②>①③④
Cognitive FIM at discharge	29±5.4	31.0±4.2	23.9±5.5	31.6±4.5	<0.01	①②④>③, ④>①
Motor benefit of FIM	10.6±7.8	9.3±7.9	13.9±8.5	11.4±7.5	0.13	

*FTU: Formal Therapy Unit One unit is equivalent of 20minute rehabilitation.
†p value for one way analysis of variance.
‡multiple comparison: digits refer to group numbers (Tukey multiple comparison procedure).

commonly used algorithm of classification tree analysis that employed multi-contingency tables of Chi-squared significant test to identify optimal splits [12]. In order to avoid over fitting, we specified the growing depth of 3 with the parent node having at least 100 subjects and a child node at least 50 subjects. Gains and index charts were constructed to identify the nodes with a relatively high probability. The statistics of misclassification risk was used to assess the prediction results. Primary outcomes to evaluate the effectiveness of additional training was motor FIM at discharge. Motor FIM on admission, the motor FIM at discharge were automatically divided into three ordinal scales (lower tertile; ≦55, mid tertile; 56–79, upper tertile; 80≦) in order for the calculations to fit into the decision tree created. To ensure the validity of the analysis, split-sample validation method was adopted in the present study. In brief, subjects were randomly divided into two groups. Decision trees analysis was carried out in one group and whether the equation obtained in the study group can be applicable in another group (validation group) was examined. All the analyses were carried out using a statistical software package (SPSS version 19.0 for Windows, Chicago IL, USA) and a p value of <0.05 was adopted to show statistical significances. All the personal data were coded deleting any information related to personal identification in order to secure anonymity of the study and the study protocol was approved by the ethical committee of the Japan Society for Rehabilitation Medicine.

Results

1. Group Comparison

Table 1 compares variables of subjects stratified into three groups depending on the motor FIM at admission (≦28, 29~56, ≥57). Subjects who scored 28 or less showed significant inter-group differences in the type of stroke, age and the interval between the onset and admission. A post-hoc analysis indicated that dual training group was younger and had shorter interval between the onset and admission relative to self-initiated training group and training by ward staff group. Subjects who scored between 29 and 56 showed similar trend in variables examined with those with lower tertile. Meanwhile in subjects who scored 57 or more on the motor FIM at admission, types of stroke and age showed inter-group differences with self-initiated training group and dual additional training group being younger relative to no additional training group.

Table 2 shows comparison of variables stratified by the motor FIM at admission. Significant inter-group differences were observed in all items examined within the subgroup who scored 28 or less. A post-hoc analysis revealed that dual training group showed better outcomes compared with training by ward staff group, and dual training group were superior to no additional training group in all parameters apart from the length of stay. Inter-group differences were also observed in a subgroup whose motor FIM at admission were between 29 and 56, and a post-hoc analysis indicated similar results showing that dual training group had better outcomes than training by ward staff group. Meanwhile no such trends were observed by post-hoc analysis in the group who scored 57 or more (upper tertile) compared with those who scored less.

2. Decision Tree Analysis using ECHAID

Figure 2 shows a decision tree created based upon ECHAID method. Overall risk estimate for the model in the study group was 0.32, while that in the validation group was 0.31, therefore the analysis was considered appropriate. The variables chosen in the decision tree were the motor FIM at admission, additional trainings, the cognitive FIM at admission. The motor FIM at admission were chosen in the first node, therefore considered most influential on the motor FIM at discharge. For those who scored 56 or less on the motor FIM at admission, no additional training group, training by ward staff and dual training group, self-initiated training group were divided. Meanwhile better cognitive FIM at admission (>28) emerged as a variable to determine improved motor FIM at discharge in those who scored 57 or more on the motor FIM at admission.

Discussion

The main purpose of the present study was to clarify the effect of additional training other than formal therapy by qualified therapists (PT, OT, ST) on motor FIM at discharge in post-stroke patients. The study utilized multi-center DB of stroke patients and the samples were randomly assigned to either study or validation group. Decision tree analyses were carried out and risk estimates for both groups were compared with an aim to examine whether the model obtained in the study group can be extrapolated in the validation group as well. To date most of studies using decision tree analysis adopt cross validation, which uses random sample out of all subjects for examining validity of the analysis implemented [13,14]. The limitation about this method is that sampled subjects for validation are included in actual analysis for creating decision tree, and therefore not quite independent. The present analysis was a result from over 1000 cases and was validated by equal

number of subjects. Therefore the decision tree created can be considered to exceed in external validity compared with results obtained from conventional methods. The results indicated that in both groups whose motor FIM at admission were either less than 28 or between 29 and 56, those who received both self-initiated training and training by ward staff showed better cognitive and motor FIM at discharge. Furthermore, the decision tree analysis, after adjusting for other possible factors that might affect motor FIM at discharge, also confirmed that implementations of additional training were beneficial in terms of improved outcomes at discharge for those whose motor FIM at admission were below 56. In principle, a factor that appears in the first node has the strongest explanatory power in the decision tree analysis. Thus it was the motor FIM at admission that was most strongly related to the motor FIM at discharge, followed by the implementation of additional training for those in the lower and mid tertile groups of baseline motor FIM. Meanwhile in the upper tertile group, cognitive profiles at admission were more strongly related to the outcomes at discharge than the implementation of additional training. In the upper tertile group, whose overall functional impairment was relatively mild compared with other groups, cognitive capacity affecting attention or concentration to the training assigned may have stronger impact on the efficacy of training than the volume of training. Overall the results suggest that implementation of self-initiated training together with training by ward staff or at least self-initiated training alone might contribute to improved outcomes assessed by motor FIM at discharge, albeit actual contents of off-hours rehabilitation were

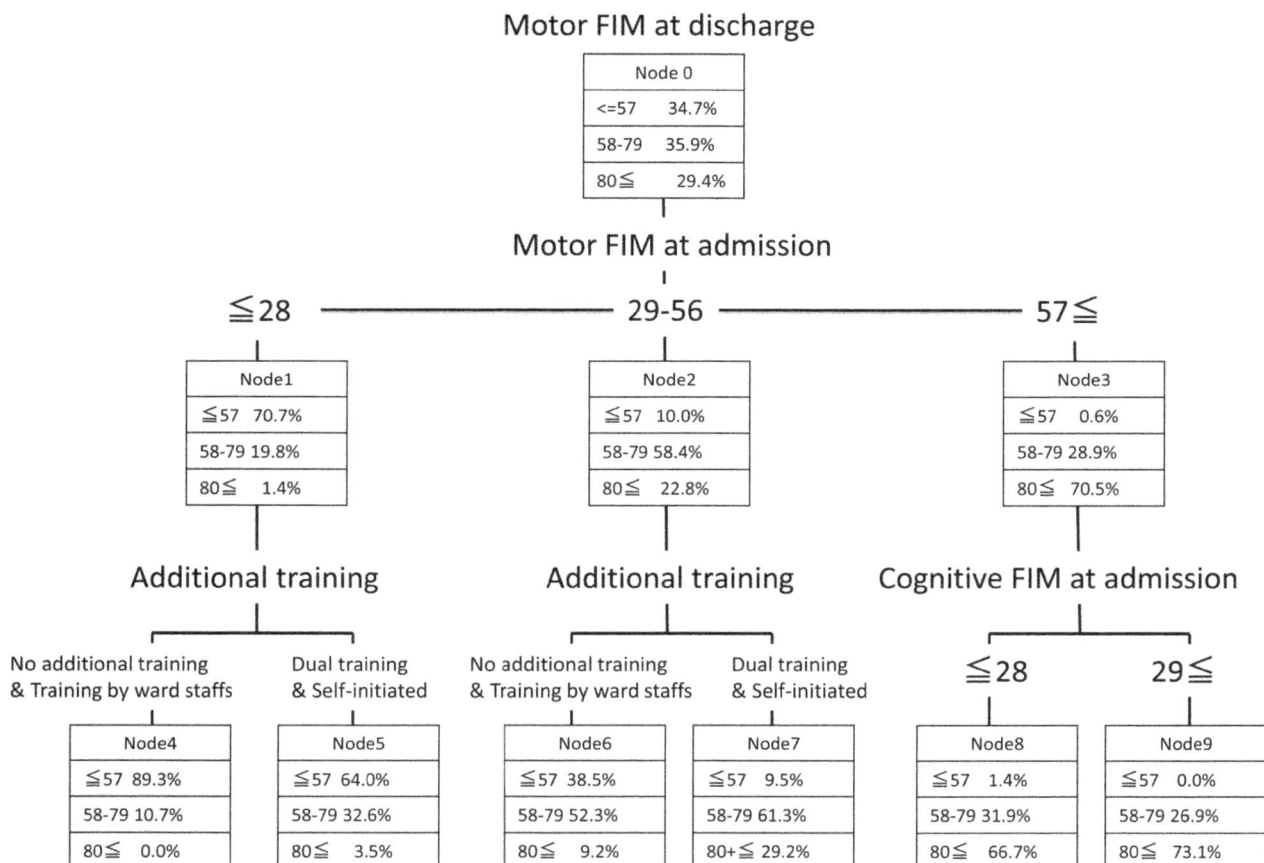

Figure 2. Decision tree for Functional Independence Measure among 1233 stroke patients (Validation Group).

not available to obtain from the DB. However, given small sample size of patients who implemented self-initiated training, the present results must be interpreted with caution. A previous study by Galvin et al [15].employing a randomized controlled trial (RCT) on the effect of self-initiated training confirmed the improvement of ADLs or easing stress experienced by family. Another report also stressed the efficacy of self-initiated training assisted by patients' family for improved physical functions of lower extremities and ADLs [7]. A systematic review by Meheroz et al [6]. have demonstrated that off hours repeated use of upper extremities may contribute to improved functions. Previous studies including RCT [15–17] that investigated the effect of self-initiated training targeted particular conditions such as first onset, no episode of dementia or restricted severity of hemiparesis, therefore the findings can be applied to conditions meeting inclusion criterion. Meanwhile the results obtained in the present study can be applied to patients with broad conditions of stroke. Regarding the effect of training by ward staff, Indredavik et al [18] stated that one of the advantages of stroke unit compared with general ward is the preventive approaches of secondary complications or disuse syndromes by staff nurses. Studies of stroke unit have shown that multidisciplinary interventions might lead to beneficial outcomes. Likewise, the present study suggested the importance of close collaborations of multidisciplinary staffs by having demonstrated that the implementation of either both self-initiated training and additional training by ward staff or self-initiated training alone was found to be beneficial for improving motor outcomes in post stroke patients admitted to recovery phase rehabilitation ward although the findings cannot directly be applied to any ward accommodating post stroke patients. Possibly due to insufficient availability of physiotherapist, average total time of regular rehabilitation per day in the present study was approximately 70 minutes, which figures fall far short of upper limit of 90 minutes. Additional training can compensate for the shortage, which therefore must

have worked effectively for the improvement of motor function as suggested in previous reports [1,19].

Even though every possible confounding factors had been considered in the present analyses, so-called reverse causality of having chosen subjects who were expected to improve cannot completely be eliminated, which serves as a limitation of the present study. Further analyses adopting propensity score, instrumental variables or RCT would be necessary to control reverse causality. Due to restriction of data availability, actual amount of time and intensity of self-initiated training and training by ward staff were not considered. Comparison of efficacy betweenthe two off hours training groups favored self-initiated training. Elevated motivation of patients themselves, leading to proactive participation to the training, may explain the observed difference although such possible reason remains a speculation under the absence of detailed information about off hours training. Despite external validity of this multi-center study having been warranted, given that many institutions participated in the DB registration had specialists of rehabilitation medicine, and had elevated motivation represented by relatively higher implementation rate of training by ward staff, the present results need to be interpreted with caution. Nonetheless, we believe that the present multi-center study using stroke DB suggested the significance of additional (self-initiated, by ward staff or both) training at least for patients whose ADLs at admission are classified as more than moderately impaired.

Author Contributions

Conceived and designed the experiments: NS DM SJ MS KK. Performed the experiments: NS DM SJ MS. Analyzed the data: NS YS. Contributed reagents/materials/analysis tools: NS. Wrote the paper: NS YS. Supervised the entire experiments: MK.

References

1. Langhorne P, Bernhardt J, Kwakkel G (2011) Stroke rehabilitation. The Lancet 377: 1693–1702.
2. Kawano T, Hatakenaka M, Mihara M, Hattori N, Hino T, et al. (2011) Neurorehabilitation after stroke. Sogo Rihabiriteshon 39: 1151–1156.
3. Langhorne P, Pollock A, Collaboration iCwTSUT (2002) What are the components of effective stroke unit care? Age And Ageing 31: 365–371.
4. Indredavik B, Bakke F, Slordahl SA, Rokseth R, Haheim LL (1999) Stroke Unit Treatment : 10-Year Follow-Up. Stroke 30: 1524–1527.
5. GE G, PW D, WB S (1995) Post-Stroke Rehabilitation: United States Government Printing Office.
6. Rabadi MH (2011) review of the randomized clinical stroke rehabilitation trials in 2009. Medical science monitor 17: RA25–43.
7. Maeshima S, Ueyoshi A, Osawa A, Ishida K, Kunimoto K, et al. (2003) Mobility and Muscle Strength Contralateral to Hemiplegia from Stroke: Benefit from Self-Training with Family Support. American journal of physical medicine & rehabilitation 82: 456–462.
8. Quinn TJ, Paolucci S, Sunnerhagen KS, Sivenius J, Walker MF, et al. (2009) Evidence-based stroke rehabilitation: an expanded guidance document from the european stroke organisation (ESO) guidelines for management of ischaemic stroke and transient ischaemic attack 2008. J Rehabil Med 41.
9. Kondo K, Yamagichi A (2005) The potential and challenges of large databanks toward EBM. Sogo Rihabiriteshon 33: 1119–1124.
10. Miyakoshi K, Iai S, Hadeishi H (2008) Factors affecting functional outcome in patients with acute subarachnoid hemorrhage. Nosotchu 30: 69–71.
11. Kondo K (2004) Impact of Recovery Phase Rehabilitation Ward : A Policy Evaluation (Recovery Phase Rehabilitation Ward and Patient Management)

(40th Annual Meeting of the Japanese Association of Rehabilitation Medicine). Jpn J Rehabil Med 41: 214–218.
12. Gan X-m, Xu Y-h, Liu L, Huang S-q, Xie D-s, et al. (2011) Predicting the incidence risk of ischemic stroke in a hospital population of southern China: A classification tree analysis. Journal of the Neurological Sciences 306: 108–114.
13. Skidmore ER, Rogers JC, Chandler LS, Holm MB (2006) Dynamic interactions between impairment and activity after stroke: examining the utility of decision analysis methods. Clinical Rehabilitation 20: 523–535.
14. Suzuki E, Majima M, Tsurukawa T, Imai T, Hishinuma A (2004) A Case-mix Study of Stroke Patients in the Post Acute Stage. Jpn J Rehabil Med 41.
15. Galvin R, Cusack T, O'Grady E, Murphy TB, Stokes E (2011) Family-Mediated Exercise Intervention (FAME): Evaluation of a Novel Form of Exercise Delivery After Stroke. Stroke 42: 681–686.
16. Duncan P, Richards L, Wallace D, Stoker-Yates J, Pohl P, et al. (1998) A Randomized, Controlled Pilot Study of a Home-Based Exercise Program for Individuals With Mild and Moderate Stroke. stroke 29: 6.
17. Dobkin BH, Plummer-D'Amato P, Elashoff R, Lee J, Group S (2010) International randomized clinical trial, stroke inpatient rehabilitation with reinforcement of walking speed (SIRROWS), improves outcomes. Neurorehabil Neural Repair 24: 235–242.
18. Indredavik B, Bakke F, Slordahl SA, Rokseth R, Haheim LL (1999) Treatment in a Combined Acute and Rehabilitation Stroke Unit : Which Aspects Are Most Important? Stroke 30: 917–923.
19. Kwakkel G, van Peppen R, Wagenaar RC, Wood Dauphinee S, Richards C, et al. (2004) Effects of augmented exercise therapy time after stroke: a meta-analysis. Stroke 35: 2529–2539.

23

Peak Oxygen Uptake after Cardiac Rehabilitation: A Randomized Controlled Trial of a 12-Month Maintenance Program versus Usual Care

Erik Madssen[1,2], Ingerid Arbo[1], Ingrid Granøien[3], Liv Walderhaug[3], Trine Moholdt[1,4]*

1 K.G. Jebsen Center of Exercise in Medicine, Department of Circulation and Medical Imaging, Faculty of Medicine, Norwegian University of Science and Technology, Trondheim, Norway, 2 Department of Pulmonary Medicine, St. Olavs Hospital, Trondheim, Norway, 3 Ålesund Hospital, Ålesund, Norway, 4 Women's Clinic, St. Olavs Hospital, Trondheim, Norway

Abstract

Background: Exercise capacity is a strong predictor of survival in patients with coronary artery disease (CAD). Exercise capacity improves after cardiac rehabilitation exercise training, but previous studies have demonstrated a decline in peak oxygen uptake after ending a formal rehabilitation program. There is a lack of knowledge on how long-term exercise adherence can be achieved in CAD patients. We therefore assessed if a 12-month maintenance program following cardiac rehabilitation would lead to increased adherence to exercise and increased exercise capacity compared to usual care.

Materials and Methods: Two-centre, open, parallel randomized controlled trial with 12 months follow-up comparing usual care to a maintenance program. The maintenance program consisted of one monthly supervised high intensity interval training session, a written exercise program and exercise diary, and a maximum exercise test every third month during follow-up. Forty-nine patients (15 women) on optimal medical treatment were included following discharge from cardiac rehabilitation. The primary endpoint was change in peak oxygen uptake at follow-up; secondary endpoints were physical activity level, quality of life and blood markers of cardiovascular risk.

Results: There was no change in peak oxygen uptake from baseline to follow-up in either group (intervention group 27.9 ($\pm$4.7) to 28.8 ($\pm$5.6) mL·kg (-1) min (-1), control group 32.0 ($\pm$6.2) to 32.8 ($\pm$5.8) mL·kg (-1) min (-1), with no between-group difference, $p = 0.22$). Quality of life and blood biomarkers remained essentially unchanged, and both self-reported and measured physical activity levels were similar between groups after 12 months.

Conclusions: A maintenance exercise program for 12 months did not improve adherence to exercise or peak oxygen uptake in CAD patients after discharge from cardiac rehabilitation compared to usual care. This suggests that infrequent supervised high intensity interval training sessions are inadequate to improve peak oxygen uptake in this patient group.

Trial Registration: ClinicalTrials.gov NCT01246570

Editor: Terence J. Quinn, University of Glasgow, United Kingdom

Funding: Authors were supported by funds from the Liaison Committee for Central Norway Regional Health Authority and the Norwegian University of Science and Technology, Funds for Medical Research at St. Olavs University Hospital, and the Norwegian Fund for Post-Graduate Training in Physiotherapy. The funders had no role in study design, data collection and analysis, decision to publish, or preparation of the manuscript.

Competing Interests: The authors have declared that no competing interests exist.

* Email: trine.moholdt@ntnu.no

Introduction

Exercise-based rehabilitation in patients with coronary artery disease (CAD) reduces mortality [1–4], and cardiorespiratory fitness is a strong, independent predictor of both cardiac- and all-cause mortality in patients with CAD [5,6]. Therefore, it is important to establish effective exercise programs that patients can adhere to in this patient group. Unfortunately, most beneficial effects from physical activity are lost quite rapidly if regular exercise is discontinued. In line with this, peak oxygen uptake (VO_{2peak}) has been found to decline at six months, and more so at 30 months, after discharge from cardiac rehabilitation in patients with CAD [7]. Thus, there is a need for studies to assess

interventions that may help patients adhere to regular and effective exercise training after ending a formalized cardiac rehabilitation exercise program [8]. It is known that high intensity interval training (HIIT) is more effective than continuous training with low-to-moderate intensity with respect to increasing VO_{2peak} in patients with CAD [9], but there is a lack of knowledge regarding long-term effects of HIIT interventions.

The primary aim of this study was therefore to assess if a 12-month maintenance program following discharge from formal cardiac rehabilitation would improve adherence to physical activity and peak oxygen uptake We hypothesized that the maintenance program would lead to an attenuated decline in VO_{2peak} 12 months after ending the formal cardiac rehabilitation, compared with patients in usual care. Secondary endpoints were physical activity level, quality of life and blood markers of cardiovascular risk.

Materials and Methods

Design

The protocol for this trial and supporting CONSORT checklist are available as supporting information; see Checklist S1 and Protocol S1. This was a two-centre, open, parallel randomized controlled trial. The study was approved by the Regional Committee for Medical and Health Research Ethics in Middle-Norway (REK-Midt 2010/86), and registered at clinicaltrials.gov (NCT01246570). Patients gave their informed, written consent before entering the study, and we performed the study according to the Helsinki declaration for medical research. After acquisition of all baseline data, patients were randomized stratified by centre the same day, using a web-based randomization tool, developed and administered by Unit of Applied Clinical Research, Department of Cancer Research and Molecular Medicine, Norwegian University of Science and Technology, Trondheim. Stratified for study centre, patients were randomized either to a maintenance exercise program or to usual care for 12 months with a 1:1 allocation ratio (Figure 1).

Participants

We recruited optimal medically treated patients above 18 years of age from the cardiac rehabilitation centres at St. Olav's University Hospital in Trondheim, and Ålesund Hospital, both in central Norway. Inclusion criteria were completion of a 12-week organized in-hospital cardiac rehabilitation program, consisting of 2 exercise sessions per week, including both HIIT and moderate continuous exercise. Patients were included in the current study 1–2 weeks after ending the formal cardiac rehabilitation program. Patients were excluded if they fulfilled one or more of the following criteria; unstable angina pectoris (chest pain at light physical activity), hemodynamic significant valvular disease (valvular disease confirmed by echocardiography and dyspnoea at light physical activity), chronic obstructive pulmonary disease or chronic heart failure with symptoms at rest or in light physical activity, uncontrolled arterial hypertension (hypertension grade 2 despite medical treatment) chronic renal failure (serum creatinine>140 µmol/L), or pregnancy.

Interventions

Maintenance program group. Patients in the maintenance program group received a written exercise program with the aim of three sessions of high intensity interval training (HIIT) per week, and were invited to attend a monthly supervised exercise session at

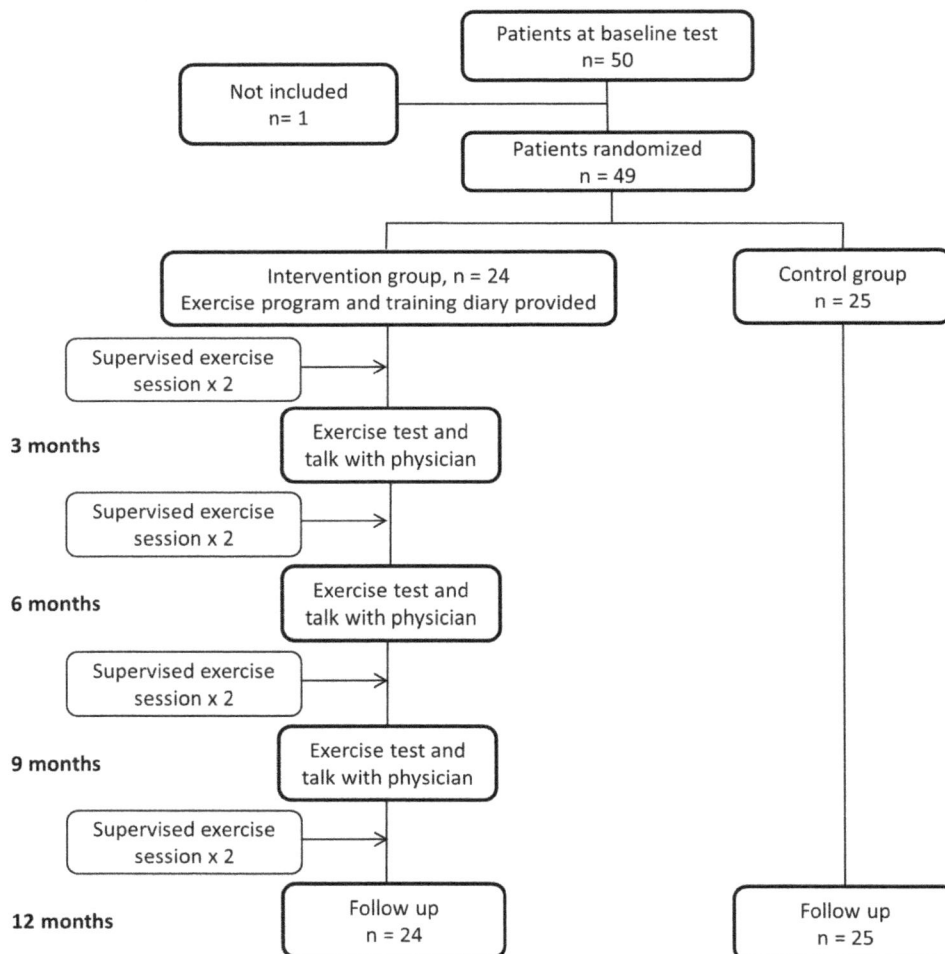

Figure 1. Flow chart of participants throughout the study.

the hospital. The HIIT program was based on protocols from previous studies [10–14], and consisted of 8–10 minutes of warm-up, followed by four times four minutes intervals, with an active pause of three minutes in-between intervals and at the end. The target heart rate was 85–95% of the maximum heart rate as measured at the initial exercise test in intervals, and 70% of maximum heart rate in the active pauses.

During the supervised exercise sessions once per month, patients walked or ran on treadmills (Woodway PPS55, Weil am Rhein, Germany), wearing heart rate monitors (Polar Electro, Kempele, Finland) to ensure that they reached target heart rate. An experienced physiotherapist and/or exercise physiologist instruct-ed and motivated the patients on how to perform HIIT, and patients were asked about their home exercise training and encouraged to maintain a high level of activity. Such instructions have previously been found to be enough to give an acceptable adherence to exercise training during 6 months [10]. The written exercise program also explained in detail how to perform the HIIT, and patients were instructed to perform HIIT as home-based exercise training, as activities which engaged large muscle groups, i.e. walking uphill, running, cross-country skiing, or bicycling. Patients were told to either use a heart rate monitor to ensure that the intensity was adequate, or to exercise with an intensity making them breathe heavily during home exercise training. We gave no advice regarding diet or other lifestyle factors during the follow-up period.

Every third month, patients in the maintenance group did a maximum exercise test as described below. These tests were done to monitor their exercise capacity; to give patients individualized feedback on their VO_{2peak} level, and to ensure them that maximal effort was well tolerated.

Control group. Patients in the control group received no instructions in how to exercise apart from what was given by the rehabilitation staff at the hospitals as usual care. In the two participating hospitals, CAD patients are encouraged to be physically active but are not given any concise exercise prescrip-tion. The control group attended baseline and 12 months follow-up tests as described below, without any other contact with the study or hospital personnel.

Outcomes and follow-up

The primary outcome measure was change in VO_{2peak} between baseline and 12 months follow-up. Secondary outcome measures were physical activity level, resting blood pressure, health-related quality of life, cardiometabolic blood markers and anthropometric measurements. In the original study protocol, endothelial function measurements (flow mediated dilatation of the brachial artery) were described. Due to technical issues at one of the participating hospitals, endothelial function could not be included in the study. Physical activity registration was not pre-specified in the original protocol, but during the preparation phase of the study it became clear that such data would be needed and thus physical activity questionnaires and activity monitors were included into the protocol.

Peak oxygen uptake. All patients performed a treadmill cardiopulmonary maximum exercise test at baseline and at follow-up after 12 months, without discontinuation of prescribed medication. Gas exchange data was analysed (Oxycon Pro, Jaeger, Hoechberg, Germany) continuously using mixing chamber, and patients were monitored with a 12-lead electrocardiogram during maximum exercise tests. After 10 minutes of warm-up, we individually adjusted a ramp protocol, by increasing the incline and speed of the treadmill, for the test to last 8–12 minutes as recommended [15]. The test was terminated when the patients

reported to be exhausted, or if clinical symptoms occurred. Peak oxygen uptake (VO_{2peak}) was calculated as the mean of the three highest VO_2 measurements during the test, each obtained over a 10-sec average. Peak heart rate was recorded at the end of the test and was not compared to age predicted values as the patients were taking betablockers. We did not use a threshold value of respiratory exchange ratio (RER) as a criterion for reaching VO_{2peak}, but average RER-values obtained during the tests are outlined in the results. Heart rate recovery was defined as the change in heart rate from the peak heart rate to the heart rate after one minute of rest standing on the treadmill.

Physical activity level. All patients reported physical activity level by questionnaires. They were asked how often they exercised (≤ 1, 2–3, ≥ 4 sessions per week), the mean duration of each exercise session (< 30, 30–45, 45–60, > 60 minutes per session), and the mean intensity-level during sessions (light, medium or hard intensity). In a subgroup of patients (n = 18, 37%), everyday physical activity level was measured with an on-body activity monitoring system (Sensewear, Bodymedia Inc., Pittsburgh, PA, USA) worn for 3–7 days during the first 1–3 weeks and repeated during the last 1–3 weeks in the follow-up period. We measured the numbers of steps taken per day, and the time spent in different activity level zones defined by metabolic equivalents (METs). Sedentary time was defined as activity < 3 METs, moderate physical activity was defined as activity ≥ 3 and < 6 METs, and vigorous physical activity was defined as ≥ 6 METs.

Resting blood pressure and resting heart rate. Resting systolic and diastolic blood pressure was measured sitting after 10 minutes of rest with a calibrated automated blood pressure monitor (Welch Allyn, Germany). Blood pressure was automati-cally measured three times by the monitor, and the average value of the two last measurements was used. Resting heart rate was measured, after 10 minutes of rest in supine position, using electrocardiogram. Height was measured to the nearest centimetre and body weight was measured to the nearest 0.1 kg using a Seca 877 scale (Seca Corp, Germany). Body mass index was calculated as body weight in kilograms divided by the square of height in meter. Waist circumference was measured to the nearest half centimetre, using a measuring tape at the height of the umbilicus.

Blood markers. Venous blood samples were drawn after 12 hours of fasting, and analysed using accredited in-hospital procedures for serum glucose, total cholesterol, low-density lipoprotein cholesterol, high-density lipoprotein cholesterol, tri-glycerides, and high-sensitive C-reactive protein (all using standard commercial kits on a Roche Modular P, Roche, Basel, Switzer-land), and glycosylated haemoglobin (Roche Cobas Integra 400).

Health related quality of life. Health related quality of life was measured by MacNew Heart Disease Health-Related Quality of Life Questionnaire [16]. This is a disease-specific questionnaire with a validated Norwegian translation [17]. The questionnaire assesses social, emotional, and physical quality of life using a 1–7 scale. Higher scores indicated better quality of life and a change of 0.5 is found to be clinically significant [16].

Sample size and statistics

A decline in VO_{2peak} of 2.0 $mL \cdot kg^{-1} \cdot min^{-1}$ (SD 4.0) could be expected after 12 months without formal rehabilitation [18]. We anticipated that the intervention program would give an increase of 2.0 $mL \cdot kg^{-1} \cdot min^{-1}$ after 12 months, giving a difference of 4.0 $mL \cdot kg^{-1} \cdot min^{-1}$ compared to usual care. This yields a standardised difference of 4/4 = 1. With a two-tailed t-test for independent samples at a power (1-β) of 0.9 and α = 0.05, a total of 44 subjects had to be enrolled [19]. To allow for an expected 10% drop out, we aimed at including 48 patients. The actual statistical analysis performed takes within-person correlation into account and thereby improves power.

Observed data are given as frequencies with percentages in parenthesis, or means ± standard deviation (SD). Baseline characteristics were compared using the chi square test, Mann-Whitney U-test or student t-test where appropriate. Changes from baseline to follow-up are reported with 95% confidence intervals (CI) using a univariate general linear model in the analyses. To test for differences between groups, we used a univariate general linear model analysis of covariance (ANCOVA) with Bonferroni adjustments. In the model, the change in the outcome variable (Δ-values) was the dependent variable, with group as fixed factor and baseline values of the outcome variable as covariates [20]. Between-group differences are reported with 95% CIs and p-values. Within- and between-group differences were considered significant if the 95% CI did not include zero [21]. Physical activity data are only presented as descriptive statistics. All statistical analyses were performed using SPSS (version 20.0, IBM, Chicago, IL, USA).

Results

Forty-nine patients (15 women) were recruited from January 2011 to March 2012 at St.Olav's Hospital and from November 2011 to June 2012 at Ålesund Hospital. Patient characteristics at baseline can be found in Table 1. All registered variables at baseline were comparable between groups except for age, which was lower in the control group (p<0.05, Table 1), and VO_{2peak}, which was higher in the control group (p<0.01, Table 2).

We experienced no adverse events during maximum exercise testing or training sessions. All participants completed scheduled tests, and the mean attendance at training sessions was 7.8 out of 8

sessions in the intervention group. None of the patients changed their medication use during the study period. During follow-up, two patients in each group were hospitalized. In the intervention group, one patient was diagnosed with a duodenal ulcer and atrial fibrillation, and one patient was diagnosed with chronic lymphatic leukaemia. In the control group, one patient experienced a tibia fracture and one patient underwent surgical treatment for breast carcinoma.

We found no within-group changes in VO_{2peak} from baseline to follow-up, and no between-group difference ($p = 0.22$, Table 2). In the intervention group, VO_{2peak} was at its highest at the third maximum exercise test, and declined slightly at test number four and five (Figure 2). We found no changes in resting heart rate, heart rate recovery, blood pressure, neither within- or between-groups from baseline to follow-up. Blood markers did not change during follow-up in any group (Table 2). Quality of life (social domain) was increased in the control group, but there was no between-group difference ($p = 0.39$).

Self-reported physical activity level is summarized in Table 3. In the intervention group, all patients reported some regular physical activity both at baseline and follow-up, whereas 5 patients in the control group reported no regular physical activity at follow-up. The majority of patients in both groups reported that they had been physically active 2–3 times per week, with duration of 45–60 minutes and with a medium intensity. Physical activity level was adequately monitored in 18 patients (37%). The mean number of steps taken per day was 7024 in the intervention group (10 patients), and 9338 in the control group (8 patients). The mean time spent in sedentary, moderate and vigorous activity level zones per day was 1333 minutes, 58 minutes and 3 minutes in the intervention group. The corresponding numbers in the control

Table 1. Patient characteristics and medication use at baseline.

	Intervention group (n = 24)	Control group (n = 25)
Sex, male/female	18/6	18/7
Age, years (range)	64.4 (47–78)	58.5 (42–71)*
Treatment qualifying for referral to rehabilitation		
PCI	15 (63)	15 (60)
CABG	7 (29)	7 (28)
Valve replacement	2 (8)	1 (4)
Cardiomyopathy	0 (0)	2 (8)
Co-morbidity		
Heart failure	3 (13)	4 (16)
PAD	0 (0)	1 (4)
Hypertension	11 (46)	13 (52)
Diabetes	4 (17)	3 (12)
Medication at baseline		
Aspirin	24 (100)	25 (100)
Clopidogrel	18 (75)	16 (64)
Warfarin	1 (4)	1 (4)
Betablockers	19 (79)	19 (76)
Statins	23 (96)	25 (100)
ACE/ARA	9 (38)	11 (44)

Data are given as numbers with percentages in parenthesis when not otherwise specified. PCI; percutaneous coronary intervention, CABG; coronary artery bypass grafting, PAD; peripheral artery disease, ACE; angiotensin converting enzyme inhibitors, ARA; angiotensin II receptor antagonists. * Between group difference at baseline (p = 0.02).

Table 2. Outcome measures at baseline and after 12 months follow-up.

	Intervention group (n = 24)			Control group (n = 25)			ANCOVA	
	Baseline	12 months	Change scores (95% CI)	Baseline	12 months	Change scores (95% CI)	Between-group difference (95% CI)	P value
Exercise test								
VO$_{2peak}$ ml·kg^{-1}·min^{-1}	27.9±4.7	28.8±5.6	0.9 (−0.6, 2.4)	32.0±6.2	32.8±5.8	0.8 (−0.5, 2.2)	0.6 (−1.5, 2.7)	0.58
VO$_{2peak}$ ml·min^{-1}	2405±517	2533±576	129 (−18, 275)	2535±760	2614±734	79 (−45, 203)	−0.04 (−0.2, 0.2)	0.70
RER$_{peak}$	1.09±0.07	1.09±0.09	0.004 (−0.03, 0.04)	1.10±0.07	1.09±0.06	−0.01 (−0.04, 0.01)	−0.01 (−0.05, 0.03)	0.71
HR$_{peak}$, beats	154.7±13.1	155.8±15.9	1.1 (−5.1, 7.3)	160.6±11.3	161.6±13.1	1.0 (−2.3, 4.2)	1.4 (−5.5, 8.3)	0.68
HR recovery, beats	27.7±11.2	31.2±14.6	3.5 (−1.9, 8.9)	28.9±10.0	30.1±10.2	1.2 (−2.9, 5.4)	−1.7 (−8.3, 4.9)	0.60
Resting measurements								
HR, beats/min	64.0±10.2	65.7±11.6	1.6 (−1.5, 4.8)	61.2±11.5	63.2±11.1	2.0 (−1.4, 5.4)	−0.2 (−4.8, 4.4)	0.92
Systolic BP, mmHg	132.8±14.7	133.7±16.4	0.9 (−4.4, 6.2)	131.3±14.5	134.3±14.0	3.0 (−2.3, 8.2)	1.4 (−5.9, 8.8)	0.69
Diastolic BP, mmHG	78.8±7.2	79.3±7.5	0.5 (−2.1, 3.1)	75.1±10.7	77.5±10.0	2.4 (−1.5, 6.2)	−0.08 (−4.8, 4.6)	0.97
Anthropometric measurements								
Weight, kg	86.8±15.6	89.0±16.5	2.1 (0.8, 3.5)*	79.2±17.8	79.9±17.3	0.7 (−0.8, 2.2)	−1.5 (−3.6, 0.5)	0.14
BMI, kg/m^2	28.0±3.9	28.7±4.1	0.7 (0.2, 1.1)*	25.8±3.3	26.1±3.2	0.3 (−0.2, 0.7)	−0.5 (−1.2, 0.2)	0.16
Waist, cm	101.4±12.1	103.2±11.7	1.8 (0.1, 3.5)*	92.6±9.8	93.0±9.4	0.3 (−0.8, 1.5)	−2.2 (−4.2, −0.1)‡	0.04
Quality of life								
Emotional domain	6.0±0.8	6.0±0.6	0.1 (−0.2, 0.3)	5.7±0.8	6.1±0.8	0.4 (−0.2, 0.7)	0.1 (−0.4, 0.6)	0.69
Physical domain	6.2±0.7	6.3±0.6	0.1 (−0.2, 0.4)	6.3±0.6	6.4±0.5	0.1 (−0.1, 0.3)	0.1 (−0.2, 0.5)	0.40
Social domain	6.4±0.6	6.5±0.4	0.1 (−0.1, 0.3)	6.4±0.6	6.7±0.4	0.3 (0.1, 0.5)*	0.1 (−0.1, 0.4)	0.37
Blood markers								
hsCPR, mg/L	1.09±0.9	1.07±0.6	−0.02 (−0.3, 0.3)	1.2±0.9	1.5±2.5	0.3 (−0.7, 1.3)	0.4 (−0.7, 1.4)	0.51
Cholesterol, mmol/L	4.3±1.0	4.3±0.8	−0.08 (−0.4, 0.2)	3.9±0.6	3.9±0.8	−0.02 (−0.2, 0.2)	−0.1 (−0.5, 0.3)	0.57
LDL, mmol/L	2.2±0.9	2.2±0.7	−0.03 (−0.3, 0.2)	2.0±0.5	2.0±0.6	0.01 (−0.2, 0.2)	−0.0 (−0.4, 0.2)	0.70
HDL, mmol/L	1.5±0.4	1.5±0.4	0.05 (−0.02, 0.13)	1.3±0.4	1.3±0.4	0.004 (−0.05, 0.05)	−0.04 (−0.1, 0.04)	0.34
TG, mmol/L	1.4±0.8	1.2±0.7	−0.19 (−0.4, 0.01)	1.2±0.6	1.3±1.1	0.07 (−0.3, 0.4)	0.2 (−0.2, 0.6)	0.24
Glucose, mmol/L	6.7±3.7	6.4±2.2	−0.3 (−0.6, 0.1)	6.0±1.8	6.2±2.4	0.2 (−0.2, 0.6)	0.3 (−0.4, 1.0)	0.43
HbA1c, %	6.1±1.2	6.0±1.0	−0.1 (−0.2, −0.01)*	6.1±0.7	6.2±1.4	0.1 (−0.1, 0.4)	0.2 (−0.1, 0.6)	0.21

VO$_{2peak}$; peak oxygen uptake, RER$_{peak}$; respiratory exchange ratio at peak oxygen uptake, HR$_{peak}$; peak heart rate, HRR, 1 min; heart rate recovery the first minute after ending an exercise test, HR; resting heart rate, SBP; systolic blood pressure, DBP; diastolic blood pressure, BMI; body mass index, hsCRP; high-sensitive C-reactive protein, LDLc; low-density lipoprotein cholesterol, HDLc; high-density lipoprotein cholesterol, TG; triglycerides, HbA1c; glycosylated haemoglobin.
* indicates within-group changes from baseline to 12 months,
‡ indicates between groups changes in mean difference.

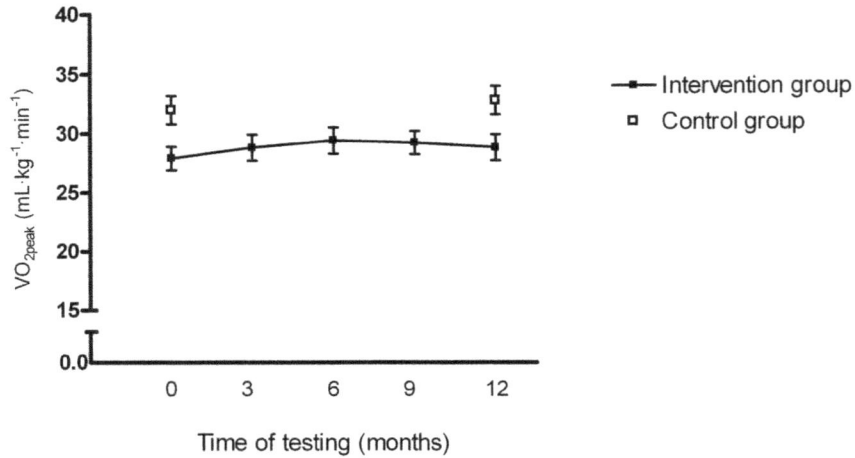

Figure 2. Peak oxygen uptake in the intervention group at baseline, after 3, 6 and 9 months, and at follow-up, and peak oxygen uptake in the control group at baseline and follow-up. The bars represent ± standard error of mean.

group were 1288 minutes, 111 minutes, and 7 minutes, respectively.

Discussion

In this randomized trial we assessed whether patients with CAD discharged from cardiac rehabilitation would benefit with respect to VO_{2peak} by attending a maintenance exercise program for 12 months compared to usual care of no formal follow-up. Our main finding was that the maintenance program did not improve VO_{2peak} compared to usual care. However, neither group deteriorated with respect to exercise capacity during follow-up.

This was to us unexpected as exercise capacity has been found to decrease in CAD patients after discharge from formal rehabilitation when the patients were not aware of the last follow-up test [18].

We can only suggest some potential explanations for our findings. Participants enrolled in clinical exercise studies may be highly motivated to perform exercise, especially when they are aware of future follow-up tests. This was illustrated by Gupta et al. [22] who found an increased level of physical activity and 6-minute walking distance at 12 months after discharge from cardiac rehabilitation. Also Izawa et al. [23] demonstrated high exercise maintenance in patients with myocardial infarction 18 months

Table 3. Self-reported physical activity.

Self-reported	Intervention group (n = 24)		Control group (n = 25)	
	Baseline	Follow-up	Baseline	Follow-up
	n = 19*	n = 21*	n = 22*	n = 22*
Frequency				
No exercise	0 (0)	0 (0)	1 (5)	5 (23)
<1/week	1 (5)	0 (0)	0 (0)	0 (0)
1/week	0 (0)	1 (5)	0 (0)	2 (9)
2–3/week	12 (63)	16 (76)	17 (77)	14 (64)
≥4/week	6 (32)	4 (19)	4 (18)	1 (4)
Duration				
<30 min	0 (0)	1 (5)	1 (5)	0 (0)
30–45 min	6 (31.5)	6 (28.5)	2 (9)	5 (29.5)
45–60 min	10 (52.5)	8 (38)	11 (50)	5 (29.5)
>60 min	3 (16)	6 (28.5)	7 (36)	7 (41)
Intensity				
Low	1 (5)	1 (5)	1 (5)	1 (6)
Medium	16 (84)	11 (52)	13 (62)	10 (59)
High	2 (11)	9 (43)	7 (33)	6 (35)

Data are given as numbers with percentages in parenthesis.
* Valid questionnaires for 19 patients at baseline and 21 patients at follow-up in the intervention group, and 22 patients at baseline and follow-up in the control group.

after cardiac rehabilitation. Both these studies had an observational design without strategies to improve exercise adherence after ending formal rehabilitation, and with patients being aware of future follow-ups. We argue that the knowledge of future follow-up tests by cardiac rehabilitation units may act as a motivation for increased levels of physical activity. This may have also been the case in our study. In fact, the objectively measured physical activity indicated that patients in the control group spent more time in the moderate activity level zone and had a higher daily step count than the patients in the intervention group. Patients randomized to the intervention group were on average 6 years older than in the control group, possibly explaining the tendency for lower level of physical activity in the intervention group. Previous studies have found adherence to physical activity to decline with age [24,25]. However, a previous study found no significant effect of age on improvement in VO_{2peak} after HIIT in patients with CAD [26]. We therefore think that the potential effect of age was on the adherence to exercise rather than on the physiological adaptations to HIIT. Of note, all included patients had some knowledge of HIIT, as this was included in the cardiac rehabilitation program prior to study inclusion.

Several studies have demonstrated that HIIT is superior to moderate continuous exercise in improving VO_{2peak} in patients with CAD [12,27,28] without compromising safety [29]. In the current study, patients in the intervention group were invited to attend a monthly supervised HIIT session at the hospital. However, one monthly session of HIIT is obviously not enough to improve or maintain exercise capacity, and therefore patients also received a training program with the aim of three sessions of HIIT per week. A previous study [10] of home-based HIIT after coronary artery bypass grafting has shown good adherence to such exercise prescription. According to the self-reported physical activity data in the current study, however, only about one third of patients in the intervention group reported that they exercised with high-intensity 2–3 times a week. Thus, a lack of adherence to prescribed exercise at home in the maintenance group is probably the single most important explanation to the lack of VO_{2peak} improvement at 12 months.

Our study may have implications for clinical rehabilitation units. We argue that all patients with CAD enrolled in a rehabilitation program should be offered one or several follow-up sessions, and that a maximum exercise testing should preferably be a part of this follow-up. Our data implies that this type of follow-up may be sufficient to prevent deterioration with respect to VO_{2peak}. However, follow-up programs of infrequent supervised exercise sessions seemed not to be effective. It is possible that a maintenance program with more frequent supervised exercise could have resulted in improvements in VO_{2peak}. In a study of patients with congestive heart failure, Prescott et al. [30] found a small beneficial effect in patients that followed a low-cost maintenance training program with group training sessions every two weeks, indicating that supervised sessions must be more frequent than in our study to result in increased work capacity.

The complete follow-up testing of patients and the high adherence to the supervised exercise are regarded as strengths of our study. Our study is however limited by the fact that the study group consisted of relatively young patients, who probably were quite motivated to exercise without formal follow-up during 12 months. Thus, our results may not be valid for older and less motivated patients with established CAD. Also, neither investigators nor participants were blinded for the study endpoints, which could raise concerns regarding objectivity of testing. However, all patients were told to exercise to complete exhaustion at every exercise test. Further, there was no difference in peak heart rate or peak RER achieved during the baseline and the follow-up test. We also chose to inform the patients in the intervention group about their VO_{2peak} at intermediate tests as we considered it to act motivating for sustained or increase levels of exercise training.

Conclusions

A 12-month maintenance exercise program consisting of infrequent supervised HIIT sessions, a home-based HIIT program and regular exercise testing did not result in improved adherence to exercise or increased VO_{2peak} in CAD patients compared to usual care. However, both the intervention and the control group sustained their VO_{2peak} 12 months after discharge from formal cardiac rehabilitation.

Author Contributions

Conceived and designed the experiments: TM EM IA. Performed the experiments: TM EM IA LW IG. Analyzed the data: TM EM. Contributed reagents/materials/analysis tools: IG LW IA TM EM. Wrote the paper: EM TM. Collected all data at Åelsund Hospital: IG LW.

References

1. Jolliffe JA, Rees K, Taylor RS, Thompson D, Oldridge N, et al. (2001) Exercise-based rehabilitation for coronary heart disease. Cochrane Database Syst Rev: CD001800.
2. Taylor RS, Brown A, Ebrahim S, Jolliffe J, Noorani H, et al. (2004) Exercise-based rehabilitation for patients with coronary heart disease: systematic review and meta-analysis of randomized controlled trials. American Journal of Medicine 116: 682–692.
3. Clark AM, Hartling L, Vandermeer B, McAlister FA (2005) Meta-analysis: secondary prevention programs for patients with coronary artery disease. Annals of Internal Medicine 143: 659–672.
4. O'Connor GT, Buring JE, Yusuf S, Goldhaber SZ, Olmstead EM, et al. (1989) An overview of randomized trials of rehabilitation with exercise after myocardial infarction. Circulation 80: 234–244.
5. Myers J, Prakash M, Froelicher V, Do D, Partington S, et al. (2002) Exercise capacity and mortality among men referred for exercise testing. New England Journal of Medicine 346: 793–801.
6. Keteyian SJ, Brawner CA, Savage PD, Ehrman JK, Schairer J, et al. (2008) Peak aerobic capacity predicts prognosis in patients with coronary heart disease. American Heart Journal 156: 292–300.
7. Moholdt T, Aamot IL, Granoien I, Gjerde L, Myklebust G, et al. (2011) Long-term follow-up after cardiac rehabilitation: a randomized study of usual care exercise training versus aerobic interval training after myocardial infarction. International Journal of Cardiology 152: 388–390.
8. Fletcher GF (2007) Cardiac rehabilitation: Something old—something new—more to do. J Cardiopulm Rehabil Prev 27: 21–23.
9. Weston KS, Wisloff U, Coombes JS (2013) High-intensity interval training in patients with lifestyle-induced cardiometabolic disease: a systematic review and meta-analysis. Br J Sports Med. 48: 1227–1234
10. Moholdt T, Bekken Vold M, Grimsmo J, Slordahl SA, Wisloff U (2012) Home-based aerobic interval training improves peak oxygen uptake equal to residential cardiac rehabilitation: a randomized, controlled trial. PLoS One 7: e41199.
11. Moholdt T, Aamot IL, Granoien I, Gjerde L, Myklebust G, et al. (2012) Aerobic interval training increases peak oxygen uptake more than usual care exercise training in myocardial infarction patients: a randomized controlled study. Clin Rehabil 26: 33–44.
12. Rognmo O, Hetland E, Helgerud J, Hoff J, Slordahl SA (2004) High intensity aerobic interval exercise is superior to moderate intensity exercise for increasing aerobic capacity in patients with coronary artery disease. Eur J Cardiovasc Prev Rehabil 11: 216–222.

13. Wisloff U, Stoylen A, Loennechen JP, Bruvold M, Rognmo O, et al. (2007) Superior cardiovascular effect of aerobic interval training versus moderate continuous training in heart failure patients: a randomized study. Circulation 115: 3086–3094.

14. Aamot IL, Forbord SH, Gustad K, Lockra V, Stensen A, et al. (2013) Home-based versus hospital-based high-intensity interval training in cardiac rehabilitation: a randomized study. Eur J Prev Cardiol. doi: 10.1177/2047487313488299

15. Froelicher V, Myers J (2006) Exercise and the heart. 5th edn. Philadelphia: Saunders Elsevier.

16. Hofer S, Lim L, Guyatt G, Oldridge N (2004) The MacNew Heart Disease health-related quality of life instrument: a summary. Health Qual Life Outcomes 2: 3.

17. Hiller A, Helvik AS, Kaasa S, Slordahl SA (2010) Psychometric properties of the Norwegian MacNew Heart Disease health-related quality of life inventory. Eur J Cardiovasc Nurs 9: 146–152.

18. Moholdt T, Aamot IL, Granoien I, Gjerde L, Myklebust G, et al. (2011) Long-term follow-up after cardiac rehabilitation A randomized study of usual care exercise training versus aerobic interval training after myocardial infarction. Int J Cardiol 152: 388–390.

19. Machin D (1997) Sample size tables for clinical studies. 2nd edn. Oxford: Blackwell Science.

20. Vickers AJ, Altman DG (2001) Statistics notes: Analysing controlled trials with baseline and follow up measurements. BMJ 323: 1123–1124.

21. Gardner MJ, Altman DG (1986) Confidence intervals rather than P values: estimation rather than hypothesis testing. Br Med J (Clin Res Ed) 292: 746–750.

22. Gupta R, Sanderson BK, Bittner V (2007) Outcomes at one-year follow-up of women and men with coronary artery disease discharged from cardiac rehabilitation: what benefits are maintained? J Cardiopulm Rehabil Prev 27: 11–18.

23. Izawa KP, Yamada S, Oka K, Watanabe S, Omiya K, et al. (2004) Long-term exercise maintenance, physical activity, and health-related quality of life after cardiac rehabilitation. American Journal of Physical Medicine and Rehabilitation 83: 884–892.

24. Jefferis BJ, Sartini C, Lee IM, Choi M, Amuzu A, et al. (2014) Adherence to physical activity guidelines in older adults, using objectively measured physical activity in a population-based study. BMC Public Health 14: 382.

25. Lohne-Seiler H, Hansen BH, Kolle E, Anderssen SA (2014) Accelerometer-determined physical activity and self-reported health in a population of older adults (65-85 years): a cross-sectional study. BMC Public Health 14: 284.

26. Moholdt T, Madssen E, Rognmo O, Aamot IL (2013) The higher the better? Interval training intensity in coronary heart disease. J Sci Med Sport. doi: 10.1016/j.jsams.2013.07.007

27. Moholdt TT, Amundsen BH, Rustad LA, Wahba A, Lovo KT, et al. (2009) Aerobic interval training versus continuous moderate exercise after coronary artery bypass surgery: a randomized study of cardiovascular effects and quality of life. American Heart Journal 158: 1031–1037.

28. Moholdt T, Aamot IL, Granoien I, Gjerde L, Myklebust G, et al. (2012) Aerobic interval training increases peak oxygen uptake more than usual care exercise training in myocardial infarction patients: a randomized controlled study. Clinical Rehabilitation 26: 33–44.

29. Rognmo O, Moholdt T, Bakken H, Hole T, Molstad P, et al. (2012) Cardiovascular risk of high- versus moderate-intensity aerobic exercise in coronary heart disease patients. Circulation 126: 1436–1440.

30. Prescott E, Hjardem-Hansen R, Dela F, Orkild B, Teisner AS, et al. (2009) Effects of a 14-month low-cost maintenance training program in patients with chronic systolic heart failure: a randomized study. Eur J Cardiovasc Prev Rehabil 16: 430–437.

24

Relationship between Neural Rhythm Generation Disorders and Physical Disabilities in Parkinson's Disease Patients' Walking

Leo Ota[1]*, Hirotaka Uchitomi[1], Ken-ichiro Ogawa[1], Satoshi Orimo[2], Yoshihiro Miyake[1]

1 Department of Computational Intelligence and Systems Science, Tokyo Institute of Technology, Yokohama, Kanagawa, Japan, 2 Department of Neurology, Kanto Central Hospital, Setagaya, Tokyo, Japan

Abstract

Walking is generated by the interaction between neural rhythmic and physical activities. In fact, Parkinson's disease (PD), which is an example of disease, causes not only neural rhythm generation disorders but also physical disabilities. However, the relationship between neural rhythm generation disorders and physical disabilities has not been determined. The aim of this study was to identify the mechanism of gait rhythm generation. In former research, neural rhythm generation disorders in PD patients' walking were characterized by stride intervals, which are more variable and fluctuate randomly. The variability and fluctuation property were quantified using the coefficient of variation (CV) and scaling exponent α. Conversely, because walking is a dynamic process, postural reflex disorder (PRD) is considered the best way to estimate physical disabilities in walking. Therefore, we classified the severity of PRD using CV and α. Specifically, PD patients and healthy elderly were classified into three groups: no-PRD, mild-PRD, and obvious-PRD. We compared the contributions of CV and α to the accuracy of this classification. In this study, 45 PD patients and 17 healthy elderly people walked 200 m. The severity of PRD was determined using the modified Hoehn–Yahr scale (mH-Y). People with mH-Y scores of 2.5 and 3 had mild-PRD and obvious-PRD, respectively. As a result, CV differentiated no-PRD from PRD, indicating the correlation between CV and PRD. Considering that PRD is independent of neural rhythm generation, this result suggests the existence of feedback process from physical activities to neural rhythmic activities. Moreover, α differentiated obvious-PRD from mild-PRD. Considering α reflects the intensity of interaction between factors, this result suggests the change of the interaction. Therefore, the interaction between neural rhythmic and physical activities is thought to plays an important role for gait rhythm generation. These characteristics have potential to evaluate the symptoms of PD.

Editor: Oscar Arias-Carrion, Hospital General Dr. Manuel Gea González, Mexico

Funding: This work was supported by the Ministry of Education, Culture, Sports, Science and Technology (MEXT) Grant-in-Aid for Scientific Research (B) to Dr. Miyake (MEXT KAKENHI Grant Number 23300209, URL: http://www.mext.go.jp/english/). The funders had no role in study design, data collection and analysis, decision to publish, or preparation of the manuscript.

Competing Interests: The authors have declared that no competing interests exist.

* Email: ohta@myk.dis.titech.ac.jp

Introduction

Walking is one of the most fundamental factors in our daily behaviors. The gait dynamics is thought to be generated by the interaction between neural rhythmic activity and physical activity [1,2]. However, because this interaction is difficult to estimate in healthy gait dynamics, we focused on the patients with Parkinson's disease (PD) (as a typical example of neurodegenerative disease) [3], which causes not only neural rhythm generation disorders, but also physical disabilities. To identify the mechanism of gait rhythm generation, we attempted to examine the relationship between neural rhythmic activity and physical activity in PD patients.

In previous studies, two symptoms were reported as neural rhythm generation disorders in PD patients' walking. One symptom was the increase in the variability of gait rhythm [4,5], and the other symptom was a change in the fluctuation property of gait rhythm from the normal $1/f$-like fluctuation property [6–8]. In healthy young people, gait rhythm is not constant; rather, it changes subtly. This change can be described by a pair of physical measures. One is the coefficient of variation (CV), which

represents the variability of gait rhythm. The other is the scaling exponent α, which represents the fluctuation property of gait rhythm and can be calculated by detrended fluctuation analysis (DFA). In particular, the fluctuation in gait rhythm is an important feature of walking. In healthy young people, the gait rhythm exhibits small variation and $1/f$-like fluctuation properties [9].

For each of these symptoms, two types of gait rehabilitation methods using sensory cues have been proposed. One is gait training with rhythmic stimuli, which is based on forced entrainment for human, including rhythmic auditory stimulation (RAS) gait training [10] and treadmill training [11]. The other is gait training with rhythmic stimuli, which is based on mutual entrainment with human, such as WalkMate gait training [12]. In RAS gait training, fixed-tempo rhythmic auditory stimuli are input to PD patients [10]. This type of rehabilitation improves mainly the variability of gait rhythm. In other words, RAS gait training decreases CV but does not change α much [8,13]. We have been developing the WalkMate system [12]. In WalkMate gait training, rhythmic auditory stimuli mutually entrained with the gait rhythm of PD patients [14]. This type of rehabilitation improves mainly the fluctuation property of gait rhythm [14]. In one study, α improved substantially, but CV did not change much after four consecutive days of WalkMate gait training [15]. These findings suggest that RAS gait training and WalkMate gait training improve different features of neural rhythm generation disorders in PD patients' walking.

Conversely, PD patients often also show physical disabilities. Postural instability is one of the main motor symptoms of physical disability in PD, and its clinical manifestations are a festinant and shuffling gait, poor postural alignment, and defective postural reflexes. There are many tests for assessing the postural instability and balance control related to the risk of falling [16]. Regarding gait dynamics, the pull test [17], which is a test of postural reflex disorder (PRD), is the most suitable to evaluate physical disabilities during a dynamic state, such as walking.

However, it is not clear whether CV and α, which evaluates the different features of neural rhythm generation disorders, are related to PRD, which evaluate physical disabilities. The purpose of this study was to examine the relationship between the set of CV and α, and PRD on a platform aimed at evaluating the gait rhythm in PD patients, to identify the mechanism of gait rhythm generation. To construct this evaluation platform, we focused on a combination of CV and α, because it can be considered as a feature amount that represents neural rhythm generation disorders. Subsequently, we classified the subjects according to the presence or absence of PRD using the platform for gait rhythm. Furthermore, the severity of PRD in a group of PD patients was classified using the platform for gait rhythm. The modified Hoehn–Yahr (mH-Y) scale [18,19] was used as the method of evaluation of the clinical signs of PRD.

In the Methods section, we describe the demographic information of participants, gait task, and the method of measurement of stride interval. Then, we explain the calculation of two dynamic indicators: the variability of the stride interval (CV) and the fluctuation property of the stride interval (α). We mention a linear discriminant analysis using a combination of CV and α, and the classification of PRD using mH-Y. In the Results section, the results of the two classifications are shown, and the accuracy and contribution of CV or α to the classifications are reported. In the Discussion section, we discuss the mechanism underlying neural rhythm generation disorders in PD patients' walking and a potential application of this platform to evaluate the motor symptoms of PD.

Methods

Participants

Forty-five patients (21 men, 24 women; mean age ± SD, 69.8±8.2 years) with PD and 17 age-matched healthy people (10 men, seven women; mean age, 70.2±2.8 years) participated in this study (Table 1). The mean disease duration (± SD) was 4.7±3.9 years. The mH-Y classifications and number of subjects were mH-Y 1–2 ($n = 19$), mH-Y 2.5 ($n = 11$), and mH-Y 3 ($n = 15$). All patients were taking at least one of antiparkinsonian medications during the experiment. The antiparkinsonian medications included levodopa/carbidopa, dopamine receptor agonist, selegiline, amantadine, and anticholinergics. Those were taken at maximum two hours before the start time of measurement. All participants could walk without a cane or walker. These experimental procedures were approved by the Kanto Central Hospital Ethics Committee. Before the experiment, we obtained written informed consent from the participants.

Gait tasks and measurement of stride interval

Participants walked at their preferred pace along a 200 m round course. We measured gait rhythm once for each participant and calculated the stride interval time series. Stride interval is defined as the time duration between two consecutive foot contacts on the same side. Foot switches (OT-21BP-G, Ojiden, Japan) were attached under the shoes and were used to detect the gait rhythm. The mean number (± SD) of stride intervals was 154±23 strides for the 200 m. Data for foot contact timing were sent to a laptop PC (CF-W5AWDBJR, Panasonic, Japan) via a wireless transmitter (S-1019M1F, Smart Sensor Technology, Japan). The sampling frequency was 100 Hz. We used only the data obtained for the left side because no significant differences between stride interval were observed between the left and right sides (left side: mean = 1.06±0.09 s, CV = 2.73% ±1.09%, α = 0.80±0.21; right side: mean = 1.06±0.09 s, CV = 2.78% ±1.62%, α = 0.81±0.22; P-values based on Welch's two-sample t test: $P = 0.97$ for mean, $P = 0.82$ for CV, $P = 0.92$ for α). We analyzed the data obtained for the right side in only one patient because a high noise level was observed in the data for the left side. To assess only the stable stride interval phase, the first 10 strides and last five strides (i.e., the transient stride interval phase) were not analyzed.

CV

We focused on the CV as a dynamic indicator to evaluate the variability of stride interval in the participants. CV represents the variability of time-series data, and is calculated as the standard deviation normalized to the mean value: $CV = SD/Mean \times 100$ [%]. The CV of healthy people is 1%–2.5%, and the CV of PD patients is 2.5%–4% [6].

DFA

We focused on the scaling exponent α as the other dynamic indicator to evaluate the fluctuation property. The scaling exponent α can be quantified by DFA as a long-range correlation in time series data [20,21]. We selected this method because it can also be applied to relatively short intervals [22].

If the α is nearly equal to 0.5, the time series is characterized by white noise. On the other hand, if α is near 1.0, the series is characterized by $1/f$ fluctuation and is suggested to be generated by chaos dynamics or limit cycle dynamics coupled with noise [23–26]. The α of the stride interval at the preferred pace has been reported as 0.50–0.85 in PD patients [6,8] and as 0.8–1.2 in healthy young people [27,28]. In healthy elderly people, the α of the stride interval is decreased to 0.7–0.9, although the CV remains unchanged [7,28,29].

Linear discriminant analysis

Fisher's linear discriminant analysis was used with a combination of CV and α to obtain a function for dividing the measured data into two groups [30].

The leave-one-out cross-validation method was used to estimate the classification rate, and the following were calculated: (1) accuracy, the rate of truly classified data among all data; (2) sensitivity, the accuracy rate for identifying positive data (participants with more severe symptoms); and (3) specificity, the accuracy rate for identifying negative data (participants with mild symptoms). To compare the individual contribution to the classification of CV and α, these two variables were normalized using a Z score, and the angle between the normalized CV axis and the boundary line was calculated by a linear discriminant function.

Table 1. Characteristics of the participants.

Classification	Difference between PRD and no-PRD			Difference between obvious-PRD and mild-PRD		
Positive/Negative	Positive (PRD, $n=26$)	Negative (no-PRD, $n=36$)	P	Positive (obvious-PRD, $n=15$)	Negative (mild-PRD, $n=11$)	P
Age (years, mean ± SD)	72.7±7.0	68.1±6.9	0.01	72.5±6.7	72.4±7.5	0.83
Sex (male:female)	15:11	16:20	0.31	8:7	7:4	0.61
Disease duration (years, mean ± SD)	4.9±4.6	2.3±3.1	0.01	6.2±5.5	4.0±2.8	0.35
mH-Y score in "on" state (median, range)	3, 2.5–3	1.25, 0–2	–	3, 3	2.5, 2.5	–

P values were calculated using Welch's two-sample t test.
PRD, postural reflex disorder; mH-Y, modified Hoehn–Yahr scale.

Classification of PRD

Walking is controlled in parallel with posture and muscle-tone control [31–34]. Postural instability, which is one of the physical disabilities, can be often evaluated by the Berg Balance Test [16]. However, when considering gait dynamics, the pull test (30th item in the Unified Parkinson's Disease Rating Scale) is the most suitable for estimating the ability of physical activities in walking [17]. Therefore, we focused on the pull test to identify the presence or absence of PRD and its severity. In the pull test, the shoulder of a PD patient is pulled backward and forward while the patient remains standing. An overview of the classification is shown in Figure 1. Performance on the pull test is associated with mH-Y, which is one of the clinical indicators used for the assessment of motor symptoms of PD [19].

The scores in the original H-Y range from 1 to 5, in increments of 1. The mH-Y includes added stages 1.5, and 2.5 [19]. We separated participants into three groups based on their mH-Y score and performance on the pull test: mH-Y score of 2 or less with no problems on the pull test (no-PRD), mH-Y = 2.5 with signs of mild disorder on the pull test (mild-PRD), and mH-Y = 3 with obvious signs of disorder on the pull test (obvious-PRD). No-PRD was determined by a normal postural reflex in the pull test. Mild-PRD was defined by very mild postural impairment (suggestive, but not diagnostic; usually one or two steps before recovery from a postural threat) [19]. Obvious-PRD was determined by the presence of retropulsion, which is defined by (1) the appearance of more than three backward steps during the pull test, followed by unaided recovery, (2) the absence of postural reflex, or (3) the indication of falling if the examinee is not supported [17]. Although the examiner's decision regarding need of support in the pull test is subjective, we paid careful attention to the classification of PRD. All participants were examined by the same doctor in the same environment. Furthermore, the doctor is a PD expert who is authorized by the Japanese Society of Neurology. Therefore, the results of the mH-Y staging were reproducible.

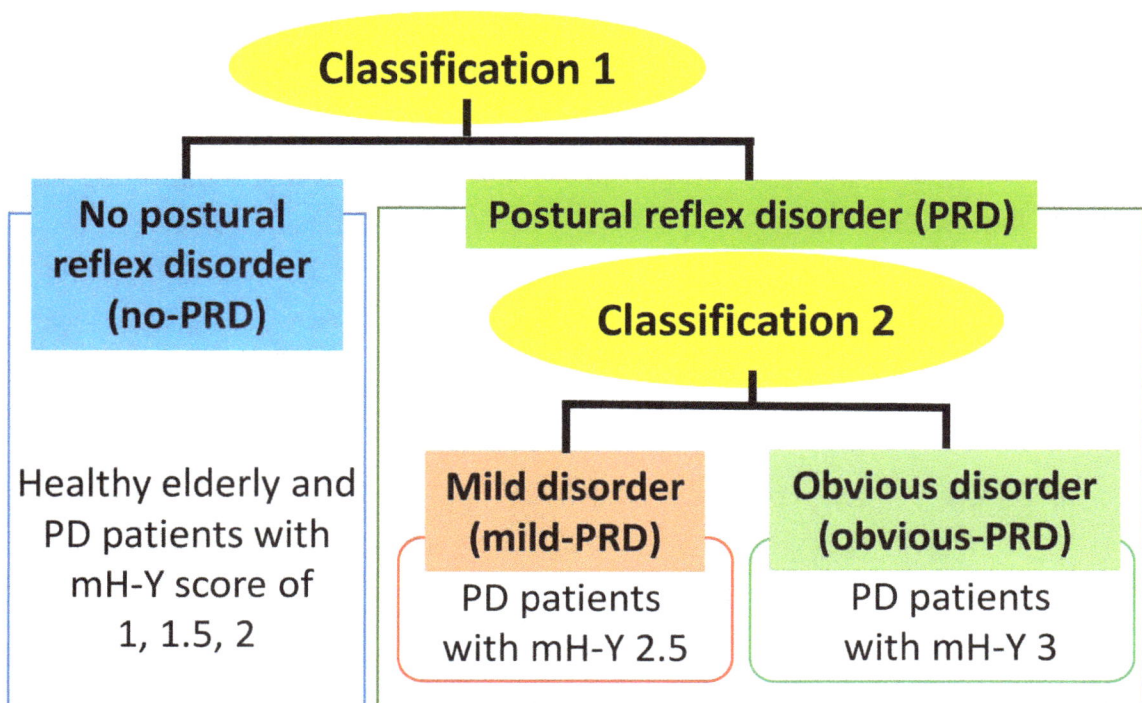

Figure 1. Classification of the severity of postural reflex disorder (PRD).

We first classified participants according to the presence and absence of PRD (Classification 1 in Figure 1, see Table 1). This classification segregated the no-PRD group (17 healthy elderly people and two PD patients, one with an mH-Y score of 1 and one with a score of 1.5) from the PRD group. We then divided the PRD group of patients into the mild-PRD and obvious-PRD groups (Classification 2 in Figure 1, see Table 1).

Results

Figure 2 shows a sample result of the gait analysis, including the stride interval time series and the result of DFA. The CV of the stride interval was larger in PD patients with PRD (Figure 2A, B) than in healthy people (Figure 2C). The α of the stride interval (Figure 2A) was lower in PD patients with obvious-PRD than in PD patients with mild-PRD (Figure 2B), in PD patients with no-PRD (Figure 2C), or in healthy elderly people (Figure 2D).

Classification 1: The presence or absence of PRD

First, we classified the PD patients and healthy elderly people into two groups according to the presence or absence of PRD. The no-PRD group comprised healthy elderly participants and PD patients with an mH-Y score of 1–2, and the PRD group comprised PD patients with an mH-Y score of 2.5–3. Figure 3A shows the distribution of all participants' data for the feature space configured by CV and α of the stride interval; namely, (CV, α) plane. The x-axis represents CV, and the y-axis represents α. The blue points represent the data for the no-PRD group, and the green points represent the data for the PRD group. On the y-axis of α in Figure 3A, the data for each group overlapped between 0.5 and 1.0. In contrast, the no-PRD group data were distributed in a

scattered pattern in the low-CV area, and the data for the PRD group were scattered in the high-CV area.

Figure 3B shows the distribution of normalized data, to indicate which axis contributes to the classification of the two groups regardless of the variation in each axis. The solid line represents the boundary line between the two groups. When we defined the no-PRD group as negative and the PRD group as positive, the accuracy was 74%, the sensitivity was 50%, and the specificity was 92%. The angle between the normalized CV axis and the boundary line shown in Figure 3B was 91°. The large angle observed between the normalized CV axis and the boundary line suggests that the CV can be used to differentiate between presence and absence of PRD.

Classification 2: Obvious-PRD or mild-PRD

Next, we focused on the two PRD groups: obvious-PRD and mild-PRD. The mild-PRD group comprised PD patients with an mH-Y score of 2.5, and the obvious-PRD group comprised PD patients with an mH-Y score of 3. Figure 4A shows the distribution of data of the PRD group in CV, α) plane. The red points represent the data for the mild-PRD group, and the light-green points represent the data for the obvious-PRD group. On the x-axis of CV in Figure 4A, the data for both groups overlap between 2.5 and 6.0. By contrast, the α for the mild-PRD group tended to scatter near 1.0 (i.e., the $1/f$-like fluctuation property was observed), and the α for the obvious-PRD group tended to scatter around 0.6 (i.e., the $1/f$-like fluctuation property was detected less often).

When we defined the mild-PRD group as negative and the obvious-PRD group as positive, the accuracy was 69%, the

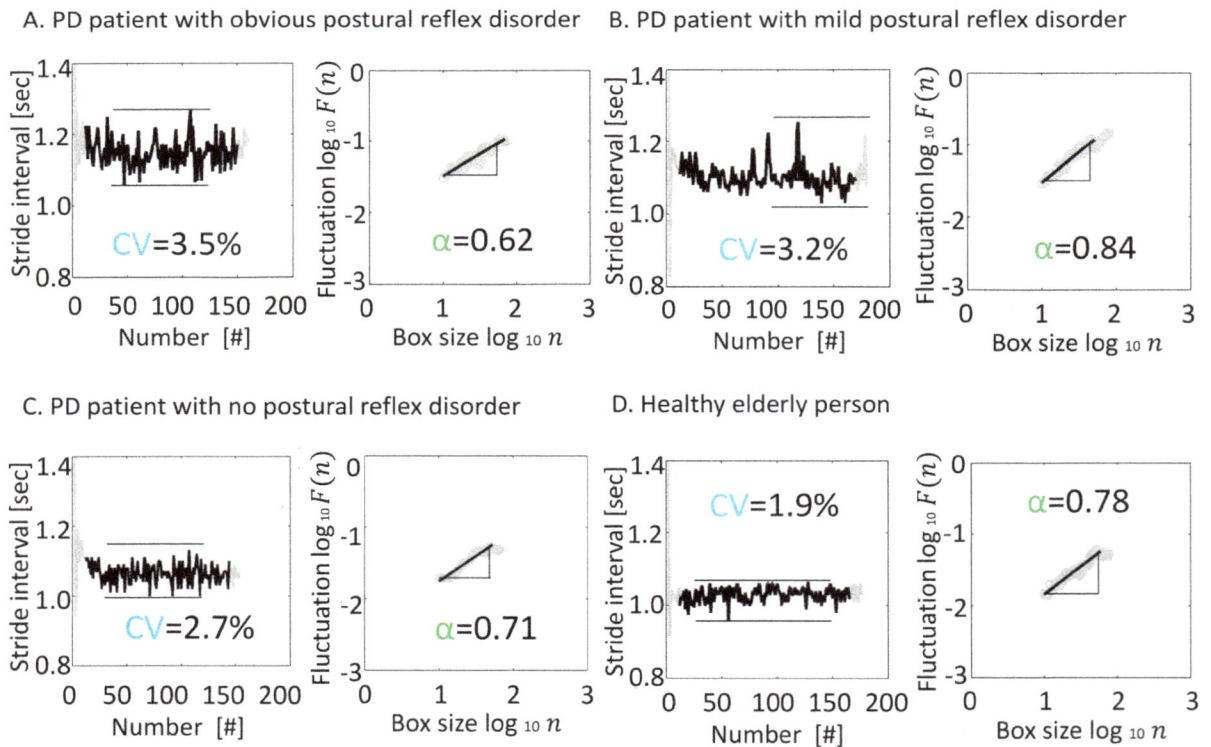

Figure 2. A sample of the stride interval and the fluctuation relative to box size. (A) PD patient with obvious postural reflex disorder (mH-Y score, 3; age 76 years; male). (B) PD patient with mild postural reflex disorder (mH-Y score, 2.5; age, 70 years; male). (C) PD patient with no postural reflex disorder (mH-Y score, 2; age, 76 years; male). (D) Healthy elderly person (age. 71 years; male).

A

B

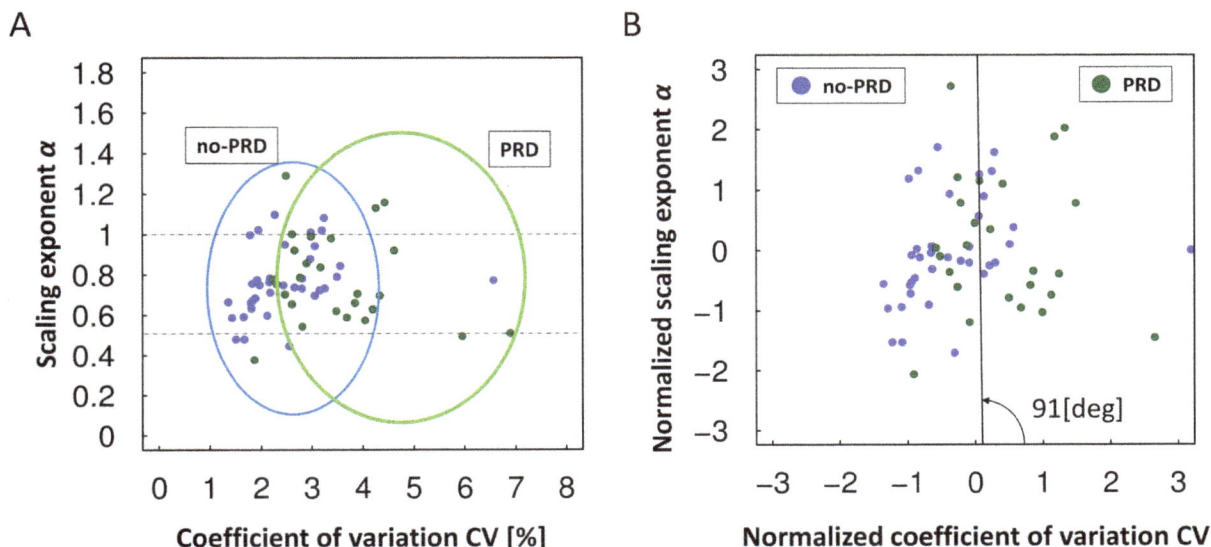

Figure 3. Classification according to the presence or absence of postural reflex disorder. The no postural reflex disorder group (no-PRD) is indicated by blue points, and the postural reflex disorder group (PRD) is indicated by green points. The x-axis represents the CV, and the y-axis represents α. The data for the no-PRD group are distributed in a small CV region around 2%, whereas those for the PRD group are distributed in a large CV region roughly from 2.5% to 5%. The two groups have a wide and overlapping distribution of α. (A) Distribution of the original data. (B) Distribution of the normalized data. The solid line represents the boundary between the no-PRD group and the PRD group.

sensitivity was 80%, and the specificity was 55%. The solid line represents the boundary line between the two groups, and the dashed line represents a horizontal line that corresponds to the average level of the original value of α. The angle between the normalized CV axis and the boundary line shown in Figure 4B was 5.7°. The small angle observed between the normalized CV axis and the boundary line suggests that α can be used to differentiate obvious-PRD from mild-PRD.

Discussion

In this study, we used CV to evaluate the variability of gait rhythm, and the scaling exponent α to evaluate the fluctuation property of gait rhythm. These are two important indicators of neural rhythm generation disorders in PD patients. We performed a linear discriminant analysis based on a combination of CV and α to differentiate between the presence and absence of PRD, and between obvious-PRD and mild-PRD. As a result, CV differentiated between the presence and absence of PRD, indicating the

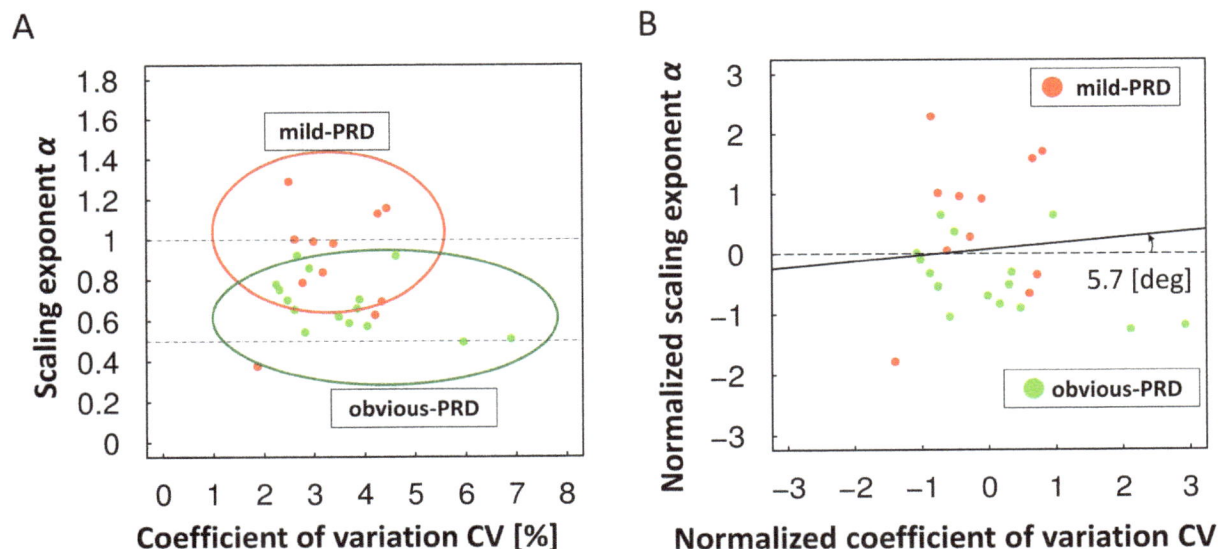

A

B

Figure 4. Classification of obvious and mild postural reflex disorder. The mild postural reflex disorder group (mild-PRD) is indicated by red points, and the obvious postural reflex disorder group (obvious-PRD) is indicated by light-green points. The x-axis represents the CV, and the y-axis represents α. (A) Distribution of the original data. (B) Distribution of the normalized data. The solid line represents the boundary between the mild-PRD and obvious-PRD groups.

strong correlation between the change of CV and symptoms of PRD. Considering that the mechanism of PRD is independent of the neural rhythmic activities, this result suggests the existence of feedback process from physical activities to neural rhythmic activities. Furthermore, α differentiated between mild-PRD and obvious-PRD. Considering α reflects the strength of interaction or relationship between factors, this result suggests the existence of interaction between physical activities and neural rhythmic activities. Therefore, the interaction between neural rhythmic activities and physical activities is thought to play an important role for gait disabilities in PD.

We now discuss the relationship between neural rhythm generation disorders and physical disabilities based on the results obtained in this study. Figure 5 summarizes the results of the classification used in this study. CV and α are dynamic indicators of neural rhythm generation disorders, and PRD is a clinical indicator of the severity of a physical disability. Area A in Figure 5 represents a low CV: i.e., the variability of the gait rhythm of the participants was small. Moreover, the participants who appeared in this area had no symptoms of PRD. Area B represents a large CV and a high α: i.e., the variability was large but the 1/f-like fluctuation property was observed. In addition, these patients had mild symptoms of PRD. Area C represents a large CV and a low α: i.e., the variability of the gait rhythm of the patients was large, and the 1/f-like fluctuation property was not observed. In addition, these patients showed obvious symptoms of PRD.

When considering the manner in which neural rhythm generation disorders progress during the transition from the healthy state to obvious-PRD, we find an important factor in walking. At first, the patient's gait rhythm tends to transfer from the area A to area B in (CV, α) plane during the transition from no-PRD to mild-PRD. This result shows that there are strong correlation between the occurrence of PRD and the increase of CV. It might be natural to be considered that the change of neural rhythm generation give rise to the disabilities for physical activity. However the mechanism of PRD is independent of development of neural rhythmic generation, because the enhancement and suppression function of the muscle tone, which is related to the occurrence of PRD, is considered to work in parallel with the function of gait rhythm generation [31–34]. Therefore, this means that physical activity is fed back to neural rhythm activity in walking. Considering the fact that neural rhythmic activity always affects the physical activity, our result suggests the existence of interaction between neural rhythmic activity and physical activity. Next, the gait rhythm tends to transfer from area B to area C during the transition from mild-PRD to PRD. This shows that there are strong correlation between progression of the severity of PRD and the decrease of α. In other words, this transition is observed as the weakening process of the 1/f fluctuation from the state we can observe the 1/f fluctuation. The 1/f fluctuation property is defined by the frequency spectrum whose power is proportional to the inverse of frequency. In general, 1/f-like

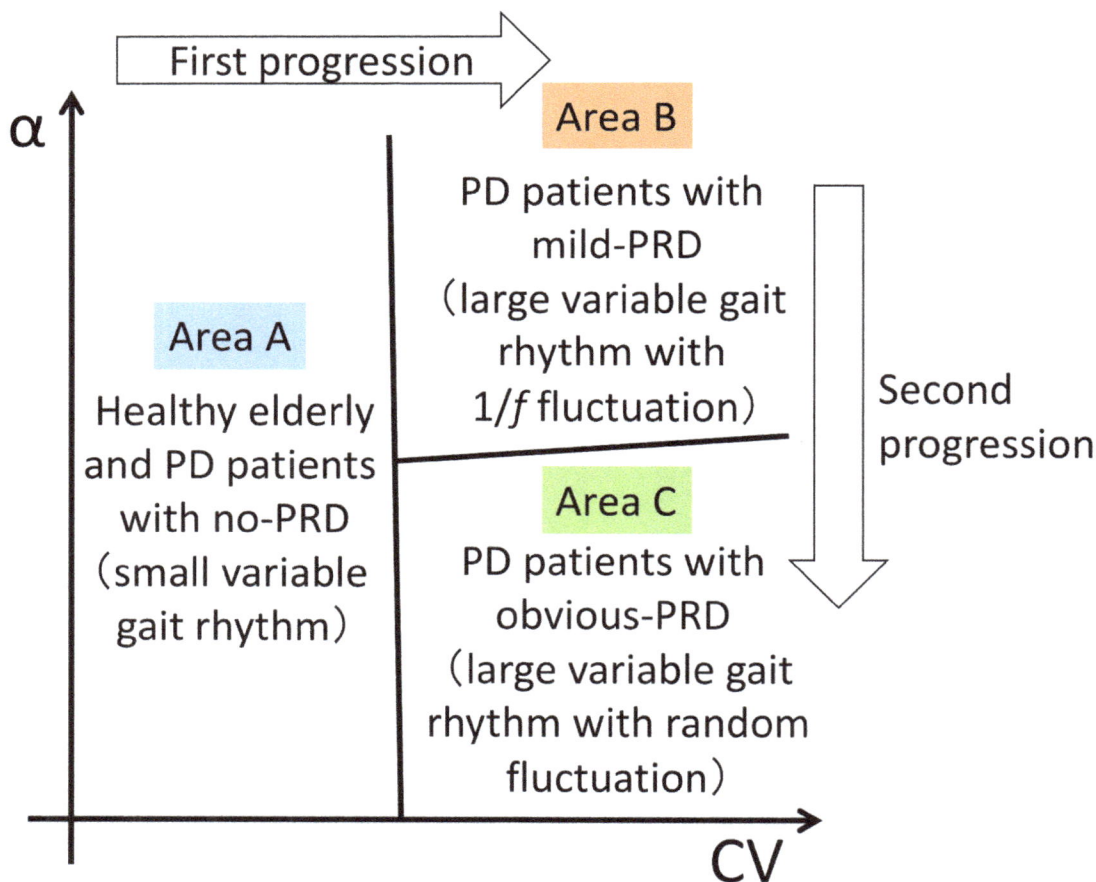

Figure 5. Concept of the evaluation platform. The x-axis is related to the CV of the stride interval, and the y-axis is related to the α of the stride interval. PRD, postural reflex disorder.

fluctuation is mainly generated by the interaction between multiple factors [9,23–28]. Therefore, the change of time series structure of the gait rhythm can be regarded as the intensity change of interaction. This result suggests that the intensity of interaction on the mechanism of gait rhythm generation is weakened by the progression of severity of PRD. This complement the fact that the interaction between neural rhythmic activity and physical activity plays an important role in gait rhythm generation.

When considering all these points, we summarize the development mechanism of gait rhythm generation disorders. The gait rhythm of the patients in area A (small CV) in Figure 5 represented the state without physical disabilities. The gait rhythm of the patients in area B (large CV, high α) represented the state that is controlled mainly by the interaction between neural rhythmic and physical activities against the physical disabilities. The gait rhythm of the patients in area C (large CV, low α) represented the destabilized state in response to weakening of the interaction between neural rhythmic and physical activities. These findings suggest that it is possible to construct an evaluation platform for neural rhythm generation disorders by combining the CV and α parameters, and to use this system to evaluate the progression of physical disabilities.

This information on Figure 5 may provide clues for evaluating the progress of PD patients during rehabilitation using RAS gait training or WalkMate gait training. RAS gait training decreases CV [8,13]. This type of gait training may improve the first progression involving variability of gait rhythm: i.e., transition from the right half-plane (area B or area C) to the left half-plane (area A) in (CV, α) plane. On the other hand, the WalkMate gait training increases the $1/f$-like fluctuation property [14,15]. This type of gait training may improve the second progression involving the fluctuation property: i.e., the transition from area C to area B. Therefore, based on this platform, we were able to extract information not only on the presence or absence of PRD, but also on the severity of PRD using (CV, α) plane for evaluating neural rhythm generation disorders. Using this system to evaluate neural rhythm generation disorders may help physical therapists to choose a rehabilitation method that fits the severity of the patients' physical disabilities.

Acknowledgments

We would like to thank all participants at the Kanto Central Hospital for their cooperation with this study. We are also grateful to the researchers who gave us useful information and to our colleagues, particularly Michael J. Hove at Harvard University and Kazuki Suzuki, Toshitaka Nomura, and Shou Itou at the Tokyo Institute of Technology for their support and for instructive comments about gait measurement and analysis.

Author Contributions

Conceived and designed the experiments: LO HU KO SO YM. Performed the experiments: LO HU SO YM. Analyzed the data: LO HU KO YM. Contributed reagents/materials/analysis tools: LO HU YM. Wrote the paper: LO HU KO SO YM. Subject recruitment: SO.

References

1. Pearson KG (2000) Neural adaptation in the generation of rhythmic behavior. Annu Rev Physiol 62: 723–753.

2. Taga G, Yamaguchi Y, Shimizu H (1991) Self-organized control of bipedal locomotion by neural oscillators in unpredictable environment. Biol Cybern 65: 147–159.

3. Jankovic J (2008) Parkinson's disease: clinical features and diagnosis. J Neurol Neurosurg Psychiatry 79: 368–376.

4. Hausdorff JM, Cudkowicz ME, Firtion R, Wei JY, Goldberger AL (1998) Gait variability and basal ganglia disorders: stride-to-stride variations of gait cycle timing in Parkinson's disease and Huntington's disease. Mov Disord 13: 428–437.

5. Schaafsma JD, Giladi N, Balash Y, Bartels AL, Gurevich T, et al. (2003) Gait dynamics in Parkinson's disease: relationship to Parkinsonian features, falls and response to levodopa. J Neurol Sci 212: 47–53.

6. Hausdorff JM, Lertratanakul A, Cudkowicz ME, Peterson AL, Kaliton D, et al. (2000) Dynamic markers of altered gait rhythm in amyotrophic lateral sclerosis. J Appl Physiol 88: 2045–2053.

7. Hausdorff JM (2007) Gait dynamics, fractals and falls: finding meaning in the stride-to-stride fluctuations of human walking. Hum Mov Sci 26: 555–589.

8. Hausdorff JM (2009) Gait dynamics in Parkinson's disease: common and distinct behavior among stride length, gait variability, and fractal-like scaling. Chaos 19: 026113. doi:10.1063/1.3147408.

9. Hausdorff JM, Peng CK, Ladin Z, Wei JY, Goldberger AL (1995) Is walking a random walk? Evidence for long-range correlations in stride interval of human gait. J Appl Physiol 78: 349–358.

10. Thaut MH, Abiru M (2010) Rhythmic auditory stimulation in rehabilitation of movement disorders: a review of the current research. Music Percept 27: 263–269.

11. Rubinstein TC, Giladi N, Haausdorff JM (2002) The power of cueing to circumvent dopamine deficits: a review of physical therapy treatment of gait disturbances in Parkinson's disease. Mov Disord 17: 1148–1160.

12. Miyake Y (2009) Interpersonal synchronization of body motion and the Walk-Mate walking support robot. Robot IEEE Trans 25: 638–644.

13. Hausdorff JM, Lowenthal J, Herman T, Gruendlinger L, Peretz C, et al. (2007) Rhythmic auditory stimulation modulates gait variability in Parkinson's disease. Eur J Neurosci 26: 2369–2375.

14. Hove MJ, Suzuki K, Uchitomi H, Orimo S, Miyake Y (2012) Interactive rhythmic auditory stimulation reinstates natural $1/f$ timing in gait of Parkinson's patients. PLoS ONE 7: e32600.

15. Uchitomi H, Ota L, Ogawa K-i, Orimo S, Miyake Y (2013) Interactive rhythmic cue facilitates gait relearning in patients with Parkinson's disease. PLoS ONE 8: e72176.

16. Thorbahn LDB, Newton RA (1996) Use of the Berg Balance Test to predict falls in elderly persons. Phys Ther 76: 576–583.

17. Bloem BR, Beckley DJ, Van Hilten BJ, Roos RAC (1998) Clinimetrics of postural instability in Parkinson's disease. J Neurol 245: 669–673.

18. Hoehn MM, Yahr MD (1967) Parkinsonism: onset, progression, and mortality. Neurology 17: 427–442.

19. Goetz CG, Poewe W, Rascol O, Sampaio C, Stebbins GT, et al. (2004) Movement Disorder Society Task Force report on the Hoehn and Yahr staging scale: status and recommendations. Mov Disord 19: 1020–1028.

20. Peng C-K, Buldyrev SV, Havlin S, Simons M, Stanley HE, et al. (1994) Mosaic organization of DNA nucleotides. Phys Rev E Stat Phys Plasmas Fluids Relat Interdiscip Topics 49: 1685–1689.

21. Peng C-K, Havlin S, Stanley HE, Goldberger AL (1995) Quantification of scaling exponents and crossover phenomena in nonstationary heartbeat time series. Chaos 5: 82–87.

22. Delignieres D, Ramdani S, Lemoine L, Torre K, Fortes M, et al. (2006) Fractal analyses for 'short' time series: a re-assessment of classical methods. J Math Psychol 50: 525–544.

23. Goldberger AL, Amaral LA, Hausdorff JM, Ivanov PC, Peng CK, et al. (2002) Fractal dynamics in physiology: alterations with disease and aging. Proc Natl Acad Sci U S A 99: 2466–2472.

24. Gates DH, Su JL, Dingwell JB (2007) Possible biomechanical origins of the long-range correlations in stride intervals of walking. Physica A 380: 259–270.

25. Ivanov PCh, Ma QDY, Bartsch RP, Hausdorff JM, Amaral LAN, et al. (2009) Levels of complexity in scale-invariant neural signals. Phys Rev E Stat Nonlin Soft Matter Phys 79: 041920.

26. Ahn J, Hogan N (2013) Long-range correlations in stride intervals may emerge from non-chaotic walking dynamics. PLoS ONE 8: e73239.

27. Hausdorff JM, Purdon PL, Peng CK, Ladin Z, Wei JY, et al. (1996) Fractal dynamics of human gait: stability of long-range correlations in stride interval fluctuation. J Appl Physiol 80: 1448–1457.

28. Hausdorff JM, Ashkenazy Y, Peng C-K, Ivanov PC, Stanley HE, et al. (2001) When human walking becomes random walking: fractal analysis and modeling of gait rhythm fluctuations. Physica A 302: 138–147.

29. Hausdorff JM, Mitchell SL, Firtion R, Peng CK, Cudkowicz ME, et al. (1997) Altered fractal dynamics of gait: reduced stride-interval correlations with aging and Huntington's disease. J Appl Physiol 82: 262–269.

30. Duda RO, Hart PE, Stork DG (2001) Pattern classification. 2nd ed. New York: Wiley. 654 p.

31. Takakusaki K, Hanaguchi T, Ohtinata-Sugimoto J, Saitoh K, Sakamoto T (2003) Basal ganglia efferents to the brainstem centers controlling postural muscle tone and locomotion: a new concept for understanding motor disorders in basal ganglia dysfunction. Neuroscience 119: 293–308.

32. Takakusaki K, Saitoh K, Harada H, Kashiwayanagi M (2004) Role of basal ganglia-brainstem pathways in the control of motor behaviors. Neurosci Res 50: 137–151.

33. Tomita N, Yano M (2007) Bipedal robot controlled by the basal ganglia and brainstem systems adjusting to indefinite environment. Proc 2007 IEEE/ICME International Conference on Complex Medical Engineering: 116–121.

34. Takakusaki K, Tomita N, Yano M (2008) Substrates for normal gait and pathophysiology of gait disturbances with respect to the basal ganglia dysfunction. J Neurol 255[Suppl 4]: 19–29.

Permissions

All chapters in this book were first published in PLOS ONE, by The Public Library of Science; hereby published with permission under the Creative Commons Attribution License or equivalent. Every chapter published in this book has been scrutinized by our experts. Their significance has been extensively debated. The topics covered herein carry significant findings which will fuel the growth of the discipline. They may even be implemented as practical applications or may be referred to as a beginning point for another development.

The contributors of this book come from diverse backgrounds, making this book a truly international effort. This book will bring forth new frontiers with its revolutionizing research information and detailed analysis of the nascent developments around the world.

We would like to thank all the contributing authors for lending their expertise to make the book truly unique. They have played a crucial role in the development of this book. Without their invaluable contributions this book wouldn't have been possible. They have made vital efforts to compile up to date information on the varied aspects of this subject to make this book a valuable addition to the collection of many professionals and students.

This book was conceptualized with the vision of imparting up-to-date information and advanced data in this field. To ensure the same, a matchless editorial board was set up. Every individual on the board went through rigorous rounds of assessment to prove their worth. After which they invested a large part of their time researching and compiling the most relevant data for our readers.

The editorial board has been involved in producing this book since its inception. They have spent rigorous hours researching and exploring the diverse topics which have resulted in the successful publishing of this book. They have passed on their knowledge of decades through this book. To expedite this challenging task, the publisher supported the team at every step. A small team of assistant editors was also appointed to further simplify the editing procedure and attain best results for the readers.

Apart from the editorial board, the designing team has also invested a significant amount of their time in understanding the subject and creating the most relevant covers. They scrutinized every image to scout for the most suitable representation of the subject and create an appropriate cover for the book.

The publishing team has been an ardent support to the editorial, designing and production team. Their endless efforts to recruit the best for this project, has resulted in the accomplishment of this book. They are a veteran in the field of academics and their pool of knowledge is as vast as their experience in printing. Their expertise and guidance has proved useful at every step. Their uncompromising quality standards have made this book an exceptional effort. Their encouragement from time to time has been an inspiration for everyone.

The publisher and the editorial board hope that this book will prove to be a valuable piece of knowledge for researchers, students, practitioners and scholars across the globe.

List of Contributors

Anne Hammarström and Arja Lehti
Department of Public Health and Clinical Medicine, Umeå University, Umeå, Sweden
Umeå Centre for Gender Studies in Medicine, Umeå University, Umeå, Sweden

Inger Haukenes
Department of Public Health and Clinical Medicine, Umeå University, Umeå, Sweden
Umeå Centre for Gender Studies in Medicine, Umeå University, Umeå, Sweden
Division of Mental Health, Department of Public Mental Health, Norwegian Institute of Public Health, Bergen, Norway

Anncristine Fjellman Wiklund and Maria Wiklund
Umeå Centre for Gender Studies in Medicine, Umeå University, Umeå, Sweden
Department of Community Medicine and Rehabilitation, Physiotherapy, Umeå University, Umeå, Sweden

Birgitta Evengård
Department of Clinical Microbiology, Division of Infectious Diseases, Umeå University, Umeå, Sweden

Britt-Marie Stålnacke
Umeå Centre for Gender Studies in Medicine, Umeå University, Umeå, Sweden
Department of Community Medicine and Rehabilitation, Rehabilitation Medicine, Umeå University, Umeå, Sweden

Michael King, Helen Killaspy and Tatiana L. Taylor
Mental Health Sciences Unit, University College London, London, United Kingdom

Sarah White, Christine Wright and Penny Turton
Division of Population Health Sciences and Education, St George's University London, London, United Kingdom

Thomas Kallert
Department of Psychiatry, Psychosomatic Medicine and Psychotherapy, Park Hospital Leipzig, Leipzig, Germany

Mirjam Schuster
University Hospital Department of Psychiatry and Psychotherapy, Dresden University of Technology, Dresden, Germany

Jorge A. Cervilla
San Cecilio University Hospital Mental Health Unit, University of Granada, Granada, Spain

Paulette Brangier
Biomedical Research Centre Mental Health Network, University of Granada, Granada, Spain

Jiri Raboch and Lucie Kalisova
Department of Psychiatry, Charles University, Prague, Czech Republic

Georgi Onchev and Spiridon Alexiev
Department of Psychiatry, Medical University Sofia, Sofia, Bulgaria

Roberto Mezzina and Pina Ridente
Department of Mental Health, Trieste Healthcare Agency, Trieste, Italy

Durk Wiersma and Ellen Visser
University Medical Center Groningen, University of Groningen, Groningen, The Netherlands

Andrzej Kiejna and Patryk Piotrowski
Department of Psychiatry, Wroclaw Medical University, Wroclaw, Poland

Dimitris Ploumpidis and Fragiskos Gonidakis
University Mental Health Research Institute, Athens, Greece

José Miguel Caldas-de-Almeida and Graça Cardoso
Faculty of Medical Science, New University of Lisbon, Lisbon, Portugal

Marco Franceschini and Patrizio Sale
Department of NeuroRehabilitation IRCCS San Raffale, Pisana, Rome

Anais Rampello and Maurizio Agosti
Department of Rehabilitation, University Hospital of Parma, Parma, Italy

Maurizio Massucci
Rehabilitation Unit, Hospital of Passignano, Passignano, Perugia, Italy

Federica Bovolenta
Medicine Rehabilitation NOCSAE Hospital AUSL of Modena, Modena, Italy

Ken Takiyama
Graduate School of Frontier Sciences, Department of Complex Science and Engineering, The University of Tokyo, Chiba, Tokyo, Japan

Masato Okada
Graduate School of Frontier Sciences, Department of Complex Science and Engineering, The University of Tokyo, Chiba, Tokyo, Japan
RIKEN Brain Science Institute,Wako, Japan

Janne Marieke Veerbeek, Erwin van Wegen and Marc Rietberg
Department of Rehabilitation Medicine, MOVE Research Institute Amsterdam, VU University Medical Center, Amsterdam, The Netherlands

Roland van Peppen
Department of Physiotherapy, University of Applied Sciences Utrecht, Utrecht, The Netherlands

Philip Jan van der Wees
Scientific Institute for Quality of Healthcare (IQ healthcare), Radboud University Nijmegen Medical Center, Nijmegen, The Netherlands

Erik Hendriks
Department of Epidemiology, Maastricht University, Maastricht, The Netherlands

Gert Kwakkel
Department of Rehabilitation Medicine, MOVE Research Institute Amsterdam, VU University Medical Center, Amsterdam, The Netherlands
Department of Neurorehabilitation, Reade Center for Rehabilitation and Rheumatology, Amsterdam, The Netherlands

Ecaterina Vasluian, Ingrid G. M. de Jong, Heleen A. Reinders-Messelink and Corry K. van der Sluis
Department of Rehabilitation Medicine, University Medical Center Groningen, University of Groningen, Groningen, The Netherlands

Wim G. M. Janssen
Department of Rehabilitation Medicine, Erasmus Medical Center Rotterdam, Rotterdam, The Netherlands

Margriet J. Poelma
Rehabilitation Center De Sint Maartenskliniek, Nijmegen, The Netherlands

Iris van Wijk
Rehabilitation Center De Hoogstraat, Utrecht, The Netherlands

Rafael A. Molina-López
Centre de Fauna Salvatge de Torreferrussa, Catalan Wildlife-Service-Forestal Catalana, Santa Perpètua de la Mogoda, Barcelona, Spain
Departament de Sanitat I Anatomia Animals, Facultat de Veterinària, Universitat Autònoma de Barcelona, Cerdanyola del Vallès, Barcelona, Spain

Jordi Casal and Laila Darwich
Departament de Sanitat I Anatomia Animals, Facultat de Veterinària, Universitat Autònoma de Barcelona, Cerdanyola del Vallès, Barcelona, Spain
Centre de Recerca en Sanitat Animal (CReSA), UAB-IRTA, Campus Universitat Autònoma de Barcelona, Cerdanyola del Vallès, Barcelona, Spain

Jinsung Wang, Yuming Lei, Khongchee Xiong and Katie Marek
Department of Kinesiology, The University of Wisconsin, Milwaukee, Wisconsin, United States of America

David E. Crane
Heart and Stroke Foundation Canadian Partnership for Stroke Recovery, Sunnybrook Research Institute, Toronto, Ontario, Canada

Bradley J. MacIntosh
Heart and Stroke Foundation Canadian Partnership for Stroke Recovery, Sunnybrook Research Institute, Toronto, Ontario, Canada
Physical Sciences, Sunnybrook Research Institute, Toronto, Ontario, Canada
Department of Medical Biophysics, University of Toronto, Toronto, Ontario, Canada

Walter Swardfager
Heart and Stroke Foundation Canadian Partnership for Stroke Recovery, Sunnybrook Research Institute, Toronto, Ontario, Canada

Neuropsychopharmacology Research Group, Sunnybrook Research Institute, Toronto, Ontario, Canada

Nipuni Ranepura and Mahwesh Saleem
Neuropsychopharmacology Research Group, Sunnybrook Research Institute, Toronto, Ontario, Canada

Nathan Herrmann
Neuropsychopharmacology Research Group, Sunnybrook Research Institute, Toronto, Ontario, Canada
Department of Psychiatry, University of Toronto, Toronto, Ontario, Canada

Paul I. Oh
Department of Clinical Pharmacology, University of Toronto, Toronto, Ontario, Canada,
Toronto Rehabilitation Institute, Toronto, Ontario, Canada

Krista L. Lanctôt
Heart and Stroke Foundation Canadian Partnership for Stroke Recovery, Sunnybrook Research Institute, Toronto, Ontario, Canada
Neuropsychopharmacology Research Group, Sunnybrook Research Institute, Toronto, Ontario, Canada
Department of Psychiatry, University of Toronto, Toronto, Ontario, Canada

Bojana Stefanovic
Heart and Stroke Foundation Canadian Partnership for Stroke Recovery, Sunnybrook Research Institute, Toronto, Ontario, Canada
Physical Sciences, Sunnybrook Research Institute, Toronto, Ontario, Canada
Neuropsychopharmacology Research Group, Sunnybrook Research Institute, Toronto, Ontario, Canada

Judith Cohen-Bittan
Université Pierre et Marie Curie (UMRS 956, UMRS 1158), Paris, France

Jacques Boddaert and Marc Verny
Université Pierre et Marie Curie (UMRS 956, UMRS 1158), Paris, France
Department of Geriatrics, Groupe hospitalier (GH) Pitié-Salpêtrière, Assistance Publique Hôpitaux de Paris (APHP), Paris, France

Frédéric Khiami
Department of Orthopedic Surgery and Trauma, GH Pitié-Salpêtrière, APHP, Paris, France,

Yannick Le Manach
Departments of Anesthesia & Clinical Epidemiology and Biostatistics, Michael DeGroote School of Medicine, Faculty of Health Sciences, McMaster University, Hamilton, Ontario, Canada

Jean-Yves Beinis
Department of Rehabilitation, Groupe Hospitalier Charles Foix, APHP, Ivry-sur-Seine, France

Mathieu Raux
Université Pierre et Marie Curie (UMRS 956, UMRS 1158), Paris, France
Department of Anesthesiology and Critical Care, GH Pitié-Salpêtrière, APHP, Paris, France
Institut national de la santéet de la recherche mèdicale (UMRS 956, UMRS 1158, UMR 689), Paris, France

Bruno Riou
Université Pierre et Marie Curie (UMRS 956, UMRS 1158), Paris, France
Department of Emergency Medicine and Surgery, GH Pitié-Salpêtrière, APHP, Paris, France Institut national de la santéet de la recherche mèdicale (UMRS 956, UMRS 1158, UMR 689), Paris, France

Xia Zhang and Jianan Li
The First Affiliated Hospital of Nanjing Medical University, Nanjing, People's Republic of China
World Health Organization Liaison Sub–Committee on Rehabilitation Disaster Relief of the International Society of Physical and Rehabilitation Medicine, Geneva, Switzerland

James E. Gosney
World Health Organization Liaison Sub–Committee on Rehabilitation Disaster Relief of the International Society of Physical and Rehabilitation Medicine, Geneva, Switzerland

Jan D. Reinhardt
World Health Organization Liaison Sub–Committee on Rehabilitation Disaster Relief of the International Society of Physical and Rehabilitation Medicine, Geneva, Switzerland
Swiss Paraplegic Research, Nottwil, Switzerland
Department of Health Sciences and Health Policy, University of Lucerne, Lucerne, Switzerland

Gail F. Forrest
Human Performance and Engineering Laboratory, Kessler Foundation Research Center, West Orange, New Jersey, United States of America
Department of Physical Medicine and Rehabilitation, Rutgers, New Jersey Medical School, Newark, New Jersey, United States of America

Karen Hutchinson
Department of Physical Therapy and Athletic Training, Boston University, Boston, Massachusetts, United States of America

Douglas J. Lorenz
Department of Bioinformatics and Biostatistics, School of Public Health and Information Sciences, University of Louisville, Louisville, Kentucky, United States of America
Kentucky Spinal Cord Research Center, University of Louisville, Louisville, Kentucky, United States of America

Jeffrey J. Buehner
Wexner Medical Center at the Ohio State University-Dodd Hall, Columbus, Ohio, United States of America

Leslie R. VanHiel
Hulse Spinal Cord Injury Lab and Crawford Research Institute, Shepherd Center, Atlanta, Georgia, United States of America

Sue Ann Sisto
State University of New York at Stony Brook, School of Health Technology and Management, Research and Development Park, Rehabilitation Research and Movement Performance Laboratory, Stony Brook, New York, United States of America

D. Michele Basso
The Ohio State University, School of Allied Medical Professions, Center for Brain and Spinal Cord Repair, Columbus, Ohio, United States of America

Shuching Hsieh
Cardiovascular Research Methods Centre, University of Ottawa Heart Institute, Ottawa, Canada

George A. Wells and Ahmed Kotb
Department of Epidemiology and Community Medicine, University of Ottawa, Ottawa, Canada
Cardiovascular Research Methods Centre, University of Ottawa Heart Institute, Ottawa, Canada

Keith R. Lohse
School of Kinesiology, Auburn University, Auburn, Alabama, United States of America
School of Kinesiology, University of British Columbia, Vancouver, British Columbia, Canada

Courtney G. E. Hilderman and Katharine L. Cheung
Department of Physical Therapy, University of British Columbia, Vancouver, British Columbia, Canada

Sandy Tatla
Department of Occupational Science and Occupational Therapy, University of British Columbia, Vancouver, British Columbia, Canada

H. F. Machiel Van der Loos
Department of Mechanical Engineering, University of British Columbia, Vancouver, British Columbia, Canada

Natália de Almeida Carvalho Duarte
Master Program in Rehabilitation Sciences, Movement Analysis Lab, University Nove de Julho, São Paulo, São Paulo, Brazil

Luanda André Collange Grecco
Doctoral Program in Rehabilitation Sciences, Movement Analysis Lab, University Nove de Julho, São Paulo, São Paulo, Brazil

Manuela Galli
Dept. of Electronic Information and Bioengineering, Politecnico di Milano and IRCCS San Raffaele Pisana, Rome

Felipe Fregni
Laboratory of Neuromodulation & Center of Clinical Research Learning, Department of Physical Medicine & Rehabilitation, Spaulding Rehabilitation Hospital and Massachusetts General Hospital, Harvard Medical School, Boston, MA, United States of America

Cláudia Santos Oliveira
Professor, Master and Doctoral Programs in Rehabilitation Sciences, Movement Analysis Lab, University Nove de Julho, São Paulo, São Paulo, Brazil

Bianca M. Buurman, Elisabeth A. van Gemert and Sophia E. de Rooij
Department of Internal Medicine and Geriatrics, Academic Medical Center, Amsterdam, The Netherlands

Jita G. Hoogerduijn
Research Group Care for the Chronically Ill, Faculty of Health Care, Hogeschool Utrecht, University of Applied Sciences Utrecht, Utrecht, The Netherlands

Rob J. de Haan
Clinical Research Unit, Academic Medical Center, Amsterdam, The Netherlands

Marieke J. Schuurmans
Research Group Care for the Chronically Ill, Faculty of Health Care, Hogeschool Utrecht, University of Applied Sciences Utrecht, Utrecht, The Netherlands
Department of Nursing Science, University Medical Center, Utrecht, The Netherlands

Bruno Roza da Costa and Anne Wilhelmina Saskia Rutjes
Division of Clinical Epidemiology and Biostatistics, Institute of Social and Preventive Medicine, University of Bern, Bern, Switzerland

Angelico Mendy
Department of Epidemiology and Biostatistics, Robert Stempel School of Public Health, Florida International University, Miami, Florida, United States of America

Rosalie Freund-Heritage
Glenrose Rehabilitation Hospital, Edmonton, Alberta, Canada

Edgar Ramos Vieira
Glenrose Rehabilitation Hospital, Edmonton, Alberta, Canada
Department of Physical Therapy, Florida International University, Miami, Florida, United States of America

Jane M. Lawrence-Dewar, Lee A. Baugh and Jonathan J. Marotta
Perception and Action Laboratory, Department of Psychology, University of Manitoba, Winnipeg, Manitoba, Canada

David A. Alter
The Institute for Clinical Evaluative Sciences, Toronto, Ontario, Canada
The Cardiac Rehabilitation and Secondary Prevention Program, Toronto Rehabilitation Institute, Toronto, Ontario, Canada
The Li Ka Shing Knowledge Institute of St. Michaels' Hospital, Toronto, Ontario, Canada

Department of Medicine, University of Toronto, Toronto, Ontario, Canada
Department of Health Policy, Management and Evaluation, University of Toronto, Toronto, Ontario, Canada

Paul I. Oh
The Cardiac Rehabilitation and Secondary Prevention Program, Toronto Rehabilitation Institute, Toronto, Ontario, Canada

Jack V. Tu and Dennis T. Ko
The Institute for Clinical Evaluative Sciences, Toronto, Ontario, Canada
The Schulich Heart Centre and the Clinical Epidemiology Unit of Sunnybrook Health Science Centre, Toronto, Ontario, Canada
Department of Health Policy, Management and Evaluation, University of Toronto, Toronto, Ontario, Canada

Peter C. Austin, Douglas S. Lee and Therese A. Stukel
The Institute for Clinical Evaluative Sciences, Toronto, Ontario, Canada
Department of Health Policy, Management and Evaluation, University of Toronto, Toronto, Ontario, Canada

Barry Franklin
Cardiac Rehabilitation and Exercise Laboratories, William Beaumont Hospital, Royal Oak, Michigan, United States of America

Philippe Terrier
IRR, Institut de Recherche en Réadaptation, Sion, Switzerland
Clinique romande de réadaptation SuvaCare, Sion, Switzerland

Kjerstin Torre
Movement to Health Laboratory, Montpellier-1 University, EuroMov, Montpellier, France

Vivien Marmelat
Movement to Health Laboratory, Montpellier-1 University, EuroMov, Montpellier, France MOVE Research Institute Amsterdam, Faculty of Human Movement Sciences, VU University Amsterdam, Amsterdam, Netherlands

Andreas Daffertshofer
MOVE Research Institute Amsterdam, Faculty of Human Movement Sciences, VU University Amsterdam, Amsterdam, Netherlands

Peter J. Beek
MOVE Research Institute Amsterdam, Faculty of Human Movement Sciences, VU University Amsterdam, Amsterdam, Netherlands
School for Sport and Education, Brunel University, Uxbridge, Middlesex, United Kingdom

Masafumi Kuzuya
Department of Geriatrics, Medicine in Growth and Aging, Program in Health and Community Medicine, Nagoya University Graduate School of Medicine, Nagoya, Japan

Nariaki Shiraishi
Department of Geriatrics, Medicine in Growth and Aging, Program in Health and Community Medicine, Nagoya University Graduate School of Medicine, Nagoya, Japan
Department of Rehabilitation, Faculty of Health Science, Nihon Fukushi University, Nagoya, Japan

Yusuke Suzuki
Department of Comprehensive Community Care Systems, Nagoya University Graduate School of Medicine, Nagoya, Japan

Daisuke Matsumoto
Department of Physical Therapy, Faculty of Health Science, Kio University, Koryo, Japan

Seungwon Jeong
Department of Social Science Center for Gerontology and Social Science, Chubu Rosai Hospital, Nagoya, Japan

Motoya Sugiyama
Department of Rehabilitation, Chubu Rosai Hospital, Nagoya, Japan

Katsunori Kondo
Center for Well-being and Society, Nihon Fukushi University, Nagoya, Japan

Ingerid Arbo
K.G. Jebsen Center of Exercise in Medicine, Department of Circulation and Medical Imaging, Faculty of Medicine, Norwegian University of Science and Technology, Trondheim, Norway

Erik Madssen
K.G. Jebsen Center of Exercise in Medicine, Department of Circulation and Medical Imaging, Faculty of Medicine, Norwegian University of Science and Technology, Trondheim, Norway
Department of Pulmonary Medicine, St. Olavs Hospital, Trondheim, Norway

Ingrid Granøien and Liv Walderhaug
Ålesund Hospital, Ålesund, Norway

Trine Moholdt
K.G. Jebsen Center of Exercise in Medicine, Department of Circulation and Medical Imaging, Faculty of Medicine, Norwegian University of Science and Technology, Trondheim, Norway
Women's Clinic, St. Olavs Hospital, Trondheim, Norway

Leo Ota, Hirotaka Uchitomi, Ken-ichiro Ogawa and Yoshihiro Miyake
Department of Computational Intelligence and Systems Science, Tokyo Institute of Technology, Yokohama, Kanagawa, Japan

Satoshi Orimo
Department of Neurology, Kanto Central Hospital, Setagaya, Tokyo, Japan

Index